DAVID HOFFMAN
MICROVASIVE ENDOSCOPY
MARKETING

AF697416

INTERVENTIONAL PULMONOLOGY

NOTICE

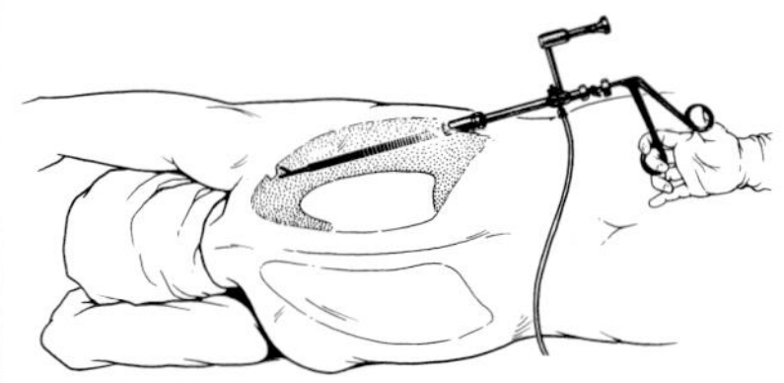

INTERVENTIONAL PULMONOLOGY

EDITORS

John F. Beamis, Jr., M.D.

Pulmonary and Critical Care Medicine
Lahey Clinic Medical Center
Burlington, Massachusetts

AND

Praveen N. Mathur, M.D.

Associate Professor of Medicine
Division of Pulmonary and Critical Care Medicine
Indiana University Medical Center
Indianapolis, Indiana

McGraw-Hill
Health Professions Division

New York St. Louis San Francisco Auckland Bogotá Caracas Lisbon London Madrid
Mexico City Milan Montreal New Delhi San Juan Singapore Sydney Tokyo Toronto

McGraw-Hill

A Division of The ***McGraw-Hill*** *Companies*

INTERVENTIONAL PULMONOLOGY

1234567890 1IMP1IMP 998

ISBN 0-07-005207-7

This book was set in Palatino by York Graphics, Inc.
The editors were Joseph Hefta and Steven Melvin;
the production supervisor was Richard Ruzycka.
Text and cover were designed by Marsha Cohen/Parallelogram.
The index was prepared by Geraldine Beckford.

Printed and bound through Imago (U.S.A.), Inc. in Singapore.

Library of Congress Cataloging-in-Publication Data

Interventional pulmonology / editors, John F. Beamis, Jr., Praveen N. Mathur.

p. cm.

Includes bibliographical references and index.

ISBN 0–07–005207–7

1. Lungs—Diseases—Diagnosis. 2. Lungs—Diseases—Treatment. 3. Bronchoscopy. 4. Thoracoscopy. 5. Lungs—Endoscopic surgery. I. Beamis, John F.

[DNLM: 1. Lung Diseases—diagnosis. 2. Lung Diseases—therapy. 3. Bronchoscopy—methods. 4. Thoracoscopy—methods. 5. Surgical Procedures, Endoscopic—methods. 6. Radiography, Interventional—methods. WF 600 I618 1999]

RD539.I55 1999

616.2'4—DC21

DNLM/DLC

for Library of Congress 98-15847

This book is dedicated to our families

Pratima, Anubhav, and Anita

and

Kazuko, Eileen, and Ann

We thank them for their love and support throughout this project
and all our varied undertakings.

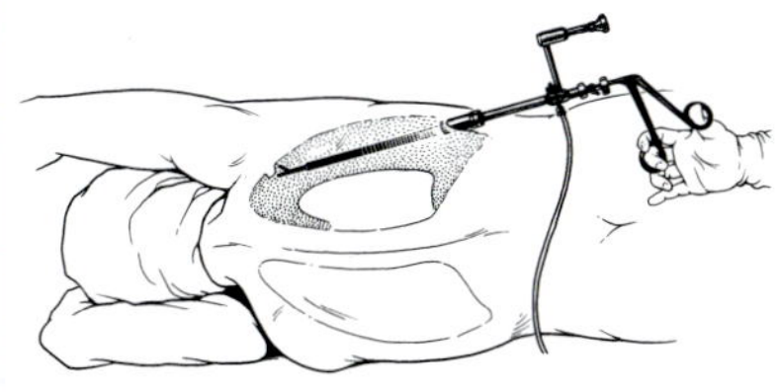

CONTENTS

PART I

THERAPEUTIC BRONCHOSCOPY

CHAPTER 1 OVERVIEW OF BRONCHOSCOPY 3
Paul A. Kvale

CHAPTER 2 PREVENTION OF DAMAGE AND MAINTENANCE OF A FLEXIBLE BRONCHOSCOPE 9
Atul C. Mehta, Ather J. Siddiqi, and Alice Walsh

CHAPTER 3 RIGID BRONCHOSCOPY 17
John F. Beamis, Jr.

CHAPTER 4 ENDOSCOPIC MANAGEMENT OF BENIGN AIRWAY STENOSIS 29
Prasoon Jain and Atul C. Mehta

CHAPTER 5 LASER BRONCHOSCOPY 43
James J. Fenton and John F. Beamis, Jr.

CHAPTER 6 CRYOTHERAPY IN ENDOBRONCHIAL DISORDERS 69
Jean-Paul Homasson and Praveen N. Mathur

CHAPTER 7 ENDOBRONCHIAL ELECTROCAUTERY 83
Tom G. Sutedja and Pieter E. Postmus

CHAPTER 8 SILICONE AIRWAY STENTS 97
Henri G. Colt

CHAPTER 9 EXPANDABLE ENDOBRONCHIAL STENTS 113
Chris T. Bellinger and Praveen N. Mathur

CHAPTER 10 BALLOON DILATION OF BENIGN TRACHEOBRONCHIAL STENOSIS 129
Francis D. Sheski and Praveen N. Mathur

CHAPTER 11 ENDOBRONCHIAL BRACHYTHERAPY 141
Andrew G. Villanueva, Anthony W. Gray, Jr., and Theodore C. M. Lo

PART II

MEDICAL THORACOSCOPY

CHAPTER 12 CHEST TUBE PLACEMENT 153
Karen M. Wolf, David C. Mares, and Praveen N. Mathur

CHAPTER 13 MEDICAL THORACOSCOPY: ROLE IN PLEURAL AND LUNG DISEASES 169
Praveen N. Mathur and Robert Loddenkemper

CHAPTER 14 THE ROLE OF THORACOSCOPY FOR THE DIAGNOSIS AND TREATMENT OF PLEURAL CANCERS 185
P. Astoul and C. Boutin

CHAPTER 15 THORACOSCOPIC MANAGEMENT OF PNEUMOTHORAX 207
Henri G. Colt

PART III

OTHER PROCEDURES

CHAPTER 16 THORACENTESIS AND CLOSED PLEURAL BIOPSY 223
Raja G. Ogirala and Fiona Meller Azrieli

CHAPTER 17 TRANSBRONCHIAL NEEDLE ASPIRATION 241
Atul C. Meha, Asok Dasgupta, and Ko-Pen Wang

CHAPTER 18 TRANSTRACHEAL OXYGEN THERAPY 255
Sanjiv Tewari, Kay Stelmach, and Atul C. Mehta

CHAPTER 19 PERCUTANEOUS THORACIC NEEDLE BIOPSY 269
Robert D. Tarver, Lynn S. Broderick, and Dewey J. Conces, Jr.

CHAPTER 20 PERCUTANEOUS TRACHEOSTOMY 285
Paul F. Dellaripa

CHAPTER 21 ANESTHESIA FOR ENDOSCOPIC PROCEDURES OF THE AIRWAY 295
Michael H. Entrup

CHAPTER 22 BRONCHOSCOPIC IMAGING FOR EARLY LUNG CANCER 313
Stephen C. T. Lam

INDEX 321

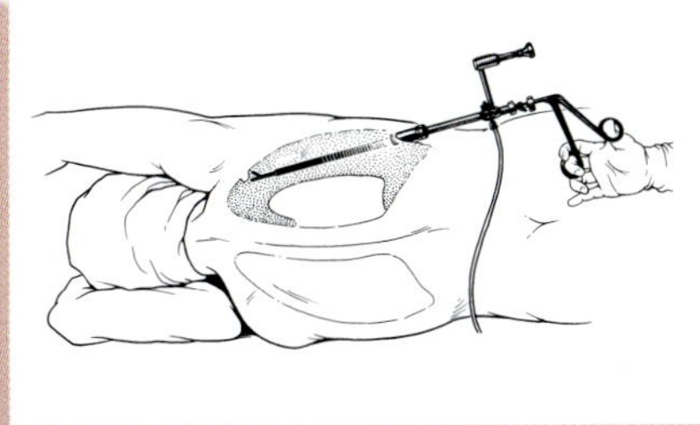

CONTRIBUTORS

P. Astoul, M.D. [14]
Department of Pulmology
Hôpital de la Conception
Marseille, France

Fiona Meller Azrieli, M.D. [16]
Assistant Professor of Medicine
Albert Einstein College of Medicine
Jacobi Medical Center
Bronx, New York

John F. Beamis, Jr., M.D. [3, 5]
Section of Pulmonary and Critical Care Medicine
Lahey Clinic Medical Center
Burlington, Massachusetts

Chris T. Bolliger, M.D. [9]
Respiratory Division
University Hospital Petersgraben
Basel, Switzerland

C. Boutin, M.D. [14]
Département of Pulmology
Hôpital de la Conception
Marseille, France

Lynn S. Broderick, M.D. [19]
Assistant Professor of Radiology
Indiana University of School of Medicine
University Hospital
Indianapolis, Indiana

Henri G. Colt, M.D. [8, 15]
Associate Professor of Medicine
Associate Director, Pulmonary Special Procedures and Nd:YAG Laser Unit
University of California Medical Center, San Diego
San Diego, California

Dewey J. Conces, Jr., M.D. [19]
Professor of Radiology
Indiana University School of Medicine
University Hospital
Indianapolis, Indiana

Asok Dasgupta, M.B., B.S., M.R.C.P. [17]
Fellow, Department of Pulmonary and Critical Care Medicine
Cleveland Clinic Foundation
Cleveland, Ohio

Paul F. DellaRipa, M.D. [20]
Staff Physician, Medical Intensive Care Unit
Lahey Clinic
Burlington, Massachusetts
and
Clinical Instructor in Medicine
Harvard Medical School
Boston, Massachusetts

Michael H. Entrup, M.D. [21]
Senior Staff Anesthesiologist and Director, Cardiac Anesthesia
Lahey Clinic
Burlington, Massachusetts
and
Assistant Clinical Professor of Anesthesiology
Tufts University School of Medicine
Boston, Massachusetts

James J. Fenton, M.D. [5]
Section of Pulmonary and Critical Care Medicine
Lahey Clinic Medical Center
Burlington, Massachusetts

Anthony W. Gray, Jr., M.D. [11]
Section of Pulmonary and Critical Care Medicine
Lahey Clinic Medical Center
Burlington, Massachusetts

Jean-Paul Homasson, M.D. [6]
Centre Hospitalier Specialise en Pneumologie
Chevilly-Laure, France

Prasoon Jain, M.D. [4]
Section of Bronchology
Department of Pulmonary and Critical Care Medicine
The Cleveland Clinic Foundation
Cleveland, Ohio

Paul A. Kvale, M.D. [1]
Senior Staff Physician, Division of Pulmonary and Critical Care Medicine
Henry Ford Hospital
and
Professor of Medicine
Case Western Reserve University School of Medicine
and
Clinical Professor of Medicine
University of Michigan School of Medicine
Detroit, Michigan

STEPHEN C. T. LAM, M.D., F.R.C.P.C. [22]
Division of Pulmonary Disease
University of British Columbia
Vancouver, British Columbia
Canada

THEODORE C. M. LO, M.D. [11]
Department of Radiation Oncology
Lahey Clinic Medical Center
Burlington, Massachusetts

ROBERT LODDENKEMPER, M.D. [13]
Department of Pneumology II
Chest Hospital Heckeshorn
Berlin, Germany

DAVID C. MARES, M.D. [12]
Division of Pulmonary, Critical Care, and Occupational Medicine
Department of Medicine
Indiana University Medical Center
Indianapolis, Indiana

PRAVEEN N. MATHUR, M.B., B.S. [6, 9, 10, 12, 13]
Division of Pulmonary, Critical Care, and Occupational Medicine
Department of Medicine
Indiana University Medical Center
Indianapolis, Indiana

ATUL C. MEHTA, M.D., F.A.C.P., F.C.C.P. [2, 4, 17, 18]
Head, Section of Bronchology
Department of Pulmonary and Critical Care Medicine
The Cleveland Clinic Foundation
Cleveland, Ohio

RAJA G. OGIRALA, M.D. [16]
Clinical Assistant Professor of Medicine
Albert Einstein College of Medicine
Montefiore Medical Center
Bronx, New York

PIETER E. POSTMUS, M.D., PH.D., F.C.C.P. [7]
Department of Pulmonology
Free University Hospital
Amsterdam, The Netherlands

FRANCIS D. SHESKI, M.D. [10]
Division of Pulmonary, Critical Care, and Occupational Medicine
Department of Medicine
Indiana University Medical Center
Indianapolis, Indiana

ATHER J. SIDDIQI [2]
Department of Pulmonary and Critical Care Medicine
Baylor College of Medicine
Houston, Texas

KAY STELMACH, R.N., R.R.T. [18]
Section of Bronchology
Department of Pulmonary and Critical Care Medicine
The Cleveland Clinic Foundation
Cleveland, Ohio

TOM G. SUTEDJA, M.D., PH.D., F.C.C.P. [7]
Department of Pulmonology
Free University Hospital
Amsterdam, The Netherlands

ROBERT D. TARVER, M.D. [19]
Professor of Radiology
Indiana University School of Medicine
Department of Radiology
Wishard Memorial Hospital
Indiana, Indiana

SANJIV TEWARI, M.D. [18]
Section of Bronchology
Department of Pulmonary and Critical Care Medicine
The Cleveland Clinic Foundation
Cleveland, Ohio

ANDREW G. VILLANUEVA, M.D. [11]
Section of Pulmonary and Critical Care Medicine
Lahey Clinic Medical Center
Burlington, Massachusetts

ALICE WALSH, R.N. [2]
Department of Pulmonary and Critical Care Medicine
The Cleveland Clinic Foundation
Cleveland, Ohio

KO-PEN WANG, M.D., F.C.C.P. [17]
Director, Chest Diagnostic Center
and
Director, Interventional Bronchology
Johns Hopkins Bayview Medical Center
Baltimore, Maryland

KAREN M. WOLF, M.D. [12]
Division of Pulmonary Critical Care and Occupational Medicine
Department of Medicine
Indiana University Medical Center
Indianapolis, Indiana

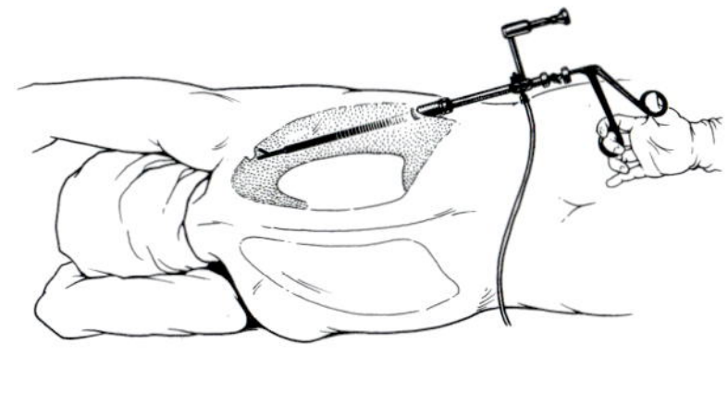

PREFACE

Advances in endoscopic and video technologies and increasing numbers of patients presenting with advanced airway obstruction and pleural diseases have stimulated the development of a new arena in pulmonary medicine called *Interventional Pulmonology.* In many ways modern pulmonary medicine practice has been defined by procedures such as flexible bronchoscopy and the numerous procedures involved in the practice of Critical Care Medicine. While the vast majority of pulmonologists perform flexible bronchoscopy, thoracentesis, and ICU procedures, only a small number perform the procedures currently included within *Interventional Pulmonology.*

What is Interventional Pulmonology? As this book goes to print a combined American Thoracic Society–European Respiratory Society task force is in the process of defining this area of pulmonary medicine. The definition that has evolved states that Interventional Pulmonology is the "the art and science of medicine related to the performance of invasive therapeutic and diagnostic procedures that requires additional training and expertise beyond that required within a standard pulmonary training program. Disease processes encompassed within this discipline include complex airway management problems, benign and malignant central airway obstruction, and pleural diseases. Diagnostic and therapeutic procedures pertaining to these areas include but are not limited to rigid bronchoscopic resection and dilatation, laser bronchoscopy, electrocautery, cryotherapy, airway stent insertion, balloon bronchoplasty and dilatational techniques, endobronchial radiation (brachytherapy), endobronchial ultrasound, percutaneous needle aspiration and biopsy, percutaneous dilatational tracheostomy, transtracheal oxygen cather insertion, transbronchial needle aspiration, and thoracoscopy."

This book addresses many of the procedures outlined in the ATS-ERS Task Force's definition of Interventional Pulmonology. Authors of the various chapters are internationally recognized experts in the performance of these procedures and many of them have been instrumental in establishing the "state of the art" in their respective fields. With comprehensive reviews of each procedure and special "How I Do It" sections in which experts share their technique, we hope that this book will serve as a reference for those interested in joining the growing numbers of interventional pulmonologists. We also feel this book will be useful for pulmonologists who will not be performing these procedures but who might refer patients to colleagues. The clinical problems that are addressed in this book can be encountered by any pulmonologist, and thus it is important that the indications, contraindications, and risks of these procedures are generally appreciated.

We wish to thank McGraw-Hill for allowing us to undertake this project and are especially appreciative of the editorial assistance provided by Joseph Hefta and Steven Melvin of McGraw-Hill. We thank James Millerick of the Medical Art Department at Lahey Clinic for producing many of the drawings of the various procedures and interventional pulmonology equipment.

We thank all of the authors for their contributions. Many of these authors are personal friends and colleagues and we appreciate their support of this project. We consider several of the authors to be our mentors and are particularly grateful for the contributions that Jean-Francois Dumon, Christian Boutin, and Robert Loddenkemper have made to this book and our medical careers.

INTERVENTIONAL PULMONOLOGY

PART I

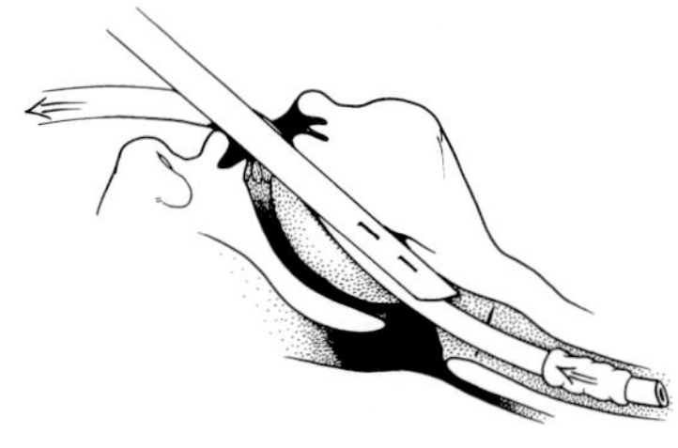

BRONCHOSCOPY

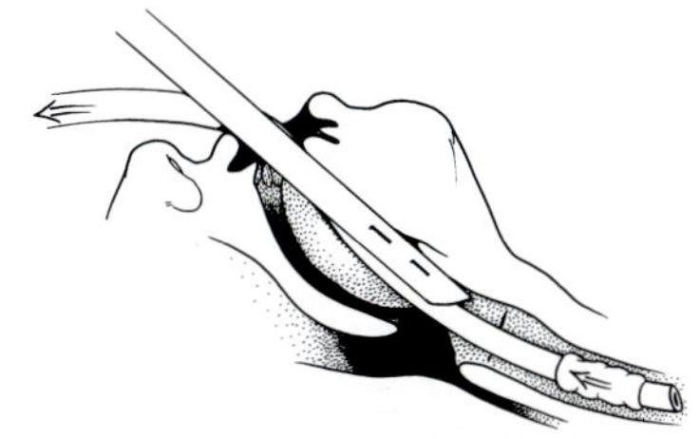

CHAPTER 1

OVERVIEW OF BRONCHOSCOPY

Paul A. Kvale

The notion that the airways could be visually inspected by use of mirrors and indirect illumination can be traced to the early nineteenth century. Horace Green began to catheterize the airways in an effort to remove foreign bodies; when he presented his work to the Surgical Society of New York in 1847, he was immediately asked to resign! As his work was expanded, other physicians began to accept the concept of bronchoscopy as a viable practice option. By 1885 Joseph O'Dwyer had developed a tube for dilating the larynx stenosed by diphtheria. Thus, interventional bronchoscopy is not a new concept; physicians have used bronchoscopes to *treat* airway disorders for more than 100 years.

Near the turn of the century, the tubes that O'Dwyer had developed were used by Kirstein and by Gustav Killian to intubate the trachea and remove foreign bodies. About the same time, Chevalier Jackson began similar work in the United States. Stimulated by the English laryngologist Morell Mackensie, Jackson conceptualized an instrument and technique for use in peroral endoscopy with which he could safely and effectively remove foreign objects from a tubular structure. His esophagoscope proved useful for the removal of objects from the esophagus, but produced calamitous results when used by unskilled hands. As a result, Jackson developed safety protocols and insisted on rigorous incremental training in the use of his esophagoscope. Jackson found that his instrument was highly successful in the dilation of esophageal strictures—a common occurrence at the time found in children who had ingested lye.

In the early part of the twentieth century, Jackson developed his own bronchoscope and a technique for insertion. With his usual diligence, he applied his esophagoscope safety and training protocols to the new bronchoscope and demonstrated its safe and effective use in viewing the tracheobronchial tree. He also developed instruments for grasping foreign bodies and performing biopsies. Unable to clearly see the distal portions of the bronchus, Jackson modified the bronchoscope so that illumination at the distal tip of the instrument was possible.

For the next 70 years of bronchoscopic practice, rigid or open-tube bronchoscopes were the only bronchoscopes available. Many complimentary instruments were introduced, including telescopes for magnifying the image and photographic equipment to document the findings. In the early part of the century the only uses of the bronchoscope were to remove foreign bodies and dilate strictures, but physicians later began to identify new applications for this remarkable instrument. Secretions could be aspirated to relieve atelectasis; the site and sometimes the cause of hemoptysis could be identified; occasionally hemoptysis could be managed exclusively by tamponade with a bronchoscope or by packing the bleeding airway. Diagnosis of malignancy became important as the incidence of lung cancer began to rise with increasing consumption of cigarettes. In 1965 Anderson and coworkers reported that lung tissue could be obtained when small, peripheral carinal spurs were biopsied; this led to the use of the bronchoscope for the diagnosis of diffuse lung diseases.[1]

Fiberoptic bronchoscopes were introduced into clinical practice by Shigeto Ikeda and coworkers in the late 1960s.[2] However, the fact that an image could be conducted through a glass fiber had been recognized nearly a century earlier. Glass fibers arranged in bundles must be coated with glass of a lower refractive index so that the image is conducted through the full length of the fiber without distortion. The use of this concept for medical instrumentation in a hollow organ was initially introduced for visualization of the stomach.[3] When Ikeda expanded this concept to bronchoscopy, it became possible to visualize smaller and more peripheral airways than was possible with rigid bronchoscopes. The newest development in flexible bronchoscopes is the introduction of a miniature camera-like device (charge coupled device, or CCD) into the tip of the instrument, thus replacing the fiberoptic bundles. The quality of the image is superior to that which can be obtained with glass fibers, and the image can be digitally manipulated for a variety of purposes.

Differences between Bronchoscopes

Rigid bronchoscopes are referred to as "open-tube bronchoscopes" for the duration of this chapter. Open-tube bronchoscopes are made from stainless steel, and they are manufactured by many different companies. All are hollow, which allows the patient to ventilate *through* them. The resistance to airflow through such an instrument is minimal. Because the airways of small children are also small in diameter, open-tube bronchoscopes are usually regarded as the instrument of choice for managing airway problems in the pediatric age group (generally under the age of 12 years). Patients must breathe *around* flexible bronchoscopes; since there is only a given size to the airway lumen, those with small airways, such as pediatric patients, may find it difficult to exchange air adequately when a flexible bronchoscope is inserted.

There are a variety of lengths and diameters of open-tube bronchoscopes available; typically, the experienced bronchoscopist will choose a length and diameter of bronchoscope size-suited for the individual patient. Some pediatric pulmonologists advocate use of a pediatric-size flexible bronchoscope for inspection of the airways, even in preterm infants. If secretions are to be aspirated and removed from small children with a flexible bronchoscope, an adaptation with a suction catheter taped alongside the bronchoscope[4] may be required because the suction channel within the small fiberoptic bronchoscopes is ineffective in the setting of thick, inspissated secretions.

A number of open-tube bronchoscopes are available for use with the adult population. Many different modifications help to make a specific instrument suitable for one or another application, such as laser bronchoscopy or insertion of stents. The rigid telescope that is passed through open-tube bronchoscopes has much better optical properties than flexible fiberoptic bronchoscopes and videobronchoscopes that utilize a CCD. A ventilating sidearm is an integral part of modern open-tube bronchoscopes, since general anesthesia is typically required because of the discomfort of peroral insertion of such an instrument. Spontaneous ventilation can still occur, but most interventional procedures done through an open-tube bronchoscope are of sufficient duration that full muscle paralysis and general anesthesia are desirable.

Flexible bronchoscopes are the instrument of choice for most adult *diagnostic* bronchoscopy. As compared with open-tube bronchoscopes, flexible bronchoscopes are easier to insert, more comfortable for the patient, and associated with fewer complications. The ability to control the direction of the tip of a flexible bronchoscope enables entry into smaller bronchi, including upper-lobe bronchi. Flexible bronchoscopes are appreciably more expensive than open-tube bronchoscopes, and the maintenance cost from damage is considerable.[5] Damage to flexible bronchoscopes may occur from a tear of the inner sheath of the suction and instrument channel, which is most common when a transbronchial needle is inserted to perform mediastinal lymph node biopsy with this device. However, similar tears of the inner sheath also can occur from other instruments, including laser fibers or by introducing wires for brachytherapy. If the flexible bronchoscope is inserted perorally, as opposed to a transnasal approach, an awake patient with teeth can bite and damage the shaft. This is a particular problem for flexible bronchoscopes with fiberoptic imaging systems, because the delicate glass fibers are especially prone to breakage.

Another major difference between open-tube and flexible bronchoscopes is the efficiency of suctioning. The working channel through a flexible bronchoscope, which is suitable for most adult bronchoscopy, is usually 2.0 to 2.5 mm in diameter. The optical lens is situated at the distal tip approximately 1 to 1.5 mm away from the channel through which blood and secretions can be suctioned. This separation between the optical lens and the channel which is used to suction blood and mucus can create a problem for keeping the lens clear for visualizing what is being done with the instrument. The distance between the working channel and the locus of the CCD for flexible videobronchoscopes is slightly greater than that for flexible fiberoptic bronchoscopes. This greater separation between the CCD and the suction channel compounds the problem of keeping the image clear with a videobronchoscope as compared with a fiberoptic bronchoscope. Whereas the CCD or lens can often be cleared by suctioning, instilling saline through the working channel, and "wiping" the CCD or lens against a nearby spur or wall of a bronchus, these maneuvers are not always effective for clearing the CCD or lens of the blood and mucus. This can make visualization difficult or impossible, necessitating removal of the fiberoptic bronchoscope in its entirety to clean the distal tip and restore the ability to visualize the interior of the airway.

If bleeding is severe and the flexible instrument has been passed transnasally instead of through an orotracheal tube, there can be inadequate control of the airway with the potential for asphyxiation. Some flexible bronchoscopes, particularly those which are used for laser-assisted bronchoscopy, have larger channels (2.6 to 3.0 mm in diameter). Even flexible bronchoscopes with these larger suction channels are not as efficient for clearing blood when bleeding is brisk as are open-tube bronchoscopes. The rigid rod telescope lens may also become covered with blood and mucus at times, making visualization difficult or impossible. However, the telescope can be removed for cleaning without removing the open-tube bronchoscope. Thus, with rigid bronchoscopy, the safety margin is much greater for maintaining a clear airway and avoiding asphyxiation when a major bleed occurs. Furthermore, multiple suction catheters can be introduced through an open-tube bronchoscope to remove blood and secretions rapidly. The open-tube bronchoscope can be pushed into either the left or right main bronchus to isolate the opposite side from which bleeding is occurring. This allows the patient to continue to be ventilated. The shaft of the open-tube bronchoscope is often an efficient instrument to tamponade and stop bleeding.

Choosing Bronchoscopes for Interventional Procedures

This book is written for those who perform or are learning to perform interventional bronchoscopy. The various types of interventional bronchoscopy discussed include laser-assisted ablation of abnormal tissue, such as tumors or areas of stenosis which obstruct the airways; endobronchial radiation therapy as an adjunct for managing patients with airway malignancies; insertion of stents to improve or maintain airway patency; balloon or mechanical dilation of narrow airways; airway cryotherapy; and electrocautery. Open-tube and flexible bronchoscopes are used in each of these situations, but there are cogent reasons to select one type of bronchoscope over another, depending on the type of interventional procedure planned (Table 1-1).

LASER BRONCHOSCOPY

Ablation of abnormal tissue that obstructs the airway can be accomplished with carbon dioxide (CO_2) lasers, yttrium-aluminum-garnet (YAG) lasers, and YAG lasers with frequency doubling of the wavelength after passing the light through a crystal made from potassium triphosphate (commonly called a KTP laser). Other wavelengths of laser light are likely to be developed for use in the future, depending on the ease of finding a medium to generate the specific wavelength desired and the interaction of the particular wavelength with the tissues in the airways.

CO_2 lasers are excellent cutting instruments. This wavelength cannot be conducted through fiberoptic bundles; consequently, it must be used with an open-tube bronchoscope or a laryngoscope for any application in the airways. CO_2 lasers do not coagulate blood vessels much larger than capillaries; hence, they are primarily used for microsurgery of laryngeal lesions and occasionally for squamous epithelial papillomata in the trachea or main bronchi. They may also be of value in making radial incisions of scar tissue or otherwise managing subglottic or high tracheal stenoses.

YAG and KTP lasers have much better photocoagulating properties than do CO_2 lasers. Each wavelength can be transmitted through fiberoptic bundles. Both have particular value in laser-assisted ablation of malignancies in the distal trachea or beyond. Either open-tube bronchoscopes or fiberoptic bronchoscopes can be used with YAG and KTP lasers. Interventional bronchoscopists who perform larger numbers of procedures generally choose open-tube bronchoscopes for most laser-assisted ablation of malignancies. Although flexible bronchoscopes are preferred by a few bronchoscopists who have high-volume practices, the choice of a flexible bronchoscope for laser bronchoscopy usually reflects a lack of experience with open-tube bronchoscopes and low-volume laser bronchoscopy practice.

For YAG and KTP laser bronchoscopy, open-tube instruments offer a number of distinct advantages. The laser is generally regarded as an adjunct to mechanical debridement of neoplastic or granulation tissue. Tissue may be desiccated or photocoagulated with laser energy, but bulky tissue can be quickly and easily removed by using the open-tube bronchoscope in an "apple-core" technique to avulse a large piece of tissue. Forceps used with open-tube bronchoscopes are larger and are suitable to extract such large pieces of tissue or to avulse the tissue itself in piecemeal fashion without the apple-core method. The laser can then be used to photocoagulate any bleeding vessels that may result from the mechanical removal of tissue with forceps or the open-tube bronchoscope itself. As discussed earlier, the ability to manage bleeding when it does occur is easier and more efficient through an open-tube bronchoscope than with a flexible bronchoscope. The entire process of opening the airway is typically much faster when open-tube bronchoscopes are chosen than if laser bronchoscopy is attempted through a flexible bronchoscope. There are a few conditions, such as high tracheal or subglottic laryngeal lesions, which may be more easily approached with a flexible bronchoscope for laser-assisted ablation. Most patients who will benefit from laser bronchoscopy are managed better with an open-tube bronchoscope, however.

Table 1-1
PREFERRED BRONCHOSCOPES FOR SPECIFIC INTERVENTIONAL PROCEDURES

Interventional Procedure	*Preferred Bronchoscope*	*Additional Equipment Needed*
CO_2 laser bronchoscopy	Open tube	CO_2 laser
YAG or KTP laser bronchoscopy	Open tube	YAG or KTP laser
Phototherapy	Flexible	Argon and tuneable dye lasers; various tips for fibers; photosensitizing agent
Brachytherapy	Flexible	Radioactive sources (Usually iridium 191)
Silastic stent insertion	Open tube	Specialized open-tube bronchoscopes; introducer and retrieval forceps; various sizes of stents
Metallic stent insertion	Flexible	Various metallic stents
Mechanical or balloon dilation	Open tube (mechanical)	Progressive sizes of open tube bronchoscopes
	Open tube or flexible (balloon)	Various sizes and lengths of balloons with high-pressure inflating syringe

ENDOBRONCHIAL RADIATION THERAPY

The preferred radioisotope for endobronchial radiation treatment is iridium 191. This isotope emits sufficient energy that its placement within the airway is temporary. Treatment can be done with a string of radioactive "seeds" which are low intensity, requiring hours or days of residence in the airway, or with high-intensity pellets and remote afterloading into previously placed airway catheters over a period of minutes. Flexible bronchoscopes are suitable for either type of endobronchial radiation; the catheters or strings of seeds are sufficiently small that an open-tube bronchoscope is not required for placement.

Other radioisotopes that are still occasionally used are those of gold and iodine. Typically, these radioactive seeds are inserted directly into malignant tissue with instruments that are adapted for use with an open-tube bronchoscope.

INSERTION OF STENTS

Silastic stents are more commonly used to improve or maintain airway patency in patients with rapidly recurring malignancies or with some situations of benign tracheal or bronchial narrowing. The instruments required to introduce a silastic stent are adapted for open-tube bronchoscopes, and they cannot be inserted through flexible bronchoscopes. Metallic stents, such as Gianturco or Wallstent devices, can be inserted through either flexible or open-tube bronchoscopes. The methods of using each type of stent are discussed in subsequent chapters.

PHOTOTHERAPY

Certain drugs such as hematoporphyrin derivative or dihematoporphyrin ethers concentrate in rapidly dividing tissues to a greater extent than in cells, which divide at a normal rate. When these drugs are injected intravenously, a gradient between malignant and normal tissue occurs. When exposed to laser light of a particular wavelength, such as an argon-driven dye laser (632 nm), toxic oxygen radicals are produced, which cause cell necrosis and death. Optical fibers that can be passed through flexible bronchoscopes are used to deliver the laser light to the target tissues the bronchoscopist intends to treat.

MECHANICAL DILATION OF AIRWAYS

Patients with stenosis of the subglottic larynx or trachea can undergo simple mechanical dilation of the narrow segment with a succession of gradually enlarging open-tube bronchoscopes. The same dilation can be accomplished with smaller and then larger orotracheal tubes or bougies, but the rigidity of an open-tube bronchoscope and the ability to simultaneously ventilate the patient through such bronchoscopes makes them particularly suitable for this purpose.

Balloons of various diameters and lengths have been developed for dilating strictures of the esophagus, pylorus, or other areas of narrowing of the gastrointestinal tract. They have been adapted by bronchoscopists for similar applications in the airways. Although the balloons can be inserted through flexible bronchoscopes with large instrument channels, they are more easily inserted through an open-tube bronchoscope. Moreover, they are typically inflated within the airway for approximately 2 min at a time, totally occluding the airway during the time of inflation. Using these balloons for "bronchoplasty" is generally better tolerated with the patient anesthetized and with an open-tube bronchoscope.

Training in Bronchoscopy

Physicians from four different disciplines are usually those who learn and continue to perform bronchoscopy as a part of their practices. Most diagnostic bronchoscopy is now done by pulmonary internists. Although anesthesiologists often become adept at use of a flexible bronchoscope, their use of this instrument is typically for placement of endotracheal tubes and positioning of double-lumen endotracheal or endobronchial tubes for single-lung ventilation during thoracic surgical procedures. Otolaryngology and thoracic surgery residency programs are required to offer training in flexible bronchoscopy and open-tube bronchoscopy. Many such residency programs have difficulty in meeting minimal training requirements for residents to develop adequate skills in the use of either type of instrument, primarily because most diagnostic bronchoscopy is done by pulmonologists. On the other hand, skill with open-tube bronchoscopes is generally not acquired during fellowships in pulmonary medicine. This may result in pulmonary physicians who desire to perform a few laser bronchoscopies as part of a "complete pulmonary practice" avoiding acquisition of the necessary expertise in the use of open-tube bronchoscopes.

Any technical skill has several essential steps necessary for the operator to avoid failure. One of the most important aspects of acquiring and maintaining a technical skill is practice. Practice should begin with models and then be transferred to living human patients. Practice is an ongoing requirement, even after the initial skill has been attained. If a particular type of bronchoscope is not used for many months between cases, the operator will lose proficiency. The greatest danger in this regard is the occasional use of an open-tube bronchoscope for interventional procedures, if the volume in a physician's practice does not lend itself to continued application of a skill that was once acquired.

FLEXIBLE BRONCHOSCOPY

A minimum of 50 diagnostic procedures is generally regarded as necessary to develop the requisite skills for flexible bronchoscopy.[6] Some trainees have better manual dexterity and hand-eye coordination skills than others; the choice of 50 procedures should therefore be regarded as an average number for minimal expertise. Cognitive skills must be acquired as well as technical skills; this includes the ability to decide when bronchoscopy is indicated as well as the relative and absolute contraindications to the performance of flexible bronchoscopy. Moreover, the trainee must be able to discriminate between those situations where open-tube bronchoscopy is preferred over flexible bronchoscopy. The various hand-eye or technical requirements for flexible bronchoscopy are enumerated in a report generated by the Section on Bronchoscopy of the American College of Chest Physicians.[6] It is emphasized that the trainee must be able to manage complications that might occur during the performance of diagnostic flexible bronchoscopy. It may well be that 50 procedures does not equip the average trainee with sufficient experience to develop all the manipulative skills to accomplish this goal.

OPEN-TUBE BRONCHOSCOPY

Becoming proficient in the use of open-tube bronchoscopes has become much more difficult since the advent of flexible bronchoscopes. In a British survey of bronchoscopies performed between 1974 and 1986, only 2 percent of nearly 40,000 procedures were done with open-tube bronchoscopes, and more than 90 percent of the open-tube procedures were done by surgeons.[7] Similar data for bronchoscopic practice in North America reveal than only 8 percent of bronchoscopists (who were mostly pulmonary physicians) perform open-tube bronchoscopy.[8]

Residency program requirements for otolaryngology and thoracic surgery include training in open-tube bronchoscopy. This is generally not the case for pulmonary fellowship training programs. The greater versatility of flexible bronchoscopy has led to its adoption by surgeons also. By and large, the skills needed for open-tube bronchoscopy are learned only by bronchoscopists who intend to perform interventional procedures. All these facts, plus the reduced number of experts available for teaching open-tube bronchoscopy has made it difficult to adequately train more than a few individuals in any given locale.

Attempts to learn open-tube bronchoscopy typically do not occur until more than 100 flexible procedures have been performed by the trainee. Supervised training by an expert open-tube bronchoscopist for many months is needed for proper development of the skills needed, given the relative infrequency for performing open-tube bronchoscopy. Only then will the interested trainee have sufficient volume of patient material to become adept at inserting and manipulating an open-tube bronchoscope. The need for safe use of an open-tube bronchoscope was an issue of great concern to Jackson, as students learned from him. Safety and efficient use of the instrument remains a guiding principle for today's teachers and students of open-tube bronchoscopy.

INTERVENTIONAL BRONCHOSCOPY

Not all training programs offer residents and fellows opportunities to learn interventional procedures. Even in those programs where interventional bronchoscopy is performed regularly, not all residents and fellows receive training in interventional procedures. Furthermore, many bronchoscopists who entered clinical practice before interventional bronchoscopy became so readily available have desired training after their residencies or fellowships were completed. As a consequence, short courses in laser bronchoscopy and stent placement have been offered and will probably continue to be offered to the interested bronchoscopist.

Short courses include didactic presentations as well as hands-on experience with animal models. Excellent models have been developed for the simulation of tumors that obstruct the airways and are amenable to laser-assisted debulking of such tissue.[9] Similar practical experience with animal models can facilitate the acquisition of the basic skills for inserting stents into airways. However, introducing an open-tube bronchoscope into an animal model (usually a dog or a goat) is a rather different procedure than performing bronchoscopy on a human subject. The potential for bleeding and other complications with humans is quite different from that with the models.

Attendance at a short course for interventional bronchoscopy can serve only to introduce and acquaint the student with the procedure's indications, contraindications, and the like. It is appropriate for the would-be interventional bronchoscopist to consider the volume of interventional bronchoscopy procedures that might be encountered. If a nearby facility is not taxed in its ability to meet the demand for interventional procedures, it is not appropriate to replicate this service when the volume of activity is anticipated to be so low that skills cannot be maintained. In a survey of attendees at laser bronchoscopy courses 24 months after completing the course, only 20 percent were performing this procedure more frequently than once every 3 months.[10] It was proposed that a minimum of 50 interventional procedures per year at a given institution and at least 25 per year for each bronchoscopist would assure the maintenance of proficiency to assure optimal patient care and safety.[10] Such a proposal, if adopted at the local level, might be expanded to include all interventional bronchoscopic procedures rather than just laser bronchoscopy. The important part of this recommendation is that any such procedure must be repeated sufficiently often for the bronchoscopist to maintain sufficient skill for optimal results and in the interest of patient safety. Whereas short courses may still be needed to introduce a bronchoscopist to interventional bronchoscopy, such courses are not an adequate substitute for lengthy training during a residency or fellowship program that can offer ample time and case material to become truly proficient.

Acknowledgment

The author is grateful for editorial assistance from Marsha Kelter in the preparation of this effort.

REFERENCES

1. Anderson HA, et al: Transbronchoscopic lung biopsy in diffuse pulmonary disease. *Dis Chest* 1965; 48:187–192.
2. Ikeda S, et al: Flexible bronchofiberscope. *Keio J Med* 1968; 1:17.
3. Hirschowitz BL, et al: Demonstration of a new gastroscope, the "fiberscope." *Gastroenterology* 1958; 35:50–53.
4. Wood RE, Fink RJ: Applications of flexible fiberoptic bronchoscopes in infants and children. *Chest* 1978; 73:737S–740S.
5. Mehta AC, et al: The high price of bronchoscopy: Maintenance and repair of the flexible fiberoptic bronchoscope. *Chest* 1990; 98:448–454.
6. Anonymous: Guidelines for competency and training in fiberoptic bronchoscopy. Section on Bronchoscopy, American College of Chest Physicians. *Chest* 1982; 81:739.
7. Simpson FG, et al: Postal survey of bronchoscopic practice by physicians in the United Kingdom. *Thorax* 1986; 41:311–317.
8. Prakash UBS, et al: Bronchoscopy in North America: The ACCP survey. *Chest* 1991; 100:1668–1675.
9. Beamis JF Jr, et al: Teaching models for Nd:YAG laser bronchoscopy. *Chest* 1989; 95:1316–1318.
10. Kvale PA: Training in laser bronchoscopy and proposals for credentialling. *Chest* 1990; 97:983–989.

CHAPTER 2

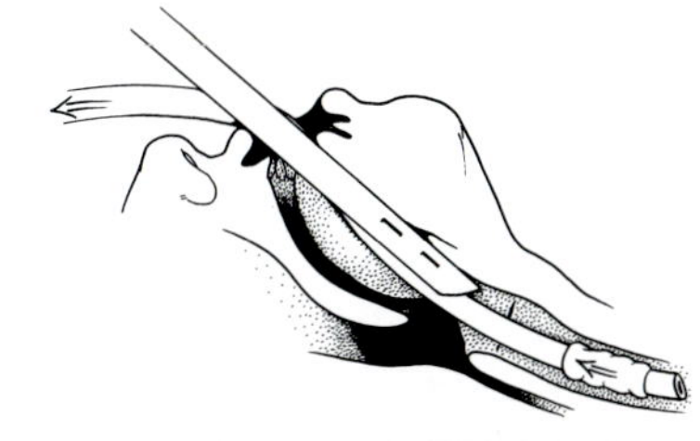

PREVENTION OF DAMAGE AND MAINTENANCE OF A FLEXIBLE BRONCHOSCOPE

Atul C. Mehta, Ather J. Siddiqi, and Alice Walsh

Flexible bronchoscopy is a well-established diagnostic, therapeutic, and palliative procedure in pulmonary medicine. Its applications range from airway examination to laser photoresection of airway lesions. Ikeda and coworkers first reported the use of a flexible bronchoscope (FB) in 1968.[1] Since then, the instrument has undergone major technical revisions and design modifications; this has also resulted in its increasing cost. Today the average cost of a FB is around $12,000 in the United States; light source, forceps, and other accessories are not included in this basic price.

The FB contains light transmitting and viewing glass fiber bundles. There are usually two light transmitting bundles and one viewing bundle. Each bundle contains 20,000 to 30,000 fine glass fibers 8 to 15 μm in diameter. Light enters at either end of the glass fiber and is internally reflected and emitted at the opposite end. The precise alignment of these optical glass fibers with eyepiece and objective lens provides proper visualization and magnification of the endobronchial tree.

The videobronchoscope (VBS) is a new evolution of the FB. In this instrument, the viewing bundle is replaced by the charge coupled device (CCD). The CCD is an image sensor that operates on electrical potential wells, each representing a pixel of total image. Each CCD has 1,000,000 pixels, which produce better quality images than the fiberoptic bronchoscope. The VBS has further increased the cost of the equipment. Thorough knowledge to prevent damage and to provide proper maintenance is mandatory prior to the use of this delicate instrument; otherwise, the repair cost could be exorbitant.

This chapter focuses on the care of the FB. For prevention of the damage, the manufacturer's instruction manual is a valuable source.[2,3] It is recommended that staff involved with FB familiarize themselves with the manual and make it readily available in their bronchoscopy suites.

Routine care of the FB is discussed under the following headings:

1. Cleaning
2. Disinfection
3. Storage
4. Transportation

Cleaning

The FB is a delicate instrument and has a limited tolerance to thermal, chemical, or physical insult. After each use, its surface should be wiped with a moist cotton gauze. The working channel is flushed and cleaned by drawing up tap water or saline. Then a "leak test" is carried out according to the manufacturer's guidelines.[3] This test detects any damage to the outer surface or inner working channel of the FB. Ideally, this test should be carried out after each procedure, especially after neodymium:yttrium-aluminum-garnet (Nd:YAG) laser photoresection and transbronchial needle aspiration (TBNA). The leak tester should never be connected or disconnected under water, because it may cause leakage into the tester or the FB. If the air leak is from the surface of the FB, then the damage is to the outer sheath (Fig. 2-1). Regular wear and tear and abrading the FB against a sharp edge are the most common causes for this type of damage, and the repair cost is around $400. If the air leak is through the working channel, it indicates a perforation in the inner plastic lining. This kind of damage is usually due to repeated excessive flexing of the FB, use of damaged endobronchial accessories, and improper handling of the laser fiber or transbronchial aspiration needle.[2] The repair of the working channel is much more costly ($4800) than the repair of the external surface of the FB.

If the leak test is positive, the instrument should be immediately removed from the wash basin, dried, and returned to the manufacturer for repair. If the leak test is negative, the FB should be submerged in warm enzymatic detergent after removing the suction valve and placing a soaking cap over the electrical pins. The amount of soaking time should be determined according to the detergent manufacturer's advice.

The working channel is scrubbed gently with a cleaning brush and after reattaching the suction valve, clean water is aspirated for 10 s followed by air suction for 30 s. Although most of the current models of FB are fully submersible, it should be remembered that the older, nonsubmersible models may require special care to the eyepiece and the umbilical cord.

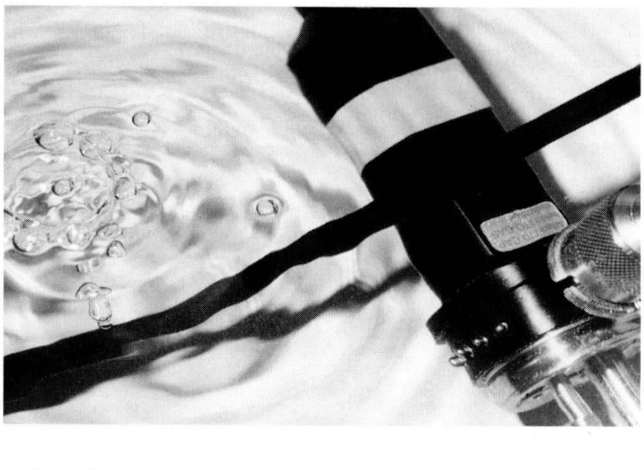

Figure 2-1

Positive leak test. Note air leak from the outer surface of the flexible bronchoscope.

Disinfection

Since the emergence of HIV infection, the concern over disinfecting procedures has become a major issue. Cidex, Glutarex, and Sporicidin are alkaline-based glutaraldehyde chemicals commonly used for disinfection. After thorough cleansing as described above, it is recommended that the equipment be immersed for 20 min in 2% glutaraldehyde solution. This destroys most bacteria, viruses, and mycobacteria. For total eradication of all mycobacteria, a 45-min soak at 25°C is required. Such long soaking times could affect turnaround time in most practices and, therefore, unless contamination with *Mycobacterium* is suspected, a 20-min immersion period is adequate.[4]

It should be noted that individuals frequently exposed to glutaraldehyde can develop sensitivity reactions such as dermatitis and conjunctivitis; therefore, undue exposure should be avoided and its use should be contained within well-ventilated areas. Due to the corrosive properties of glutaraldehyde, contact of the metal components of the FB for more than 24 h should be avoided. In high concentrations, glutaraldehyde could be toxic to aquatics. Local environmental guidelines for its disposal should be followed, since they may vary from state to state.

Other less toxic disinfectants such as phenol and isopropyl alcohol are less sporicidal then glutaraldehyde. If iodine (Betadine) is used for disinfection, care should be taken to clean the optical lens and eyepiece of the FB, since it may leave a yellowish discoloration. The FB should never be boiled, autoclaved, or placed in an ultrasonic device.[5]

Sterilization

Ethylene oxide (ETO) gas is the most common agent used for sterilization of the FB and should be employed after the bronchoscope is used in patients with HIV or hepatitis.[6] ETO gas penetrates the inaccessible areas of the FB. During the sterilization process, the manufacturer's guidelines regarding temperature, humidity, and pressure settings must be followed for the desired results and to prevent damage to the instrument. The ETO venting cap must be properly placed to equalize the pressures between the exterior and interior of the submersible FB prior to sterilization. This prevents damage to the outer sheath of the FB (Figs. 2-2 and 2-3).

Peracetic acid solution in a computerized automated device has also been used for sterilization of the FB. This requires immersion of the instrument in buffered peracetic acid solution for approximately 12 min (Steris System I, Steris Incorporated, Mentor, Ohio). This device has a simple push button operation with a self-diagnostic and monitoring system (chemi-

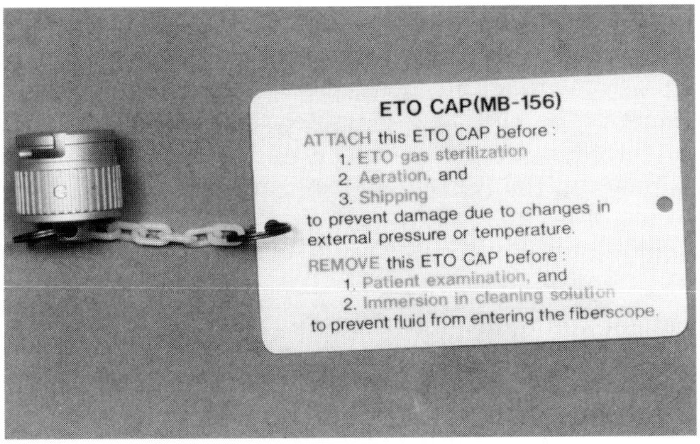

Figure 2-2

Ethylene oxide venting cap.

cal and bacteriological). Effectiveness of this system has been proved in a prospective fashion.[7]

Storage

The FB should be stored in a cabinet in a neutral and vertical position with the angle lock lever released. The storage facility itself should be dry, ventilated, and sheltered from direct sunlight and extremes of temperature. The cabinet should be shielded from fluoroscopic or roentgenographic equipment to avoid undue radiation, which may cause yellowish discoloration and darkening of the fiberoptic bundles.

Transportation

The instrument carrying case with the FB placed in its protective recessed mold is the ideal means of transporting the instrument. Catching the FB between the lids of the case can cause severe damage to the instrument (Fig. 2-4), with black spots appearing in the field of vision suggesting breakage of the fiberoptic bundles. The ETO venting cap must be used during high-altitude flights to equalize the pressure within the body of the submersible FB. The carrying case should not be used for storage of the FB, because it causes bacterial contamination of the instrument.

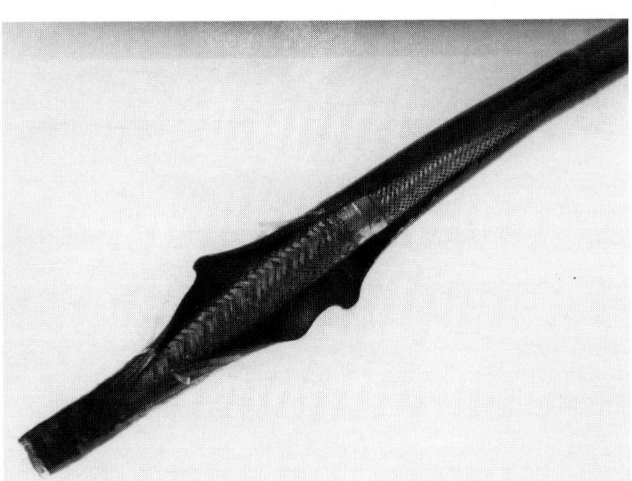

Figure 2-3

Ruptured external rubber sheath of the flexible bronchoscope from ethylene oxide gas sterilization without using the ETO venting cap. *(From Mehta et al,[2] with permission.)*

Prevention of Damage

Prevention of damage to the FB should be an integral part of teaching and learning bronchoscopy. Damage to the FB can be prevented several ways, each of which are discussed under the following headings.

1. Proper handling and lubrication
2. Optimal anesthesia
3. Special procedures

PROPER HANDLING AND LUBRICATION

The three most common maneuvers used during bronchoscopy are (1) in-and-out (push-and-pull) movement, (2) flexion and extension at the tip, and (3) clockwise and counterclockwise rotation on its long axis. Excessive angulation of the FB during any of these maneuvers can lead to breakage of the quartz fibers. The FB should always be in a neutral position while inserting it through the nose, mouth, or endotracheal tube. Excessive angulation of the instrument at its most proximal flexible portion can be avoided by keeping an adequate distance between the operator and the pa-

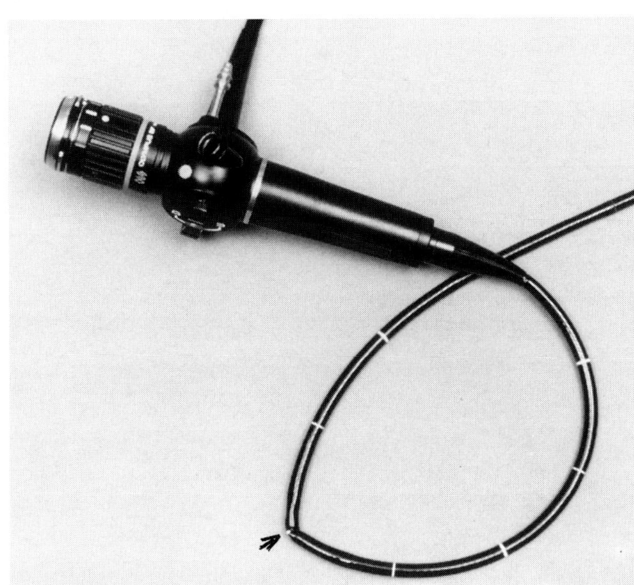

Figure 2-4

Severe damage to the flexible scope caused by accidentally catching the instrument between the lids of the carrying case.

tient. Rotation of its long axis should be carried out by the flexion and extension of the wrist and when the instrument is as straight as possible. This minimizes torque applied to the FB (Fig. 2-5).

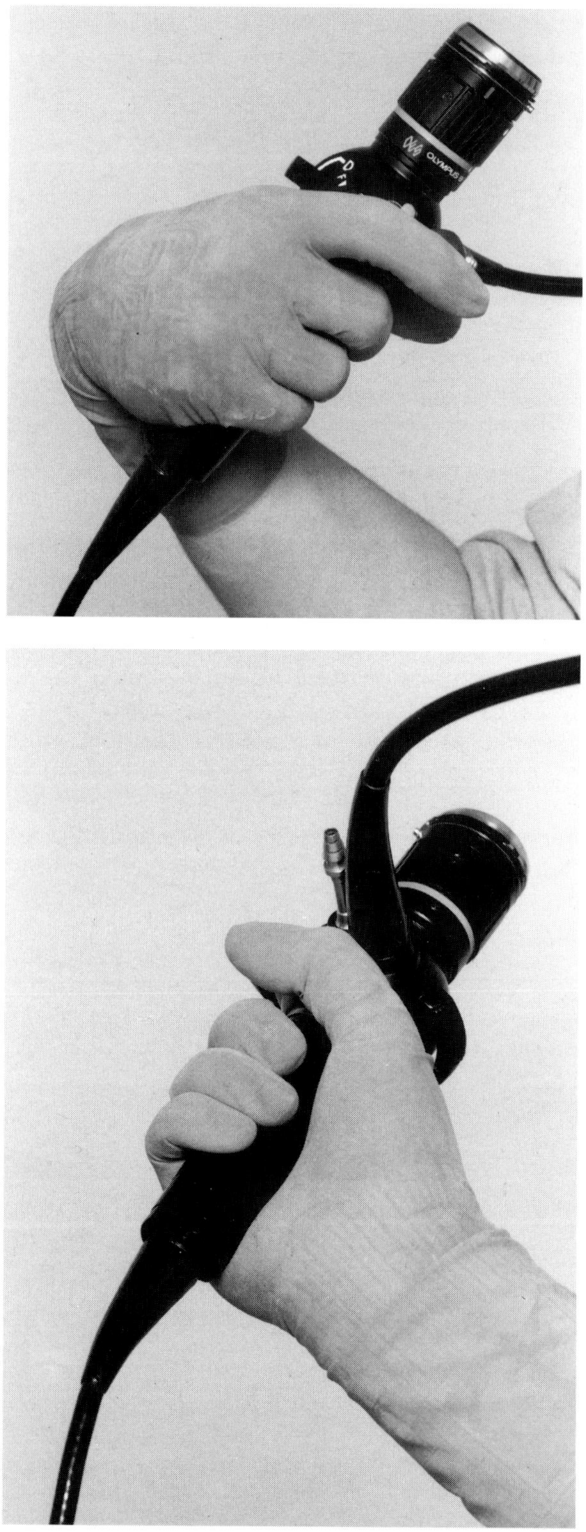

A

B

Figure 2-5

Rotation at the long axis of the instrument should be carried out by flexion or extension of the wrist. *(From Mehta et al,[2] with permission.)*

Passage of an inadequately lubricated FB through an undersized endotracheal tube (ETT) or a tracheostomy tube can cause serious damage to the outer lining of the FB (Fig. 2-6). Water soluble lubricants are preferred, since petroleum-based lubricants can cause damage to the outer distal rubber sheath. The use of an adult FB requires an ETT of at least 8 mm in diameter. For a smaller ETT, a pediatric FB should be used. Failure to do so may cause respiratory distress to the patient and damage to the bronchoscope.

OPTIMAL ANESTHESIA

To prevent damage to the FB, patients should be adequately anesthetized. There are various combinations of drugs that can be used for this purpose. If no contraindication exists for premedication, a combination

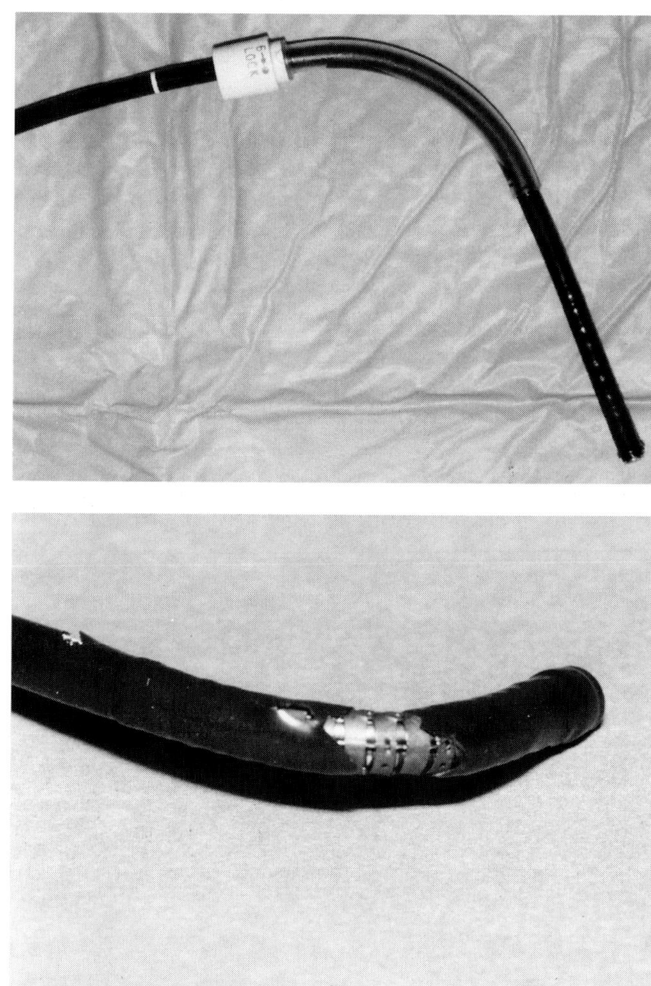

A

B

Figure 2-6

A. Insertion of the flexible scope through an improper size tracheostomy tube leading to obstruction within the tube and causing patient distress. *B*. Forceful removal of the scope through the tracheostomy tube causing severe damage to its external surface. *[From Stelck MH, et al: Maintenance of bronchoscope and bronchoscopy equipment. In Prakash UBS (ed): Bronchoscopy, New York, Raven, 1994.]*

of intramuscular meperidine, hydroxyzine, and atropine for their sedating, antiemetic, and anxiolytic properties, respectively, is recommended. Intravenous midazolam can be used as needed during the procedure. The vocal cords and bronchial tree are anesthetized by 2% lidocaine, which can also be used topically on the pharyngeal mucosa and larynx. Lidocaine jelly is used to anesthetize the nasal mucosa. The goal is to have well anesthetized patients who will not pull or bite and damage the FB. The transnasal route is preferred to prevent patients from biting the FB. If the transoral route is to be used or if the procedure is being performed through the ETT, a bite guard must be in place. Excessive use of topical lidocaine can cause grand mal seizures, which may inadvertently lead to biting of the orally inserted FB and cause damage (Fig. 2-7). Therefore, endobronchial instillation of lidocaine should be carried out judiciously, especially in the pediatric and geriatric populations.

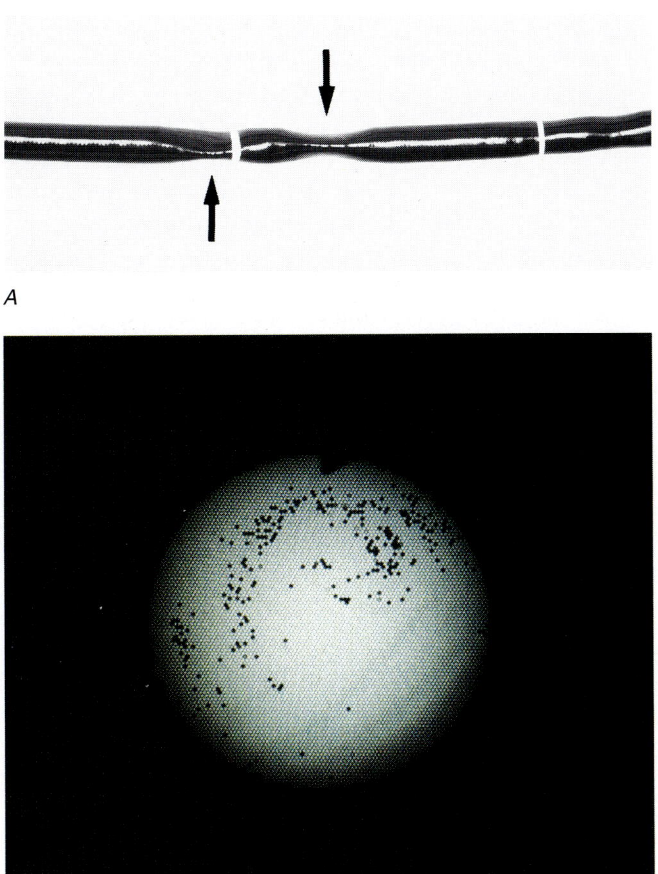

A

B

Figure 2-7

A. Damage to the exterior of the bronchoscope by the patient's biting it during the procedure. *B.* Each dark spot on the view field represents a broken fiberoptic bundle caused by the patient biting the instrument. *(From Mehta et al,[2] with permission.)*

SPECIAL PROCEDURES

Transbronchial Needle Aspiration

Transbronchial needle aspiration (TBNA) for cytology and histology specimens has significantly increased the diagnostic yield of FB.[8–11] However, if improperly used, it can cause severe damage to the instrument.[2,12] The working channel of the FB is made up of a thin plastic tubing to achieve greater flexibility. Damage to this tubing by improper use of the needle can cause seepage of fluids into the fiberoptic bundles, affecting the quality of the image (Fig. 2-8). New, retractable needles have reduced the incidence of damage to the FB, and the nonretractable version has become obsolete.[11,12] During insertion of the retractable needles, the beveled end must be withdrawn completely within the protecting metal hub at the distal end of the plastic catheter. The beveled end of the needle should not be placed proximal to the hub, otherwise, during its forward thrust, it may pierce its own plastic catheter and in turn may cause damage to the working channel of the FB (Fig. 2-9). During insertion of the needle catheter through the working channel, the FB should be kept as straight as possible and in a forward viewing, neutral position. The needle must not be extended out of the catheter until its distal tip is visualized beyond the tip of the FB. After TBNA, the FB should be positioned as for needle insertion, and the catheter withdrawn in one swift motion back through the channel without retracting the needle back into its catheter. A leak test is mandatory following each TBNA. It is also recommended that TBNA should be performed only by an experienced bronchoscopist.

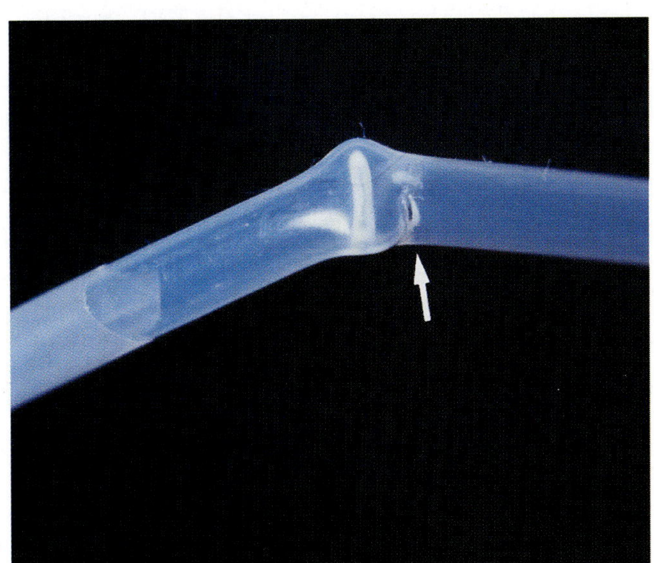

Figure 2-8

Working channel of the flexible bronchoscope retrieved during its repair. Note perforation of the channel during TBNA. Kink in the catheter corresponds to proximal flexible portion of the scope and represents excessive bending. *(From Mehta et al,[2] with permission.)*

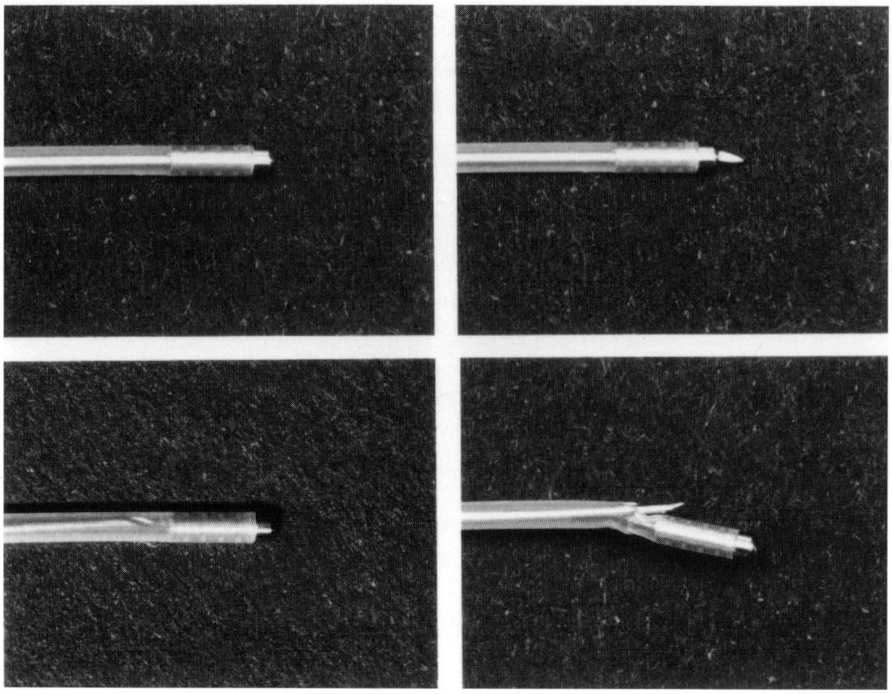

Figure 2-9

Top left: Proper method of TBNA: Note the beveled end of the needle is placed within the metal hub. *Top right:* The beveled end of the needle jutting out of the hub. If the catheter is inserted in the FB in this position, it can cause severe damage to the working channel. *Bottom left:* Note the needle position. It is pulled back proximal to the hub. *Bottom right:* With a forward thrust, it can penetrate its own catheter and in turn damage the scope. *[From Stelck MH, et al: Maintenance of bronchoscope and bronchoscopy equipment. In Prakash UBS (ed): Bronchoscopy, New York, Raven, 1994.]*

Nd:YAG Laser Photoresection

Nd:YAG laser photoresection has been used with the bronchoscope since 1979.[13] Endobronchial Nd:YAG laser resection of lung tumors provides an excellent palliation and improved survival when combined with brachytherapy and radiation therapy in selected patients.[14–19] Procedures can be safely performed through the FB. There is, however, always a risk of endobronchial ignition. While using FB, extreme care should be taken to avoid such a complication (Table 2-1).[20,21] The distal end of the ETT should be kept at least 4 cm from the treatment site. The laser fiber should protrude at least 4 mm from the distal end of the FB and should remain at least 4 mm away from the lesion (noncontact technique). The FI_{O_2} delivered during the procedure should be kept below 40 percent. For maximum safety, single pulse mode should always be used, and interrupted or continuous pulse mode should be avoided. We usually start at 0.4-s pulse duration and adjust according to the tissue reaction. A low power density and short pulse duration minimize the chances of ignition. For a noncontact fiber an initial setting of 40 W and for synthetic sapphire crystal probes 4 to 5 W (contact techniques) are recommended. We pause every 40 pulses to remove and clean any blood or tissue debris sitting on the laser fiber tip. This further prevents endobronchial combustion and damage to the FB.[22] The laser fiber should be properly inspected for any damage prior to its use. Insertion of the damaged portion of the fiber through the FB can cause severe damage to the instrument. In this regard, safety of reusable bare laser fibers with FB has not been established, and such practice should be avoided (Fig. 2-10). Coaxial coolant, either gas (atmospheric air) or saline, should always be used to keep the fire tip cool and clean. A hot metal tip can damage the working channel of the FB. On occasion, a laser procedure may take 2 to 3 h. To prevent fatigue-induced accidents, we recommend that operating room time be limited to less than 4 h. Using designated team members

Table 2-1

"RULE OF FOUR" TO PREVENT LASER-INDUCED DAMAGE TO THE FLEXIBLE BRONCHOSCOPE[a]

Distance	ETT to lesion	>4 cm
	Fiber tip to lesion	>4 mm
	FFB to fiber tip	>4 mm
FI_{O_2}		<40%
Initial setting (W)	Noncontact technique	40 W
	Contact technique	4 W
Pulse duration		0.4 s
Number of pulses between cleaning		40
Operating room time		<4 h
Laser team		4

[a]See text.

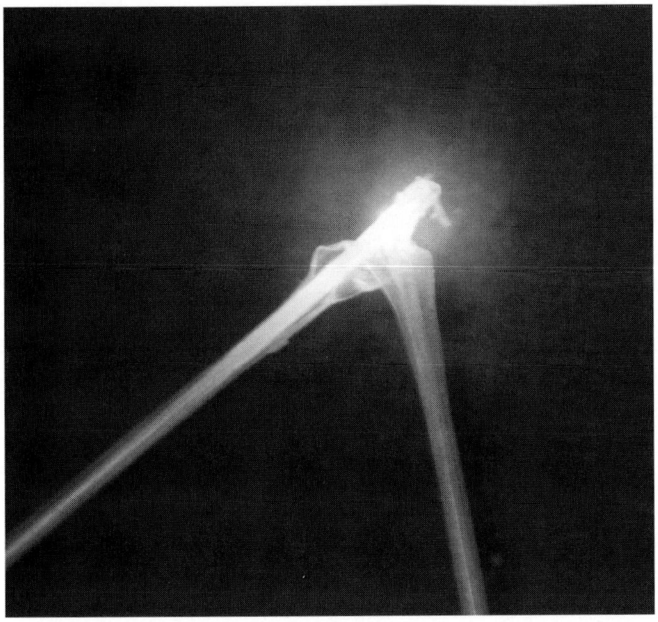

Figure 2-10

Cracked reusable laser fiber. Note seepage of the laser beam through the damaged portion causing melting of its protective sheath. *[From Stelck MH, et al: Maintenance of bronchoscope and bronchoscopy equipment. In Prakash UBS (ed): Bronchoscopy, New York, Raven, 1994.]*

(bronchoscopist, anesthesiologist, operating room nurse, and bronchoscopy assistant) familiar with the procedure further minimizes the risk. Combustible anesthetic agents should be avoided during the laser procedure. It should be noted that the manufacturers of the FB may not include laser procedures as one of the indicated uses of the instrument and may not provide warranty repairs for laser-related damage.

Electrosurgery

The use of FB as an electrosurgical tool has been overshadowed by the advent of laser therapy. The real pioneers of electrocautery through fiberoptic endoscopes are gastrointestinal endoscopists. The successful use of the FB for endobronchial electrocautery has been reported in selected situations.[23–25] The two most common methods used are excision of tumors with a diathermy snare and electrodestruction of tumors with a cautery probe.

An electrocautery unit consists of two electrodes connected to the terminal on a high-frequency alternating current generator. One electrode acts as an active instrument with a small surface area and high current density. The other, dispersive electrode is a larger surface area grounding plate with a low current density, and this is attached to the patient's back. Heat is generated by electrical resistance causing tissue interaction ranging from drying to vaporization.[26]

Unlike the flexible gastroscope, the FB is not a grounded instrument. If a wire loop snare or a cautery probe touches the distal metal tip of the FB, it can cause endobronchial ignition, damage to the instrument and injury to the patient.[23] This can be minimized by using bipolar cautery, keeping the inspired oxygen concentration below 30%, and maintaining a good distance between the endotracheal tube and the probe or snare.[27] If the operator's glove is perforated, a contact between the distal tip of the FB and the probe can deliver an electrical shock to the operator.

Accessories

We recommend replacement rather than repair of the damaged FB accessories such as biopsy forceps, cytology brushes, or cleaning brushes to prevent damage to the working channel of the FB. In our opinion, accessories of larger diameter and those without Teflon coating are more traumatic to the working channel than are smaller diameter and Teflon coated accessories.

Summary

The FB is a delicate instrument and is vulnerable to damage during various steps of the procedure. Repair cost could run in the thousands of dollars per incident. The manufacturer's instruction manual details areas for proper handling of the instrument and should be carefully studied and adhered to by all staff members involved with bronchoscopy. In our survey, it was apparent that more than 80 percent of damage to the FB was due to improper technique and was preventable. Proper maintenance can reduce the repair cost by 50 percent, from $40 to less than $20 per procedure.[2]

REFERENCES

1. Ikeda S, et al: Flexible bronchoscope, *Keo J Med* 1968; 17:16–18.
2. Mehta AC, et al: The high price of bronchoscopy. Maintenance and repair of the flexible fiberoptic bronchoscopy. *Chest* 1990; 98:448–454.
3. Pentax Bronchofiberscopes Owners Manual. 1992: pp 25–26.
4. Lee FYW, Mehta AC: Care and maintenance of the flexible bronchoscope, In Feinsilver SH, Fein AM (eds): *Text Book of Bronchoscopy.* Baltimore, Williams & Wilkins, 1995:100–108.
5. Elford B: Care and cleansing of the fiberoptic bronchoscope. *Chest* 1978; 73:761–763.
6. Hanson PJV, et al: Recovery of the human immunodeficiency virus from the fiberoptic bronchoscope. *Thorax* 1991; 6:410–412.
7. Seballos RJ, et al: Clinical evaluation of a liquid chemical sterilization system for the flexible bronchoscope. *J Bronchology* 1995; 2:192–199.
8. Mehta AC, et al: Newer procedures using the fiberoptic bronchoscope in diagnosing lung cancer. *Cleve Clin J Med* 1987; 54:195–203.
9. Shure D, Fedullo PF: Transbronchial needle aspiration in the diagnosis of submucosal and peribronchial bronchogenic carcinoma. *Chest* 1985; 88:49–51.

10. Wang KP, Terry PP: Transbronchial needle aspiration in diagnosis and staging of bronchogenic carcinoma. *Am Rev Respir Dis* 1983; 127:344–347.
11. Wang KP: Flexible TBNA biopsy for histological specimen. *Chest* 1985:860–863.
12. Kelly SJ, Wang KP: Transbronchial aspiration. *J Thorac Imaging* 1987; 2:330–334.
13. Dumon JF, et al: Bronchofiberscope et laser YAG Neodyme. *Rev Fr Mal Resp* 1981; 9:76.
14. Mehta AC, et al: Flexible bronchoscopy and use of lasers. In Wang KP, Mehta AC (eds): *Flexible Bronchoscopy.* Cambridge MA, Blackwell Scientific 247–274, 1995.
15. Desai SJ, et al: Survival experience following ND:YAG laser photoresection for primary bronchogenic carcinoma. *Chest* 1988; 94:939–944.
16. Mehta AC, et al: Palliative treatment of malignant airway obstruction by Nd:YAG laser. *Cleve Clin J Med* 1985; 52:513–524.
17. Livingston DR, et al: Palliation of malignant tracheobronchial obstruction by Nd:YAG laser: An update of experience at the Cleveland Clinic Foundation. *J Am Osteopath Assoc* 1987; 87:226–233.
18. Brutinel WM, et al: A two year experience with neodymium-YAG laser in endobronchial obstruction. *Chest* 1987; 91:159–165.
19. Ross DJ, et al: Survival characteristic after neodymium-YAG laser photo resection in advanced stage lung cancer. *Chest* 1990; 98:581–585.
20. Casey KR, et al: Intratracheal fire ignited by the Nd:YAG laser during treatment of tracheal stenosis. *Chest* 1983; 84:295–296.
21. Kwartz S, et al: Nd:YAG laser induced burn. Management and long-term follow-up. *Chest* 1989; 95:916–918.
22. Mehta AC, et al: Loss of the fiberoptic laser tip. *Chest* 1985; 88:796.
23. Hooper RG, Jackson FN: Endobronchial electrocautery. *Chest* 1985; 87:712–714.
24. Gerasin VA, Shafirovsky BB: Endobronchial electrosurgery. *Chest* 1988; 93:270–274.
25. Hooper RG, Jackson FN: Endobronchial electrocautery. *Chest* 1988; 94:595–598.
26. Barlow DE: Endoscopic application of electrocautery; A review of basic principles. *Gastrointest Endosc* 1982; 28:73–76.
27. Marsh BR: Bipolar cautery for the fiberoptic bronchoscope. *Ann Otol Rhinol Laryngol* 1987; 96:120–121.

CHAPTER 3

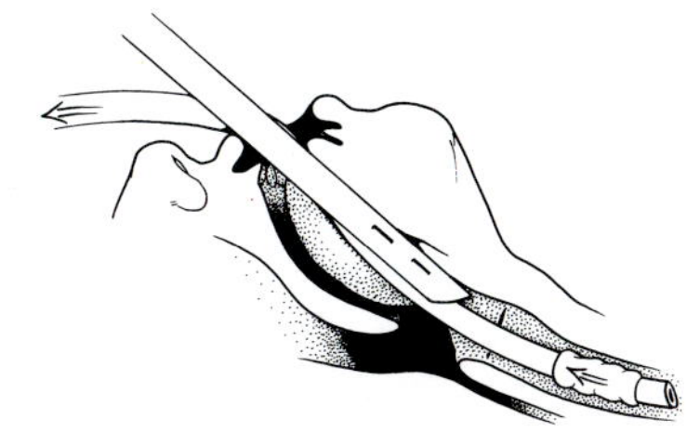

RIGID BRONCHOSCOPY

John F. Beamis, Jr.

The bronchi enlarge and elongate at each inspiration, diminish and shorten during expiration. The heart at each beat dinges in the bronchial wall or pushes the whole bronchial tube sidewise; the thumping is transmitted to the fingers holding the inserted [rigid] bronchoscope. One gets the impression of being in the midst of the machinery of life itself.

Chevalier Jackson
The Life of Chevalier Jackson: An Autobiography

Slightly more than a century ago, the first translaryngeal rigid bronchoscopy was performed by Gustov Killian of the University of Freiburg, Germany.[1] For more than 80 years, this remarkable instrument was the main access to the lower airway for diagnostic and therapeutic interventions. During this time, rigid bronchoscopies were performed primarily by our surgical colleagues in otolaryngology and thoracic surgery. Killian, an otolaryngologist, developed an international reputation because of his skills in removing foreign bodies from the lower airway. In the United States, Chevalier Jackson, also an otolaryngologist, improved on Killian's techniques, advanced the design of the bronchoscope and supporting instruments, and developed procedural and safety protocols that continue to be used today.[2] Jackson trained generations of thoracic endoscopists and is considered the father of American bronchoesophagology. The invention of the flexible bronchoscope in the late 1960s by Ikeda dramatically changed the world of bronchoscopy.

Ikeda's invention provided visualization of the more distal airways, permitted bronchoscopy to be performed comfortably in a patient under local anesthesia, and opened the field of bronchoscopy to the pulmonary internist. The rapid and widespread application of the flexible bronchoscope dramatically reduced the need for rigid bronchoscopy. The number of rigid and flexible bronchoscopies performed at the Mayo Clinic between 1969 and 1985 and the effect of the flexible bronchoscope on the field of rigid bronchoscopy are depicted in Fig. 3-1. Although the use of rigid bronchoscopy took a downturn with the introduction of the flexible bronchoscope, rigid bronchoscopy is not a dying art. As seen in Fig. 3-1, a moderate but significant increase in the use of the rigid bronchoscope has occurred since 1981. This is the result of interventional pulmonology for, at this time, Mayo pulmonologists began performing laser bronchoscopy and later bronchial stent placement—two procedures that employed the rigid bronchoscope. It has been a worldwide experience that the introduction of modern interventional procedures has reaffirmed the use of the rigid bronchoscope. As will be mentioned in later chapters, rigid bronchoscopy is considered by many to be the preferred bronchoscope for procedures, such as laser and cryotherapy applications and insertion of silicone stents. Once a procedure only performed by surgeons, rigid bronchoscopy is probably more commonly performed by pulmonologists at this time.

Indications

From the days of Killian and Jackson until the beginning of the lung cancer epidemic of the 1960s, foreign body retrieval was the most common indication for rigid bronchoscopy. Other indications included dilation of strictures caused by diphtheria and tuberculous stenosis and in cleaning out airway secretions in patients with bronchiectasis. Endobronchial cancer therapy with the rigid bronchoscope was performed in a few centers where radioactive seeds were inserted into airway tumors through the scope.[3] This method resulted in considerable radiation exposure to the bronchoscopists and was abandoned when improved techniques for external radiation therapy were developed.

Figure 3-1

Number of rigid and flexible bronchoscopy procedures performed at Mayo Clinic 1969–1985. (Courtesy of Denis Cortese, MD, Mayo Clinic, Jacksonville, FL.)

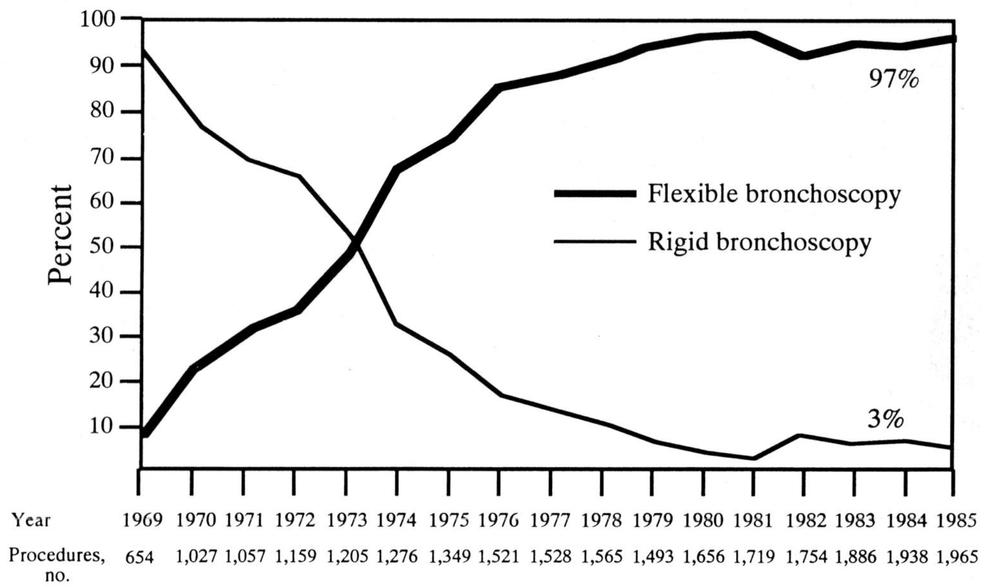

Current indications for rigid bronchoscopy in adults emphasize the therapeutic use of this instrument (Table 3-1). The scope itself and simple accessories, such as suction tubes and biopsy and alligator forceps are sufficient to clean the airways of clots and blood in the diagnosis and management of massive hemoptysis. Often a flexible bronchoscope can then be passed through the rigid scope to perform a complete diagnostic study. Despite the ability to visualize the origin of all lobar bronchi and lower lobe segmental bronchi with the rigid bronchoscope, the flexible bronchoscope has replaced the rigid instrument for nearly all diagnostic indications. Occasionally, a deep bronchial wall biopsy with the rigid instrument can be helpful if a submucosal lesion cannot be reached by the smaller biopsy forceps used through the flexible bronchoscope. This indication can often be obviated by the use of transbronchial needle aspiration by means of a flexible bronchoscope (Chap. 17). The excellent optics provided by the telescopes used with rigid bronchoscopy permit excellent photographic documentation with still or video photography.

Table 3-1
CURRENT INDICATIONS FOR RIGID BRONCHOSCOPY

Diagnostic
Deep biopsy
Photographic documentation
Therapeutic
Massive hemoptysis
Dilation of stenosis
Laser therapy
Stent insertion
Foreign body removal
Tumor resection
Cryotherapy
Electrocautery

The vast majority of indications for modern rigid bronchoscopy are therapeutic. Thoracic endoscopists currently have a number of tools that can be used to treat various tracheobronchial disorders (Table 3-2). A number of these therapies—laser, cryotherapy, stents, and electrocautery—will be discussed in later chapters. Facility with a rigid bronchoscope makes many of these procedures easier and quicker for the bronchoscopist and safer for the patient. It can be argued that many of these procedures can be performed with either rigid or flexible bronchoscopy, and what ultimately determines the technique is the bronchoscopist's experience, expertise, and preference. There has been little objective comparison of the two techniques for specific therapeutic applications. Chan and colleagues[4] compared rigid and flexible bronchoscopy for neodymium:yttrium-aluminum-garnet (Nd:YAG) laser applications and found little overall difference in outcome; however, the authors suggested that rigid bronchoscopy is more efficacious for central lesions, whereas the flexible bronchoscope is preferred for more distal laser applications. This conclusion could also be applied to bronchoscopic cryotherapy and electrocautery. Currently, silicone stents must be inserted through a rigid bronchoscope, whereas self-expandable metal stents can be inserted with either bronchoscope.

Table 3-2
ENDOBRONCHIAL THERAPIES

Tool	Scope	Rapid Effect	Repeatable	Complication: Immediate	Complication: Delayed	Lesion
Laser	Rigid/flexible	++++	++++	++	+	Endobronchial
Brachytherapy	Flexible[a]	+	+	+	+++	Endobronchial/submucosal
Cryotherapy	Rigid/flexible	++	++++	++	++	Endobronchial
Balloon dilation	Rigid/flexible	++++	++++	+++	+	Submucosal/external compression
Photodynamic therapy	Flexible[a]	++	+++	+	+++	Endobronchial/submucosal
Electrocautery	Rigid/flexible	+++	++++	++	++	Endobronchial
Stent	Rigid/flexible[b]	++++	+++	++	+++	External compression

[a]Preferred method.
[b]Silicone stents require rigid scope; self-expandable metal stents require fluoroscopy.

Mechanical resection of endobronchial tumors with a rigid bronchoscope is a classic technique still performed by many rigid bronchoscopists. Mathisen and Grillo[5] described the "time-honored" method of clearing out endobronchial tumors with the bevel tip of a rigid bronchoscope, and they believe ancillary therapy, such as lasers, is not necessary to accomplish airway opening and results in increased cost and risk. These surgeons first biopsy a tumor to assess its consistency and vascularity, and then they advance the bronchoscope in a corkscrew manner, shearing the tumor off the airway wall. The resected tumor is removed with forceps. Bleeding from the base is controlled with tamponade by the bronchoscope. Diluted epinephrine or epinephrine pledgets are used to stop oozing from the base of the tumor. Although the technique described is respected, many therapeutic bronchoscopists prefer to devascularize the tumor with adjunctive therapies, such as laser, cryotherapy, and electrocautery, to minimize bleeding.[6] After a tumor has been treated, it can be cored out with the rigid bronchoscope.

The extraction of foreign bodies remains a valid indication for rigid bronchoscopy; however, at this time, the rigid bronchoscope must be considered second-line therapy. Many bronchoscopists would at least attempt most foreign body removals with a flexible bronchoscope.[7] If the foreign body cannot be extracted with a flexible bronchoscope, the rigid bronchoscope can be employed.[8] Currently, many prefer the rigid bronchoscope for removal of foreign bodies in children.[9]

The rigid bronchoscope is an excellent tool to dilate benign tracheal and bronchial stenosis, either idiopathic in etiology or following tuberculosis, endotracheal intubation, or tracheostomy.[10] The operator must begin with bronchoscopes of small diameter and gradually progress to scopes of larger diameter that will dilate the airway to near-normal caliber. During each dilation, the bevel of the bronchoscope is inserted into the stenotic lumen, and, with a gentle corkscrew motion, the scope is advanced through the stenosis. Several passes are made with each diameter bronchoscope until the scope passes freely through the stenosis. If the stenosis is too narrow to admit the tip of the bronchoscope at the initial maneuver, ancillary therapies, such as bougies or laser, can be used to widen the stenosis until the bronchoscope can be admitted.

As a therapeutic instrument with or without ancillary therapies, such as laser or cryotherapy, the rigid bronchoscope is associated with a number of distinct advantages, including the ability to use large-bore suction catheters to control hemorrhage, the ability to tamponade hemorrhagic areas with the wall of the bronchoscope, better control of the airway to maintain ventilation in patients who have high-grade obstruction, the ability to obtain tactile information regarding the mobility of the airway and surrounding tumors, the use of large forceps to obtain deep biopsy specimens, the ability to shear off and remove large pieces of tumor or foreign bodies with grasping or foreign body forceps, and the excellent optical characteristics of the telescopic lens, which permit superb photographic documentation.

The Instrument

The modern rigid bronchoscope consists of an open metal tube, whose distal end is smooth and beveled (Fig. 3-2). For use in adults, the diameter of the tube varies in width from 9 to 13 mm. A typical rigid bronchoscope has several openings on the side of the barrel to permit ventilation of the opposite lung if the tube is passed deep into the airway on one side. A tracheoscope has no side holes and should be used only for diagnostic or therapeutic indications between the vocal cords and the carina. A standard rigid bronchoscope is 40 cm in length. Some bronchoscopes have light carriers or suction channels built into the internal wall. The proximal end of the rigid bronchoscope contains side ports, which may be used to administer oxygen or supply assisted Venturi jet ventilation (Fig. 3-2C). The excellent optics of rigid bronchoscopy are achieved by inserting a telescopic lens through the bronchoscope tube. The classic telescope is a series of lenses within a stainless tube offering a wide angle view with a mild degree of magnification. Various accessories can be inserted through specially designed ports (Fig. 3-3) or through the open tube alongside the telescopic lens. These include rigid and semi-rigid suction catheters, biopsy forceps, foreign body forceps, bougies, transbronchial needles for aspiration, laser fibers, cryotherapy probes, and electrocautery wires (Fig. 3-4).

Ventilation Techniques

The classic technique of rigid bronchoscopy as described by Jackson for removal of foreign bodies and biopsy of bronchial lesions was often performed with the patient apneic after breathing 100% oxygen, giving the bronchoscopist precious few seconds to perform a therapeutic and diagnostic procedure. After the in-

Figure 3-2

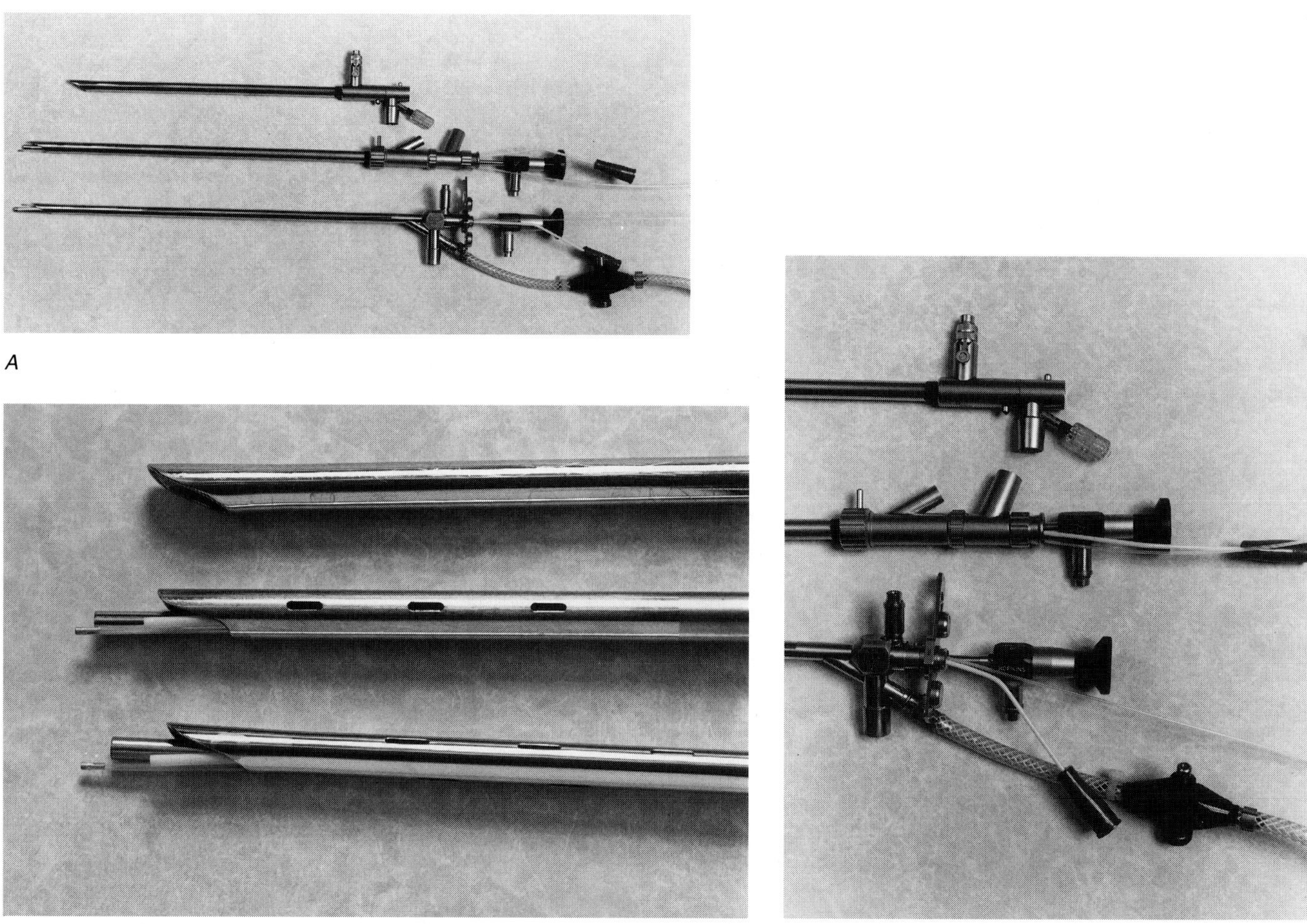

A B C

A. Rigid bronchoscopes used at Lahey Clinic Medical Center. *Top,* Storz tracheoscope for tracheal lesions (Karl Storz Endoscopy-America, Culver City, CA). *Middle,* Dumon-Harrell universal bronchoscope with suction catheter, telescope, and laser fiber (Bryon Corp, Woburn, MA). *Bottom,* Storz ventilating bronchoscope with suction catheter, telescope, laser fiber, and Venturi jet adapter (Karl Storz Endoscopy-America). *B.* Closeup of bronchoscopic barrels. The tracheoscope has no side holes. *C.* Proximal end of bronchoscopes with usual orientation of telescopes and suction catheters.

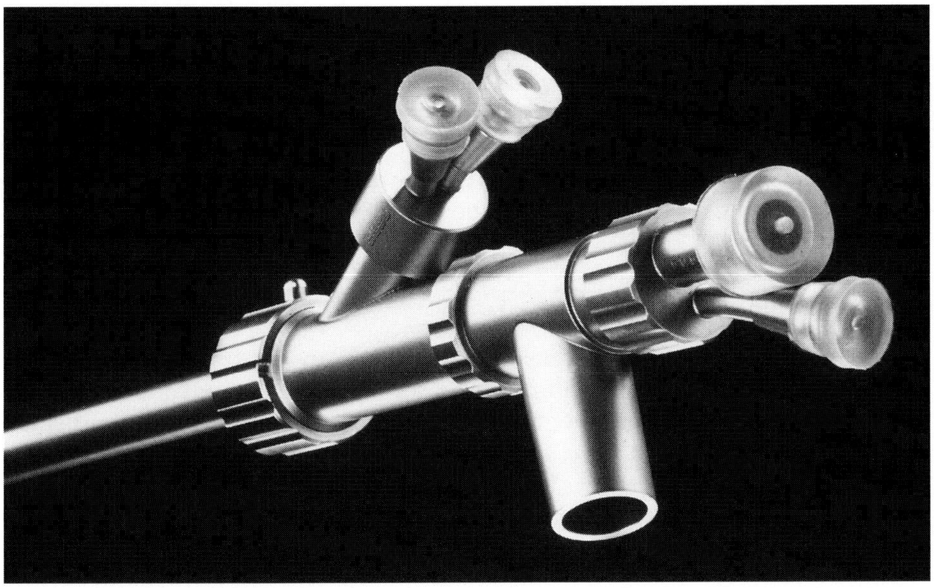

Figure 3-3

Proximal end of universal head of Dumon-Harrell bronchoscope showing ports for suction catheters, laser fiber, telescope, and ventilation.

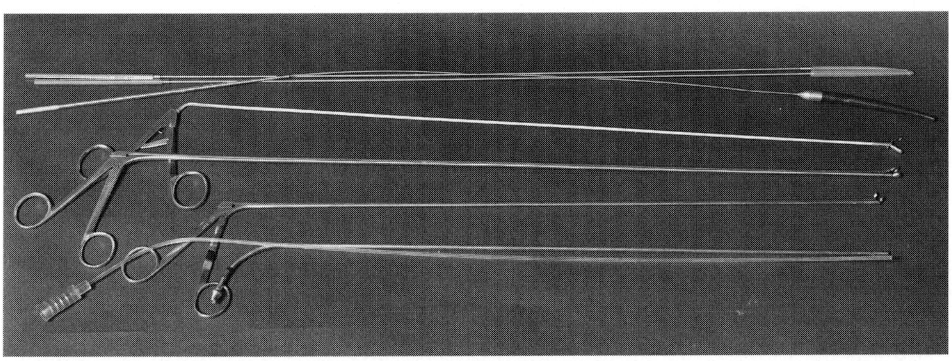

A

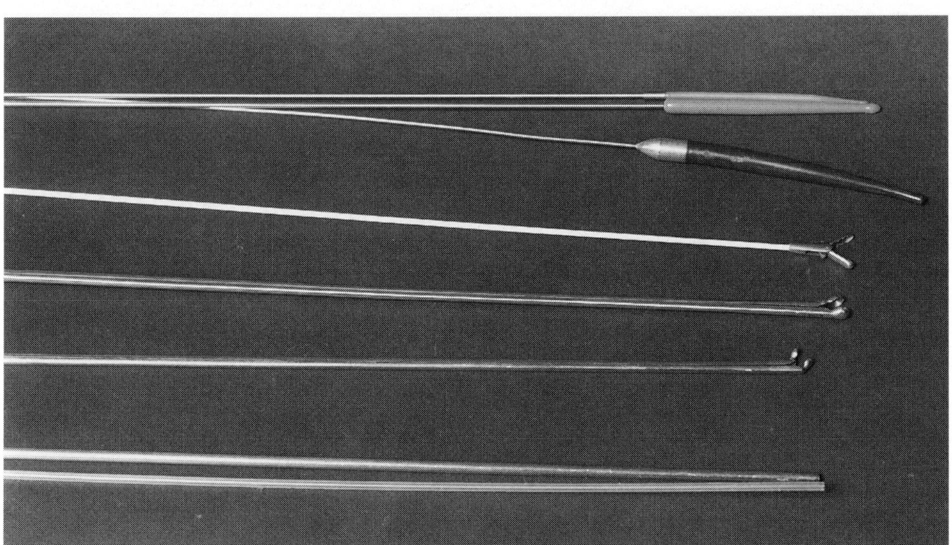

B

Figure 3-4

A and *B*. Accessory instruments for rigid bronchoscopy. *Top to bottom*, Several sizes of Jackson dilators, alligator forceps, standard biopsy forceps, up-biting biopsy forceps, rigid suction tube, and plastic suction tube.

struments were out of the tube, the bronchoscope was capped, enabling the anesthesiologist to ventilate the patient. Modern techniques of laser bronchoscopy and placement of stents require longer procedures, and thus other ventilatory techniques must be employed (Table 3-3). Spontaneous ventilation is occasionally sufficient to achieve adequate gas exchange during rigid bronchoscopy. However, patients with airway obstruction, when sedated to the degree to permit intubation, may not adequately ventilate during a lengthy procedure. Perrin and coworkers[11] described the technique of spontaneous assisted ventilation during which the patient is anesthetized to the point where spontaneous ventilation is preserved. Frequent assisted breaths are provided by the anesthesiologist. This method leads to rapid awakening after the procedure but is often insufficient to control cough during the procedure. Controlled ventilation requires the use of muscle relaxants or deeper anesthesia. Venturi jet ventilation, which permits the use of an open tube, is an effective method to maintain gas exchange during long procedures. Our method is similar to that described by Godden and colleagues[12] and Stradling[13] and involves "injecting" 100% oxygen at 50 psi into the side port of the bronchoscope. Adequate ventilation is determined by the movement of the chest with each injected breath. Room air is entrained through the open end of the scope, resulting in an inspired oxygen concentration of considerably less than 100%. Adequacy of oxygenation is monitored with pulse oximetry. Closed circuit ventilation systems for rigid bronchoscopy have also been employed. These systems require controlling air leaks by packing the mouth with gauze or by placing an inflatable cuff around the barrel of the tube. These methods are cumbersome at best and at times dangerous since high airway pressures may build up during assisted breathing. These methods permit the use of inhalational anesthetic agents. Some bronchoscopists place a small endotracheal tube through the larynx to ventilate the patient and then pass the rigid bronchoscope alongside the endotracheal tube.[14] The size of the larynx limits the diameter of the rigid tube that can be used with this technique.

Table 3-3
VENTILATION AND ANESTHESIA FOR RIGID BRONCHOSCOPY

- Ventilation options
  - Apnea
  - Spontaneous
  - Spontaneous/assist
  - Controlled
    - Closed system
    - Open system—jet ventilation
  - Via endotracheal tube
- Anesthetic techniques
  - Topical/sedation
  - General
    - Inhalational
    - Intravenous

Anesthesia

Unlike flexible bronchoscopy, most patients undergoing rigid bronchoscopy require general anesthesia. Patients with high-grade tracheal obstruction and some elderly and debilitated patients may tolerate the procedure under local anesthesia with topical lidocaine and conscious sedation with midazolam or a narcotic or both. Most bronchoscopists prefer that the patient receive general anesthesia with an intravenous agent. Currently, excellent intravenous anesthetics and narcotics are available that provide rapid onset of action, comfortable anesthesia, and rapid awakening of the patient. Anesthesia for rigid bronchoscopy is discussed in Chap. 21.

Contraindications

Because most patients undergo rigid bronchoscopy under general anesthesia, any contraindications to anesthetic agents, such as severe hemodynamic instability or respiratory failure with refractory hypoxemia, would prohibit the use of rigid bronchoscopy. Patients with an unstable cervical spine or diminished range of motion of the cervical spine caused by spondylosis should not undergo rigid bronchoscopy. Occasionally, maxillofacial trauma or oral disease prevents opening of the jaw to admit the bronchoscope. Laryngeal disease, such as stenosis or obstructing neoplasms, may prevent translaryngeal passage of the scope without inducing further trauma. Patients who have undergone total laryngectomy can actually undergo bronchoscopy easily through the tracheostomy stoma.

Complications

With good technique and safe anesthesia, complications associated with rigid bronchoscopy should be minimal.[15] Injury to the teeth and gums is most common, especially in the patient with a short, thick neck and micrognathia. Rupture of the tracheal or bronchial wall is always a possibility with aggressive dilatation. Minor or massive bleeding can occur during resection of the tumor. Fortunately, complications associated with rigid bronchoscopy are rare and can usually be avoided with proper technique and following the safety precautions outlined years ago by Jackson.

Future of Rigid Bronchoscopy

Although not exactly a forgotten art in the United States, rigid bronchoscopy is performed by a minority of pulmonologists. Tape and coworkers[16] surveyed 1000 pulmonologist members of the American College of Physicians and found that 8 percent performed rigid bronchoscopy, whereas 96 percent performed fiberoptic bronchoscopy. Prakash and colleagues[17] polled 1700 members of the American College of Chest Physicians who were pulmonologists and found that only 8.4 percent used rigid bronchoscopy. It is easy to understand why many pulmonologists in the United States insist on the use of flexible bronchoscopy for all airway endoscopic indications: They have had no experience with the rigid bronchoscope and may not be able to obtain proper training. Now that most bronchoscopies are performed by pulmonologists, newly trained cardiothoracic surgeons and otolaryngologists have not received exposure to rigid bronchoscopy—a procedure that was once an important part of their practice. In the United Kingdom, nearly 20 percent of bronchoscopists have performed rigid bronchoscopy, and 4.3 percent of bronchoscopies performed by internists involve rigid bronchoscopy.[18] In the Netherlands, where most bronchoscopists have training in both rigid and flexible bronchoscopy and where "the majority [of bronchoscopists] still regard the skill to perform rigid bronchoscopy a *must*," only 4.8 percent of bronchoscopies involve use of the rigid bronchoscope.[19] Throughout the world, the vast majority of rigid bronchoscopies are performed in association with interventional procedures, such as laser, placement of stents, electrocautery, and cryotherapy. These interventions will continue to stimulate the interest of some bronchoscopists to learn the skill and art of rigid bronchoscopy.

Achieving training in rigid bronchoscopy is often difficult. Such training is not an integral part of current pulmonary and critical care medicine fellowships. Access to rigid bronchoscopic equipment, operating room privileges, and expensive equipment for interventions may be difficult for most pulmonologists to obtain. Attracting a sufficient volume of cases to maintain one's skills and to stimulate interest of anesthesiologists and bronchoscopic team members may be difficult. The problems involved in training for laser bronchoscopy outlined by Kvale[20] are often encountered in training for rigid bronchoscopy. Attendance at postgraduate courses and practice with teaching models[21] are helpful but do not give the physicians sufficient experience to use the instrument on patients. Achieving extensive experience and expertise with flexible bronchoscopy and working closely with a recognized expert during fellowship or in the post-training years remain the best methods of achieving skills in performing rigid bronchoscopy. Stradling[13] stated "no physician specializing in respiratory medicine today is considered adequately trained unless competent with the bronchoscope: The problem is learning the art." A similar statement can be applied to interventional pulmonology: No physician specializing in interventional pulmonology today is considered adequately trained unless competent with the rigid bronchoscope: The problem is learning the art.

HOW I DO IT

At our institution, almost all patients undergoing rigid bronchoscopy receive general anesthesia. For this reason, they undergo standard preoperative evaluation and testing. Laboratory tests include complete blood count, electrocardiography, measurement of oxygen saturation or arterial blood gases, and other more detailed testing as warranted by the patient's underlying condition. Invariably, chest roentgenography and computed tomography have been performed because of the patient's pulmonary condition. Informed consent is obtained by the bronchoscopist and by the anesthesiologist. In the operating suite, the patient is placed in the supine position with the head supported to keep the neck slightly flexed. General intravenous anesthesia is induced, and intravenous muscle relaxation is administered. The anesthesiologist remains in control of the ventilation and attempts to achieve oxygen saturation of 100%. The upper teeth are protected with a disposable tooth guard, and the pharynx is suctioned clear. Three techniques can be used to intubate the patient with the rigid bronchoscope. The choice of these techniques depends on the state of the patient and the skill of the operator.

INTUBATION OVER ENDOTRACHEAL TUBE

This method is best used for patients who come to rigid bronchoscopy already intubated, and it is a safe technique for the novice in rigid bronchoscopy because it ensures adequate oxygenation and ventilation of the patient throughout the intubation process. The patient is brought to the operating suite intubated, and general anesthesia and muscle relaxation are administered; in the initially nonintubated patient, general anesthesia and muscle relaxation are administered, and the patient is intubated. The endotracheal tube is left untaped and is held toward the left side of the mouth by the anesthesiologist. A tooth guard is applied and the pharynx suctioned. The mouth is held open by the fingers of the operator's left hand, and the bronchoscope is inserted into the back of the mouth (Fig. 3-5*A*). Visualization is accomplished by looking directly down the barrel of a bronchoscope, which has its own inner light source, or by using the telescope with or without a video adapter. With the distal bevel of the bronchoscope held against the tongue, the bronchoscope is advanced and positioned slightly anterior to the endotracheal tube. The endotracheal tube must be visualized throughout the maneuver. Gradually, the bronchoscope is advanced from the right side of the mouth along the path of the endotracheal tube to a position in which the left vocal cord can be visualized. At this point, the operator can see the anterior aspect of the left cord and the endotracheal tube passing through the vocal cords (Fig. 3-5*B*). Secretions around the vocal cords can be suctioned using the rigid or flexible suction instruments. The anesthesiologist is asked to let down the endotracheal tube balloon cuff. Air bubbles up through the cords when the cuff relaxes. The anesthesiologist is asked to pull the endotracheal tube out very slowly. The bronchoscopist must never lose sight of the endotracheal tube as it is being withdrawn. After the deflated cuff has passed above the vocal cords, the bronchoscope is rotated 90 degrees, the proximal end of the bronchoscope is moved from the right side of the mouth toward the midline, and the scope is advanced gently under direct vision into the upper trachea (Fig. 3-5*C*). When the bevel of the scope has passed through the vocal cords, the scope is

Figure 3-5

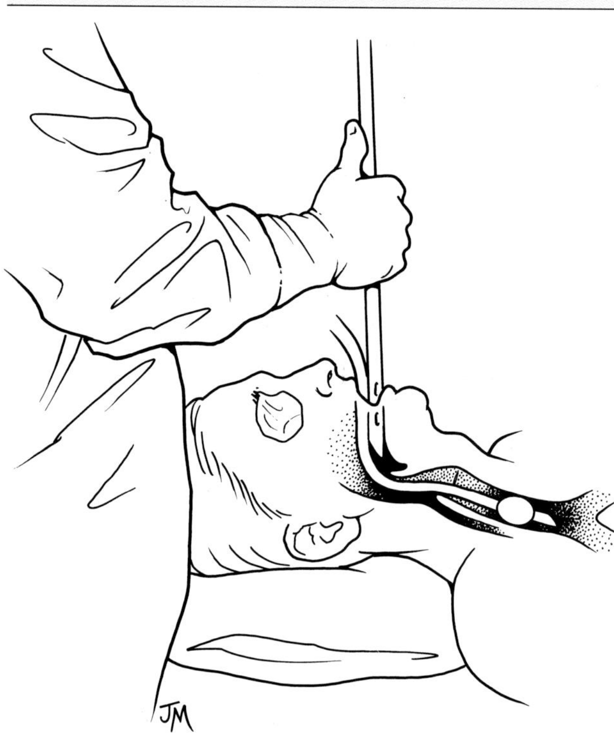

A

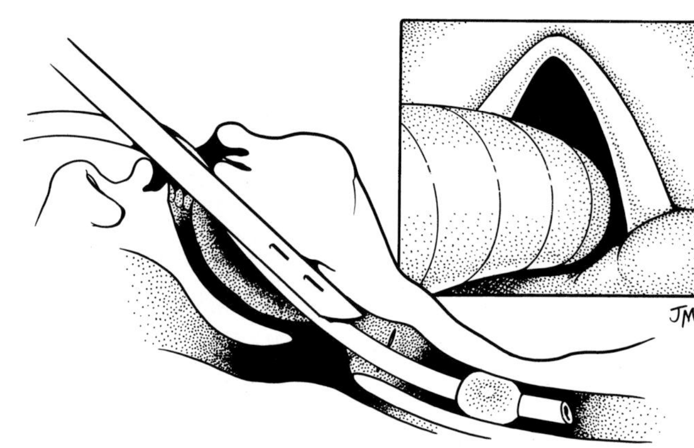

B

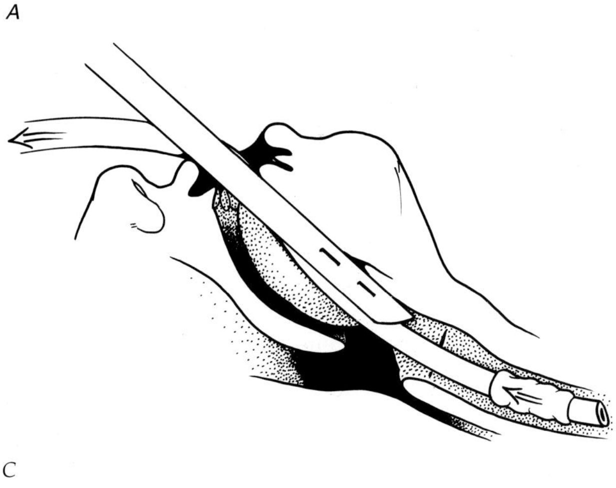

C

Rigid bronchoscope intubation over an endotracheal tube. *A*. Initial position of the bronchoscope. *B*. Position of bronchoscope and endoscope viewed in supraglottic pharynx. *C*. Rigid bronchoscope is advanced as endotracheal tube is withdrawn.

turned 90 degrees back toward its initial position and advanced down the trachea. As the bronchoscope passes the midtrachea, it is usually necessary to remove any pillows under the patient, permitting the patient's neck to be full extended. If the telescopic lens has not been used during the intubation process, it is now placed within the bronchoscope to permit maximum visualization of the airway and the mucosa. It is best to advance the scope with a gentle side-to-side twisting motion rather than pushing straight ahead. When the bronchoscope is in the trachea, manual jet ventilation is begun through the bronchoscope. The jet is powered by 100% oxygen at 50 psi pressure through an oxygen blender. Adequate ventilation is determined by movement of the chest wall with each breath.

To visualize the distal airways and to advance the scope into the main bronchi requires advancing the scope in a twisting motion and maintaining the patient's head in the proper position. To advance the scope into the right main bronchus, the patient's head is turned toward the left shoulder. To visualize the left main bronchus, the head is rotated toward the right. After the bronchoscope has been advanced to the proper position, various diagnostic and therapeutic procedures can be carried out.

INTUBATION USING A LARYNGOSCOPE

This method is useful for the bronchoscopist who has advanced beyond the novice stage but who continues to have problems locating the larynx without some assistance. The operator uses a laryngoscope with a straight blade in the standard manner to visualize the epiglottis (Fig. 3-6*A*). After the epiglottis has been visualized, the bronchoscope, which is held in the right hand, is passed under direct vision. The tip of the bronchoscope bevel is placed just under the epiglottis. The bronchoscopist begins to look down the barrel of the bronchoscope and lifts the epiglottis anteriorly with the tip of the bronchoscope as the laryngoscope is withdrawn. Care must be taken not to advance the blade of the laryngoscope into the vallecula or under the epiglottis since the two instruments are too large to be within the glottis at one time (Fig. 3-6*B1,2*). Often the epiglottis can be visualized simply by using the blade of the laryngoscope at the level of the base of the tongue. After the tip of the rigid bronchoscope has been placed under the epiglottis, the vocal cords are usually quickly seen as the scope is tipped anteriorly. When the laryngoscope is removed from the mouth, the head of the bronchoscope is rotated toward the midline, keeping the vocal cords in view. The scope is turned 90 degrees clockwise so that the bevel of the scope will pass through the vocal cords. The scope is advanced into the trachea (Fig. 3-6*B3*) and then rotated 90 degrees counterclockwise to the midposition. The trachea and lower bronchial tree are then visualized. This technique is also useful for the patient with a short neck and for the patient with excessive redundant tissue within the posterior pharynx. It permits more rapid visualization of the larynx than the classic method. The initial position of the patient is the same as described earlier, with the neck in a slightly flexed position. The patient is fully asleep, and muscle relaxants have been administered before insertion of the laryngoscope.

CLASSIC TECHNIQUE

The classic technique of intubating with a rigid bronchoscope involves no tools to assist the bronchoscopist. The patient is fully anesthetized, and muscle relaxants have been administered. Depending on the patient's pulmonary reserve, the bronchoscopist has approximately 30 to 60 s to achieve intubation and restore ventilation. Thus, this technique is not for the novice and requires considerable practice. The procedure begins with the tooth guard placed over the patient's upper teeth and the oral cavity suctioned clear. The rigid bronchoscope is held with the right hand. The thumb of the left hand is placed against the upper teeth. The third, fourth, and fifth fingers are placed in the mouth, and slight pressure is applied on the bottom teeth. The barrel of the bronchoscope is held as a pool stick between the tips of the thumb and second finger of the left hand. The procedure begins with the bevel of the scope facing anteriorly (Fig. 3-7*A*). It is imperative that the scope be kept exactly in the midline. The scope is advanced into the mouth perpendicular to the operating table. The anterior wall of the bronchoscope is placed along the dorsum of the tongue. The bronchoscopist looks directly down the barrel of the bronchoscope or places a telescope into the bronchoscope and uses a video camera. The first structure that is seen is the uvula, which should be at the 6 o'clock position. With the base of the tongue as a fulcrum, the head of the bronchoscope is lowered to approximately a 45-degree angle from the table. As the scope is gently advanced using a twisting motion, the epiglottis will come into view. The tip of the bevel of the bronchoscope is used to lift the tip of the epiglottis anteriorly to pass the scope under the epiglottis. After the scope has been passed under the epiglottis and has been advanced approximately 1 cm, the vocal cords should come into view. The bronchoscope is gently advanced; when it reaches a position immediately above the vocal cords, the head of the bronchoscope is rotated 90 degrees clockwise. The scope is advanced through the vocal cords (Fig. 3-7*B*). The bronchoscope is advanced to the midtracheal level to be sure that the side holes of the bronchoscope have passed through vocal cords. The Venturi jet ventilator is hooked up at this point and the patient ventilated. Bronchoscopy is carried out as described earlier (Fig. 3-7*C*).

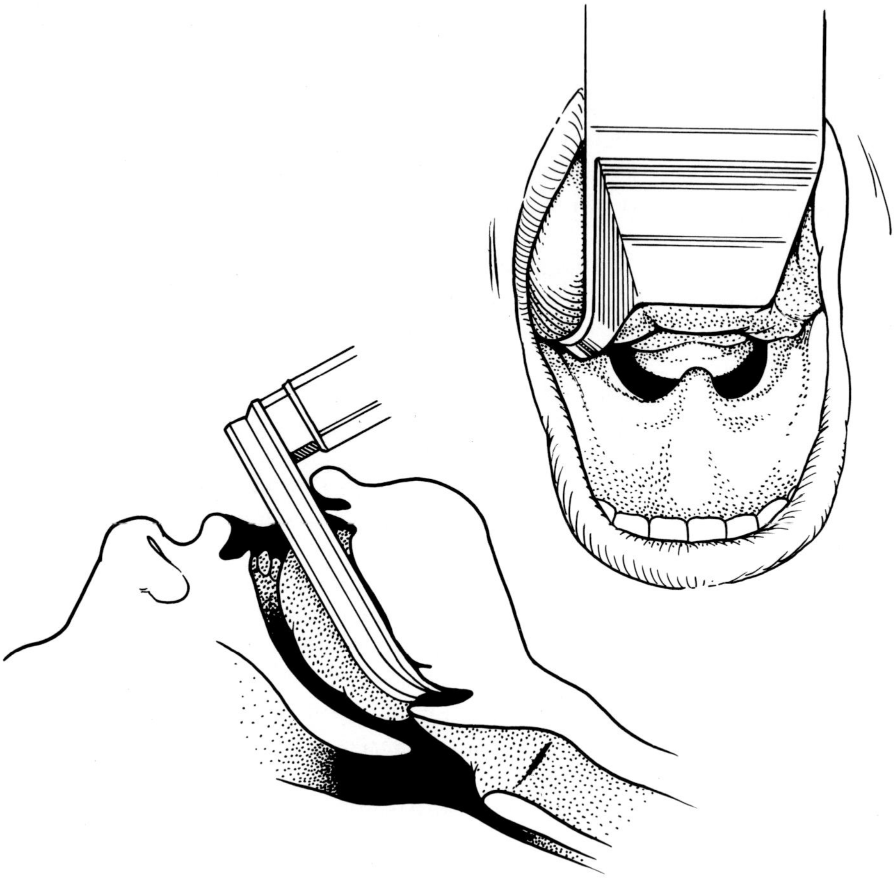

A

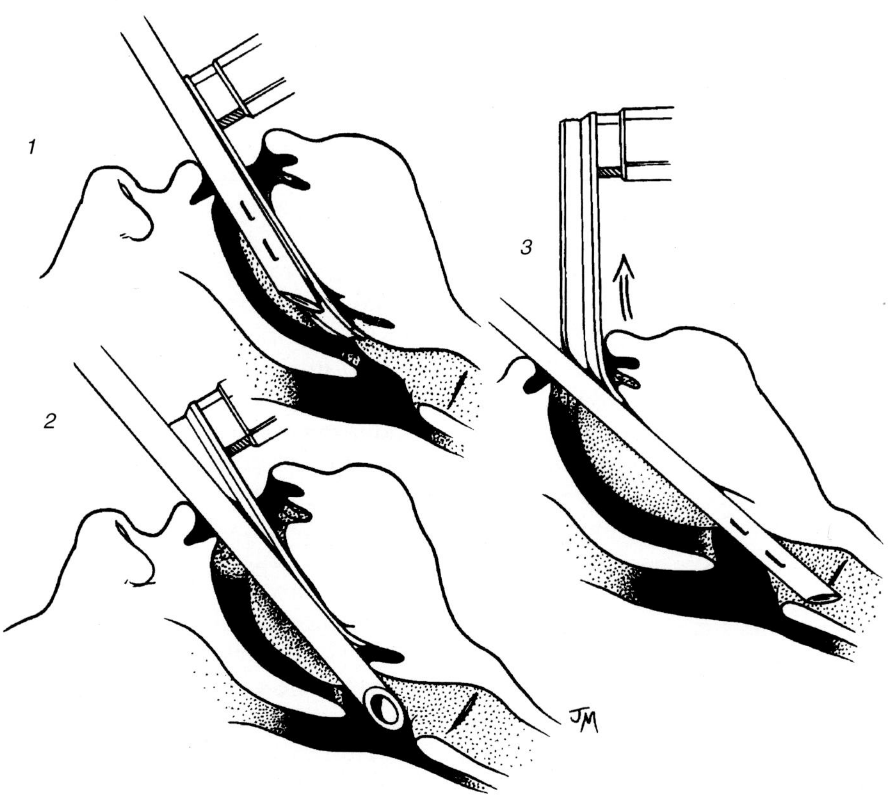

B

Figure 3-6

Rigid bronchoscope intubation using a laryngoscope. *A*. Laryngoscope positioned to visualize epiglottis. *B.(1)* A laryngoscope and bronchoscope in posterior pharynx. *(2)* Bronchoscope advanced under epiglottis and rotated 90 degrees. *(3)* Bronchoscope advanced through vocal cords as laryngoscope is withdrawn.

Figure 3-7

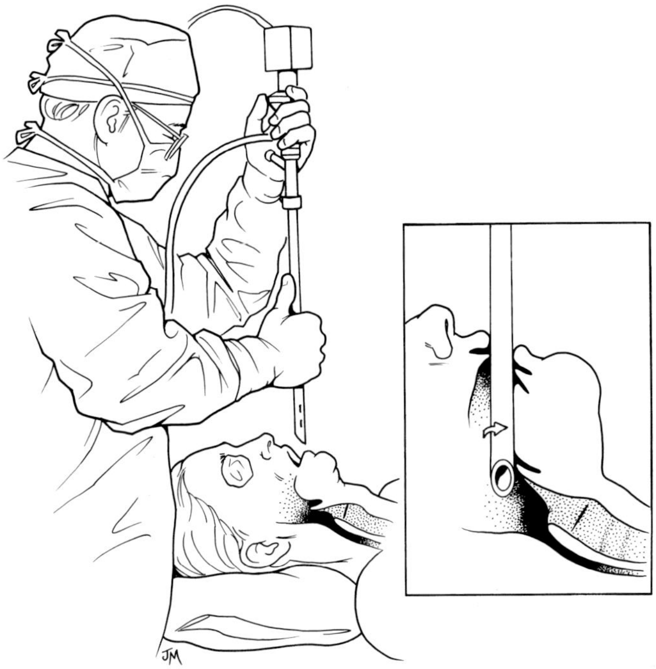

A

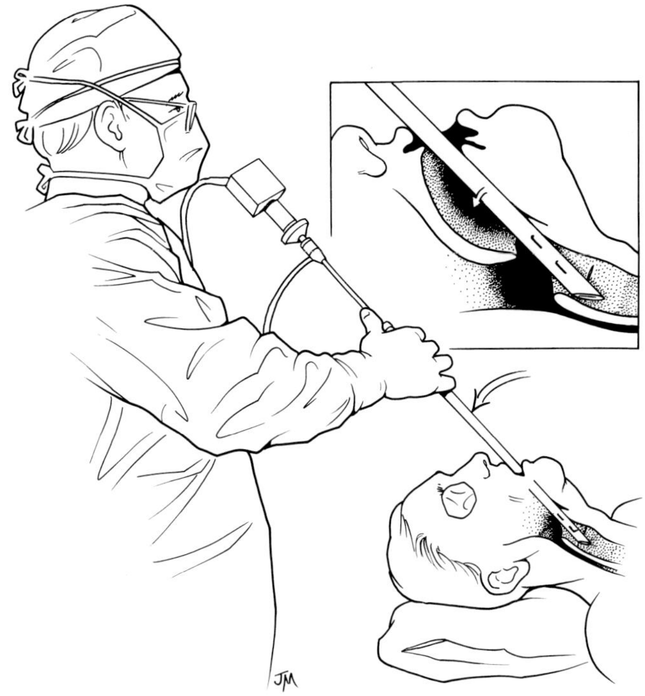

B

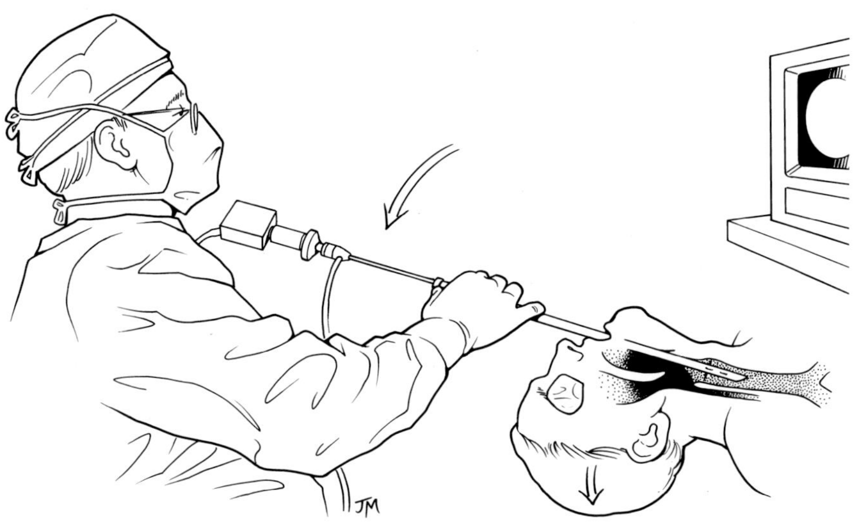

C

Classic technique of intubation with rigid bronchoscope. *A.* "Sniff position" with neck slightly flexed and head extended. Bronchoscope is in midline with bevel anterior. At entrance of glottis, bronchoscope is rotated 90 degrees. *B.* When bevel is through the vocal cords, bronchoscope is rotated back 90 degrees, and proximal end of bronchoscope is lowered. *C.* Patient's neck is extended as bronchoscope enters lower airways.

It took me a number of months and many attempts before I was able to intubate a patient using the classic technique. Now, I find the classic technique quicker and sufficient for most patients. The first two techniques are often faster for the inexperienced bronchoscopist. Intubation along an endotrachael tube has the advantage of ensuring adequate oxygenation and ventilation during the intubation process. Laryngoscopic intubation and the classic technique are performed with the patient apneic and must be successful within a matter of seconds. For this reason, use of the laryngoscope is often preferred by bronchoscopists in training because it closely resembles endotracheal intubation. Whatever technique is used, the goal is to intubate the trachea with the rigid bronchoscope quickly and with minimal trauma to the laryngeal structures and rapidly enough to prevent the development of hypoxemia.

REFERENCES

1. Becker HD: Gustov Killian: A biological sketch. *J Bronchol* 1995; 2:77–83.
2. Boyd AD: Chevalier Jackson: The father of American bronchoesophagoscopy. *Ann Thorac Surg* 1994; 57:502–505.
3. Yankauer S: Lung tumor treated bronchoscopically. *N Y Med J* 1922; 115:741–742.
4. Chan AL, Tharratt RS, Siefkin AD, Albertson TE, Volz WG, Allen RP: Nd:YAG laser bronchoscopy: Rigid or fiberoptic mode? *Chest* 1990; 98:271–275.
5. Mathisen DJ, Grillo HC: Endoscopic relief of malignant airway obstruction. *Ann Thorac Surg* 1989; 48:469–473.
6. Prakash UB: Options in the bronchoscopic therapy of airway neoplasms. *J Bronchol* 1997; 4:497–500.
7. Mehta AC, Dasgupta A: Bronchoscopic approach to tracheal bronchial foreign bodies in adults: Pro flexible bronchoscopy *J Bronchol* 1997; 4:173.
8. Diaz-Jimenez JP: Bronchoscopic approach to tracheal bronchial foreign bodies in adults: Pro rigid bronchoscopy. *J Bronchol* 1997; 4:168–172.
9. Holinger LD: Pediatric bronchoscopy: Rigid versus flexible bronchoscopy. Pro rigid bronchoscopy. *J Bronchol* 1996; 3:153–155.
10. Helmers RA, Sanderson DR: Rigid bronchoscopy: The forgotten art. *Clin Chest Med* 1995; 16:393–399.
11. Perrin G, Colt HG, Martin C, Mak MA, Dumon JF, Gouin F: Safety of interventional rigid bronchoscopy using intravenous anesthesia and spontaneous assisted ventilation: A prospective study. *Chest* 1992; 102:1526–1530.
12. Godden DJ, Wiley RF, Fergusson RJ, Wright DJ, Crompton GK, Grant IW: Rigid bronchoscopy under intravenous general anesthesia with oxygen Venturi ventilation. *Thorax* 1982; 37:532–534.
13. Stradling P: *Diagnostic Bronchoscopy: A Teaching Manual,* 5th ed. London: Churchill Livingstone; 1986:175–177.
14. Shulman MS, Madoff IM: Rigid bronchoscopy revisited (letter). *J Cardiothorac Vasc Anesth* 1991; 5:303.
15. Miller JI Jr: Rigid bronchoscopy. *Chest Surg Clin North Am* 1996; 6:161–167.
16. Tape TG, Blank LL, Wigton RS: Procedural skills of practicing pulmonologists: A national survey of 1,000 members of the American College of Physicians. *Am J Respir Crit Care Med* 1995; 151:282–287.
17. Prakash UB, Offord KP, Stubbs SE: Bronchoscopy in North America: The ACCP survey. *Chest* 1991; 100:1668–1675.
18. Simpson FG, Arnold AG, Purvis A, Belfield BW, Muers MF, Cooke NJ: Postal Survey of bronchoscopic practice by physicians in the United Kingdom. *Thorac* 1986; 41:311–317.
19. Sutedja T, Festen J, Vanderschueren R, Jansen J, Postmus P: A postal survey of bronchoscopic practice in the Netherlands. *J Bronchol* 1996; 3:17–21.
20. Kvale PA: Training in laser bronchoscopy and proposals for credentialing. *Chest* 1990; 97:983–989.
21. Beamis JF Jr, Shapshay SM, Setzer S, Dumon JF: Teaching models for Nd:YAG laser bronchoscopy. *Chest* 1989; 95:1316–1318.

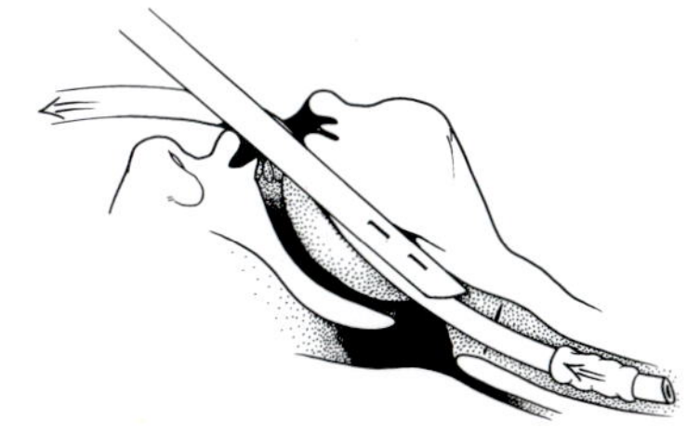

ENDOSCOPIC MANAGEMENT OF BENIGN AIRWAY STENOSIS

Prasoon Jain and Atul C. Mehta

Benign airway stenosis is a well-known complication of endotracheal intubation and tracheostomy.[1] More recently, other causes of subglottic stenosis have been identified.[2] The clinical manifestations vary from an asymptomatic to a life-threatening situation, depending on the severity of stenosis and the patient's cardiopulmonary reserve.

Traditionally, surgery has been the mainstay of treatment.[3] However, the procedure is not without risks, and adequate relief from disabling symptoms is not achieved in all cases. Moreover, many patients are unable to undergo a surgical procedure because of underlying cardiopulmonary limitations. Recent advances in endoscopic techniques and laser therapy have provided an effective and less invasive therapeutic option for some of these patients.

Earlier attempts of endoscopic interventions such as electrocautery, cryotherapy, and mechanical dilation caused considerable mucosal trauma, resulting in unpredictable healing, restenosis, and a high failure rate. To minimize the mechanical and thermal injury to the mucosa, most interventional pulmonologists have now adopted the less traumatic endoscopic approaches. Our approach is to use laser photodissection (LPD) and gentle dilation (GD) with or without placement of airway stents in a carefully selected subset of patients with benign airway stenosis.[4]

The objectives of this chapter are to describe the clinical features, approach to the patient, and currently available endoscopic therapies for patients with benign airway stenosis. In addition, we describe our method of managing these patients at Cleveland Clinic Foundation. Open surgical options are briefly discussed.

Causes of Benign Airway Stenosis

The causes of benign airway stenosis are listed in Table 4-1 and are discussed in detail elsewhere.[5] Congenital anomalies are the most common cause of airway narrowing in the pediatric population. Indeed, congenital subglottic stenosis ranks among the three most common congenital malformations involving the upper airway.[6]

Congenital tracheal stenosis is usually due to a developmental defect in which the membranous portion of the trachea is deficient and the cartilaginous rings extend along the entire circumference of the tracheal wall. Congenital tracheomalacia is the other important cause of airway compromise in infants and children.[7] The management of these patients is difficult because of the frequent association with other congenital anomalies such as esophageal atresia. Weblike tracheal stenosis occurs in 10 percent of patients with congenital airway obstruction.[8] Endoscopic therapy is an effective alternative to surgery in these patients. Occasionally, vascular malformations cause symptomatic airway obstruction in the pediatric population.[9]

Postintubation injury is by far the most common benign cause of airway stenosis in adults. Prospective studies have shown that 63 to 94 percent of patients

Table 4-1
CAUSES OF BENIGN SUBGLOTTIC AND TRACHEAL STENOSIS

Congenital
- Closed first ring
- Tracheomalacia
- Membranous web
- Cartilage deformity
- Vascular anomaly

Acquired
- Internal trauma
  - Endotracheal intubation
  - Tracheostomy
  - Prior endoscopic therapy
- External trauma
- Systemic diseases
  - Wegener's granulomatosis
  - Tuberculosis
  - Amyloidosis
  - Papillomatosis
  - Fibrosing mediastinitis
- Thermal injury
- Idiopathic

sustain some form of laryngeal injury after endotracheal intubation.[10,11] The most common lesions are vocal cord ulceration, granuloma, and laryngeal edema. Usually, the lesions resolve spontaneously in 8 to 12 weeks. Some patients, however, develop laryngeal scarring and subglottic or tracheal stenosis. In a prospective study, Stauffer and coworkers detected tracheal stenosis in 5 of 27 (19 percent) patients after endotracheal intubation.[12] In this study, tracheal stenosis was defined as greater than 10 percent reduction in the transverse air column in a distinct short segment of trachea. In another study, Whited reported a 12 percent incidence of chronic laryngotracheal stenosis among patients intubated for longer than 10 days.[13]

Airway stenosis is a well established complication of tracheostomy performed by the standard surgical approach.[14–16] Preliminary reports indicate that symptomatic upper airway stenosis may also occur after the percutaneous tracheostomy technique.[17] Careful radiologic examination reveals some degree of stenosis in as many as two-thirds of patients with tracheostomy.[12] However, clinically significant stenosis is encountered in a smaller proportion of patients.[14,18] In one series, severe symptomatic stenosis occurred in 8 percent of patients with tracheostomy.[19]

The mechanisms of endotracheal intubation or tracheostomy-induced airway injury are diverse.[20] An important factor is mucosal ischemia caused by the inflated cuff. The use of high-pressure cuffs in the past was associated with a significantly higher risk of mucosal injury. These cuffs are no longer in use. The risk of cuff injury is considerably lower with currently used low-pressure, high-volume cuffs.

Many factors are implicated in the development of stomal stenosis after tracheostomy. Pressure and leverage due to the tracheostomy tube cause ulceration near the stomal site. Moreover, pooling of infected secretions above the inflated tracheostomy cuff promotes inflammation and fibrosis.[21,22] The use of large-diameter tubes is associated with higher risk of developing stomal stenosis.[1,22] Some studies have shown a positive correlation between the duration of intubation and the incidence of airway stenosis.[13] However, others have failed to confirm any such association.[10,12]

Various systemic infections and diseases of unknown etiology cause upper airway stenosis. In a series of 158 cases with Wegener's granulomatosis followed at the National Institutes of Health, Hoffman and coworkers reported symptomatic upper airway stenosis in as many as 16 percent of patients.[23] Nearly half of these patients had severe tracheal stenosis and presented with stridor that required tracheostomy.

Strictures of the upper airway caused by burns have distinctive features.[24] Typically, the stenosis develops at multiple levels in the trancheobronchial tree. These patients, thus, pose a difficult therapeutic challenge. The initial insult is a combined chemical and thermal injury to the mucosa resulting in intense inflammation. A significant proportion of these patients requires intubation for airway maintenance. Many patients follow a protracted course and need prolonged ventilatory support. As a result, the relative contributions of inhalation and intubation in causing airway injury are difficult to separate. However, simultaneous airway involvement at multiple levels is very suggestive of inhalation injury as the dominant factor responsible for airway stenosis.

In some cases, upper airway stenosis occurs without any apparent predisposing cause.[25–28] In a recent report, Grillo and coworkers described 49 patients with idiopathic laryngotracheal stenosis.[25] Forty-six of forty-nine (94 percent) patients were females. Workup to detect an underlying systemic illness was unrevealing. None of the patients had prior intubation. Radiologic studies demonstrated circumferential narrowing between the cricoid cartilage and the trachea. Bronchoscopic examination revealed subglottic stenosis beginning immediately below the vocal cords with injected mucosa and friable submucosal scarring.

Histopathologic examination showed dense fibrosis with thickened lamina propria. The underlying tracheal cartilage was spared. Most patients underwent surgery with good results.

Recent data suggest that gastroesophageal reflux disease is the cause of "idiopathic" subglottic stenosis in some cases.[29–31] In an uncontrolled study, many patients with subglottic stenosis reported heartburn.[29] In some cases, ambulatory esophageal pH monitoring showed abnormalities suggestive of gastroesophageal reflux. It is interesting that antireflux measures improved the treatment outcome in some patients.

Signs and Symptoms

The clinical presentation of airway stenosis depends on the severity and location of airway obstruction. In the majority of cases, symptoms develop within 3 months of extubation. The initial presentation varies from an asymptomatic radiologic abnormality to a life-threatening upper airway obstruction. The usual symptoms are shortness of breath, hoarseness, and wheezing. Occasionally, an unusually difficult or failed intubation suggests the presence of airway stenosis. Some patients remain asymptomatic until an additional insult further compromises an already narrowed airway. In these cases, a viral upper respiratory tract infection may produce life-threatening airway obstruction.

The severity of symptoms roughly correlates with the degree of stenosis. An obstruction causing narrowing of the airway lumen to less than 50 percent of normal results in dyspnea only with significant exertion. Disabling dyspnea and stridor occur when stenosis affects more than 75 percent of the tracheal lumen. These patients are at high risk of life-threatening upper airway obstruction due to an inability to clear secretions.

Previous history of endotracheal intubation or tracheostomy should raise the index of suspicion. However, absence of such history or systemic diseases known to cause subglottic stenosis do not exclude the diagnosis. In some cases of idiopathic subglottic stenosis, a careful history may suggest gastroesophageal reflux disease.

Investigations

FLOW VOLUME LOOP

Abnormalities on the flow volume loop frequently precede clinical symptoms. The patients with fixed upper airway obstruction due to airway stenosis demonstrate plateaus during both inspiratory and expiratory phases of the flow volume loop (Fig. 4-1). The abnormalities resolve after successful endoscopic or surgical therapy. Therefore, this simple noninvasive study is invaluable in the initial evaluation and follow-up of these patients.

IMAGING STUDIES

The aim of noninvasive imaging is to determine the length, location, and extent of airway compromise before fiberoptic bronchoscopy. Occasionally, marked narrowing precludes passage of the bronchoscope past the stenotic area. Radiologic evaluation of the tracheobronchial tree distal to a stenosis is very useful in these patients.

A plain chest roentgenogram is the usual initial radiologic examination.[32] Chest radiography is accurate for differentiating focal from diffuse airway disease. However, its utility is limited by low sensitivity.[33] Currently, computed tomography (CT) is widely used for evaluation of the central airways.[34] The advantages of CT scanning are clarity of anatomic details on cross-sectional imaging and the ability to evaluate surrounding mediastinal structures.[35] Comparative studies have shown that the CT scan is more sensitive than the chest roentgenogram in detecting tracheal diseases.[33] However, certain limitations of a chest CT scan should be noted. First, the length of the stenotic segment is not well appreciated on axial imaging. Moreover, tracheomalacia can not be detected with conventional CT scans.

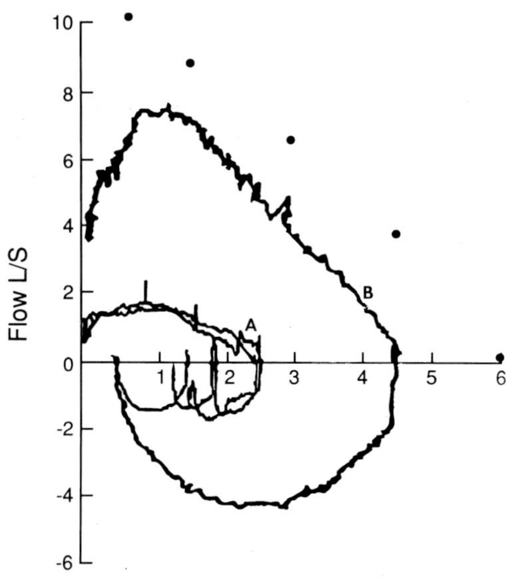

Figure 4-1

Flow volume loop study demonstrating abnormality in both inspiratory and expiratory component in a patient with tracheal stenosis (*smaller loop*). Following laser photodissection and gentle dilation, the flow volume loop is nearly normal (*larger loop*). Dots denote predicted values.

To overcome some of these limitations, investigators have studied certain modified CT techniques for evaluating upper airway stenosis. Cine CT can demonstrate nonfixed upper airway obstruction.[36] In a prospective study, the results of cine CT were compared with the endoscopic findings in 17 patients with suspected upper airway stenosis.[37] Cine CT detected all four cases of endoscopically proven tracheomalacia. However, in five cases focal stenosis was misinterpreted as tracheomalacia, indicating a low specificity. The acquisition of cine CT data is technically difficult.[38] Motion artifacts prevent use of this technique in patients with respiratory distress. Nonavailability of this technology further limits the utility of cine CT.

More recently, helical computerized tomography with multiplanar reconstruction (MPR) has been used to image the central airway.[39–41] In this technique, CT data are used to reconstruct images of the airway in both coronal and sagittal planes. Quint and associates compared conventional CT with helical CT/MPR for the evaluation of the upper airway.[42] The results demonstrated similar accuracy of axial CT scan and CT with MPR for detecting tracheal and main-stem bronchial stenosis. However, CT images with MPR were superior in estimating the length of stenotic segments. In one case, CT with MPR detected a thin horizontal web missed by the axial CT imaging. Moreover, mild degrees of airway stenosis were better visualized with MPR. At Cleveland Clinic Foundation we now routinely use helical CT with MPR for the evaluation of subglottic and tracheal stenosis (Fig. 4-2). In our experience, the information provided often influences the therapeutic approach.

Magnetic resonance imaging (MRI) is emerging as an important imaging technique for upper airway diseases.[43] The main advantage of MRI is the ability to image airways in three planes without employing ionizing radiation or contrast agents. Magnetic resonance imaging is the examination of choice for demonstration of airway compression by vascular structures.[44] Further studies are needed to define the role of MRI in the evaluation of patients with benign airway stenosis.

FLEXIBLE BRONCHOSCOPY

Flexible bronchoscopy (FB) is the single most crucial step in the evaluation of patients with suspected airway stenosis. Direct visualization provides useful information about the cause and severity of airway compromise. Airway collapse with forced respiratory maneuvers during the bronchoscopic examination is diagnostic of tracheomalacia.

Certain limitations of bronchoscopy should be noted. Assessment of the length of the stenotic segment is subjective and therefore prone to error, especially when the procedure is performed by an inexperienced operator. Occasionally, marked narrowing prevents the passage of the bronchoscope past the stenotic area. In these cases, endoscopic evaluation of the distal airway is not possible.

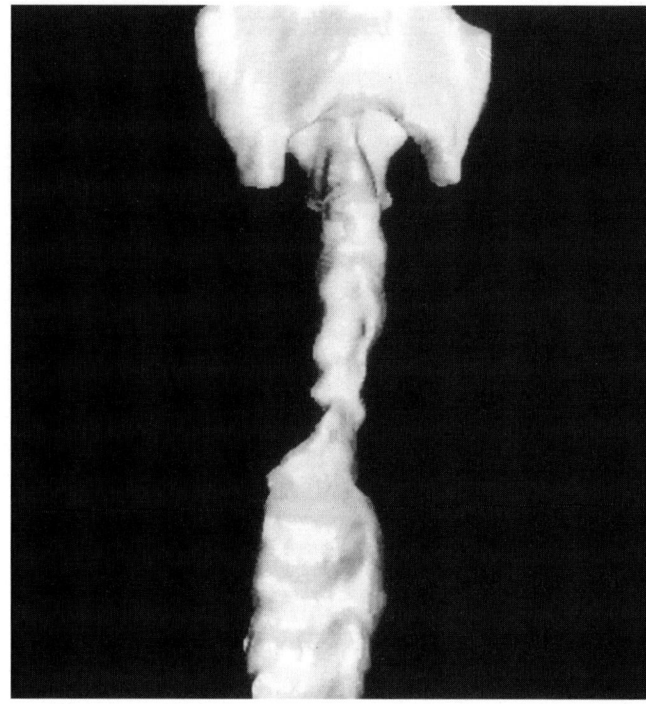

Figure 4-2

Helical CT scan with multiplanar reconstruction of images in a patient with tracheal stenosis with tracheomalacia.

Mechanical trauma to an already compromised airway during the bronchoscopy may precipitate life-threatening airway obstruction. Therefore, the airway examination should be as gentle as possible. No attempts should be made to force the bronchoscope through a critically narrowed segment of the airway. Preferably, this procedure should be performed by the most experienced operator.

Treatment of Benign Airway Stenosis

The management of benign airway stenosis is challenging and requires a multidisciplinary approach involving the interventional pulmonologist, anesthesiologist, otolaryngologist, and thoracic surgeon. The initial therapeutic approach depends on the site, severity, and length of the stenotic segment. Tracheomalacia is another important determinant of the initial choice and outcome of therapy. A review of various nonsurgical approaches follows.

DILATION

Previously, the endoscopic management of the subglottic and tracheal stenosis was limited to mechanical dilation using Jackson dilators and sequential passage of rigid bronchoscopes of increasing size through the stenotic segment. Patients managed in this manner typically required repeated dilation owing to the high incidence of recurrence of stenosis. Hawkins described his experience of managing eight patients with postintubation subglottic stenosis with endoscopic dilation.[45] The process was laborious, requiring an average of six dilations over an 8-week period.

Forceful mechanical dilation causes mucosal trauma followed by disorganized healing by second intention. Excessive fibrous tissue proliferation and scarring lead to restenosis and recurrence of symptoms. Therefore, except in unexpected and emergent situations in which acute dilation may be needed to establish airway patency,[46] a carefully planned multimodality approach should be followed in all cases.

LASER THERAPY

Over the past two decades, various advances in technology have enabled interventional pulmonologists to effectively use lasers in the management of airway obstruction.[47] Two types of laser systems applied in the tracheobronchial tree are the carbon dioxide (CO_2) laser and the neodymium: yttrium-aluminum-garnet (Nd:YAG) laser.[48–50] Specific wavelength and beam coherence capability make the CO_2 laser a more precise cutting instrument. As a result, thermal damage to the surrounding tissues is minimized. Unfortunately, application of the CO_2 laser requires rigid bronchoscopy because a suitable flexible optical fiber that is capable of transmitting CO_2 laser energy through FB has not been developed. Nd:YAG energy can pass through available flexible quartz fibers, allowing application through flexible bronchoscopes. The efficacy and safety of Nd:YAG laser use in the tracheobronchial tree is well established.[51–53] However, interaction of the Nd:YAG laser beam with tissue produces a high degree of scattering of energy, leading to tissue vaporization and photocoagulation.[48] As a result, the effect of the Nd:YAG laser on soft tissue is somewhat unpredictable. Therefore, the procedure needs to be performed with very careful attention to technical details. At all times, the laser beam should be directed parallel to the tracheal wall, skimming the surface of the target tissue to avoid damage to the underlying tissues and the cartilaginous rings.

The availability of the laser technology has provided an effective alternative mode of endoscopic therapy for patients with benign airway stenosis.[54–60] In the past decade, many investigators have emphasized the importance of minimizing mucosal trauma during the laser photocoagulation. In 1984, Dedo and Sooy described their innovative "microtrapdoor" mucosal flap technique in the management of tracheal and posterior glottic stenosis.[56] The procedure involved the use of a CO_2 laser to make an incision in the superior surface of the scar. A thin flap of epithelium was carefully elevated. The underlying scar tissue was vaporized using the CO_2 laser. The mucosal flap was placed back to facilitate rapid epithelialization of the raw underlying tissues. The authors used this technique in nine patients with posterior glottic stenosis and ten patients with subglottic or tracheal stenosis. Success was measured by the ability to decanulate and by relief of dyspnea on exertion. Success was reported in 8 of 9 patients (89 percent) with posterior glottic stenosis and 9 of 10 patients (90 percent) with subglottic or tracheal stenosis. The average increase in the cross-sectional diameter was 279 percent. Prior attempts of endoscopic dilation had been unsuccessful in four of these patients. The success of this technique was attributed to the mucosal preservation that facilitated rapid reepithelialization, thus preventing exuberant scar tissue formation.

In 1987, Shapshay and associates reported their experience of managing five patients with severe fibrous subglottic and tracheal stenosis.[58] The tracheal lumen was narrowed to 3 mm in three patients and 4 mm in the other two patients. Radial incisions were made through the epithelium and the underlying scar tissue using either a CO_2 or Nd:YAG laser. The power settings were carefully chosen to vaporize and not to coagulate the soft tissues. Laser application was followed by dilation using a 8.5-mm rigid bronchoscope. A successful outcome was defined as resolution of symptoms and an increase in the size of the tracheal lumen for at least 1 year. Their technique proved useful in all patients; however, three patients required more than one laser treatment. The authors emphasized the importance of preserving islands of epithelium between the radial laser incisions which rapidly reepithelialized the tracheal wall after the dilation.

Recently, Rebeiz and coworkers have confirmed the efficacy of this endoscopic approach for patients with benign airway stenosis.[61] Twenty-one patients with laryngotracheal stenosis underwent laser excision and dilation. Immediate patency of the airway was achieved in all patients. Of 21 patients 16 (76 percent) remained asymptomatic during a 1- to 6-year follow-up. The remaining five patients underwent tracheal sleeve operation with good results. Seven patients with dense scarring and longer than 1-cm stenosis had several recurrences after 3 to 16 months that required between three and five additional sessions of laser treatment.

In 1993, Mehta and coworkers reported successful application of a mucosal sparing technique using laser photocoagulation and gentle dilation in 18 patients with weblike concentric tracheal stenosis.[60] In nine patients, the stenosis was located in the subglottic area; in seven, it was located in the upper trachea; and in the remaining two patients, the mid- or lower trachea was involved. The Nd:YAG laser was utilized to produce radial incisions through the entire length of stenotic segment. Thereafter, "gentle dilation" was performed using a single insertion of the largest possible rigid bronchoscope that the patient's trachea could accommodate after the laser photodissection. The follow-up period ranged from 2 to 85 months, with a mean of 32 months. Symptomatic improvement and near normalization of the flow volume loop indicated a successful outcome. Overall, the therapeutic goal was achieved in 12 of 18 of the patients (67 percent). Of these, eight required a single treatment, whereas four needed two or more treatments. Presence of tracheomalacia and scars longer than 1 cm predicted therapeutic failure.

In summary, the mucosal sparing technique using a laser is emerging as an effective alternative to surgical therapy in a carefully selected group of patients with benign subglottic and tracheal stenosis. Refinements in laser technology and recognition of the importance of minimizing mucosal trauma have contributed to the increasing success rate in recent years. Scarring longer than 1 cm and tracheomalacia predict treatment failure. These patients frequently need placement of an intraluminal stent or surgery for symptomatic relief.

INTRALUMINAL STENTING

Airway stents are frequently employed for the palliative treatment of large airway obstruction secondary to extrinsic compression or malignant strictures.[62–66] Their precise role in the management of benign airway stenosis remains to be defined. Primarily, airway stents are utilized when bronchoscopic evaluation discloses significant tracheomalacia. Another important indication is failure of laser therapy in patients who are not surgical candidates. Some patients continue to require mechanical support by airway stents for a variable time after the surgery. Occasionally, stents are placed while patients are awaiting definitive surgical therapy.

Presently, a variety of intraluminal stents are available and are described in detail elsewhere.[67] A commonly used stent is the Montgomery T-tube silicone stent, which serves as both a stent and a tracheostomy tube. The external limb of the stent facilitates cleaning and suction of secretions.[68] The stent has ridges and grooves along the extraluminal limb, allowing application of a ring washer, which prevents posterior dislocation of the tube.[69] The major disadvantage of the Montgomery tube is the continued need for maintaining a tracheostomy, which is unacceptable to many patients. Laryngeal edema is another potential complication.

The Montgomery T tube has been effectively used in the management of both benign and malignant airway stenosis.[70,71] Cooper and associates described the use of silicone T tubes in 36 patients with benign airway stenosis.[72] In 12 patients, the T tube was the sole treatment. Extubation was successful in 9 of 12 patients (75 percent). The prosthesis was kept in place for an average of 8.5 months. In six patients, the T tube was placed prior to definitive resection and in nine, as an adjunct to primary resection. In nine other patients, the T tube was placed after failure of surgical therapy.

The other frequently used prosthesis is a "dedicated tracheobronchial stent" devised by Dumon.[73] This stent is made of molded silicone and has regularly placed studs on the outer surface to prevent displacement. The insertion is facilitated by a specially designed stent introducer system (EFER, La Ciotat, France) placed through a rigid bronchoscope. Between 1987 and 1989, Dumon placed 118 prosthesis in 66 patients, of whom 23 had tracheal stenosis. All but two patients experienced immediate symptomatic relief. Obstruction of the prosthesis by dried secretions was recorded in two patients. In two other cases, injury to the vocal cords during insertion caused aphonia. Granuloma formed in 10 patients.

In 1994, Vergnon and associates placed either silicone endoxane stents or Novastent prostheses using Dumon's technique in 16 patients with benign tracheal stenosis.[74] After stent placement, most patients exhibited a marked improvement in dyspnea. Pulmonary function tests showed a statistically significant improvement in the immediate postoperative period and 10 months after the stent placement. Stent removal or readjustment was needed in four patients.

Stent displacement or migration is the most troublesome problem with the use of silicone stents. Dumon encountered this complication 12 times in his original series of 66 patients. Migration is less likely in patients with malignant stenosis because extrinsic compression prevents the Dumon stent from slipping. Since such mechanical support is missing in patients with benign airway stenosis the risk of displacement is higher. Stents placed within 2 cm of the vocal cords are particularly prone to migrate from their original location. Moreover, migration is more likely when a short stent is placed in a conical stenosis.[62] External fixation may reduce the risk of migration of the stent from its original position.[75,76]

In 1986 Wallace and associates described the first successful application of self-expandable Gianturco metallic stents in the tracheobronchial tree in humans.[77] Since then, numerous experimental and clinical studies have established the feasibility of using expandable stents in patients with extrinsic airway compression.[78–82] Some investigators have placed Gianturco stents after laser photocoagulation of intraluminal tumors. Recently, some investigators have employed Gianturco expanding wire stents in the management of benign airway stenosis.[83–86]

Nashef and coworkers placed 28 Gianturco stents in 15 patients with nonneoplastic airway narrowing.[87] The pretreatment abnormalities were classified as pure fibrous stenosis in six patients, fibroinflammatory stenosis in four patients, and tracheomalacia in five patients. Five of six patients with fibrous stenosis and three of five patients with tracheomalacia had good functional outcome. Results were suboptimal in patients with fibroinflammatory stenosis. Self-limiting irritating cough and hemoptysis occurred in all cases. One patient suffered from fatal hemoptysis due to erosion into the pulmonary artery 10 days after the stent placement. A granulomatous inflammatory reaction appeared in five patients who required laser photodissection. Entrapment of a suction catheter in the wire of the stent and dysphagia each occurred in one patient.

The advantages of metallic stents over silicone stents include ease of placement and greater stability of the stent in the tracheobronchial tree. Retention of secretions is not a problem. However, the use of metal stents is not without risks. The reported complications of expandable stents in the tracheobronchial tree include hemoptysis, wire fracture, and unraveling of the metal wires, causing considerable trauma to the airway. Furthermore, endoscopic removal of Gianturco stents is difficult.[88] After placement in the airway, Gianturco stents gradually expand and are incorporated in the tracheal wall. Follow-up bronchoscopy reveals mucosal growth over the wires. Forceful attempts at endoscopic retrieval may result in significant airway injury. Although Wallace and coworkers have reported successful removal of this stent in four patients without any untoward sequel, once deployed, these stents should be considered irretrievable. For this reason, the use of Gianturco stents is best avoided in patients with benign airway stenosis.

To sum up, intraluminal stent placement is an important component of the endoscopic management of patients with benign airway stenosis. Mechanical support to the collapsing airway is particularly beneficial in patients with trancheomalacia. Many patients with previously failed endoscopic and surgical therapies may achieve sustained symptomatic relief after stent placement.

MULTIMODALITY APPROACH

In the recent years, various components of endoscopic therapy have gradually evolved into a multimodality approach.[55–61] Centers specializing in managing this difficult problem have developed their own protocols. However, the essential components remain the same: use of laser photodissection, dilation, and intraluminal stent placement. In 1982, Simpson and colleagues retrospectively analyzed the outcome of endoscopic therapy in 60 patients with upper airway stenosis.[55] The treatment protocol included laser dissection, dilation, and stent placement whenever needed. Carbon dioxide lasers coupled to a Zeiss microscope were used to vaporize a scar or granulation tissue. Intraluminal stents were placed in 39 of 60 patients (65 percent). Overall, 41 of 60 patients (68 percent) were successfully managed. The endoscopic therapy was successful in 25 of 31 patients (80.6 percent) with subglottic stenosis. Soft silicone stents were employed in 21 of 25 successfully managed patients (84 percent).

More recently, Shapshay and associates treated 12 patients with total cervical tracheal stenosis, by endoscopic laser excision, bronchoscopic dilation, and prolonged stenting with a silicone T tube.[89] Carbon dioxide or Nd:YAG laser systems were used to make radial incisions. Laser therapy was followed by dilation of the stenotic segment with the rigid bronchoscope. In each case, a 12- to 14-mm silicone T-tube airway stent was placed. The treatment was successful in 8 of 12 patients (67 percent). Six of eight successfully treated patients, however, required additional laser treatments over a follow-up period of 1 to 6 years. Of three patients with suboptimal initial results, two underwent sleeve resection of the trachea with good final results.

Adjuvant Therapy

The role of adjuvant therapies such as corticosteroids and antibiotics after the endoscopic management remains unclear.[4] Koufman and associates used systemic or local steroids in 13 patients managed endoscopically with a CO_2 laser and dilation.[54] The treatment was successful in 10 of 13 patients. This study, however, was uncontrolled. Therefore, no conclusions can be drawn regarding the beneficial effects of steroids in these patients. Available data indicate that corticosteroids delay epithelial migration and possibly increase scar tissue formation.[90] Therefore, many investigators have cautioned against the routine use of corticosteroids in this setting.[61,89] To date, there is no consensus on the proper use of corticosteroids or their net effect on patient outcome. We use steroids only in patients with bronchospastic disease and when procedure-related laryngeal edema is suspected.

Similarly, the role of systemic antibiotics is controversial. In an animal model, Sakasi and coworkers showed that infection predisposes to increased scar formation, delayed wound healing, and worsened airway stenosis.[21] Unfortunately, no controlled clinical studies are available. Still, some investigators have used prophylactic antibiotics for all patients undergoing endoscopic therapy.[47,55] In these studies, broad spectrum antibiotics were given for 2 to 3 weeks. In contrast, we use antibiotics only if mucopurulent secretions are identified during the procedure.[60] Randomized studies are needed to clarify the role of antibiotics and their effect on patient outcome.

Additional postoperative adjuncts to treatment include humidified oxygen and careful suctioning. For this purpose, soft rubber catheters are preferred over stiff suction catheters, especially when Gianturco stents are placed. Saline nebulization is recommended after airway stent placement to facilitate the removal of retained secretions. Inhaled acetylcysteine may further aid in bronchopulmonary toilet after stent placement. The inside of Montgomery tubes can be cleaned with cotton tipped applicators dipped in hydrogen peroxide.[69]

Predictive Features for Outcome

Careful selection of patients is crucial for successful patient outcome after the endoscopic therapy. Studies indicate that scarring longer than 1 cm in vertical dimension and tracheomalacia are frequently associated with failure of endoscopic therapies and indicate the need for more invasive surgical procedures.[60] Other endoscopic features predictive of poor outcome are listed in Table 4-2.[55,57]

Suboptimal patient selection for endoscopic therapy results in either primary treatment failure or recurrence of symptoms soon after the procedure. Typically, these patients fail repeated attempts at endoscopic therapy and ultimately require surgery. Endoscopists need to be aware of these prognostic variables. We strongly advocate an early referral to an otolaryngologist or thoracic surgeon when endoscopic features associated with poor outcome are detected.

Complications

Complications of endoscopic therapy are very few. Strong and associates reported minor infection next to the exit of the stent transfixation wire in 2 of 23 patients.[53] No major complications such as bleeding or perforation have been reported in other published series. With proper precautions, the risk of endobronchial ignition during the laser application is minimal. Complications associated with stent placement are mentioned above and are reviewed elsewhere.[67]

Table 4-2
FEATURES ASSOCIATED WITH POOR OUTCOME

Circumferential scarring with cicatrical contracture[55,57]
Scarring longer than 1 cm in vertical dimensions[55,57,60]
Tracheomalacia[55,60]
History of bacterial infection associated with tracheostomy[55]
Carinal involvement[57]
Combined laryngeal and tracheal stenosis[55]

Surgery

Surgery is indicated when unfavorable features suggest poor outcome with endoscopic therapy. Another important indication is failure of prior endoscopic intervention. Surgery is generally recommended in patients with substantial cricoid cartilage deformity. Involvement of the glottis also suggests the need for surgical therapy.[91]

The choice of surgical procedure depends on the anatomic features and preference of the surgeon.[92–94] In general, resolution of symptoms and decanulation of tracheostomy are accepted as indicators of successful outcome. Primarily, two surgical techniques are employed: segmental resection of the stenosed segment and reconstruction of the stenosed airway with bone or cartilage graft.

For simple tracheal stenosis, the standard surgical treatment is segmental resection and end-to-end anastomosis.[95,96] Another option is tracheal sleeve operation.[97] In experienced hands, a greater than 90 percent success may be expected after segmental resection and primary anastomosis.[3] The procedure is associated with a relatively low mortality and morbidity. To optimize the airway for effective ventilation during the procedure, many patients receive preoperative Nd:YAG laser photodissection.[97] In some patients tracheomalacia persists after the operation. These patients require long-term use of Montgomery tubes for mechanical support of the airway.

Segmental resection and primary anastomosis are difficult to perform when stenosis extends closer than 1.5 cm to the vocal cords. These patients require laryngotracheal reconstruction. Patients with cartilage deformity and glottis involvement need expansion laryngotracheoplasty for optimal results.[93,94,98–101] The procedure is more complicated and involves division of the cricoid and thyroid cartilage. In addition, cartilage or bony grafts are employed for structural support.

HOW I DO IT

The following section describes our method of dealing with concentric weblike tracheal stenosis using a Nd:YAG laser for mucosal sparing followed by gentle dilation.

Team Approach

Our team consists of an interventional pulmonologist, radiologist, anesthesiologist, otolaryngologist, and thoracic surgeon. In addition, experienced nurses and respiratory therapists are essential members of our team.

Patient Selection

All patients undergo a rigorous evaluation. Endoscopic therapy is chosen for the patients with a smaller than 1 cm long weblike stenosis. Patients with unfavorable features on endoscopic evaluation (Table 4-2) are referred to the otolaryngologist and/or thoracic surgeon.

Evaluation

Preoperative laboratory evaluation includes complete blood count and coagulation profile. A chest roentgenogram and spirometry with flow volume loop are performed in all cases. Recently, we have imaged the airway with a helical CT with three-dimensional multiplanar reconstruction prior to performing FB. In our experience, helical CT/MPR and FB provide complementary information and are often helpful in therapeutic decision making.

Patient Education

After the thorough evaluation we discuss various therapeutic options with the patient. Patient education is an essential component of our protocol. We discuss the procedure, outcome, potential complications, and need for close follow-up. We make sure that the patient has realistic expectations and is aware of the risk of restenosis after the therapy.

Anesthesia

Patients are independently evaluated by the anesthesiologist prior to the procedure. For several reasons, we prefer to perform the laser treatment and endoscopic dilation under general anesthesia. General anesthesia ensures maximum patient cooperation. The cough reflex is inhibited, and therefore the risk of misdirecting the laser beam is reduced. Potential complications during the procedure such as bleeding and endobronchial ignition are more easily managed in anesthetized patients. General anesthesia also facilitates the passage of the rigid bronchoscope for gentle dilation.

Ventilation

The majority of patients undergoing endoscopic management have stenotic lesions in the subglottic area or high in the trachea. Therefore, conventional ventilation using an endotracheal tube is not possible. For patients without preexisting tracheostomy, we use a specially designed triple-lumen, inverted J-shaped stainless steel jet injection cannula for maintaining ventilation during the procedure (Fig. 4-3).[102] This cannula, about 3 mm in diameter, is introduced under laryngoscopic guidance. Two lumina of this catheter open in a common proximal port. This port delivers jet ventilation. The distal end of the cannula is placed well beyond the area of stenosis (Fig. 4-4). The third port is used to measure the airway pressure. We use a jet ventilation frequency of 70 to 150 cycles per minute. Patients are carefully monitored with continuous-pulse oximetry and arterial blood-gas analysis at regular intervals. High-frequency jet ventilation provides adequate oxygenation and alveolar ventilation in the majority of our patients. The nonflammable nature of the stainless steel cannula enhances procedure safety by reducing the risk of endobronchial fire during the laser application. Using this technique, the need for a new tracheostomy for the purpose of airway maintenance and ventilation during the procedure is eliminated. For patients with preexisting tracheostomy, the stainless steel jet cannula is introduced through the stoma.

Laser Photodissection

We perform Nd:YAG laser photodissection using FB. In our experience, it is easier to direct the laser beam using an FB than with a rigid bronchoscope. As a result, the laser energy is delivered more precisely to the intended target. We employ an average power setting

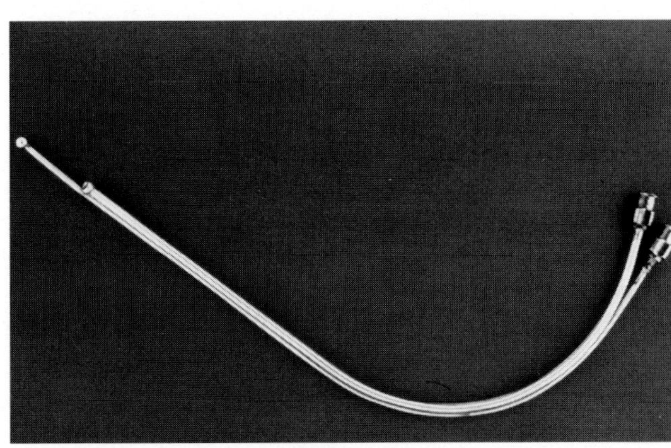

Figure 4-3

Experimental stainless steel jet injection cannula with three ports. Two of the lumina deliver jet ventilation; the third lumen is used to measure the airway pressure.

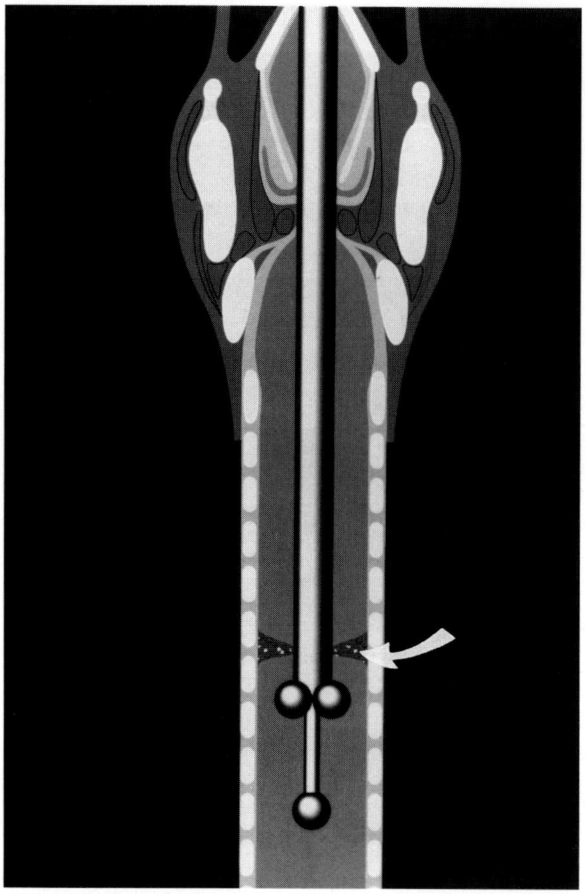

Figure 4-4

Diagrammatic representation of coronal section of the airway with a three-port ventilation system in place. The *arrow* represents stenosis. Note that the distal end of the jet cannula is placed well beyond the area of stenosis.

of 30 to 40 W with 0.4-s pulse duration in the majority of our cases. To reduce the risk of endobronchial ignition, we avoid inspired oxygen concentrations greater than 40%.

The Nd:YAG laser is utilized to produce radial incisions through the entire vertical length of the stenotic lesion, usually at 3-, 9-, and 12-o'clock positions. The Nd:YAG laser can be delivered by contact or noncontact techniques. We prefer a noncontact technique in the majority of our cases. The laser beam is directed parallel to the tracheal wall at all times, skimming the surface of the target tissue. As a result, the risk of cartilage damage and resultant tracheomalacia is minimized.

Under general anesthesia, pharyngeal muscles relax. As a result, the operator may face difficulty in locating the larynx. In these cases, the jet injection catheter works as a guide to locate the larynx with the FB. The presence of the thin stainless steel cannula does not cause any mechanical limitation during the laser photodissection. The ventilation is delivered distal to the operative site. Thus, the jet stream of air does not interfere with the photodissection. The jet injection cannula can easily be repositioned during the procedure.

Dilation

After producing radial incisions, gentle dilation is performed. For this purpose, a rigid bronchoscope is used under telescoptic guidance. To minimize mucosal trauma, we perform a single gentle dilation utilizing a size 7.0, 8.0, or 9.0 rigid bronchoscope. No attempts are made to dilate the stenotic lesion with progressively increasing sizes of rigid bronchoscopes.

Postoperative Care

The procedure is performed on an outpatient basis. Patients are carefully observed for adequacy of ventilation in the postoperative recovery room for several hours. Patients with bronchospastic disease receive steroids in the perioperative period. Steroids are also begun when there is suspicion of laryngeal trauma during the procedure. Once initiated, the corticosteroids are continued for 2 to 3 weeks. We use antibiotics only when a significant amount of mucopurulent material is noted during the procedure. The antibiotics are continued for 10 days. Inhaled β_2 agonists are used in patients with clinical evidence of wheezing.

Follow-up

Patients are followed in the office 6 to 8 weeks after the procedure. Any change in symptoms is recorded. We routinely document improvement by comparing pre- and postoperative spirometry data and flow volume loops at 6 to 8 weeks. Follow-up bronchoscopy is not performed in all patients. FB is performed when patients fail to achieve symptomatic relief and when the flow volume loop continues to demonstrate fixed upper airway obstruction. Recurrence of symptoms usually indicates restenosis, and we evaluate these patients with FB.

Recurrent Subglottic Stenosis

Our protocol limits the endoscopic therapy to three treatments. Irrespective of the presence or absence of unfavorable features, recurrence of symptoms with objective evidence of airway stenosis after the third endoscopic therapy prompts us to advise a definitive surgical procedure. However, surgery may not be an option in some patients owing to associated medical conditions. Occasionally, patients refuse surgery. In these situations we may elect to exceed our limit of three attempts and perform additional endoscopic treatments.

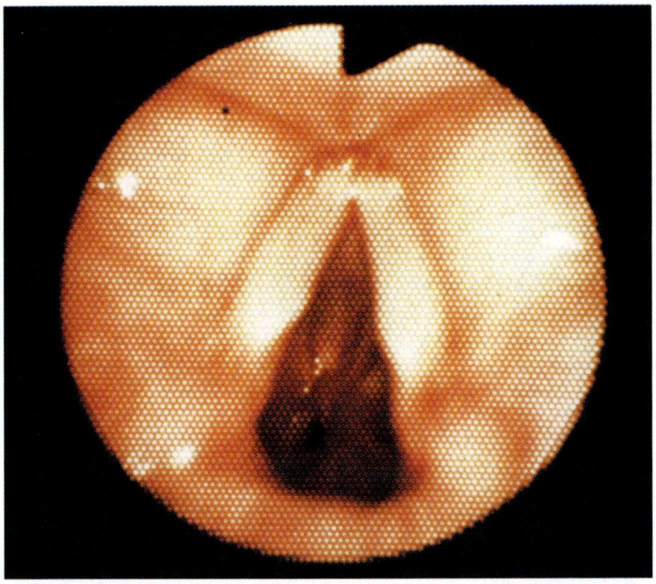

A

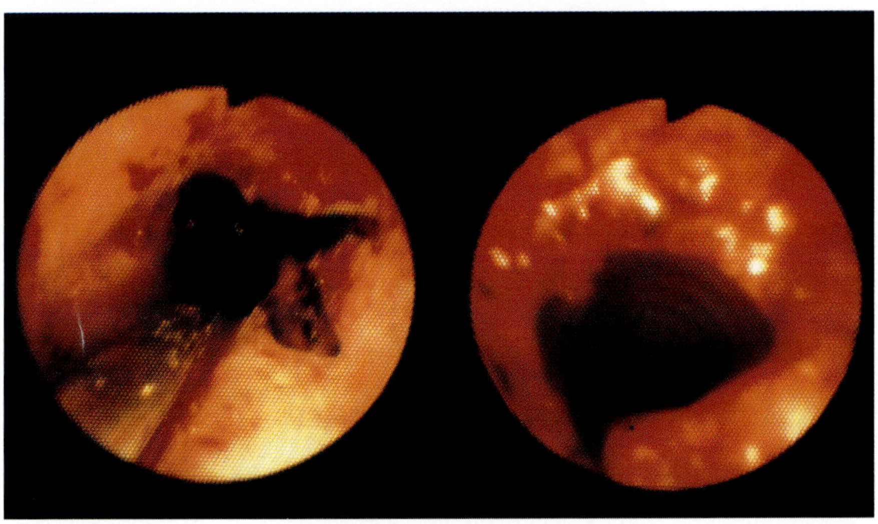

B C

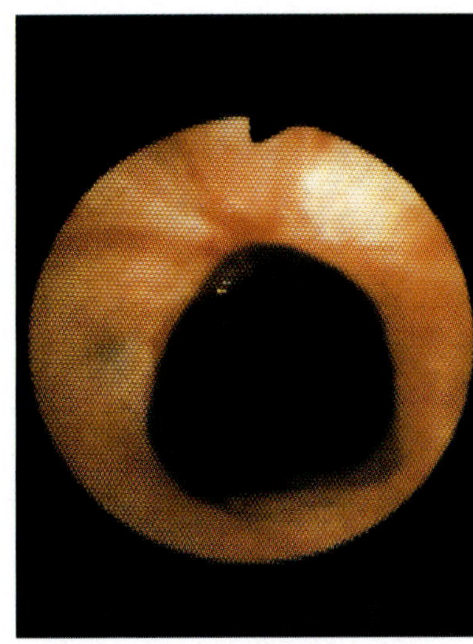

D

Figure 4-5

A. High grade subglottic stenosis on initial bronchoscopic evaluation. *B*. Intraoperative appearance of the tracheal lesion after laser photodissection. *C*. Further improvement in the tracheal lumen is seen after a single insertion of rigid bronchos cope. *D*. After 12 months, flexible bronchoscopic examination reveals near normalization of the tracheal lumen.

Results

We treated 18 patients with severe subglottic and concentric tracheal stenosis using Nd:YAG LPD and GD with the rigid bronchoscope from March 1985 to April 1992.[60] The underlying causes of stenosis were traumatic or prolonged intubation in 12 patients and prior tracheostomy in four patients. In two patients, no etiology was identified. In nine patients, the stenosis involved the subglottic area; in seven, upper trachea; and in the remaining two, mid or lower trachea. A total of 28 Nd:YAG LPD procedures (mean of 1.5 per patient) were performed. The treatment was successful in 67 percent of cases. A majority of these patients had severe and potentially life-threatening upper airway obstruction on initial bronchoscopic evaluation (Fig. 4-5*A*). Follow-up examination showed a significant improvement in airway caliber in successfully treated patients (Fig. 4-5*B*–*D*). Nonfatal respiratory complications such as infection, airway perforation, bleeding, or endobronchial ignition did not occur in any patient. Similarly, no patient developed acute upper airway obstruction during the evaluation or laser treatment.

Summary

Despite many advances in endoscopic and surgical techniques, the management of benign subglottic and tracheal stenosis remains difficult and often frustrating for both the patient and the physician. A meticulous assessment and carefully planned, individualized approach offers the best hope of a successful outcome. One of the major challenges in this regard is to recognize the candidates for initial endoscopic intervention as opposed to surgery. Successful outcome with endoscopic therapy depends on proper patient selection, atraumatic dissection, and gentle dilation of the narrowed airway segment. Experience and skill of the endoscopist and meticulous postoperative care are equally important. Further studies are needed to clarify the role of adjunctive therapies such as perioperative use of corticosteroids and antibiotics.

In the surgical literature, benign upper airway stenosis is still considered a primarily surgical disease. The studies reviewed above offer a less invasive approach for the management of these patients. Clearly, with careful patient selection, a favorable outcome is possible with endoscopic therapy. Some patients are unsuitable candidates for major surgery due to underlying cardiopulmonary limitation or other medical contraindications. A successful endoscopic therapy may avoid the need for major surgery in some of these patients. Moreover, a successful endoscopic therapy avoids the discomfort and complications associated with a major operation. Furthermore, the need for hospital admission is avoided. Although, formal cost comparison studies are not available, the immediate cost is clearly lower with endoscopic therapy. We believe that both endoscopic and surgical approaches are complimentary. In most cases, a prior failure of one neither precludes the application nor affects the outcome of the other technique.

REFERENCES

1. Streitz JM Jr, Shapshay SM: Airway injury after tracheostomy and endotracheal intubation. *Surg Clin North Am* 1991; 71:1211–1230.
2. Aboussouan LS, Stoller JK: Diagnosis and management of upper airway obstruction. *Clin Chest Med* 1994; 15:35–53.
3. Grillo HC, et al: Postintubation tracheal stenosis. Treatment and results. *J Thorac Cardiovasc Surg* 1995; 109:486–493.
4. Mehta AC, et al: Endoscopic management of benign airway stenosis. *Clin Chest Med* 1995; 16:401–413.
5. Choplin RH, et al: Diffuse lesions of trachea. *Sem Roentgenol* 1983; 18:38–50.
6. Holinger PH, et al: Subglottic stenosis in infants and children. *Ann Otol* 1976; 85:591.
7. Benjamin B: Tracheomalacia in infants and children. *Ann Otol Rhinol Laryngol* 1984; 93:438–442.
8. Shapshay SM: Laser bronchoscopy. In Davis RK (ed): *Lasers in Otolaryngology—Head and Neck Surgery.* Philadelphia, WB Saunders, 1990:85–105.
9. Fletcher BD, Cohn RD: Tracheal compression and innominate artery: MRI evaluation in infants. *Radiology* 1989; 170:103–107.
10. Kastanos N, et al: Laryngotracheal injury due to endotracheal intubation: Incidence, evolution, and predisposing factors. A prospective long-term study. *Crit Care Med* 1983; 11:362–367.
11. Colice GL, et al: Laryngeal complications of prolonged intubation. *Chest* 1989; 96:877–884.
12. Stauffer JL, et al: Complications and consequences of endotracheal intubation and tracheostomy. *Am J Med* 1981; 70:65–76.
13. Whited RE: A prospective study of laryngotracheal sequelae in long term intubation. *Laryngoscope* 1984; 94:367–377.
14. Andrews MJ, Pearson FG: Incidence and pathogenesis of tracheal injury following cuffed tube tracheostomy with assisted ventilation. *Ann Surg* 1971; 173:249–263.
15. Cooper JD, Grillo HC: The evolution of tracheal injury due to ventilatory assistance through cuffed tubes: A prospective study. *Ann Surg* 1969; 169:334–348.
16. Geffin B, et al: Stenosis following tracheostomy for respiratory care. *JAMA* 1971; 216:1984–1988.
17. Mcfarlane C, et al: Laryngotracheal stenosis: A serious complication of percutaneous tracheostomy. *Anesthesia* 1994; 49:38–40.
18. Westgate HD, Roux KL Jr: Tracheal stenosis following tracheostomy: Incidence of predisposing factors. *Anesthes Analg* 1970; 49:393–401.
19. Dane TEB, King EG: A prospective study of complications after tracheostomy for assisted ventilation. *Chest* 1975; 67:398–404.
20. Bishop MJ: Mechanisms of laryngotracheal injury following prolonged tracheal intubation. *Chest* 1989; 96:185–186.
21. Sakasi CT, et al: Tracheostomy-related subglottic stenosis: Bacteriologic pathogenesis. *Laryngoscope* 1979; 89:857–865.
22. Andrews MJ, Pearson FG: An analysis of 59 cases of tracheal stenosis following tracheostomy with cuffed tube and assisted ventilation, with special reference to diagnosis and treatment. *Br J Surg* 1973; 60:208–212.
23. Hoffman GS, et al: Wegener granulomatosis: An analysis of 158 patients. *Ann Intern Med* 1992; 116:488–498.
24. Gaissert HA, et al: Upper airway compromise after inhalation injury. *Ann Surg* 1993; 218:672–678.
25. Grillo HC, et al: Idiopathic laryngotracheal stenosis and its management. *Ann Thorac Surg* 1993; 56:80–87.
26. Maddus MA, et al: Subglottic tracheal resection and synchronous laryngeal reconstruction. *J Thorac Cardiovasc Surg* 1992; 104:1443–1450.
27. Jazbi B, et al: Idiopathic subglottic stenosis. *Ann Otolaryngol* 1977; 86:644–647.
28. Park SS, et al: Idiopathic subglottic stenosis. *Arch Otolaryngol Head Neck Surg* 1995; 121:894–897.
29. Jindal JR, et al: Gastroesophageal reflux disease as a likely cause of idiopathic subglottic stenosis. *Ann Otol Rhinol Laryngol* 1994; 103:186–191.
30. Koufman JA: The otolaryngologic manifestations of gastroesophageal reflux disease (GERD): A clinical investigation of 225 patients using ambulatory 24-hour pH monitoring and an experimental investigation of the role of acid and pepsin in the development of laryngeal injury. *Laryngoscope* 1991; 101(suppl 53).
31. Little FB, et al: Effects of gastric acid on the pathogenesis of subglottic stenosis. *Ann Otol Rhinol Laryngol* 1985; 94:516–519.
32. Shepard JO, McLoud TC: Imaging the airway. Computed tomography and magnetic resonance imaging. *Clin Chest Med* 1991; 12:151–168.
33. Kwong JS, et al: Diagnosis of diseases of the trachea and main bronchi: Chest radiography vs CT. *AJR* 1993; 161:519–522.
34. Gamsu G, Webb WR: Computed tomography of the trachea and mainstem bronchi. *Sem Roentgenol* 1983; 18:51–60.
35. Gamsu G, Webb WR: Computed tomography of the trachea: Normal and abnormal. *AJR* 1982; 139:321–326.
36. Ell SR, et al: Cine CT demonstration of nonfixed upper airway obstruction. *AJR* 1986; 146:669–677.
37. Brody AS, et al: Airway evaluation in children with use of ultrafast CT: Pitfalls and recommendations. *Radiology* 1991; 178:181–184.
38. Ell SR, et al: Cine CT technique for dynamic airway studies. *AJR* 1985; 145:35–36.
39. Newmark GM, et al: Spiral CT evaluation of the trachea and bronchi. *J Comput Assist Tomogr* 1994; 18:552–554.

40. Lacrosse M, et al: 3D spiral CT of the tracheobronchial tree. *J Comput Assist Tomogr* 1995; 19:341–347.
41. Whyte RI, et al: Helical computed tomography for the evaluation of tracheal stenosis. *Ann Thorac Surg* 1995; 60:27–31.
42. Quint LE, et al: Stenosis of the central airway: Evaluation by using helical CT with multiplanar reconstruction. *Radiology* 1995; 194:871–877.
43. Gamsu G, Sostman D: Magnetic resonance imaging of the thorax. *Am Rev Resp Dis* 1989; 139:254–274.
44. Mahboudi S, et al: Magnetic resonance imaging of airway obstruction resulting from vascular anomalies. *Int J Pediat Otorhinolaryngol* 1994; 28:111–123.
45. Hawkins DB: Glottic and subglottic stenosis from endotracheal intubation. *Laryngoscope* 1977; 87:339–346.
46. Nimmagadda UR, et al: Acute management of unsuspected subglottic stenosis by tracheal dilation. *Anesth Analg* 1995; 80:841–843.
47. Friedman EM, et al: Carbon dioxide laser management of subglottic and tracheal stenosis. *Otolaryngol Clin North Am* 1983; 16:871–877.
48. Ramser ER, Beamis JF Jr: Laser bronchoscopy. *Clin Chest Med* 1995; 16:415–426.
49. Dunccavage JA, Ossoff RH: Laser application in the tracheobronchial tree. *Otolaryngol Clin North Am* 1990; 23:67–75.
50. Shapshay SM, Beamis JF Jr: Use of CO_2 laser. *Chest* 1989; 95:449–456.
51. Dumon JF, et al: Principles for safety in application of the Nd:YAG laser in bronchology. *Chest* 1984; 86:163–168.
52. Cavaliere S, Foccoli P, Farina PL: Nd:YAG laser bronchoscopy. *Chest* 1988; 94:15–21.
53. Strong MS, et al: Endoscopic management of laryngeal stenosis. *Otolaryngol Clin North Am* 1979; 12:797–805.
54. Koufman JA, et al: Endoscopic managment of subglottic stenosis with the CO_2 surgical laser. *Otolaryngol Head Neck Surg* 1981; 89:215–220.
55. Simpson GT, et al: Predictive factors of success or failure in the endoscopic management of laryngeal and tracheal stenosis. *Ann Otol Rhinol Laryngol* 1982; 91:384–388.
56. Dedo HH, Sooy CD: Endoscopic laser repair of posterior glottic, subglottic and tracheal stenosis by division or micro-trapdoor flap. *Laryngoscope* 1984; 94:445–450.
57. Ossoff RH, et al: Efficacy of bronchoscopic carbon dioxide laser surgery for benign strictures of the trachea. *Laryngoscope* 1985; 95:1220–1223.
58. Shapshay SM, et al: Endoscopic treatment of subglottic and tracheal stenosis by radial laser incision and dilation. *Ann Otol Rhinol Laryngol* 1987; 96:661–664.
59. Beste DJ, Toohill RJ: Microtrapdoor flap repair of laryngeal and tracheal stenosis. *Ann Otol Rhinol Laryngol* 1991; 100: 420–423.
60. Mehta AC, et al: Concentric tracheal and subglottic stenosis. *Chest* 1993; 104:673–677.
61. Rebeiz EE, et al: Endoscopic laser radial incision and dilatation of laryngotracheal stenosis: A six year experience. *Trans Annu Meet Am Bronchoesophagol Assoc* 1993; 77–80.
62. Bolliger CT, et al: Silicone stents in the management of inoperable tracheobronchial stenosis. *Chest* 1993; 104: 1653–1659.
63. Insall RL, Morritt GN: Palliation of malignant tracheal strictures using silicone T tubes. *Thorax* 1991; 46:168–171.
64. Orlowski TM: Palliative intubation of the tracheobronchial tree. *J Thorac Cardiovasc Surg* 1987; 94:343–348.
65. Westaby S, et al: A bifurcated silicone rubber stent for relief of tracheobronchial obstruction. *J Thorac Cardiovasc Surg* 1982; 83:414–417.
66. Sonett JR, et al: Endobronchial management of benign, malignant, and lung transplantation airway stenosis. *Ann Thorac Surg* 1995; 59:1417–1422.
67. Colt HG, Dumon JF: Airway stents: Present and future. *Clin Chest Med* 1995; 16:465–478.
68. Montgomery WW: Current modifications of the salivary bypass tube and tracheal T-tube. *Ann Otol Rhinol Laryngol* 1986; 95:121–125.
69. Montgomery WW: Manual for the care of the Montgomery silicone tracheal T-tube. *Ann Otol Rhinol Laryngol* 1986; 95 (suppl 125):1–8.
70. Cooper JD, et al: Use of the silicone tracheal T-tubes for the management of complex tracheal injuries. *J Thorac Cardiovasc Surg* 1981; 82:559–568.
71. Whitehead E, Salam MA: Use of the carbon dioxide laser with the Montgomery T-tube in the management of extensive subglottic stenosis. *J Laryngol Otol* 1992; 106:829–831.
72. Cooper JD, et al: Use of silicone stents in the management of airway problems. *Ann Thorac Surg* 1989; 47:371–378.
73. Dumon JF: A dedicated thacheobronchial stent. *Chest* 1990; 97:328–332.
74. Vergnon JM, et al: Efficacy of tracheal and bronchial stent placement on respiratory function tests. *Chest* 1995; 107: 741–746.
75. Colt HG, et al: External fixation of subglottic tracheal stents. *Chest* 1994; 105:1653–1657.
76. Mouney DF, Lyons GD: Fixation of laryngeal stents. *Laryngoscope* 1985; 95:905–907.
77. Wallace MJ, et al: Tracheobronchial tree: Expandable metallic stents used in experimental and clinical applications. *Radiology* 1986; 158:309–312.
78. Rousseau H, et al: Self-expandable prosthesis in the tracheobronchial tree. *Radiology* 1993; 188:199–203.
79. De Souza AC, et al: Use of expandable wire stent for malignant airway obstruction. *Ann Thorac Surg* 1994; 57: 1573–1578.
80. Nomori H, et al: Indications for an expandable metallic stent for tracheobronchial stenosis. *Ann Thorac Surg* 1993; 56: 1324–1328.
81. Sawada S, et al: Malignant tracheobronchial obstructive lesions: Treatment with Gianturco expandable metallic stents. *Radiology* 1993; 188:205–208.
82. Carrasco CH, et al: Management of tracheal and bronchial stenosis with the Gianturco stents. *Ann Thorac Surg* 1994; 58:1012–1017.
83. Simonds AK, et al: Use of expandable metal stents in the treatment of bronchial obstruction. *Thorax* 1989; 44:680–681.
84. Han JK, et al: Bronchial stenosis due to endobronchial tuberculosis: Successful treatment with self-expanding metallic stent. *AJR* 1992; 159:971–972.
85. Zannini P, et al: Self expanding stents in the treatment of tracheobronchial obstruction. *Chest* 1994; 106:86–90.
86. Varela A, et al: Use of Gianturco self-expandable stents in the tracheobronchial tree. *Ann Thorac Surg* 1990; 49:806–809.
87. Nashef SAM, et al: Expanding wire stents in benign tracheobronchial diseases: Indications and complications. *Ann Thorac Surg* 1992; 54:937–940.
88. Hind CRK, Donnelly RJ: Expandable metal stents for tracheal obstruction: Permanent or temporary? A cautionary tale. *Thorax* 1992; 47:757–758.
89. Shapshay SM, Beamis JF, Dumon JF: Total cervical tracheal stenosis: Treatment by laser, dilation and stenting. *Ann Otol Rhinol Laryngol* 1989; 98:890–895.
90. Healy GB: An experimental model for the endoscopic correction of subglottic stenosis with clinical applications. *Laryngoscope* 1982; 92:1103–1115.
91. McCaffrey TV: Management of laryngotracheal stenosis on the basis of site and severity. *Otolaryngol Head Neck Surg* 1993; 109:468–473.
92. Grillo HC, Mathisen DJ: Surgical management of tracheal strictures. *Surg Clin North Am* 1988; 68:511–524.

93. McCaffrey TV: Management of subglottic stenosis in the adult. *Ann Otol Rhinol Laryngol* 1991; 100:90–94.
94. Anand VK, et al: Surgical considerations in tracheal stenosis. *Laryngoscope* 1992; 102:237–243.
95. Grillo HC: Surgical treatment of postintubation tracheal injuries. *J Thorac Cardiovasc Surg* 1979; 78:860–875.
96. Har-El G, et al: Resection of trachea with end to end anastomosis. *Ann Otol Rhinol Laryngol* 1993; 102:670–674.
97. Bisson A, et al: *J Thorac Cardiovasc Surg* 1992; 104:882–887.
98. Maddalozzo J, Holinger LD: Laryngotracheal reconstruction for subglottic stenosis in children. *Ann Otol Rhinol Laryngol* 1987; 96:665–669.
99. April MM, Marsh BR: Laryngotracheal reconstruction for subglottic stenosis. *Ann Otol Rhinol Laryngol* 1993; 102:176–181.
100. Zalzal GH: Treatment of laryngotracheal stenosis with anterior and posterior cartilage grafts. *Arch Otolaryngol Head Neck Surg* 1993; 119:82–86.
101. Rosenfield RM, Bluestone CD: Does early expansion surgery have a role in the management of congenital subglottic stenosis? *Laryngoscope* 1993; 103:286–290.
102. Mehta AC, et al: Ventilatory management during neodymium: yttrium aluminum garnet photodissection of subglottic and higher tracheal lesions. *Trans Am Broncho-Esophagol Assoc* 1986; 148–153.

C H A P T E R 5

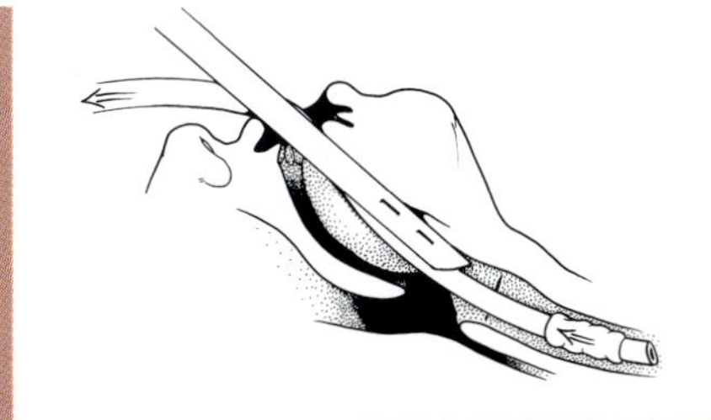

LASER BRONCHOSCOPY

James J. Fenton and John F. Beamis, Jr.

The epidemic of cancer of the lung, which developed in the 1960s, resulted in many patients having malignant obstruction of the central airways. Conventional therapy, such as external radiation therapy, chemotherapy, or dilation techniques with rigid bronchoscopy, often proved to be inadequate to relieve the symptomatic obstruction. The application of sophisticated laser technology for the treatment of various tracheobronchial obstructions, using standard rigid and flexible bronchoscopes, has proved to be a major advance in the treatment of these patients and was the original stimulus for the specialty of interventional pulmonology. The successes of laser bronchoscopy have stimulated interest in other endobronchial therapies, such as cryotherapy, electrocautery, and brachytherapy.

Laser bronchoscopists represent a significant proportion of interventional pulmonologists but a relatively small minority of bronchoscopists in general. Laser bronchoscopists must be experts in diagnostic bronchoscopy techniques, become knowledgeable in laser physics and laser tissue interaction, and be comfortable dealing with patients with respiratory insufficiency, acute hypoxemia, and airway bleeding. This chapter reviews laser physics, tissue interaction, and laser safety as it relates to bronchoscopic applications. It also addresses indications, contraindications, and techniques of laser bronchoscopy. Familiarity with this chapter will not make one a laser bronchoscopist, but we hope it will serve as a basis for beginning clinical application.

Laser Light

A *light amplification* by *stimulated emission* of *radiation* (LASER) beam is an intense form of electromagnetic energy channeled into parallel, synchronized rays of light of the same wavelength that are used for many industrial and medical applications. Light represents a portion of the electromagnetic spectrum designated with wavelengths between 100 and 20,000 nm. Included in this range is ultraviolet light, visible light, and infrared light (Fig. 5-1). Visible light is perceived by the human eye as different colors, with the shorter wavelengths of 400 nm seen as violet blue and the longer wavelengths of 700 nm seen as red light. All light is produced by the spontaneous or stimulated emission of energy by atoms, the smallest components of a molecule. The nucleus of the atom contains positively charged particles called protons and neutral particles called neutrons. Orbiting the nucleus are negatively charged electrons, which balance the positively charged protons. Each electron orbit corresponds to a certain energy level, and the greater the distance from the nucleus, the higher the energy level of the electron. Light is generated when electrons surrounding an atom spontaneously drop from an orbit with a higher energy level to one with a lower energy level (Fig. 5-2). For this release to occur, the atom must first be "excited" to the higher level by an external photon of energy. Photons are discrete particles of radiant energy that travel in waves and provide the energy necessary to form light. The energy of a photon is related to the frequency (Hz) of the wave multiplied by a constant (Planck's constant $= 6.623 \times 10^{-34}$ joule seconds) and is inversely proportional to the wavelength. This influx of energy propels the electron to a more distant orbit corresponding to a higher energy level. If an atom in an excited state is again stimulated by a photon of the same energy as the one absorbed, two photons of equal energy and frequency will be released when the electron's orbit decays to a lower level.[1] This release is termed stimulated emission of radiation and is the basis for laser light energy. When the process is ampli-

Figure 5-1

Electromagnetic spectrum.

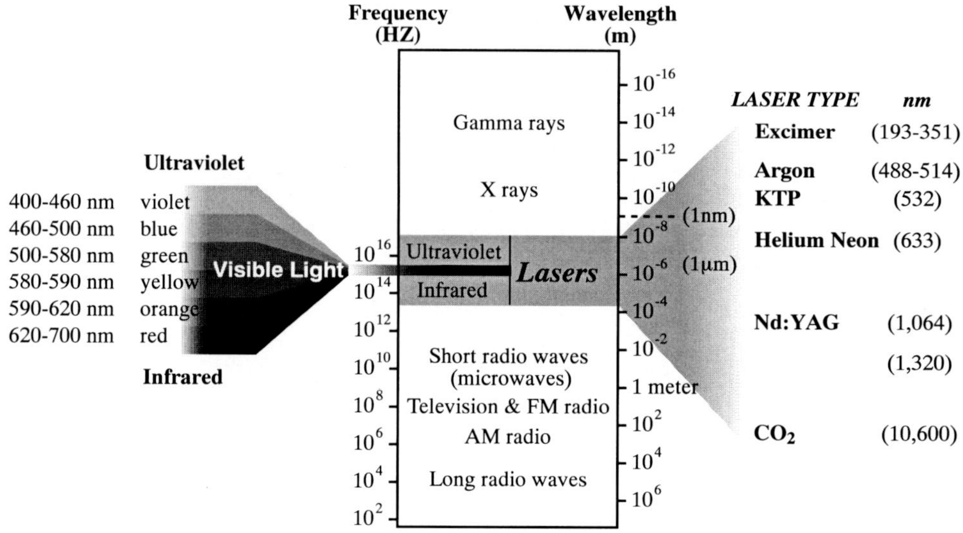

Figure 5-2

Generation of light.

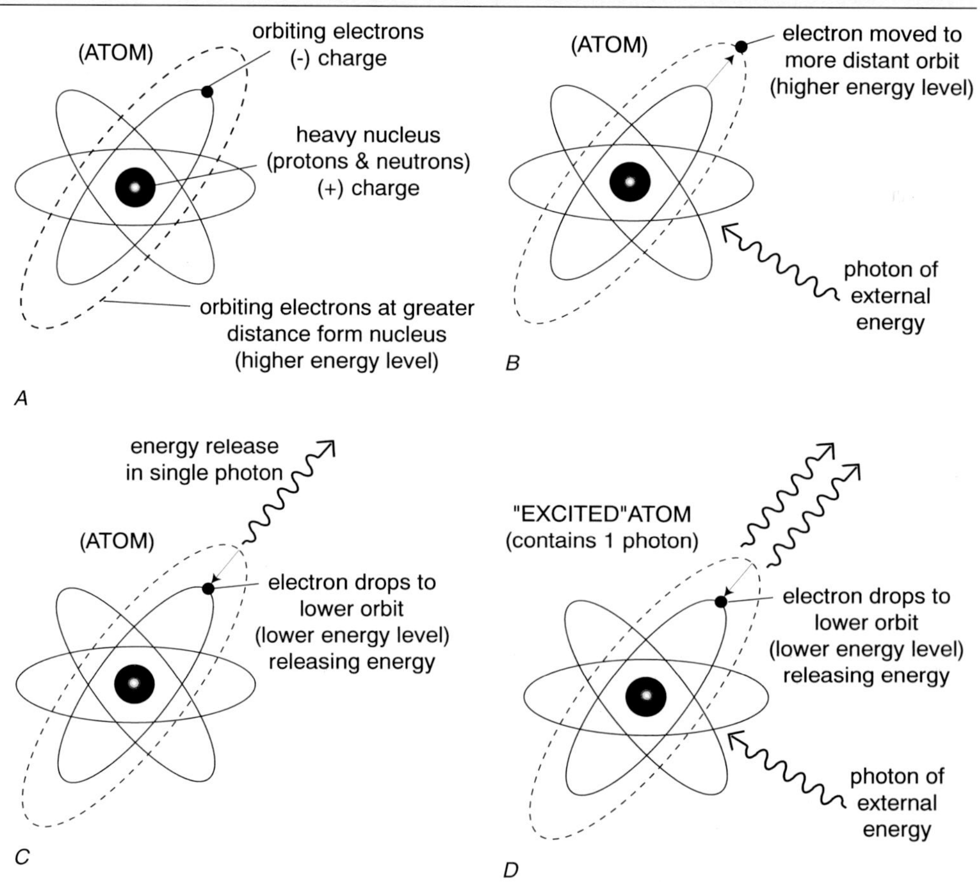

Figure 5-3

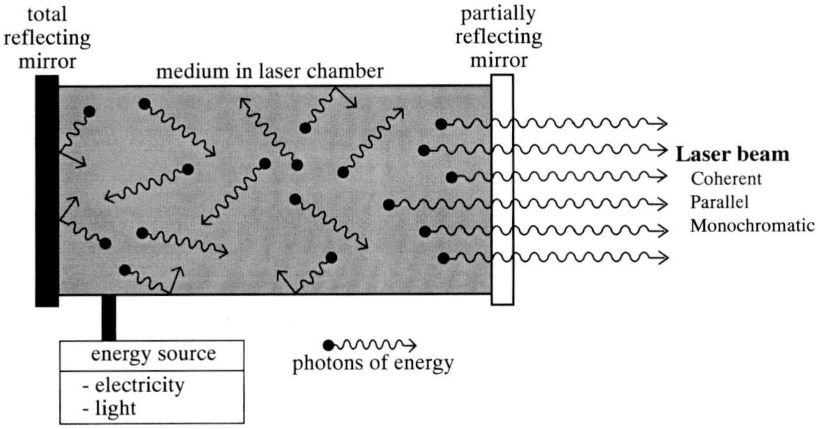

Components of a laser.

fied to an intense level by an external energy source, a specialized form of light energy is created, which we term laser light.

Lasers create their special form of light energy by using an optical cylinder containing a medium consisting of solids, gases, or dyes (Fig. 5-3). The cylinder contains a fully reflective mirror at one end and a partially reflective mirror at the other end. Atoms of the active laser medium become stimulated when an external source adds thermal, electrical, or optical energy to the system. Spontaneous emission of energy occurs as electrons change orbit around the atoms within the medium, giving off energy in various directions. As the photons of energy bounce off the walls, mirrors, and other atoms within the cylinder, intensification of the electromagnetic energy occurs. The light energy leaves through the partially transmissive mirror at a rate that is dictated by the incoming external energy source. The energy is emitted as laser light and follows the special properties of stimulated light emission.[2,3]

Three unique properties of laser light make lasers particularly useful[1,3] (Fig. 5-4). First, all waves of laser light are in phase with each other and have identical frequencies, wavelengths, and velocities as they travel through space. This property is known as coherence, and it results in a concentration of laser power at the target point. Waves of laser light are also considered monochromatic because they have nearly the same color, wavelength, and energy. This characteristic permits all of the radiant power to be centered in a narrow electromagnetic spectral band. Finally, all waves of laser light are essentially parallel and thus are considered collimated. This property permits lasers to travel great distances with minimal loss of intensity of light energy. Ordinary light energy (i.e., incandescent bulbs) will scatter in multiple directions at varied wavelengths, making it good for illumination but inadequate for more precise medical applications. Laser light, on the other hand, is emitted in a narrow, parallel bundle with minimal scatter into space,[3,4] making

Figure 5-4

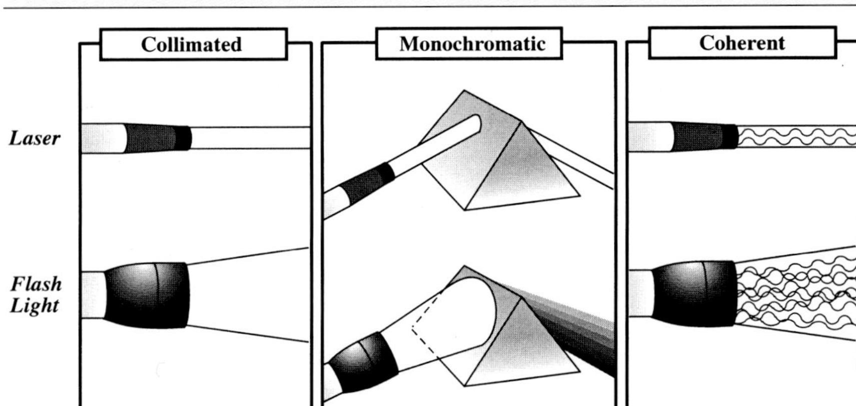

Properties of laser light

it particularly useful as a surgical tool. Compared with most other forms of light, lasers also have a high luminosity (brightness), which makes them useful for light therapy.

Two other important characteristics of laser light determine a laser's impact on a target. The transverse electromagnetic mode (TEM) is one measure of a laser's distribution of intensity in a cross-sectional dimension. Although lasers are collimated and coherent, the impact configuration on a target is not perfectly uniform, as illustrated in the ideal mode (Fig. 5-5). Instead, the actual cross-sectional impact configuration of most lasers is symmetric in a bell-shaped or gaussian distribution, with more beam intensity being concentrated in the center of the target. This impact configuration is termed basic mode.

In addition to the TEM, a laser beam's intensity is also determined by its power density, which is the concentration of power per unit of cross-sectional area of the beam. Optical lenses focus the laser beam into a small focal spot, creating a high power density in that area. For each laser, the beam focus is fixed to prevent divergence and loss of power density. The power density is a function of the size of the focal spot. The smaller the focal spot, the higher the power density (Fig. 5-6). The power density can also be intensified by increasing the incoming power of the beam, which is usually in the range of 20 to 100 watts (W) for most medical lasers.[1] Therefore, power density is proportional to incoming power and inversely proportional to the area of the focal spot. Although the power consumed by a laser is less than that of an ordinary light bulb, the intensity of a concentrated beam makes it useful for cutting, coagulating, and vaporizing tissue.

A laser's TEM and power density are important determinants of the laser beam's effect on the target tissue. Because the TEM determines the profile of the beam's effective cross-sectional area, it also determines the pattern of tissue interaction (Fig. 5-7). The tissue cavity created by laser destruction has the same configuration as the intensity profile (basic mode) of the laser beam. The extent of tissue destruction is a function of the amount of absorption, the length of exposure, and the power density of the laser beam. When laser light is applied to tissue, some of the energy penetrates into the tissue and is absorbed producing heat, whereas the rest of the energy is reflected back (Fig. 5-8). Power density at the surface of the tissue will be higher than the power density farther inside because of the partial reflection of energy. Absorption attenuates the original power density incrementally as it passes deeper into the tissues. The distance below the surface of the tissue at which the power density has decreased to a percentage of the original level (usually 1 percent) is termed the attenuation depth.[3] It is differentiated from penetration depth, which is the distance at which the laser energy no longer has significant effects on the tissue. Laser beams can still have a considerable effect on tissues even after 99 percent attenuation if the exposure is prolonged or if the power density of the original beam is very high. For instance, if the laser beam has an original power density at the surface of 100 W/cm^2, only 1 W/cm^2 will be present at the 99 percent attenuation depth. However, if the original power density at the surface is 10,000 W/cm^2, 100 W/cm^2 will be present at the 99 percent attenuation depth. The attenuation depth is a function of the tissue type and the wavelength of the laser light,

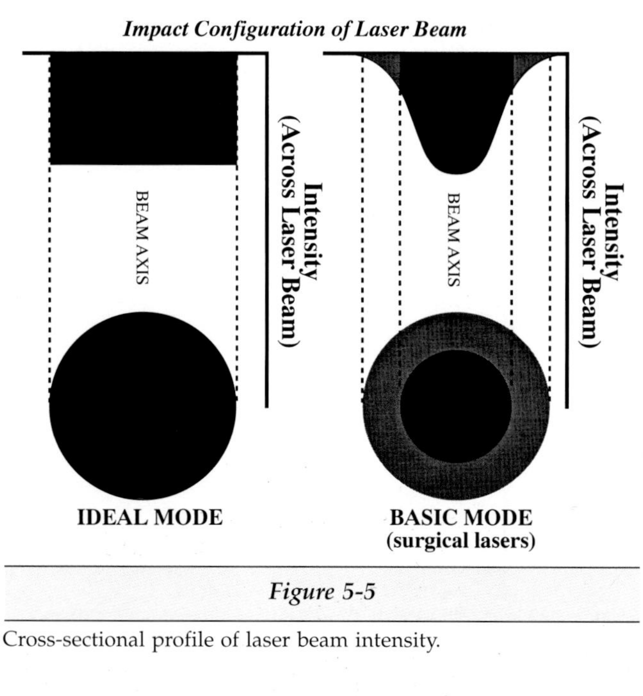

Figure 5-5

Cross-sectional profile of laser beam intensity.

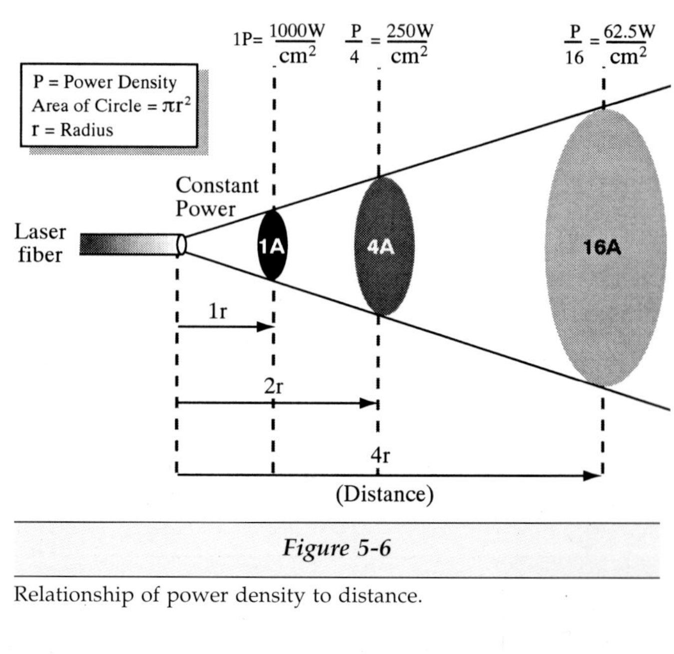

Figure 5-6

Relationship of power density to distance.

Figure 5-7

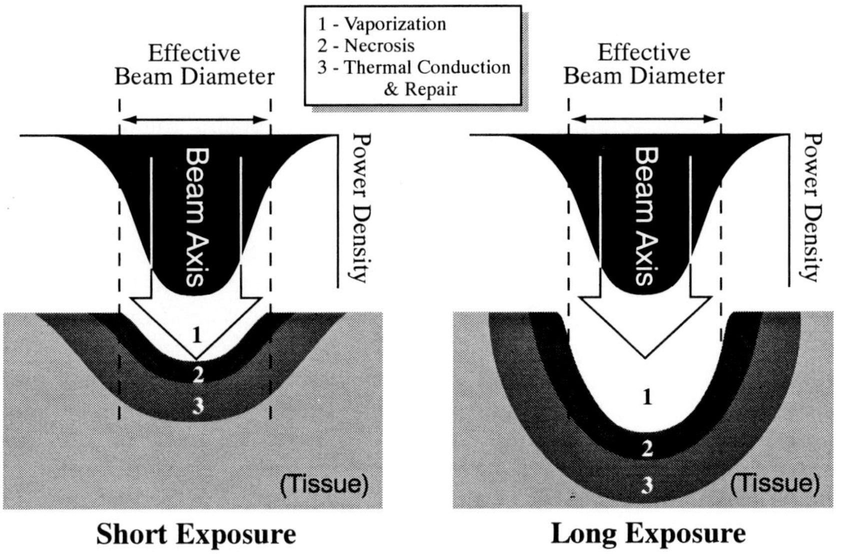

Zones of tissue injury from laser exposure.

Figure 5-8

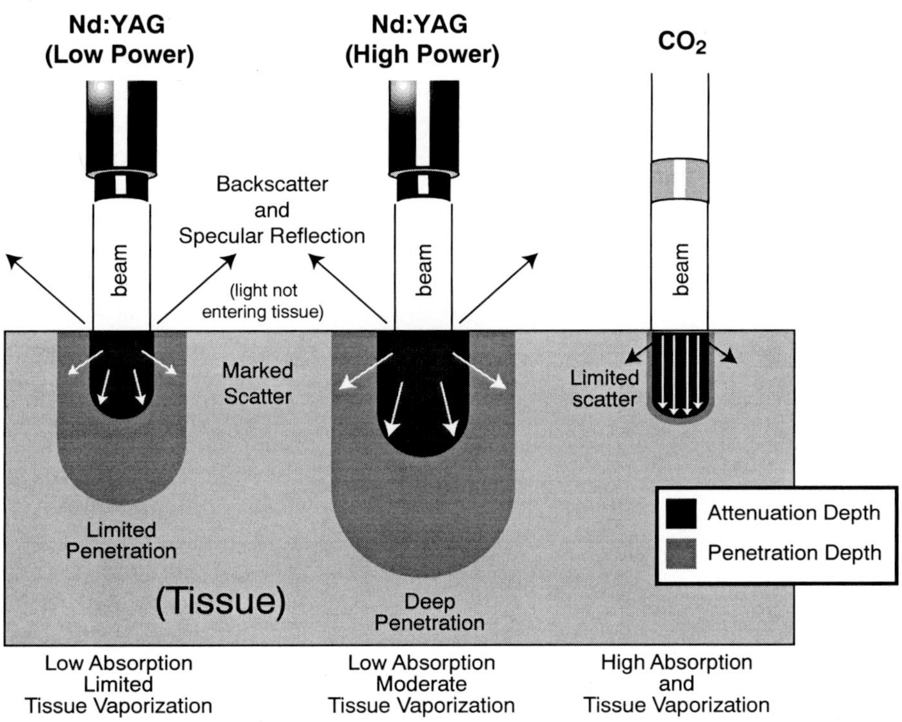

Tissue laser absorption characteristics.

whereas the penetration depth is dependent on the tissue type, wavelength, and the power density.

The amount of attenuation that occurs secondary to absorption is termed the attenuation coefficient.[3] This value is the sum of the absorption coefficient (α) and the scattering coefficient (σ) [$A = \alpha + \sigma$]. Each laser has a different scattering characteristic when the beam penetrates living tissues, but the amount of scattering within tissues is generally dependent on the tissue type and wavelength of the laser beam. Lasers that have high scatter coefficients function well as coagulators, whereas lasers that have high absorption coefficients are more useful for precision cutting. For instance, a carbon dioxide (CO_2) laser has a high absorption coefficient that produces rapid tissue vaporization and makes it an ideal cutting instrument. Its low scattering coefficient, however, limits its ability to photocoagulate bleeding tissues. In contrast, a neodymium, yttrium, aluminum, garnet (Nd:YAG) laser functions well as a coagulator because of its high scattering coefficient, but it is a relatively poor cutting instrument. Nevertheless, the Nd:YAG laser is capable of serving both functions because at higher power settings or within dark tissues, more absorption and vaporization occur. The main determinant of a laser's effect on a particular tissue is the proportion of the scattering and absorption coefficients at the wavelength of the individual laser.

Lasers can interact with living tissues in different ways.[2] Light energy is converted into heat energy, enabling the thermal effects of laser radiation to be used for cutting, vaporization, and coagulation of tissues. Because of the high water content, laser energy is readily absorbed by living tissues. This laser energy is rapidly converted into heat, which results in cell destruction. Lasers can also mechanically disrupt tissues either by pressure waves or by inducing vaporization of intracellular or extracellular water, resulting in separation of tissue layers. This interaction is useful in the removal of cataracts or intravascular atheromatous plaques. Laser light energy can also stimulate various biochemical reactions by interacting with photosensitizing chemicals absorbed by abnormal tissues. This use of laser light is termed photodynamic therapy, which is used in the diagnosis and treatment of patients with tracheobronchial malignancies.[5–8]

The performance characteristics of individual lasers are determined by the substance used as the laser medium. Each substance produces varying wavelengths of emitted light. The first laser used a synthetic ruby crystal as a laser medium; now, commonly used materials include argon, krypton, fluorescent organic dyes, gold vapor gas, helium-neon, potassium titanyl phosphate (KTP), CO_2, and a combination of erbium (Er) or Nd:YAG.

The argon gas laser has a wavelength of 514 nm in the visible blue-green spectrum of light and can be transmitted through optical fibers. Because of its blue color, however, much of its energy is absorbed in hemoglobin, which greatly limits its use in photoresection of endobronchial malignancies.[9] The gold vapor and liquid dye lasers are used to excite the photosensitizer dihematoporphyrin ether, which is selectively retained by tumor cells.[7,8] By exposing the tissue to appropriate laser light, clusters of tumor cells can easily be identified and treated. The helium-neon gas laser has no therapeutic role in laser bronchoscopy, but it produces light in the visible spectrum, making it useful as an aiming guide for other lasers, such as the CO_2 and Nd:YAG laser. The KTP laser uses a solid medium similar to the Nd:YAG laser and has been used in photocoagulation and resection of tracheobronchial stenosis.[10]

The CO_2 laser has commonly been used for lesions of the aerodigestive tract.[11] The CO_2 laser has a long wavelength of 10,600 nm, resulting in prompt absorption by most living tissues. This invisible infrared electromagnetic energy is rapidly converted to thermal energy, resulting in vaporization of the water in the tissue. If the tissue has a high water content, absorption is further enhanced and tissue destruction is more precise. The CO_2 laser's high absorption and low scatter coefficients give it a predictable depth of penetration and make it ideal for precise surgical applications.[3,12] Tonsillectomy, adenoidectomy, and uvulopalatopharyngoplasty (UPPP) have been performed with the use of the CO_2 laser.[13] Although well accepted for the treatment of benign and malignant lesions of the head and neck,[14] its use in tracheobronchial malignancies has been limited. The CO_2 laser can seal small vessels and lymphatics up to 0.5 mm in diameter,[15,16] but it is an ineffective photocoagulator and cannot reliably control bleeding from larger vessels. Another important drawback of the CO_2 laser is its cumbersome articulated mirror delivery system, which requires a micromanipulator and surgical microscope for operation. Use of this system for lower airway tumors requires precise alignment of the laser beam down the entire length of a rigid bronchoscope. This complex set-up makes resection difficult and often precludes the use of certain suction devices. At present, there is no commercially available flexible optical fiber for the CO_2 laser that allows its use with a fiberoptic bronchoscope.

The Nd:YAG laser has been used extensively for the treatment of patients with tracheobronchial malignancies because the laser beam is delivered through a quartz optical fiber, which is easily adaptable for use with either the flexible or rigid bronchoscope.[17] The Nd:YAG laser operates in the invisible near infrared range of the electromagnetic spectrum at a wavelength of 1064 nm. At this wavelength, scattering exceeds absorption for most lighter colored tissues, which makes the Nd:YAG laser effective at coagulating large amounts of tissue. If the tissue is darker pigmented or if a higher power setting is used, absorption and vaporization can be increased. The wide power range (5 to 100 W) of the Nd:YAG laser contributes to its versatility by permitting photocoagulation at low settings and vaporization at higher settings. The Nd:YAG laser penetrates to about 6 mm and will coagulate vessels of up to 2 mm in diameter. A new type of Nd:YAG laser has been developed with a wavelength of 1320 nm, which may have advantages over the current system because of slightly less tissue scatter.[9] The Nd:YAG laser fiber can be fitted with a sapphire tip to permit a contact operational mode, but because these tips limit viewing, contact probes are usually not used in tracheobronchial endoscopy.[4] Because the noncontact Nd:YAG laser is the most common laser used for tracheobronchial disease, the rest of this chapter will concentrate on the use of this laser for bronchoscopic applications.

Indications

The Nd:YAG laser has been used for more than 15 years to reestablish airway patency in patients with primary bronchogenic and metastatic malignancies, benign tumors, tracheal stenosis, and tumors of uncertain prognosis.[18] Malignant tracheobronchial obstruction from primary bronchogenic carcinoma is the most common indication for Nd:YAG laser bronchoscopy and accounts for 49 to 75 percent of the cases (Table 5-1).[18–20,22–24] The most common primary tumor cell type treated by the Nd:YAG laser is squamous cell carcinoma followed by adenocarcinoma.[19,20] Tracheobronchial obstruction as a result of endobronchial metastasis from renal, thyroid, colon, breast, and esophageal carcinomas account for between 6 and 18 percent of laser bronchoscopies and is the next most common indication for the procedure. Although they are responsible for less than 10 percent of the cases of tracheobronchial obstruction, benign tumors, such as hamartomas, fibromas, papillomas, lipomas, and amyloidomas, are an excellent indication for use of the Nd:YAG laser.[21] Benign tumors often originate from a pedicle base in the tracheobronchial mucosa and are usually not vascular, making them particularly attractive for flexible endoscopic laser resection.[22] Laser treatment of the base of lesions may help prevent recurrences, and in some cases, treatment of lesions, such as hamartomas and papillomas, can be curative. Endobronchial amyloid and tracheopathia osteoplastica are usually not curable by laser resection, but these lesions are relatively slow growing and often do not require multiple treatments.[23]

At many institutions, tracheal stenosis represents a relatively common indication for laser bronchoscopy, accounting for 10 to 27 percent of the cases. Tracheal stenosis usually occurs after translaryngeal intubation or tracheostomy, but it can occur without a known cause or in response to granulomatous or diphtherial infections. Personne and coworkers[22] have identified three main types of iatrogenic stenoses (Fig. 5-9). The diaphragm type of stenosis (type I) consists of a concentric fibrotic intraluminal stricture without involvement of the tracheal wall and is ideal for laser resection. The second type of stenosis (type II) involves extrinsic, "bottle-neck narrowing" of the trachea sec-

Table 5-1
INDICATIONS FOR LASER BRONCHOSCOPY

Author	*Year*	*Patients*	*Bronchogenic Carcinoma*	*Metastatic Carcinoma*	*Tracheal Stenosis*	*Benign Tumor*	*Uncertain Prognosis*	*Miscellaneous*
Cavaliere et al.[19]	1994	1884	1419 (75%)	105 (5.6%)	Not included	156 (8%)	143 (8%)	61 (3.2%)
Cavaliere et al.[23]	1988	1000	612 (61%)	37 (3.7%)	139 (13.9%)	59 (5.9%)	64 (6.4%)	89 (8.9%)
Brutinel et al.[24]	1987	116	71 (61%)	17 (14.7%)	Not included	9 (8%)	13 (11%)	6(5%)
Beamis et al.[20]	1991	269	200 (74%)	36 (18%)	27 (10%)	6 (2%)	Not included	Not included
Personne et al.[22]	1986	1310	643 (49%)		389 (27%)	75 (5.7%)	57 (4%)	146 (11%)
Dumon[18]	1985	544	278 (51%)		132 (24%)	31 (6%)	20 (4%)	83 (15%)[a]

[a]Suture removal, 29; hemorrhage, 20; foreign body, 4.

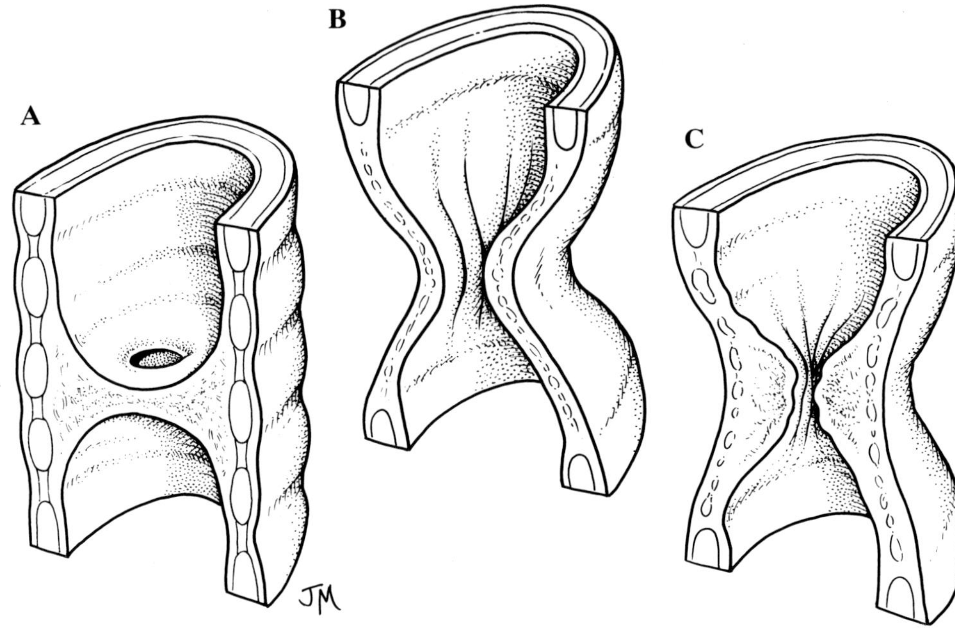

Figure 5-9

Types of tracheal stenosis. *A*, Type I; *B*, type II; *C*, type III.

ondary to collapse of the tracheal wall. Because no intraluminal component is present, use of the Nd:YAG laser for this type of narrowing is contraindicated. The last type of stenosis (type III) is a combination of the first two types and may be acceptable for laser therapy of the intraluminal fibrotic ring in certain situations. If stenosis is suitable for endoscopic therapy, the laser is used to make radial incisions in the tracheal scar before gentle rigid bronchoscopic dilation of the tracheal or subglottic stenosis.[25,26] Some patients with severe obstruction of the lower airway may require a permanent tracheostomy or implantation of a silicone stent or a Montgomery tracheal T tube to maintain patency of the airway.[27,28] If implantation of the stent fails to achieve long-term patency, tracheal sleeve resection may be necessary, but symptomatic clinical improvement after relief of tracheal obstruction using laser bronchoscopy has been well documented.[25,26,29]

A less common indication for endobronchial laser therapy is treatment of tumors of uncertain prognosis, which include carcinoid, adenoid cystic, spindle cell, mucoepidermoid, and other mixed cell types. These lesions should be resected surgically if possible, but in many instances, surgery is impossible because the lesions are widespread or the patient is a poor operative candidate. The Nd:YAG laser can be used to treat these low-grade malignant tumors effectively, which accounts for approximately 5 percent of laser bronchoscopies. Other infrequent uses for the Nd:YAG laser include treatment of tracheobronchial granulomas,[23] removal of suture threads, control of hemorrhage from biopsy sites or necrotic mucosa,[18] and even vaporization of granulation tissue surrounding an aspirated foreign body.[30]

Nd:YAG laser bronchoscopy is indicated for almost any centrally obstructing lesion within the airway lumen of the tracheobronchial tree, but some lesions are more favorable for treatment than others (Table 5.2). Tracheal and bronchial main stem lesions are more easily treated than lesions in the distal bronchi, and they represent the primary indication for laser bronchoscopy. Although location of the lesion is a primary concern, the appearance of a lesion is also important. For instance, mechanical resection of short, polypoid lesions is technically easier than resection of lesions that involve a longer portion of the airway. Because

Table 5-2
CHARACTERISTICS OF LESIONS FOR LASER BRONCHOSCOPY

Favorable lesions for laser resection	Unfavorable lesions for laser resection
Tracheal and main stem lesions	Extrinsic lesions
Polypoid lesions	Diffuse lesions with extensive submucosal involvement
Short lesion length	Upper lobe and segmental lesions
Large endobronchial involvement	Long tapering lesions
Visible distal bronchial lumen	Total bronchial obstruction
Functional lung distal to the obstruction	

much of laser bronchoscopy involves the use of the rigid bronchoscope to physically resect the tumor, long tapering lesions with extensive submucosal infiltration make the procedure technically more difficult and often reduce the chances for a successful outcome. Complete obstruction of the airway lumen also complicates the procedure because it makes it difficult to know the course of the bronchus beyond the area of obstruction. This information is crucial to avoid inadvertent perforation of the airway wall during laser resection. Most patients do not have complete airway obstruction, and a passage beyond the lesion can often be found by gently probing the area with a suction catheter or a flexible bronchoscope. If the course of the bronchus can be determined, mechanical and laser resection can proceed. Otherwise, complete obstruction of the airway lumen is a contraindication to laser bronchoscopy, and it represents the most common reason for not performing laser resection.[31]

Contraindications

Because the procedure is often used as palliative therapy for individuals with severe malignant tracheobronchial stenosis, there are actually few contraindications to laser bronchoscopy. Dumon[18] stated that "since it [laser bronchoscopy] is almost always used in a high-risk patient population, the normal limitations used for conventional bronchoscopic application must be expanded." He added that the only absolute contraindication to laser bronchoscopy is lack of an intraluminal lesion. Because lesions extrinsic to the airway are not amenable for treatment, it is important to confirm that the airway narrowing is not the result of compression from mediastinal tumors, lymphadenopathy, lobar collapse, or from type II tracheal stenosis. Failure to recognize extrinsic airway compression as a cause of airway narrowing can result in inadvertent perforation of the tracheobronchial wall. Except for extraluminal disease, there are few other reasons not to consider laser resection even in patients who are at a higher surgical risk. Personne and colleagues[22] performed laser resection on 267 patients "in extremis" with severe hypoxia or coma and recorded only a 2.7 percent mortality rate. A low rate of fatal complications of 0.3 to 3 percent has been confirmed by three other large series.[18,20,23] This low perioperative mortality rate indicates that the procedure can be an acceptable palliative treatment even for very ill patients.[22]

Although there are few absolute contraindications to laser bronchoscopy, a number of relative contraindications need to be considered (Table 5-3). A preoperative evaluation is often used to identify cardiovascular and respiratory problems that might place the patient at an unacceptably high risk for complications.

Table 5-3
CONTRAINDICATIONS TO LASER BRONCHOSCOPY

Absolute contraindications
Extraluminal disease
Relative contraindications
Cardiovascular
Recent myocardial infarction
Ventricular arrhythmias
Conduction abnormalities
Hypotension
Decompensated congestive heart failure
Respiratory
Severe obstructive lung disease
Extensive tumor involvement
Involvement of pulmonary artery
Unsalvageable lung distal to obstruction
Chronic collapse
Small cell carcinoma cell type
Posterior tracheal wall location or tracheoesophageal fistula
Extensive preprocedure radiation therapy
Electrolyte abnormalities
Bleeding diathesis
Sepsis
Tracheobronchial malacia

Postoperative myocardial infarction and cardiac arrest account for 30 to 60 percent of perioperative deaths, and respiratory insufficiency from persistent obstruction accounts for another 40 percent of fatal outcomes.[18,20,23] Although knowledge of underlying cardiopulmonary problems is important and may preclude surgery in some individuals, the palliative benefits of laser bronchoscopy frequently outweigh the small risk of postprocedural complications. In many instances, respiratory insufficiency is both the primary indication for the procedure and the reason why the patient is a higher surgical risk. For some patients, bronchoscopic laser resection represents the only chance for rapid relief of dyspnea. Failure to wean patients from mechanical ventilation after bronchoscopy is infrequent and usually occurs as a result of being unable to establish an effective airway and not from underlying obstructive lung disease.

It is important to know whether there is functional lung distal to the obstruction. Lung parenchyma that is severely damaged by radiation treatments or recurrent postobstructive pneumonia is unable to participate in gas exchange even when the obstruction is removed.[32] In addition, significant tumor involvement of the pulmonary artery can result in irreversible ventilation-perfusion inequalities, negating any effects of laser resection. Bronchography,[32] angiography,[33] and computed tomography of the chest can be helpful in evaluating lung parenchyma in the region of the obstruction. Nonfunctional lung found distal to the region of obstruction represents a strong relative contraindication to laser resection.

The type and location of the lesion may be additional relative contraindications to laser bronchoscopy because they influence the likelihood of procedural complications. Tumors involving the posterior tracheal wall can extend into the esophagus, increasing the risk of perforation or fistula formation during laser applications. Some authors[32] even suggest esophageal endoscopy before laser resection to identify patients at risk for tracheoesophageal fistula. The risk of airway erosion and perforation is also increased by extensive preprocedure radiation therapy, which can distort and soften the tracheal wall.[18] Particular caution should be taken with upper lobe lesions because laser treatment can result in excessive bleeding owing to the proximity of major vessels. The cell type of the tumor can influence the success of the procedure and may be an indication to use other methods of treatment. For example, small cell carcinoma of the lung is often diffuse and usually contains a large extrabronchial component, making the lesion unfavorable for laser resection. Bleeding related to small cell carcinoma, however, may be treated effectively with the Nd:YAG laser. Coagulopathies, electrolyte abnormalities, hypotension, and sepsis represent other obvious contraindications to laser endoscopy and should be corrected before the procedure.

Anesthesia

The method of anesthesia delivery for Nd:YAG laser bronchoscopy depends on the type of bronchoscopic technique. For flexible bronchoscopies, light intravenous conscious sedation is usually employed in a fashion similar to standard diagnostic bronchoscopy. If the patient is intubated, however, intravenous general anesthesia can be given. Anesthesia for the rigid bronchoscopic procedure is usually accomplished by a combination of intravenous agents, including midazolam, propofol, fentanyl, and occasionally a depolarizing neuromuscular blocker. If a closed rigid bronchoscopic method is preferred, ventilation is achieved through the side arm of the bronchoscope. Inhalational anesthetic agents can be used with a closed system, but there may be more potential for cardiopulmonary complications.[34] Some bronchoscopists prefer to operate through the open end of the rigid bronchoscope, and thus a different type of ventilation is required. Perrin and colleagues[35] prefer spontaneous assisted ventilation, but other authors[20,36–38] use a manual Venturi jet ventilation technique. Our system consists of an air-oxygen blender (Bird/3M, Palm Springs, CA) combined with a high pressure (50 psi) manual injector attached to the side port of the rigid bronchoscope.[39] This method of ventilation enables the surgeon to operate through the open end of the rigid bronchoscope while ventilation is maintained by manually injecting an air-oxygen mixture at 20 to 60 breaths per minute.[37,38,40] A high frequency jet ventilation technique has also been described wherein a machine delivers approximately 300 breaths per minute.[41] The effectiveness of manual Venturi jet ventilation has been well validated,[42,43] and the use of continuous CO_2 monitoring is not required. Standard O_2 pulse oximetry is recommended to avoid inadvertent desaturation events during the procedure. After rigid bronchoscopy, most patients are easily extubated in the operating room after clearance of the intravenous anesthesia. Patients usually stay a few hours in the postanesthesia care unit after which they are either transferred back to their hospital room or discharged. General anesthesia for rigid laser bronchoscopy can be performed safely through various techniques, and most elderly or debilitated patients can tolerate the intervention without difficulty. Anesthesia during rigid bronchoscopy will be described in Chap. 21.

Techniques for Laser Bronchoscopy

RIGID VERSUS FLEXIBLE BRONCHOSCOPY

The Nd:YAG laser can be used with either a flexible or rigid bronchoscope, and which instrument is better has been discussed widely.[44,45] Ironically, the original papers in the early 1980s by Toty[46] and Dumon[47] described the use of the Nd:YAG laser with both the flexible and rigid bronchoscopes. For the next few years, the flexible bronchoscope was used alone or in conjunction with an endotracheal tube or rigid scope in the majority of laser resections.[24,31,48,49] Subsequently, reports of major complications, including deaths resulting from massive hemorrhage[24,34,50] and airway fire[51] began to surface, and by the late 1980s, many authors[24,52] advocated using the rigid bronchoscope for most Nd:YAG laser resections. Despite this claim, Chan and coworkers[44] compared results of 61 Nd:YAG laser procedures performed with a flexible bronchoscope with results of 51 procedures performed through a rigid bronchoscope on 79 patients and found no difference in the complication or survival rates between the two groups. The authors suggested that the rigid scope should be used for proximal lesions and the flexible scope for distal lesions and recommended that laser bronchoscopists should be proficient in both techniques. Each method is associated with certain advantages and disadvantages.

Flexible Bronchoscopy

The major advantage of the flexible bronchoscope is its versatility and familiarity to the pulmonologist. In the 1991 Bronchoscopy Survey by the American College of Chest Physicians,[53] the flexible scope was used by more than 80 percent of responding physicians at some point in their practice. The popularity of the flexible scope for laser procedures may partly be related to the limited number of physicians who are trained in rigid bronchoscopy. In this survey, only 8.4 percent of the responders used the rigid scope in their practice. This trend away from the use of rigid bronchoscopy limits the choice of methods to apply the Nd:YAG laser, but in some instances, flexible bronchoscopy may actually be the preferred technique. The flexible scope is small and maneuverable, which permits easier access to distal airway lesions and improves visualization of the bronchial tree. Aiming the laser beam is also easier with the flexible scope because the operator has more control over the tip of the laser fiber. Because of its size and controllability, it may also be passed through the rigid bronchoscope for dissection and coagulation purposes. Usually, the flexible bronchoscope is reserved for lesions that do not have a propensity for hemorrhage, such as granulomas, papillomas, and small distal malignant tumors. The flexible laser bronchoscope is ideal for recurrent tumors and pedunculated tumors with a narrow base. The versatility and familiarity of the flexible scope make it well adapted for the safe and effective laser resection of specific lesions within the tracheobronchial tree (Table 5-4).

Other proposed advantages of flexible bronchoscopy for laser applications include potential cost savings and the avoidance of general anesthesia. Unfortunately, these probably only represent theoretical advantages. Because flexible bronchoscopy is often performed outside of an operating room setting, it can be more convenient and less costly than rigid bronchoscopy. For large obstructing lesions, however, multiple procedures are often required, frequently negating any anticipated cost savings. In one study,[54] an average of 1.97 treatments were required to obtain a response compared with only one treatment session using a rigid bronchoscope. Additionally, each procedure may be more time consuming for the operator because removal of tumor debris is less efficient through the flexible bronchoscope. The frequent need for multiple procedures and the increased investment of time minimize the proposed advantages of flexible bronchoscopy for laser photoresection.

Another theoretical advantage of the flexible bronchoscope is the potential to avoid the inherent risks of general anesthesia, including myocardial infarction, arrhythmia, hemodynamic instability, CO_2 retention, barotrauma, and prolonged neuromuscular weakness.[34,36,55] Unger and others[45,56] advocate the use of flexible bronchoscopy for most tracheobronchial laser procedures and report no significant anesthesia-related hemodynamic or ventilatory complications in more than 290 procedures performed under topical anesthesia.[57] Cardiovascular complications, such as myocardial infarction, however, can still result from flexible bronchoscopy,[54] especially if severe hemorrhage or airway compromise occurs. In fact, the only deaths in some studies using flexible bronchoscopy for laser procedures have not been the result of anesthetic complications but rather due to uncontrollable hemorrhage.[24,34,54] Although complications related to general anesthesia for rigid bronchoscopy have been well documented,[20,22,23,55] the overall rate of occurrence is exceedingly low. Cavaliere and coworkers[19] reported respiratory failure in only 0.5 percent, cardiac arrest in

Table 5-4

INDICATIONS FOR THE FLEXIBLE FIBERSCOPE IN LASER BRONCHOSCOPY

In combination with a rigid bronchoscope
Benign tumors (granulomas, papillomas)
Small malignant tumors
Distal tumors
Less than 50% obstruction of airway lumen
Recurrent tumors
Narrow based pedunculated tumors
Hemoptysis photocoagulation

SOURCE: Adapted from Ramser ER, Beamis JF Jr: Laser bronchoscopy. *Clin Chest Med* 1995; 16:415–426.

0.4 percent, and myocardial infarction in 0.2 percent of 2253 cases in which more than 90 percent were performed under general anesthesia using a rigid bronchoscope. In a separate prospective study[35] of 124 interventional rigid bronchoscopies, no cardiac complications occurred, and transient reversible hypoxemia was seen in only 15 percent of cases. Avoidance of complications from general anesthesia and potential cost savings represent only theoretical advantages of flexible bronchoscopy, but they may still be important considerations in some patients.

Rigid Bronchoscopy

Although there may be advantages to flexible bronchoscopy for certain situations, the rigid bronchoscope is now generally preferred for most large obstructing tracheobronchial lesions.[20,22,23,52] Rigid laser bronchoscopy has a number of important advantages over flexible bronchoscopy, including efficiency, effectiveness, and, most important, safety. It is usually more efficient because larger pieces of tumor material can be removed through the rigid scope, significantly reducing the time of the procedure and the total number of procedures required.[44,54] Often only one procedure is required because the barrel of the bronchoscope can be used to "core" out the obstructing endoluminal lesion and quickly reestablish airway patency. The barrel can also be used to dilate a narrowed trachea and possibly eliminate the need for surgical resection. Other advantages of rigid bronchoscopy include the ability to perform stent implantation or removal at the time of the laser intervention. Both silicone stents and self-expandable metal stents can be placed through a rigid bronchoscope.

Although improved efficiency is desirable, the most important advantage of rigid bronchoscopy is safety. Dumon and colleagues[52] commented that they could not overstress that flexible laser bronchoscopy in patients with major obstructive malignancy is dangerous, and this type of instrumentation does not have the potential for effective response in the event of a major crisis. Personne and coworkers[58] outlined three safety priorities for laser bronchoscopy—maintenance of ventilation, effective suction, and a clear visual field. They felt the rigid bronchoscope was the most effective instrument to accomplish these goals. With rigid bronchoscopy, the airway is secure, and light general anesthesia can be administered for patient comfort and surgeon convenience. Maintaining a clear field and patent airway is more easily achieved with the rigid bronchoscope because of better suctioning capabilities. With the flexible scope, suction is limited because the working channel is partially occluded by the laser fiber. Control of bleeding is also superior with the rigid bronchoscope because the barrel of the scope can be used to tamponade the hemorrhaging site. An epinephrine soaked gauze pad can even be passed through the rigid scope and placed directly on the bleeding area. Although some physicians[59] report that the bleeding rate may actually be higher with the rigid technique because of the tendency to use the scope as a shearing tool, most authors[52,53] believe the ability to maintain a patent airway and control any excessive bleeding is of paramount importance. Thus, the rigid bronchoscope is a safer instrument for laser application in patients at higher risk for procedural complications.

Both rigid and flexible bronchoscopy are associated with advantages and disadvantages that need to be considered when deciding on the best technique to employ the Nd:YAG laser. Each case should be handled individually, but the primary advantages of the rigid bronchoscope are its efficiency, effectiveness, and safety in the treatment of large malignant obstructing lesions of the tracheobronchial tree. For distal small airway lesions or nonvascular benign tumors, the flexible bronchoscope can be used safely and effectively for laser applications. Debate will likely continue as to which is the best technique for laser bronchoscopy, but the answer is more likely a factor of the type and location of the lesion rather than the actual bronchoscopic instrument used. Bronchoscopists performing laser photoresection of tracheobronchial lesions should be proficient in both techniques to assess the risks and benefits of each technique as it applies to a particular patient.

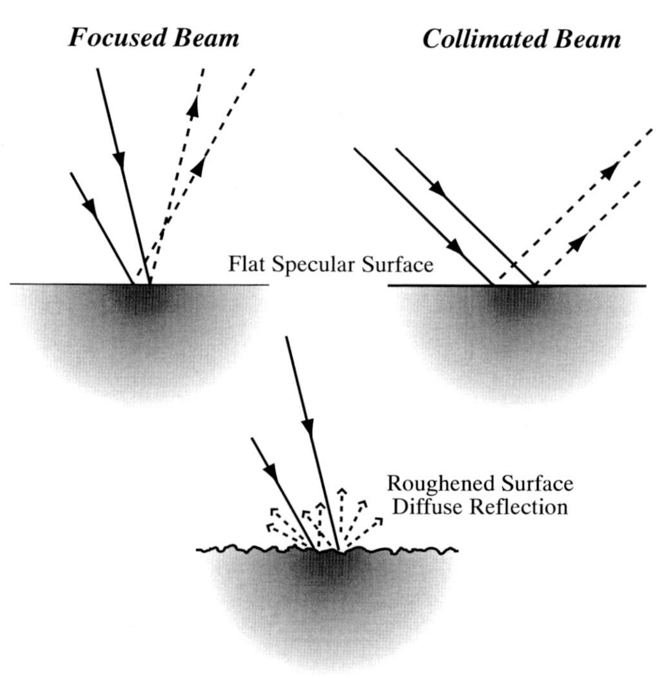

Figure 5-10

Reflection characteristics of surfaces.

Safety

Laser safety requires the knowledge of the properties of individual lasers and the potential hazards that can arise with improper use. Each laser has a different capacity for producing injury, and the American National Standards Institute (ANSI) has classified lasers (I to IV) based on the degree of their potential hazard.[60] This classification system uses an accessible emission limit (AEL) and a maximum permissible exposure (MPE) limit for various organs.[1] The AEL is the amount of laser radiation that can be collected by a specific detector per unit of area. The MPE corresponds to the total energy absorbed by the tissue and is a function of the wavelength of the laser and the duration of exposure. A class I rating is given to lasers that do not emit hazardous levels of radiation and represent the lowest risk for injury. Class II lasers are also very safe if exposure duration is limited to less than 0.25 s in the visible band of light because the natural aversion reflex of the eye is rapid enough to avoid injury by this type of laser. Their low power gives an AEL of below 1 mW, which is the arbitrary power level that separates class II lasers from the next laser class. Class III lasers have a wide power range between 1 and 500 mW and can be potentially dangerous even if viewed momentarily. Most surgical lasers are classified as class IV because they have a power output above 500 mW. The main safety risks for surgical lasers are thermal and ocular injuries related to accidental reflection of laser light.

Inadvertent injury to the patient and operating room personnel is an important safety concern with the use of class IV surgical lasers. Misdirected laser light energy can reflect off instruments and specular (shiny) surfaces located near the operating field causing corneal, retinal, and thermal injury to exposed areas (Fig. 5-10). Surgical instruments can be roughened or blackened to help diffuse and absorb these poten-

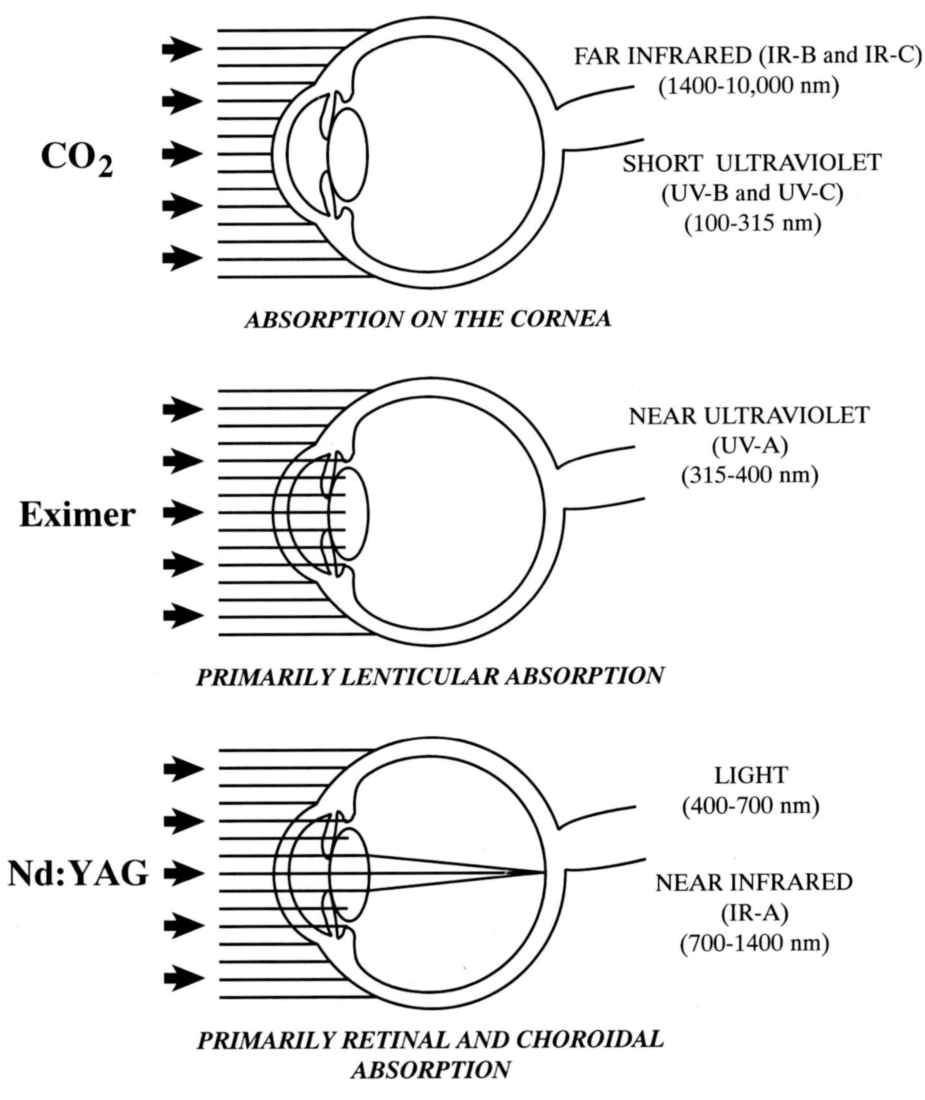

Figure 5-11

Primarily retinal and choroidal absorption.

tially dangerous reflections of laser light.[61] Even if a laser beam is reflected, it retains much of its focus and intensity because of the collimation and coherence properties of laser light.[62] The dangers of reflected laser light are often not readily apparent because Nd:YAG and CO_2 lasers have wavelengths in the invisible range of the electromagnetic spectrum. The bronchoscopist may actually be at the highest risk for injury because Nd:YAG laser light can scatter and reflect back along the endoscope. This is usually not a concern with the CO_2 laser as the optics of the system protect the operator from injury. To avoid inadvertent injury from reflected laser light, safety glasses or eye shields are mandatory for all operating room personnel as well as for the patient. In addition, the windows in the procedure room should be covered to protect anyone outside the room from becoming accidentally exposed. Signs indicating the use of laser light should also be placed on the doors entering the room. Certain built-in precautions, such as foot pedals for laser activation and a standby mode, help to avoid accidental deployment of laser energy.

One of the most well-recognized hazards of class IV surgical lasers is retinal or corneal injury. Although the eye has a natural lid aversion reflex that limits exposure to bright light, the power density of certain lasers is great enough to produce significant damage. Because of their various wavelengths, lasers affect the eye in different ways (Fig. 5-11). Laser beams with short wavelengths in the ultraviolet region (100 to 400 nm) or long wavelengths in the far infrared region (1400 to 10,000 nm) of the electromagnetic spectrum are absorbed by the cornea and lens of the eye. Lasers with wavelengths in the visible and near infrared region (400 to 1400 nm), such as the Nd:YAG laser, are more dangerous to the retina. This area of the electromagnetic spectrum has been termed the retinal hazard region because laser light of this wavelength can be focused by the lens onto the retina with a magnitude of up to 100,000 times.[62] If the beam becomes focused onto a small point on the retina, significant damage can occur from thermal effects. If the damage is in an area, such as the fovea of the macula, irreversible loss of fine vision can occur. Unfortunately, the loss of vision is usually permanent because neural tissue has limited ability to regenerate itself. For this reason, all lasers in classes II to IV should be considered potentially dangerous to the eye if adequate precautions are not taken. The type of eye protection is important because safety glasses are designed for use with lasers of a specific wavelength. Eye protection manufactured for use with one type of laser may not be protective against lasers with a different wavelength. For instance, clear plastic safety glasses are adequate for brief exposures to CO_2 laser energy because of the limited penetration of CO_2 laser light, but a Nd:YAG laser can easily penetrate plastic or glass. For protection against the Nd:YAG laser, special eye wear with an optical density of 7.0 at 1064 nm is required.

Although ocular damage is the most feared safety risk, the skin and airway mucosa are also susceptible to injury from the laser. The likelihood of injury to the skin may actually be greater than to the eye because of the larger area of exposure. Lasers in the visible and near infrared region (400 to 1400 nm), such as the Nd:YAG laser, can produce thermal injury severe enough to create third-degree burns.[62] The CO_2 laser, however, has a longer wavelength (10,600 nm) that limits skin penetration and reduces the risk of a severe burn. Nevertheless, thermal injury can still occur if exposure is prolonged or if plastic, paper, or cloth items near the surgical field are accidentally ignited by the laser. The airway mucosa is also vulnerable to thermal injury because airway fires can occur if the flexible bronchoscope, endotracheal tube, or plastic suction catheter is accidentally ignited by the laser.[51] A polyvinyl chloride (PVC) endotracheal tube should not be used with a CO_2 laser because it is flammable, and toxic gases can be released from the burned plastic. The use of a red rubber tube with aluminum wrapping can reduce the risk of airway fires caused by the CO_2 laser.[63] This special tube should not be used with a Nd:YAG laser because the darker rubber tube may actually absorb more laser energy. The risk of airway fires can also be reduced by limiting the power of the Nd:YAG laser exposure time and the $F_{I_{O_2}}$.[64] The use of a metallic rigid bronchoscope will also substantially reduce the risk of airway fires, although with proper precautions, a flexible bronchoscope or endotracheal tube can be used safely during laser applications. Although airway fires and burns are rare events, they are important safety considerations when using most types of surgical lasers.

The composition of the smoke plume generated by the laser has also recently come under investigation.[65] In 1988, a questionnaire study by Lobraico and coworkers[66] demonstrated an association between CO_2 laser treatment of papillomas and the subsequent development of these lesions in the treating physicians. Furthermore, Garden and colleagues[67] demonstrated the presence of intact human papillomavirus (HPV) DNA in the vapors of laser-treated verrucae and cautioned practitioners about the potential transmissibility of infection. Abrahamson and coworkers,[68] however, were unable to demonstrate HPV DNA present in the smoke plume from vaporization of laryngeal papillomas unless direct suction contact was made with the tissue during surgery. The presence of human immunodeficiency virus (HIV) DNA in laser smoke has also been documented, but sustained growth of the cultured cells did not occur, possibly because of damage produced by the laser energy.[69] The risk of clinical disease in surgical personnel from viral transmission has not yet been established, but special safety

Table 5-5
DUMON'S 10 COMMANDMENTS OF SAFE YAG LASER RESECTION[18]

1. Know the anatomic danger zones: Aortic arch, pulmonary artery, and esophagus being the main hazard areas.
2. Have a well-trained laser team, including an anesthetist specialized in light general anesthesia and two assistants drilled in emergency response procedures.
3. Screen patients carefully: Any endoluminal growth is amenable to laser resection, but purely external compression is beyond the reach of the technique.
4. Use the rigid bronchoscopic technique (custom-made open tube, light general anesthesia, straight telescope, and two suction catheters) for any high-grade obstruction, especially if malignancy is involved.
5. Monitor blood gases and cardiac performance. At the least sign of hypoxemia, interrupt treatment long enough to oxygenate the patient, if necessary under closed-circuit conditions.
6. Fire the laser parallel to the wall of the airway; never aim directly into it.
7. Coagulate at will but avoid using the laser at high power settings; mechanical resection after laser coagulation is preferable to laser resection alone whenever possible.
8. Do not neglect hemorrhage, for even slow bleeding will lead to hypoxemia if left unattended.
9. Terminate each procedure with a thorough laser irradiation of the resected area and a tracheobronchial toilet to remove all secretions and/or debris.
10. Keep the patient under observation in a specially outfitted recovery room for a reasonable period of time.

precautions, such as smoke evacuation systems, are recommended until further studies can be performed.

Certain guidelines need to be followed for the safe operation of the Nd:YAG laser during bronchoscopy (Table 5-5). For flexible bronchoscopy, these recommendations concentrate on the prevention of hemorrhage and airway fires (See Table 2-1). To help avoid these complications and achieve successful results, the location of the tip of the laser fiber should be known at all times. When firing the laser, the tip of the fiber should be at least 4 cm from the distal end of an endotracheal tube and at least 4 mm from the end of the bronchoscope to prevent ignition of the plastic. The concentration of inspired oxygen should also be 40 percent or less to decrease the risk of airway fires. The tip of the laser fiber is best positioned 0.4 cm to 1 cm from the lesion and should be kept clean at all times. When appropriately positioned, the laser should also be fired parallel to the airway wall in pulses of 0.4 to 1 s in duration with a setting of 20 to 40 W. The goal of Nd:YAG laser application should not be to vaporize the tumor completely but rather to photocoagulate the lesion to produce hemostasis and necrosis. Residual tumor can be removed mechanically with biopsy forceps, a balloon catheter, or vigorous suctioning, eliminating the need for vaporization. Aggressive use of laser energy should also be avoided because penetration of the Nd:YAG laser is often deeper than is apparent on the surface, and the full extent of tissue necrosis is not complete until 24 to 48 h after the procedure.[45] Instead, repeat bronchoscopy is recommended in a few days to assess the extent of the remaining tumor and need for further treatment. For smaller lesions, subsequent bronchoscopy may not be necessary, but for large obstructing lesions, a multiple stage procedure is often the safest approach. If these guidelines are followed, Nd:YAG laser bronchoscopy can safely and effectively be performed through the flexible bronchoscope with successful palliation in more than 80 percent of patients.[56]

For rigid bronchoscopy, the same Nd:YAG laser fiber is passed down the barrel of the scope along with a suction catheter and telescope. The laser fiber is aimed at the lesion by manipulating the rigid scope itself. The laser power settings remain at 20 to 40 W, with a pulse duration of 0.4 to 1 s. The metal rigid bronchoscope is nonflammable, and thus the laser fiber does not have to extend beyond the end of the scope. It is important, however, to keep the flexible suction catheter out of the laser field to avoid any chance of fire. The laser fiber should be in close proximity (<1 cm) to the lesion because laser energy disperses as it exits the tip of the fiber, and the distance to the lesion determines the effective power density. As with flexible laser bronchoscopy, the initial goal should be photocoagulation of the tumor and not vaporization. Debridement of the remaining tissue can be accomplished by alligator forceps or a suction catheter. If needed, the beveled end of the rigid bronchoscope can be also used to shear off parts of the tumor once photocoagulation has devitalized the tissue. Care must be taken not to perforate the airway wall with the rigid scope. It is always important to know the path of the distal airway before aggressively advancing the scope beyond the tumor. The flexible scope can be helpful for blunt dissection of the tumor and in evaluating the airways distal to the main obstruction. After most of the tumor has been removed by these means, hemostasis can be achieved through further laser photocoagulation.

Outcome

Although laser bronchoscopy has become more commonly used for benign and malignant tracheobronchial obstruction,[18–20,22] no randomized controlled trials exist proving a survival benefit in treated patients. Numerous studies, however, have shown a significant palliative benefit with regard to relief of dyspnea, control of hemoptysis, and facilitation of weaning from mechanical ventilation. In 1419 patients with bronchogenic carcinoma, Cavaliere and coworkers[19] achieved satisfactory immediate results corresponding to a normal airway lumen gauge or significant improvement in ventilation in 93 percent of patients. Brutinel and colleagues[24] found that airway caliber was improved in 79.7 percent of 182 sites and that even completely obstructed airways could be opened 57.7 percent of the time. In a previous study at the Lahey Clinic,[20] subjective symptomatic relief was demonstrated after 313 of 400 procedures (78.3 percent) in patients with benign and malignant disease.

Although many of the larger studies relied on subjective measurements of improvement, other studies have documented objective benefits in pulmonary function tests, performance scores, and even ventilation-perfusion scans after laser bronchoscopy. Spirometry and flow volume loops have shown immediate functional improvement, with increases in peak expiratory flow rates ranging from 26 to 512 percent.[70,71] Waller and coworkers[72] showed a mean overall improvement in FEV_1 of 27 percent and symptomatic relief in 103 of 116 patients whose main complaint was dyspnea. Gelb and Epstein[49] reported significant improvement in Karnofsky performance scores, dyspnea index, and FEF_{25-75} in 23 of 27 patients with incomplete malignant obstruction of the tracheobronchial tree. Jain and colleagues[73] also used Karnofsky scores in patients treated by Nd:YAG laser photoresection and reported an improved performance status in 13 of 15 patients lasting between 2 and 13 months. Other performance scores, such as the simple 0 to 4 symptom score used by Clarke and coworkers,[74] confirmed good symptomatic relief in 73 percent of their first 200 patients consecutively treated with laser bronchoscopy.

Ventilation-perfusion relationships have also been studied in patients undergoing laser bronchoscopy. George and colleagues[75] found that both ventilation and perfusion improved after laser treatments in 23 of 28 patients (82 percent) and that spirometric values, 6-min walking distance, Karnofsky performance index, and breathlessness scores also improved significantly. In addition, it appears that improvements are not simply transient. Although some patients with benign and malignant tracheobronchial lesions may require multiple procedures, Emslander and coworkers[76] reported complete or partial removal of tumor in 74 percent of 224 laser applications and showed that in 72 percent of the successful results, the stenoses were still open after 4 to 6 months.

Nd:YAG laser photocoagulation is also effective at controlling hemoptysis[9,73,74] from malignant endobronchial lesions, with a response rate estimated to be 60 percent.[9] Although photocoagulation for hemoptysis has shown initial success, long-term benefits were not as easily maintained as with treatment for relief of dyspnea. Clarke and coworkers[74] reported that patients who were treated principally for hemoptysis tended to have a recurrence of their symptoms within 30 days of treatment, whereas those who were treated for dyspnea or cough tended to experience recurrence much later.

Laser bronchoscopy has also been shown to be beneficial for patients with impending respiratory failure as well as for those who require mechanical ventilation. Radiation therapy can relieve cough, chest pain, and dyspnea in 60 to 80 percent of patients, but it only relieves atelectasis in 25 percent of patients, and improvement is usually delayed.[77] External beam radiation therapy is a common palliative intervention for patients with bronchogenic carcinoma, but only laser bronchoscopy provides the means for rapid resolution of symptoms. In one series,[70] laser bronchoscopy was successful at relieving breathlessness and avoiding mechanical ventilation in 11 of 14 patients who had respiratory distress on presentation. The authors[70] concluded that laser treatment provided an excellent method of resuscitating patients with life-threatening tracheal obstruction, enabling subsequent management, such as radiation therapy, chemotherapy, or tracheobronchial stenting. Laser bronchoscopy may also facilitate weaning from mechanical ventilation in patients with respiratory failure caused by endoluminal obstruction. Stanopoulos and colleagues[78] reported that laser bronchoscopy improved the clinical status of 9 of 17 mechanically ventilated patients by permitting successful extubation. This subgroup of patients had appreciably shorter requirements for mechanical ventilation and a longer survival. The initial use of Nd:YAG laser bronchoscopy for treatment of an endobronchial lesion can be debated, but the palliative use of laser therapy in an inoperable, symptomatic pa-

Table 5-6
SURVIVAL DATA OF PATIENTS WHO UNDERWENT LASER BRONCHOSCOPY

Author	*Number Patients*	*Number Primary*	*Number Metastatic*	*Percent Improved*	*Survival 3 Months*	*Survival 6 Months*	*Survival 1 Year*	*Mean*	*Median*
Cavaliere et al. [23]		333		92%	75%	50%	26%		
Beamis et al.[20]	236	200	36		60%	34%	10%		
Brutinel et al.[24]		71	17	79%	65%[a]	55%[a]	28%		
Kvale et al.[31]				92%					
Dumon[18]	278			85%					
Eichenhorn et al.[80]		19		84%	75%[a]	70%[a]	35%[a]		340 days
Clarke et al.[74]		105	12		72%	45%	25%		5.9 months
Desai et al.[79]		47			55%	42%	21%	208 days	143 days

[a]Estimate by Kaplan-Meier curve.

tient has been shown to be beneficial for relief of dyspnea, control of hemoptysis, and weaning from mechanical ventilation.

Laser bronchoscopy is clearly a valuable tool in providing immediate symptomatic relief, but its survival benefit is more difficult to demonstrate (Table 5-6). Randomized studies[79] evaluating this palliative treatment in terminal patients has been considered unethical. Although the issue of survival is a difficult one, it appears that there may be a survival advantage for patients undergoing laser resection of malignant tracheobronchial obstruction. In a preliminary study of 19 patients treated with laser photoresection, Eichenhorn and coworkers[80] found a median survival of 340 days, which was greater than 198 to 266 days found in historical control subjects using irradiation alone.[81,82] In another study using historical controls, Brutinel and colleagues[24] compared 71 patients with bronchogenic carcinoma treated with Nd:YAG laser photoresection with 25 patients who would have received laser treatment had it been available. They found that 76 percent of the control subjects were dead within 4 months, and all were dead within 7 months. By contrast, 60 percent of patients in the laser-treated group were alive at 7 months and 28 percent were alive at 1 year. Desai and colleagues[79] also found a significant increase in survival in a subgroup of patients treated with emergent laser resection compared with historical control subjects who had emergent radiation therapy alone. In mechanically ventilated patients, Stanopoulos and coworkers[78] showed an increased survival (98 days versus 8.5 days) in patients who were weaned after emergent laser resection of an obstructing lesion. The addition of brachytherapy to laser resection may also contribute to increased survival. Shea and colleagues[83] found an improved mean survival time (41 weeks versus 16 weeks) in patients treated with both endobronchial brachytherapy and Nd:YAG laser photoresection.

Although a survival advantage was suggested by these data, the retrospective design of the studies makes statistical validation difficult. Furthermore, other authors[84] failed to show any overall survival benefit for patients undergoing laser treatment. Although Desai and coworkers[79] found improved survival in a subgroup of patients treated emergently, they did not find an overall increase in survival in patients who underwent elective laser photoresection. Clarke and colleagues[74] also gave no evidence that laser treatment prolongs life and suggested that patients die of progression of their primary disease rather than obstruction of the bronchi. Nevertheless, patients on mechanical ventilation or with impending respiratory failure likely represent a subgroup of patients who may have a survival benefit from laser photoresection. A survival advantage may also be seen if endobronchial brachytherapy is combined with laser resection.

Absolute survival, however, may not be the best way to judge the importance of a palliative intervention in symptomatic patients. The rapid relief of dyspnea and improved performance provide justification for laser bronchoscopy in most patients. Laser bronchoscopy has been shown to be an effective method for immediate relief of respiratory symptoms related to both benign and malignant tracheobronchial obstruction. It is complementary to other modes of therapy, such as radiation, chemotherapy, stenting, or surgery, and often provides the time necessary to initiate these treatments. Relief of endoluminal obstruction also facilitates the treatment of postobstructive pneumonia. After 11 years and more than 1500 patients, Cavaliere and coworkers[19] concluded that laser therapy is no longer considered a treatment of last resort but instead has its own role in the therapy of cancer of the lung. Laser bronchoscopy should be an initial consideration for patients with severe tracheobronchial obstruction irrespective of survival analysis.

HOW I DO IT

TECHNIQUE OF RIGID BRONCHOSCOPY

More than 80 percent of the laser bronchoscopy procedures performed at our institution are performed using a rigid bronchoscope. This is our preferred method of laser application for patients with high-grade obstruction of the trachea, main bronchi, bronchus intermedius, and occasionally lesions at the origin of the lower lobe bronchi. Patients undergo rigid bronchoscopy as described in Chap. 3. The procedure takes place in a standard operating room. Laser safety precautions are followed strictly. Personnel in attendance include the bronchoscopist, the anesthesia team (M.D. or certified registered nurse anesthetist), a scrub nurse, a circulating nurse, and a nurse whose sole responsibility is to operate the laser. For most routine laser applications, the Storz ventilating bronchoscope (Karl Storz Endoscopy-America, Culver City, CA) is used. If use of a stent is likely, the Dumon-Harrell rigid bronchoscope (Bryan Corp, Woburn, MA) may be used. The Storz bronchoscope is preferred because it has its own inner light source and thus can be used without a telescope. This permits the use of rigid suction instruments and large biopsy and alligator forceps to remove bulky tumor fragments. The Storz bronchoscope does not have specific channels for the laser fiber and flexible suction catheter as does the Dumon-Harrell bronchoscope. We do not consider this a disadvantage because we prefer to place the laser fiber, suction catheter, and telescope through the open end of the bronchoscope. These three instruments within the barrel of the bronchoscope "stent" each other, enabling easy maneuverability. Since we prefer to use Venturi Jet ventilation, we are not concerned about air leaking from the open end of the bronchoscope. Although we initially used a beam splitter to permit direct vision down the telescope and video display, we currently perform the procedure guided solely by the image on a video monitor. A three-chip CCD video camera (Smith and Nephew, Andover, MA) produces an excellent video image, permitting the operator, the anesthesiologist, and support personnel to follow the procedure. A sketch of our standard setup for laser bronchoscopy is shown in Fig. 5-12.

As described in Chap. 3, the patient is brought to the operating room suite and administered general anesthesia and muscle relaxation. One of the three methods to intubate the trachea with a rigid bronchoscope is employed. When the bronchoscope is below the vocal cords and near the level of the lesion, the laser fiber and a plastic suction catheter are passed through the open end of the bronchoscope along with the optical telescope (Fig. 5-13). When the lesion to be treated is tracheal stenosis, the laser is used at short pulse durations and at relatively high power. A setting of 0.7-s pulse duration and 40 W of power might be used. Because the Nd:YAG laser is not a good cutting tool, it will not cut fibrotic stenosis as well as a CO_2 laser might. However, at short pulse durations and relatively high power (but never more than 50 W of power), the Nd:YAG laser becomes a fairly good cutting tool. Several cuts are made in the region of stenosis, usually at the four quadrants. Care is taken to deliver the laser energy parallel to the airway. After a laser cut has been made in the stenotic web, the tissues tend to fall apart. It may take several laser shots to heat the tissue sufficiently to produce vaporization, but when vaporization begins, the tissue usually cuts easily with minimal or no bleeding. When sufficient radial incisions have been accomplished, the rigid bronchoscope is used to dilate the area of stenosis. Often bronchoscopes of several diameters, beginning with the smallest available, must be used to dilate the airway. On occasion, we use Jackson dilators (Karl Storz Endoscopy-America, Culver City, CA) to stretch

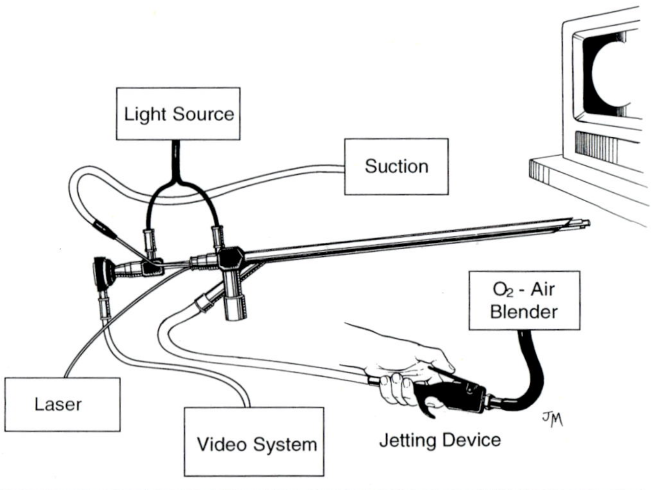

Figure 5-12

Laser bronchoscopy setup currently used at Lahey Clinic Medical Center.

Figure 5-13

Positioning of patient, bronchoscopist, and rigid bronchoscope during laser bronchoscopy.

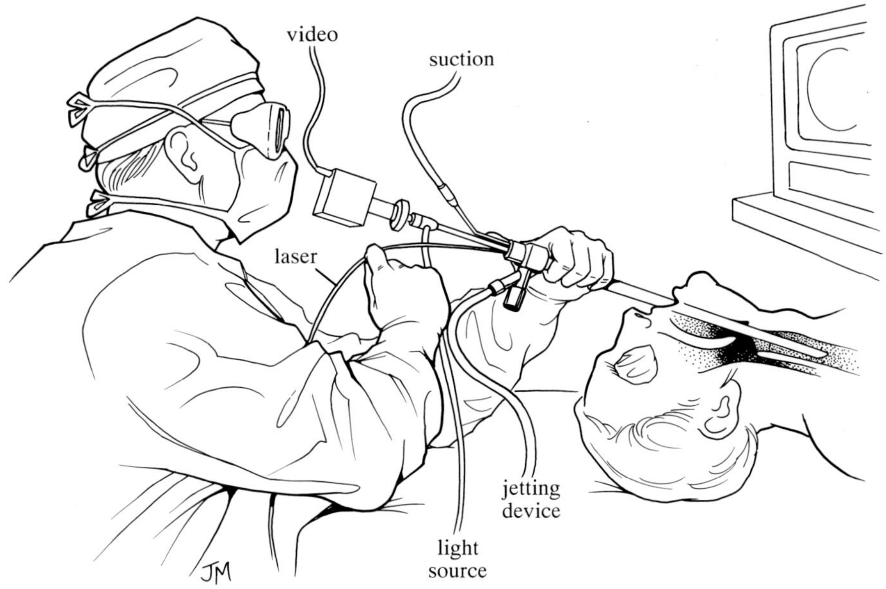

Figure 5-14

Rigid bronchoscopy technique of Nd:YAG laser bronchoscopy. *A.* Photocoagulation of lesion; suction catheter close to lesion. *B.* Lesion resected with tip of bronchoscope and delivered into barrel of scope. *C.* Distal airway is suctioned of secretions. *D.* Laser fiber passed through flexible bronchoscope within the rigid bronchoscope to treat base of tumor.

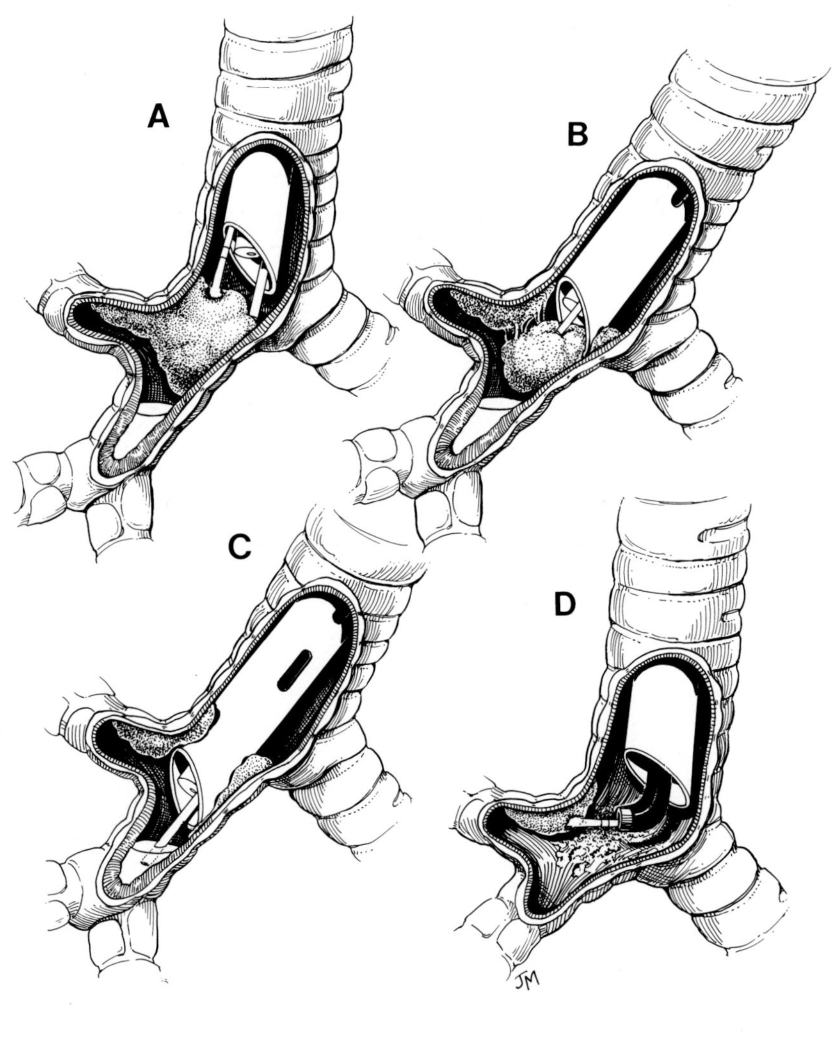

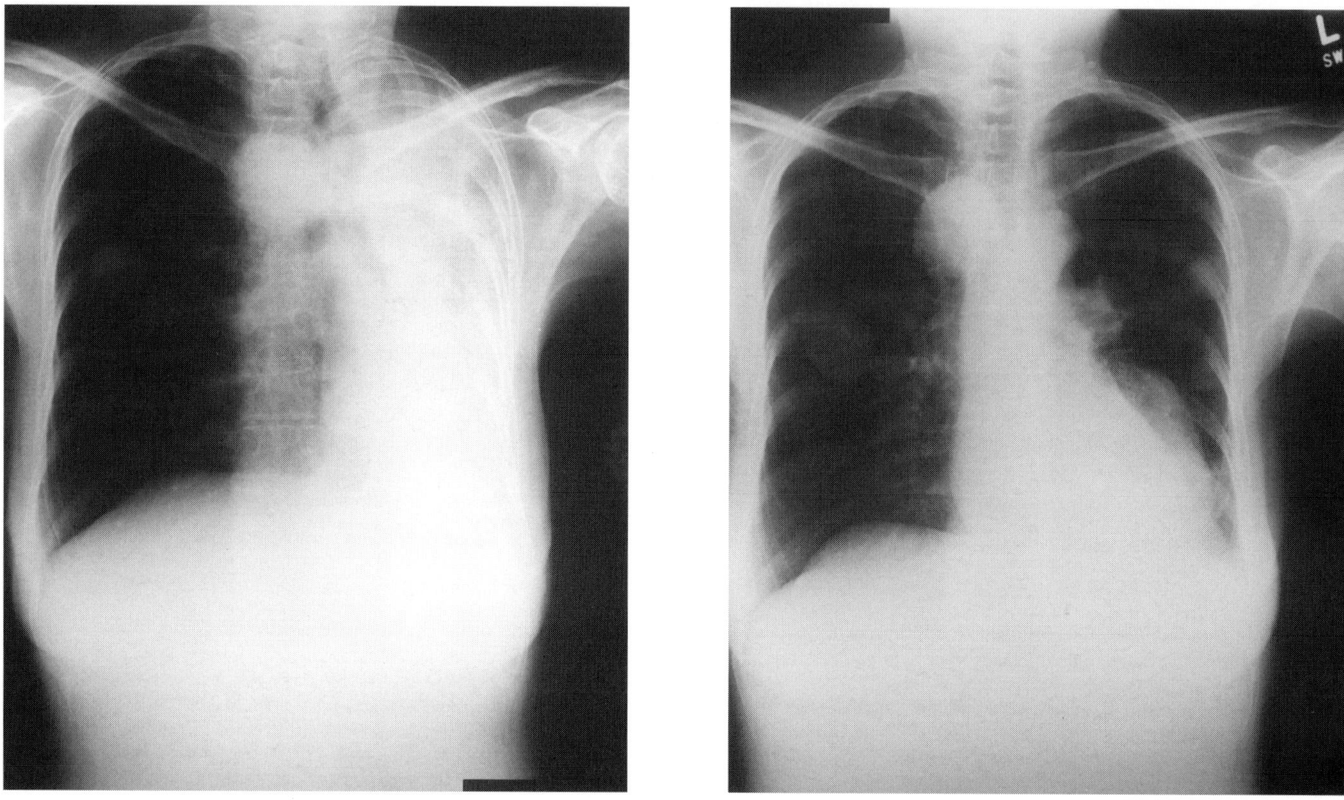

A *B*

Figure 5-15

Chest roentgenogram of patient before (*A*) and after (*B*) laser bronchoscopy for metastatic endobronchial obstruction.

the airway. The goal in the treatment of tracheal stenosis is to use as little laser energy as possible to prevent further airway inflammatory changes that might lead to restenosis.

In treating malignant endobronchial obstruction, the rigid bronchoscope is brought as close to the superior margin of the tumor as possible without irritating the tissues and producing bleeding. The laser is used at energies to promote photocoagulation rather than vaporization. Usually Nd:YAG laser power settings of 30 W at 1-s pulse duration are used. Because the blood often spatters, the tip of the telescope is kept within the barrel of the bronchoscope. The laser fiber is advanced approximately 1 cm distal to the tip of the bronchoscope. The suction catheter is held by the fingers of the right hand and is used to probe the tumor and remove any bleeding and necrotic debris from the surface of the tumor. Initially, multiple brief laser shots are used to photocoagulate the surface of the tumor. The aiming light from the laser helps direct each laser shot. An attempt is made to "paint" the entire surface of the tumor without producing vaporization. As the tumor becomes photocoagulated, it often shrinks to some degree. Again, it is important to fire the laser parallel to the direction of the airway. In near total or total obstruction, one must be careful not to fire the laser into the wall of the airway, possibly leading to perforation. When the tumor is sufficiently photocoagulated, the bronchoscope is gently advanced using the tip of the bronchoscope to shear the tumor from the bronchial wall. Knowing when the tumor has been photocoagulated sufficiently to permit safe resection takes considerable experience. The bronchoscope is advanced in a corkscrew type of motion, with any pressure being applied along the normal airway wall rather than toward the tumor bed. Permitting the tip of the bronchoscope to dig into the tumor bed could lead to airway perforation. As tumor fragments are resected, they are delivered through the barrel of the bronchoscope using the suction catheter or an alligator forceps. When the airway caliber has been established by tumor resection and dilation with the bronchoscope, the bed of the tumor is photocoagulated using brief laser shots. This technique prevents delayed bleeding. The tumor resection procedure using the rigid bronchoscope is shown in Fig. 5-14. After the airway lumen has been reestablished, secretions distal to the area of obstruction are suctioned clear. The bronchoscopist must always remember that the treatment of most endobronchial tumors is palliative treatment and that viable tumor will usually remain in the airway wall. The goal is to achieve sufficient airway caliber to permit

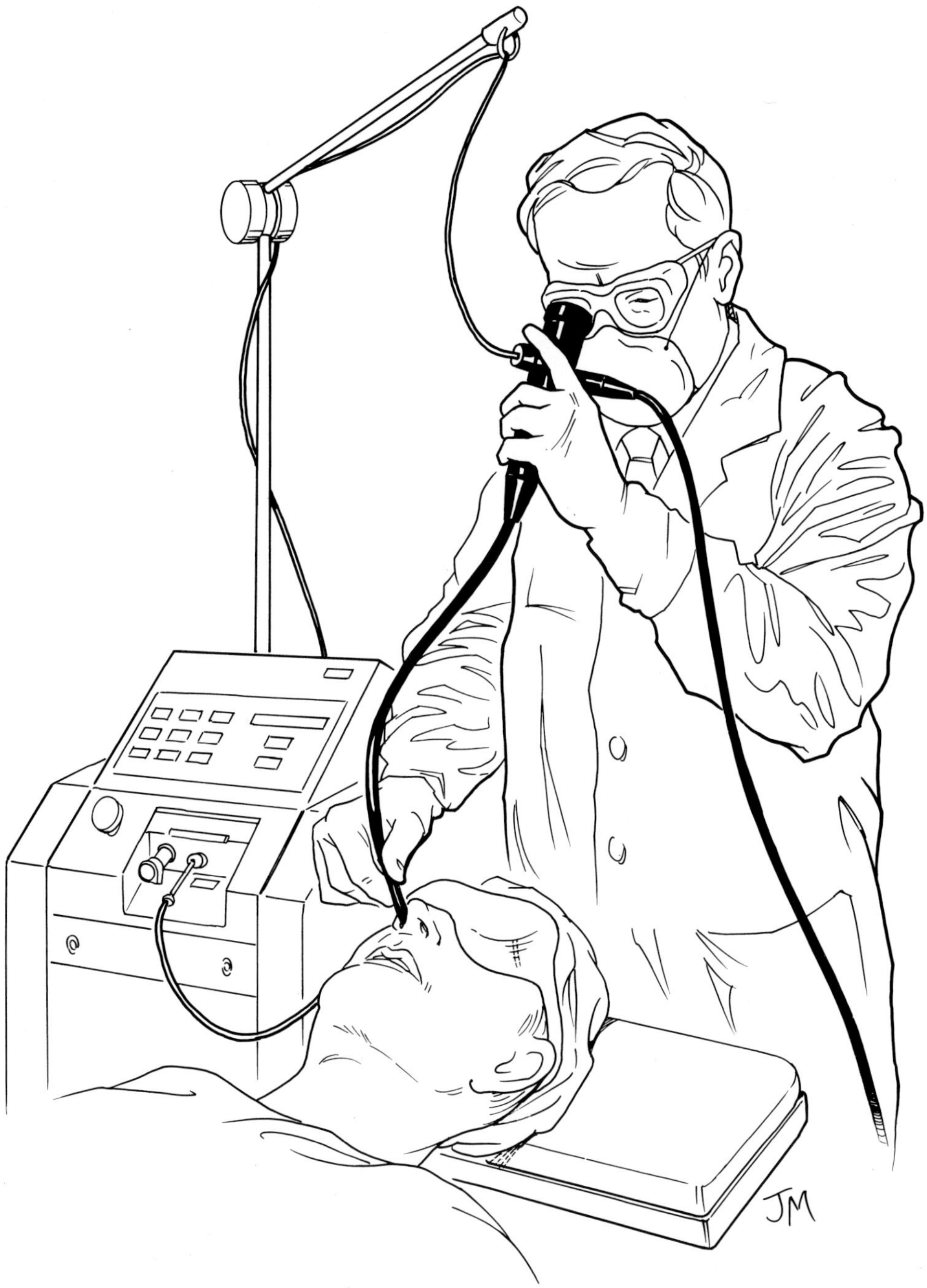

Figure 5-16

Laser bronchoscopy with flexible bronchoscope.

reestablishment of function in the distal airways and drainage of secretions without damaging the airway wall by aggressive laser or bronchoscopic manipulation (Fig. 5-15). When laser resection has been completed and the muscle relaxants are reversed, the patient is permitted to awaken from anesthesia. All attempts are made to extubate the patient in the operating suite. Because most patients are in the last stages of malignancy, it is desirable not to reintubate the patient and to have the patient leave the operating suite breathing spontaneously without need for endotracheal tube or ventilator. Patients are discharged several hours after the procedure or occasionally after one night's hospitalization. Endobronchial brachytherapy may be performed within 24 h after laser resection.

TECHNIQUE OF FLEXIBLE BRONCHOSCOPY

The 15 to 20 percent of laser procedures performed with a flexible bronchoscope (Fig. 5-16) in our institution are for lesions with less than 50 percent airway obstruction, to photocoagulate or vaporize benign lesions, or to coagulate bleeding tumors that cannot be resected. The procedure is performed in our bronchoscopy suite. A standard fiberoptic bronchoscopy technique is used, with topical anesthesia to nares and

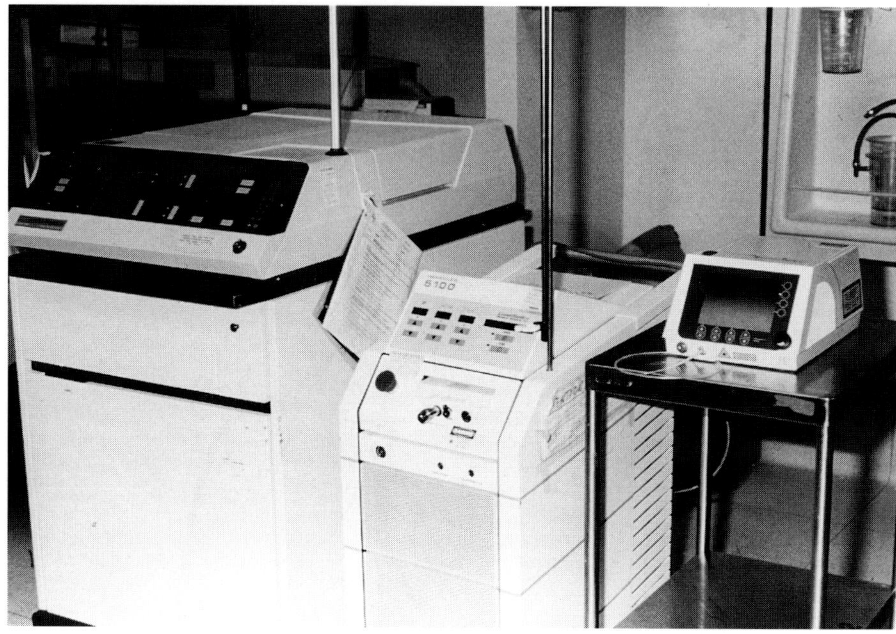

Figure 5-17

Nd:YAG lasers. *Left,* Heraeus 8900: 100-W, water-cooled laser circa 1985. *Middle,* Laser Sonics 5500: 60-W, air-cooled laser circa 1995. *Right,* Cerlas D980 NM diode laser with tissue interaction; properties similar to those of Nd:YAG laser (Ceram Opec, East Long Meadow, MA).

posterior pharynx and conscious sedation with midazolam and meperidine. The bronchoscope is passed transnasally to the level of the lesion. The laser fiber is passed down the working channel of the bronchoscope. It is important that the laser fiber tip be placed at least 1.5 to 2 cm from the tip of the bronchoscope. The laser settings are usually 1-s pulse duration with 30 W of power. Since the laser fiber occludes the bronchoscope working channel to the point that suctioning is inefficient, the procedure must be halted frequently to clean the region of any debris and char that develops from the laser heat. Firing the laser into char may set off a spark, which could lead to a disastrous airway fire. Fragments of tumor or tissue can be removed with biopsy forceps or with suction. After the procedure, the patient is observed for a brief period of time and then discharged. When the goal of the procedure is to photocoagulate the surface of a bleeding tumor, the initial laser shots are made at the base of the tumor in a circumferential manner. As the tumor shrinks and becomes devascularized, the laser shots are aimed closer to the center of the bleeding site. This method often results in effective palliation of hemoptysis for days to several weeks.

Occasionally, patients with high-grade airway obstruction are treated with fiberoptic bronchoscopic

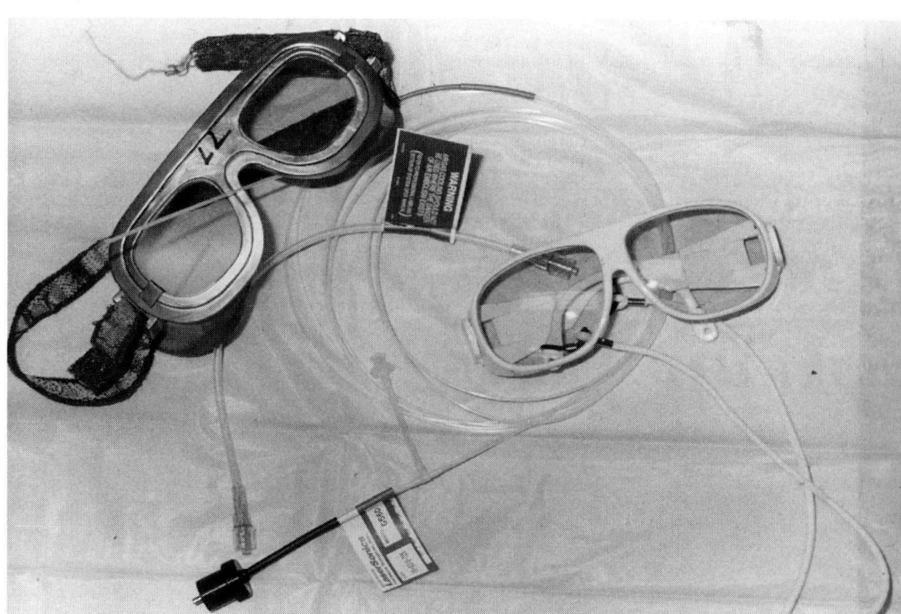

Figure 5-18

The 1.8-mm coaxial quartz fiber for Nd:YAG laser application. Protective goggles and glasses for Nd:YAG laser usage.

laser application under general anesthesia. In this instance, the patient is intubated with a large endotracheal tube (8 to 9 mm if possible), and the scope is passed into the airway through a standard swivel adapter that permits mechanical ventilation with the scope through the endotracheal tube. In this situation, Mehta's rule of 4s (see Table 2-1) must be followed. Again, the surface of the tumor is photocoagulated with the laser. Because resection is not performed as easily as with the rigid bronchoscope, the tumor must be at least partially vaporized. Tumor fragments can be removed with suction or biopsy forceps. Balloon catheters can be used to dilate and probe the airway further. Occasionally, endoscopy snares are used to remove fragments of tumor. Because it is difficult to remove large pieces of tumor, this procedure may take a considerable amount of time. Some physicians prefer to photocoagulate the lesion extensively at one setting and then to return in 24 to 48 h for removal of devitalized tumor. As with other general anesthetic techniques, all attempts are made to extubate the patient at the end of the procedure.

EQUIPMENT

Lasers used for bronchoscopy are shown in Fig. 5-17. Protective eye wear is shown in Fig. 5-18.

REFERENCES

1. Wright CV, Riopelle, MA: *Surgical CO2 Laser Fundamentals.* Houston, Biomedical Communications, 1988.
2. Beamis JF, Shapshay SM: Nd:YAG laser therapy for tracheobronchial disorders. *Postgrad Med* 1984; 75:173–180.
3. Polanyi TG: Laser physics. *Otolaryngol Clin North Am* 1983; 16:753–774.
4. Dumon JF, Corsini A: Cicatricial tracheostenosis. In: *Bronchoscopic Laser Resection Manual.* Biomedical Communications, 1989.
5. Pass HI, Pogrebniak H: Photodynamic therapy for thoracic malignancies. *Semin Surg Oncol* 1992; 8:217–225.
6. Hayata Y, Kato H, Konaka C, Ono J, Takizawa N: Hematoporphyrin derivative and laser photoradiation in the treatment of lung cancer. *Chest* 1982; 81:269–277.
7. Edell ES, Cortese DA: Bronchoscopic phototherapy with hematoporphyrin derivative for treatment of localized bronchogenic carcinoma: A 5-year experience. *Mayo Clin Proc* 1987; 62:8–14.
8. Kato H, Cortese DA: Early detection of lung cancer by means of hematoporphyrin derivative fluorescence and laser photoradiation. *Clin Chest Med* 1985; 6:237–253.
9. Hetzel MR, Smith SG: Endoscopic palliation of tracheobronchial malignancies. *Thorax* 1991; 46:325–333.
10. Rimell FL, Shapiro AM, Mitskavich MT, Modreck P, Post JC, Maisel RH: Pediatric fiberoptic laser rigid bronchoscopy. *Otolaryngol Head Neck Surg* 1996; 114:413–417.
11. Strong MS, Jako GJ, Polanyi TG, Wallace RA: Laser surgery in the aerodigestive tract. *Am J Surg* 1973; 126:529–533.
12. Polanyi TG: Physics of surgery with lasers. *Clin Chest Med* 1985; 6:179–202.
13. Ossoff RH, Coleman JA, Courey MS, Duncavage JA, Werkhaven JA, Reinisch L: Clinical applications of lasers in otolaryngology—head and neck surgery. *Lasers Surg Med* 1994; 15:217–248.
14. Coleman JA Jr, Van Duyne MJ, Ossoff RH: Laser treatment of lower airway stenosis. *Otolaryngol Clin North Am* 1995; 28:771–783.
15. Shapshay SM, Simpson GT 2d: Lasers in bronchology. *Otolaryngol Clin North Am* 1983; 16:879–886.
16. Gillis TM, Strong MS: Surgical lasers and soft tissue interactions. *Otolaryngol Clin North Am* 1983; 16:775–784.
17. Mehta AC: Laser applications in respiratory care. In Kacmarek RM, Stoller JK (eds): *Current Respiratory Care.* Toronto: BC Decker; 1988:100–106.
18. Dumon JF: *YAG Laser Bronchoscopy.* New York: Praeger Publishers; 1985.
19. Cavaliere S, Foccoli P, Toninelli C, Feijo S: Nd:YAG laser therapy in lung cancer: An 11-year experience with 2,253 applications in 1,585 patients. *J Bronchol* 1994; 1:105–111.
20. Beamis JF Jr, Vergos K, Rebeiz EE, Shapshay SM: Endoscopic laser therapy for obstructing tracheobronchial lesions. *Ann Otol Rhinol Laryngol* 1991; 100:413–419.
21. Shah H, Garbe L, Nussbaum E, Dumon JF, Chiodera PL, Cavaliere S: Benign tumors of the tracheobronchial tree: Endoscopic characteristics and role of laser resection. *Chest* 1995; 107: 1744–1751.
22. Personne C, Colchen A, Leroy M, Vourc'h G, Toty L: Indications and technique for endoscopic laser resections in bronchology: A critical analysis based upon 2,284 resections. *J Thorac Cardiovasc Surg* 1986; 91:710–715.
23. Cavaliere S, Foccoli P, Farina PL: Nd:YAG laser bronchoscopy: A five-year experience with 1,396 applications in 1,000 patients. *Chest* 1988; 94:15–21.
24. Brutinel WM, Cortese DA, McDougall JC, Gillio RG, Bergstralh EJ: A two-year experience with neodymium-YAG laser in endobronchial obstruction. *Chest* 1987; 91:159–165.
25. Shapshay SM, Beamis JF Jr, Dumon JF: Total cervical tracheal stenosis: Treatment by laser, dilation, and stenting. *Ann Otol Rhinol Laryngol* 1989; 98:890–895.
26. Mehta AC, Lee FY, Cordasco EM, Kirby T, Eliachar I, DeBoer G: Concentric tracheal and subglottic stenosis: Management using the Nd:YAG laser for mucosal sparing followed by gentle dilatation. *Chest* 1993; 104:673–677.
27. Wanamaker JR, Eliachar I: An overview of the treatment options for lower airway obstruction. *Otolaryngol Clin North Am* 1995; 28:751–770
28. Montgomery WW, Montgomery SK: Manual for use of Montgomery laryngeal, tracheal, and esophageal prostheses: Update 1990. *Ann Otol Rhinol Laryngol Suppl* 1990; 150:2–28.
29. Gelb AF, Tashkin DP, Epstein JD, Zamel N: Nd:YAG laser surgery for severe tracheal stenosis physiologically and clinically masked by severe diffuse obstructive pulmonary disease. *Chest* 1987; 91:166–170.
30. Hayashi AH, Gillis DA, Bethune D, Hughes D, O'Neil M: Management of foreign-body bronchial obstruction using endoscopic laser therapy. *J Pediatr Surg* 1990; 25:1174–1176.
31. Kvale PA, Eichenhorn MS, Radke JR, Miks V: YAG laser photoresection of lesions obstructing the central airways. *Chest* 1985; 87:283–288.
32. Dierkesmann R: Indication and results of endobronchial laser therapy. *Lung* 1990; 168 (Suppl):1095–1102.
33. Dierkesmann R, Huzly A: The significance of the pulmonary artery in endobronchial laser treatment (abstr). *Lasers Surg Med* 1983; 3:197–198.
34. Warner ME, Warner MA, Leonard PF: Anesthesia for neodymium-YAG (Nd:YAG) laser resection of major airway obstructing tumors. *Anesthesiology* 1984; 60:230–232.
35. Perrin G, Colt HG, Martin C, Mak MA, Dumon JF, Gouin F: Safety of interventional rigid bronchoscopy using intravenous anesthesia and spontaneous assisted ventilation: A prospective study. *Chest* 1992; 102:1526–1530.

36. Duckett JE, McDonnell TJ, Unger M, Parr GV: General anaesthesia for Nd:YAG laser resection of obstructing endobronchial tumours using the rigid bronchoscope. *Can Anaesth Soc J* 1985; 32:67–72.
37. Vourc'h G, Fischler MF, Michon F, Melchior JC, Seigneur F: High frequency jet ventilation v. manual jet ventilation during bronchoscopy in patients with tracheo-bronchial stenosis. *Br J Anaesth* 1983; 55:969–972.
38. Vourc'h G, Fischler MF, Michon F, Melchior JC, Seigneur F: Manual jet ventilation v. high frequency jet ventilation during laser resection of tracheo-bronchial stenosis. *Br J Anaesth* 1983; 55:973–975.
39. Sanders RD: Two ventilating attachments for bronchoscopes. *Del Med J* 1967; 39:170–175.
40. Ramser ER, Beamis JF Jr: Laser bronchoscopy. *Clin Chest Med* 1995; 16:415–426.
41. Schlenkhoff D, Droste H, Scieszka S, Vogt H: The use of high-frequency jet-ventilation in operative bronchoscopy. *Endoscopy* 1986; 18:192–194.
42. Lennon RL, Hosking MP, Warner MA, Cortese DA, McDougall JC, Brutinel WM, Leonard PF: Monitoring and analysis of oxygenation and ventilation during rigid bronchoscopic neodymium-YAG laser resection of airway tumors. *Mayo Clin Proc* 1987; 62:584–588.
43. Goldhill DR, Hill AJ, Whitburn RH, Feneck RO, George PJ, Keeling P: Carboxyhaemoglobin concentrations, pulse oximetry and arterial blood-gas tensions during jet ventilation for Nd:YAG laser bronchoscopy. *Br J Anaesth* 1990; 65:749–753.
44. Chan AL, Tharratt RS, Siefkin AD, Albertson TE, Volz WG, Allen RP: Nd:YAG laser bronchoscopy: Rigid or fiberoptic mode? *Chest* 1990; 98:271–275.
45. Unger M: Rigid vs flexible bronchoscope in laser bronchoscopy. *J Bronchol* 1994; 1:69–71.
46. Toty L, Personne C, Colchen A, Vourc'h G: Bronchoscopic management of tracheal lesions using the neodymium yttrium aluminum garnet laser. *Thorax* 1981; 36:175–178.
47. Dumon JF, Reboud E, Garbe L, Aucomte F, Meric B: Treatment of tracheobronchial lesions by laser photoresection. *Chest* 1982; 81:278–284.
48. Hetzel MR, Nixon C, Edmondstone WM, Mitchell DM, Millard FJ, Nanson EM, Woodcock AA, Bridges CE, Humberstone AM: Laser therapy in 100 tracheobronchial tumours. *Thorax* 1985; 40:341–345.
49. Gelb AF, Epstein JD: Laser in treatment of lung cancer. *Chest* 1984; 86:662–666.
50. Arabian A, Spagnolo SV: Laser therapy in patients with primary lung cancer. *Chest* 1984; 86:519–523.
51. Casey KR, Fairfax WR, Smith SJ, Dixon JA: Intratracheal fire ignited by the Nd:YAG laser during treatment of tracheal stenosis. *Chest* 1983; 84:295–296.
52. Dumon JF, Shapshay S, Bourcereau J, Cavaliere S, Meric B, Garbi N, Beamis J: Principles for safety in application of neodymium:YAG laser in bronchology. *Chest* 1984; 86:163–168.
53. Prakash UB, Offord KP, Stubbs SE: Bronchoscopy in North America: The ACCP survey. *Chest* 1991; 100:1668–1675.
54. George PJ, Garrett CP, Nixon C, Hetzel MR, Nanson EM, Millard FJ: Laser treatment for tracheobronchial tumours: Local or general anesthesia? *Thorax* 1987; 42:656–660.
55. Hanowell LH, Martin WR, Savelle JE, Foppiano LE: Complications of general anesthesia for Nd:YAG laser resection of endobronchial tumors. *Chest* 1991; 99:72–76.
56. Mehta AC, Golish JA, Ahmad M, Zurick A, Padua NS, O'Donnell J: Palliative treatment of malignant airway obstruction by Nd:YAG laser. *Cleve Clin Q* 1985; 52:513–524.
57. Unger M: Neodymium:YAG laser therapy for malignant and benign endobronchial obstructions. *Clin Chest Med* 1985; 6:227–290.
58. Personne C, Colchen A, Bonnette P, Leroy M, Bisson A: Laser in bronchology: Methods of application. *Lung* 1990; 168 (Suppl):1085–1088.
59. Unger M, Parr GV, Lugano E: Various applications of Nd:YAG laser in tracheobronchial pathology. In Ogura Y (ed): *Nd:YAG Laser in Medicine and Surgery: Fundamental and Clinical Aspects.* Tokyo: Professional Postgraduate Services; 1986:261–265.
60. American National Standards for the Safe Use of Lasers in Health Care Facilities. American National Standards Institute, Inc. Orlando, The Laser Institute of America, 1996.
61. Wood RL Jr, Sliney DH, Basye RA: Laser reflections from surgical instruments. *Lasers Surg Med* 1992, 12:675–678.
62. Sliney DH: Laser safety. *Lasers Surg Med* 1995; 16:215–225.
63. Schramm VL Jr, Mattox DE, Stool SE: Acute management of laser-ignited intratracheal explosion. *Laryngoscope* 1981; 91:1417–1426.
64. Shapshay SM, Beamis JF Jr: Safety precautions for bronchoscopic Nd:YAG laser surgery. *Otolaryngol Head Neck Surg* 1986; 94:175–180.
65. Wenig BL, Stenson KM, Wenig BM, Tracey D: Effects of plume produced by the Nd:YAG laser and electrocautery on the respiratory system. *Lasers Surg Med* 1993; 13:242–245.
66. Lobraico RV, Schifano MJ, Brader KR: A retrospective study on the hazards of the carbon dioxide laser plume. *J Laser Applicat* 1988; 1:6–8.
67. Garden JM, O'Banion MK, Shelnitz LS, Pinski KS, Bakus AD, Reichmann ME, Sundberg JP: Papillomavirus in the vapor of carbon dioxide laser-treated verrucae. *JAMA* 1988; 259:1199–1202.
68. Abramson AL, DiLorenzo TP, Steinberg BM: Is papillomavirus detectable in the plume of laser-treated laryngeal papilloma? *Arch Otolaryngol Head Neck Surg* 1990; 116:604–607.
69. Baggish MS, Poiesz BJ, Joret D, Williamson P, Refai A: Presence of human immunodeficiency virus DNA in laser smoke. *Lasers Surg Med* 1991; 11:197–203.
70. George PJ, Garrett CP, Hetzel MR: Role of the neodymium YAG laser in the management of tracheal tumours. *Thorax* 1987; 42:440–444.
71. Mohsenifar Z, Jasper AC, Koerner SK: Physiologic assessment of lung function in patients undergoing laser photoresection of tracheobronchial tumors. *Chest* 1988; 93:65–69.
72. Waller DA, Gower A, Kashyap AP, Conacher ID, Morritt GN: Carbon dioxide laser bronchoscopy—A review of its use in the treatment of malignant tracheobronchial tumours in 142 patients. *Respir Med* 1994; 88:737–741.
73. Jain PR, Dedhia HV, Lapp NL, Thompson AB, Frich JC Jr: Nd:YAG laser followed by radiation for treatment of malignant airway lesions. *Lasers Surg Med* 1985; 5:47–53.
74. Clarke CP, Ball DL, Sephton R: Follow-up of patients having Nd:YAG laser resection of bronchostenotic lesions. *J Bronchol* 1994; 1:19–22.
75. George PJ, Clarke G, Tolfree S, Garrett CP, Hetzel MR: Changes in regional ventilation and perfusion of the lung after endoscopic laser treatment. *Thorax* 1990; 45:248–253.
76. Emslander HP, Munteanu J, Prauer HJ, Heinl KW, Hinke KW, Sebenning H, Daum S: Palliative endobronchial tumor reduction by laser therapy: Procedure—immediate results—long-term results. *Respiration* 1987; 51:73–79.
77. Slawson RG, Scott RM: Radiation therapy in bronchogenic carcinoma. *Radiology* 1979; 132:175–176.
78. Stanopoulos IT, Beamis JF Jr, Martinez FJ, Vergos K, Shapshay SM: Laser bronchoscopy in respiratory failure from malignant airway obstruction. *Crit Care Med* 1993; 21:286–391.
79. Desai SJ, Mehta AC, VanderBrug Medendorp S, Golish JA, Ahmad M: Survival experience following Nd:YAG laser photoresection for primary bronchogenic carcinoma. *Chest* 1988; 94:939–944.

80. Eichenhorn MS, Kvale PA, Miks VM, Seydel HG, Horowitz B, Radke JR: Initial combination therapy with YAG laser photoresection and irradiation for inoperable non-small cell carcinoma of the lung: A preliminary report. *Chest* 1986; 89:782–785.
81. Petrovich Z, Stanley K, Cox JD, Paig C: Radiotherapy in the management of locally advanced lung cancer of all cell types: Final report of randomized trial. *Cancer* 1981; 48:1335–1340.
82. Roswit B, Patno ME, Rapp R, Veinbergs A, Feder B, Stuhlbarg J, Reid CB: The survival of patients with inoperable lung cancer: A large-scale randomized study of radiation therapy versus placebo. *Radiology* 1968; 90:688–697.
83. Shea JM, Allen RP, Tharratt RS, Chan AL, Siefkin AD: Survival of patients undergoing Nd:YAG laser therapy compared with Nd:YAG laser therapy and brachytherapy for malignant airway disease. *Chest* 1993; 103:1028–1031.
84. Quin JA, Letsou GV, Tanoue LT, Matthay RA, Higgins RS, Baldwin JC: Use of neodymium yttrium aluminum garnet laser in long-term palliation of airway lesions. *Conn Med* 1995; 59: 407–412.

C H A P T E R 6

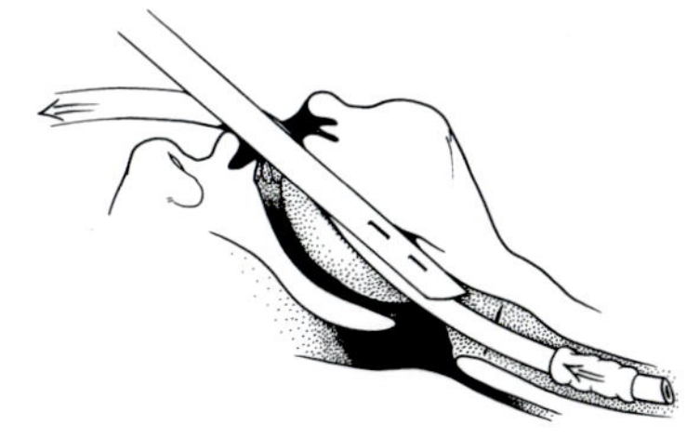

CRYOTHERAPY IN ENDOBRONCHIAL DISORDERS

Jean-Paul Homasson and Praveen N. Mathur

History of Cryosurgery

The analgesic and anti-inflammatory properties of ice have been known for several centuries,[1–3] but it was not until the mid-1800s that freezing was used for destruction of tissue. Arnott described the use of salt solutions containing crushed ice at temperatures of about −8° to −12° C to freeze advanced cancers in accessible sites, producing reduction in tumor size and pain.[4,5] The work of Carnot, Thomson, and Joule in thermodynamics involved the compression of vapors to form liquids and resulted in the invention of the refrigerator. This Joule-Thomson effect, which is the sudden expansion of a gas from a high- to a low-pressure region, explains the function of some cryoprobes, especially those used in pulmonary medicine. As freezing techniques improved, White[6,7] showed that liquid air could be used to treat various dermatologic lesions. Pusey[8] introduced carbon dioxide "snow" into clinical use for the treatment of various skin disorders, including carcinomas; Lortat-Jacob[9] mixed CO_2 gas with acetone in a special cryocauterer to make a cooling mixture. During the years 1936 to 1940, Fay[10–12] used freezing techniques in gynecology for inoperable cancers with good results in controlling pain, hemorrhage, and tumor volume. Hass and Taylor[13] described freezing local lesions in several organs; necrotic lesions were uniformly and sharply defined without evidence of suppuration or sequestration and were followed by a slow healing process. In 1959, Rowbotham and coworkers[14] employed a cryosurgical apparatus that pumped cold alcohol through a cannula. During the same period, Tytus and Ries[15] described a closed cannula and freezing mixture of acetone and solid carbon dioxide, but were unable to achieve adequate freezing.[16] The automated cryosurgical device introduced by Cooper and Lee[17] in 1961 led to a major stimulus in cryosurgery. This cryoprobe consisted of a metal tip where temperatures could reach −196° C. Initially designed for the treatment of Parkinson's disease, it was used to treat carcinomas at various sites.[18–21] During the next several years, many cryosurgical devices were developed for use in a number of surgical and medical specialties.[22–32] Owing to the relative inaccessibility of endobronchial lesions, thoracic cryosurgical techniques were late to develop. Nevertheless, following initial work by Grana and coworkers,[33] who described cryotherapy in the tracheae of healthy dogs, Thomford and coworkers[34] described the morphologic changes in canine tracheae after freezing and demonstrated the destruction of tracheal tumors without causing perforation. Initially there was inflammatory infiltration followed by vascular thrombosis, and chondrocyte depletion; then new cartilage was formed and the bronchial mucosa returned to normal. This work confirmed that freezing did not lead to perforation or fibrosis of the tracheobronchial tree. Subsequently, the same group[35] showed that freezing could destroy tracheal tumors in rats.

Neel and coworkers published similar studies on mongrel dogs.[36–38] They confirmed the destructive effect of cold followed by healing of the tracheobronchial tree without stenosis and restoration of a normal ciliated epithelium.

The first cryotherapy treatment for carcinomatous obstruction of a bronchus took place in 1968.[39] Another case was reported by Sanderson and coworkers in 1975.[40] The first reported series came from the Mayo

Clinic and consisted of 28 patients with endobronchial tumors. The authors concluded that cryotherapy served as a good alternative for palliation. Treatment of nonneoplastic stenosis of the upper airways was reported by Rodgers and coworkers.[41,42] Despite this successful early experience with cryosurgery, the technique was used by only a few teams in the United States between 1975 and 1982. The reason for this lack of acceptance is unknown. Interest virtually disappeared in favor of the Nd:YAG laser after 1980. In the 1980s, cryotherapy was rediscovered in Europe, by Homasson and coworkers in France,[43] Maiwand in England,[44] and Astesiano and coworkers in Italy.[45] During the decade 1985 to 1995, cryosurgery has undergone a renaissance, and now this technique is employed in a number of specialties, including pulmonology, dermatology, urology, and oncologic surgery. The literature has documented the efficacy of cryosurgery[43,46–51] and its utility in combination with other treatment modalities such as irradiation[52] or chemotherapy.[53] Cryotherapy is a cytotoxic procedure and thus might well be integrated into the therapeutic plan for bronchial cancers. Morasso and coworkers outlined the main advantages of this technique,[54] which were confirmed during the 9th World Congress of Cryosurgery in Paris in 1995: tracheobronchial cryosurgery is simple and efficient, easy to perform, and inexpensive, and it carries a very low morbidity. Cryotherapy should not be considered as a competitor to Nd:YAG laser for relieving bronchial obstruction, since indications may vary and at times these techniques could be complementary.

Newer cryodevices are now commercially available. Recently ultrasound imaging has been combined with freezing, leading to renewed interest in freezing tumors of the liver and prostate. The use of imaging techniques, coupled with further improvement in equipment, including thinner cryoprobes, will no doubt advance the use of cryosurgery. Further progress in the development of cryosurgery will depend on collaborative work between biologists, engineers, and clinicians, leading to a better understanding of the process and the development of improved instrumentation.

Scientific Basis of Cryosurgery

Cryosurgery deals with the destruction of biologic materials through freezing and has developed in parallel with the science of cryopreservation, which deals with attempts to use freezing for the long-term preservation of biologic materials. The fundamental processes that occur during cryosurgery were identified during research on the use of freezing to preserve biologic cells and tissues. However, the thermal parameters that affect the viability of cells frozen in suspensions may be different from those that affect the viability of cells frozen in tissue. Understanding the process of freezing and the mechanisms of damage is very important. The impact of low temperature and varying temperatures on cell and tissue structure appears to be key (Fig. 6-1). Temperature is a measure of the kinetic energy of molecular motion: as temperature lowers, molecular processes slow and may even arrest. The tissue exposed to the cryoprobe will, therefore, experience a progression of sublethal prefreeze stresses followed by lethal freezing. The tissue damage induced by freez-

Figure 6-1

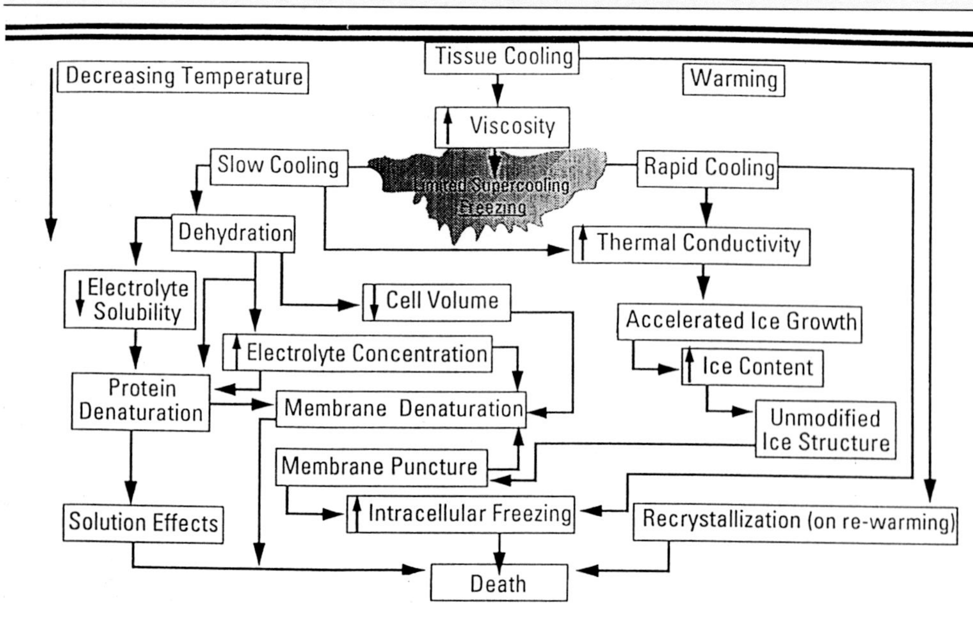

The impact of low and varying temperatures on the cell and tissue structure.

ing occurs at several levels, including the molecular, cellular, and structural levels.

The success of freeze injury is influenced by many factors; the survival of cells is dependent on the cooling rate,[55–57] the thawing rate,[58] the lowest temperature achieved,[59] and repeated freezing-thawing cycles.[59,60] Certain tissues are *cryosensitive* (skin, mucous membrane, and granulation tissue), and others are *cryoresistant* such as fat, cartilage, and fibrous or connective tissue. The cryosensitivity depends on the water content of the cells. Tumor cells may be more sensitive than normal cells.[61]

MECHANISMS OF CELLULAR DAMAGE BY FREEZING

Results of the experimental studies, including mathematical modeling of freezing processes in cells,[62,63] have shown that the mechanisms of cellular damage by freezing can be explained through heat and mass transfer. This process occurs between cells and their local environment. Using the cryomicroscope,[61,64,65] the changes in the volume of cells during freezing and the formation of intracellular ice can be observed.

According to Mazur,[66] the physical events occurring in cells in suspension during freezing are as follows:

1. At −5° C the system remains in a liquid state, despite the cytoplasmic freezing point of −2.2° C. This phenomenon is due to supercooling (any cells which remain unfrozen below −2.2° C are by definition supercooled) and to a decrease of the freezing point due to the various solutes in the suspension.
2. Between −5 and −15° C extracellular crystals form. The intracellular medium remains supercooled and unfrozen as the cell membrane provides a barrier to the propagation of ice. It is at this stage that the cooling velocity plays a determinant role. The supercooled cytoplasmic state, being thermodynamically unstable, can be abolished in two ways: by cellular dehydration or by intracellular freezing. If the cell is cooled slowly enough, dehydration of intracellular water allows the buildup of an intracellular solute concentration that eliminates intracellular freezing due to supercooling. However, if the cell is cooled rapidly, the intracellular water will not have enough time to pass through the cell membrane and crystals will form within the cell.
3. Below −15° C an isothermic transitional state occurs, during which any further increase in solute concentration results in a decrease of the freezing point of the remaining unfrozen liquids.
4. Finally, a solid state or complete crystallization is attained.

During thawing, various physicochemical phenomena are again determined by the velocity of temperature change.

After a suboptimal freezing, rapid thawing exposes the cell to a high electrolyte concentration and to an elevated temperature, which can induce a migratory intra- or extracellular recrystallization, either by the growth or aggregation of small crystals.

Slow thawing after supraoptimal freezing induces the migratory recrystallization phenomenon; this is an extremely destructive process for intracellular organelles primarily due to the grinding action of ice.[67,68] Rapid thawing avoids this recrystallization, thus preventing cellular exposure to a high, toxic electrolyte concentration and to an elevated temperature.

During this period, six factors are involved in the determination of a cellular cryolesion and cell death: extracellular crystallization that compresses and deforms the cells ("pack ice effect"), intracellular crystallization, cellular dehydration with collapse, increase in intracellular electrolyte concentration, denaturation of membranous lipoprotein, and simple thermic shock.

These factors are closely interrelated and intervene to different degrees in the determination of cellular cryolesions. Both mechanical effects due to the formation of ice crystals and more complex biochemical effects secondary to cellular dehydration occur. However, the primary determinant of the final degree of cellular damage is the cooling velocity. These principles provide the basis of the cryosurgery technique: use low-temperature instruments to create the fastest possible freezing of the target tissue and establish intracellular freezing. Slow or spontaneous thawing provides for maximal lethal physicochemical effects. The largest possible tissue volume should be frozen at its eutectic point.

In vitro studies typically present a uniform distribution of the cold source around the cellular system under study. This is not the case in live cryosurgery, where the factors of cellular tissue cohesion and vascularization also come into play.

FREEZING OF TISSUE

The effects of cooling rates on cell viability determined from experiments with cells in suspension may not be the same when cells are frozen in tissue during cryosurgery.[69] The process of freezing depends on the interaction between ice crystals, the solution surrounding the ice crystals, and the cells. Tissue sensitivity to cold is dependent on the existence of a microcirculation. After cryosurgery a clear line of demarcation develops between tissue that was frozen and tissue that was not frozen.[70] Following cryosurgery, the cells in the frozen region have a disrupted structure. Cryolesions of ischemia and infarction appear a few minutes to several hours after treatment. Circulation stops rapidly after thawing. This cryo-induced thrombosis seems to result from several factors: vasoconstriction of arterioles and venules that occurs during mild hypothermia, modification of the vascular endothelium, an increase in the permeability of the vascular walls, an increase in the blood viscosity, a lowering of the intracapillary hydrostatic pressure, a decrease in blood flow, and formation of platelet plugs. These vascular effects explain the hemostatic effect of cryosurgery. At the borders of the frozen region, hypothermia has a heterogenous effect, and it is in these areas that chemotherapy or radiotherapy has a complementary destructive effect. This explains the larger volume of the "combined therapeutic area" (Fig. 6-2) often seen with the addition of chemotherapy.[53,71,72] At slow cooling rates, anticancer drugs are trapped in the damaged tumor and in areas immediately surrounding the frozen tissue. The small blood vessels expand, and the cells dehydrate. This expansion, which is a result of the heat and mass transfer during freezing, damages blood vessels at the outer edge of the frozen region and deprives cells within of their blood supply. Consequently, ischemic damage occurs in the entire region that was frozen. The result of these cellular changes in the days following cryotherapy is cellular necrosis. An acidophilic slough forms (Figs. 6-3 and 6-4), and tumor tissue is no longer viable and is therefore destroyed. Histopathologic findings, however, are not modified by freezing if biopsies are made immediately after cryosurgery. At this time, cryolesions are visible only under an electron microscope. The mechanism of cellular and tissue damage following cryosurgery explains the delayed effect of this technique and is the reason cryosurgery is often not useful in cases of acute respiratory distress from airway obstruction. Besides these physical and vascular effects of cryosurgery, there have been many references to a cryoimmunologic mechanism.[73–75] At present, there are no definite conclusions regarding this possible mode of action, and further study is needed.

Clinical Basis for Cryotherapy

The results of cryotherapy have been evaluated by different means, including endoscopic appearance, clinical criteria, radiologic changes, changes in respiratory function, and histologic appearance. Walsh and coworkers[47] studied the effects of cryotherapy on dyspnea, hemoptysis, cough, and stridor. In this study, symptoms, lung function, chest radiography, and bronchoscopic findings were recorded serially before and after 81 cryotherapy sessions in 33 consecutive patients. Most patients showed improvement in overall symptoms, stridor, hemoptysis, and dyspnea. Homasson[43] showed that hemoptysis ceased in 80 percent of patients. Improvement in dyspnea is variably reported but occurs in about 50 percent of patients.[50] Other symptoms that may improve are wheeze, cough, and thoracic pain. Maiwand also reported an improvement in cough.[44]

Figure 6-2

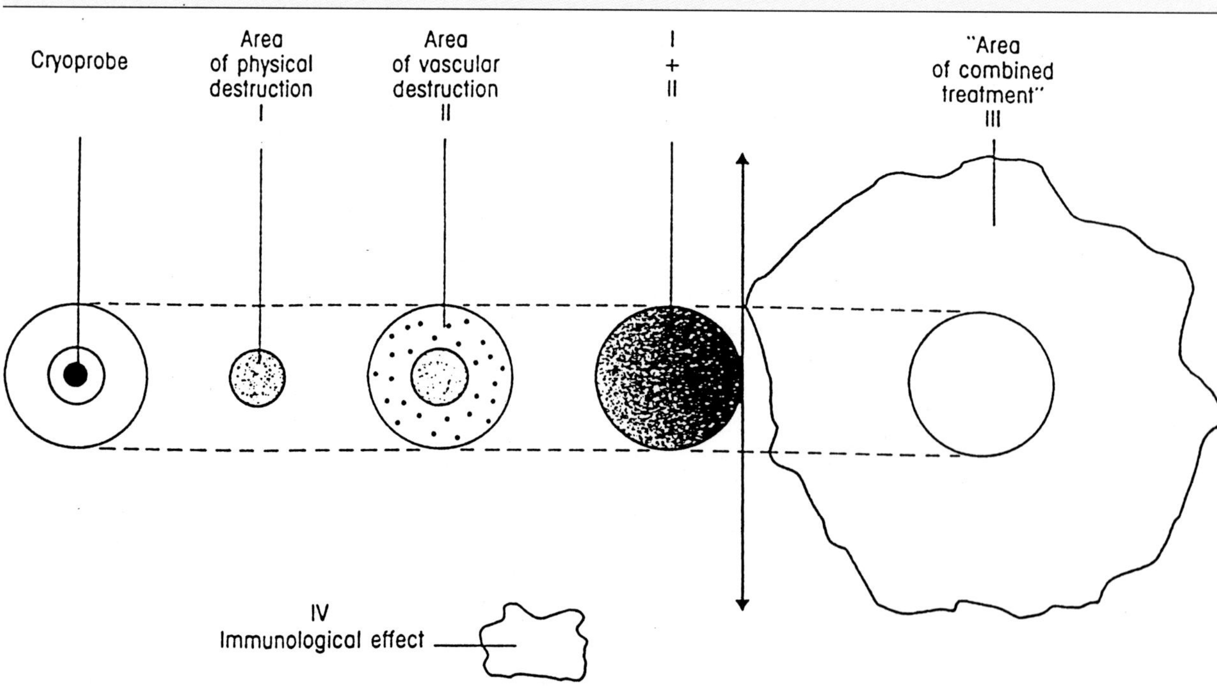

Schematic illustration of the cryolesion.

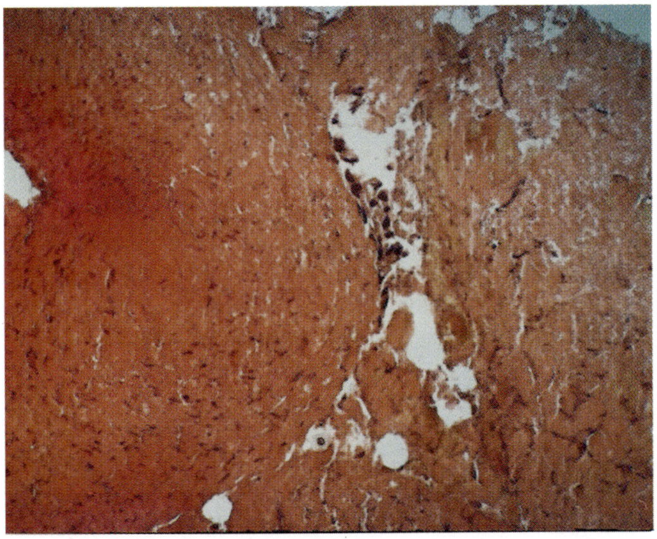

Figure 6-3

Acidophilic slough. (Hematoxylin & eosin × 250)

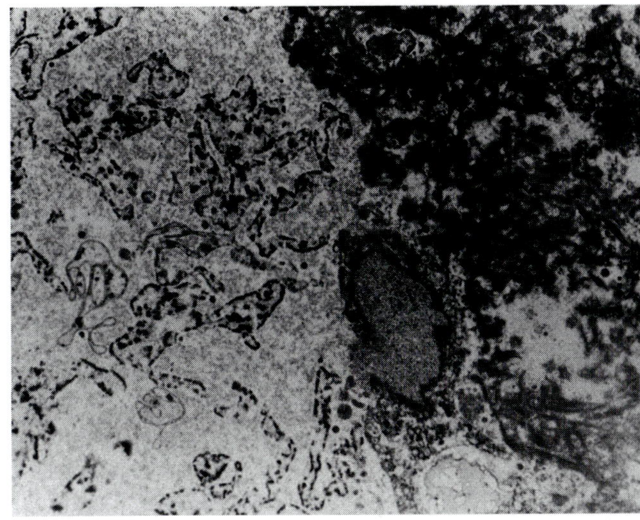

Figure 6-4

Bronchus cellular fragments of a squamous cell carcinoma with fibrin. (EM, × 4500)

Objective improvement of pulmonary function has been demonstrated in 58 percent of patients, and Walsh and coworkers have shown that these changes in lung function correlate with symptoms.[47] Benign lesions, particularly granulation tissue, have also been treated with cryotherapy with very good results with no recurrence months or even years after treatment. Tumors of low or intermediate malignancy are rare, and very few have been treated with cryosurgery. Nevertheless, when surgery is not possible for these tumors, treatment with cryotherapy can yield good results. A number of cases of carcinoid tumors, cylindromas, mucoid squamous tumors, and laryngotracheal papillomas have been successfully treated.

Cryotherapy destroys only the visible endobronchial portion of malignant tumors. Therefore, therapeutic results are difficult to assess and depend on various criteria measured, such as endoscopic appearance, tumor histology, or symptoms. Cryotherapy is a palliative treatment. Overall, the results have been favorable in 70 to 80 percent of patients treated, regardless of the criteria used to measure performance. Cryotherapy invariably improves the quality of life by reducing the unpleasant symptoms of bronchial obstruction. Significant improvement in survival has not been demonstrated.

ASSOCIATIONS OF CRYOTHERAPY WITH CHEMOTHERAPY OR RADIOTHERAPY

Chemotherapy has been shown to be more effective following cryotherapy.[71] Anticancer drugs appear to accumulate in the tumor site immediately following cryotherapy. Using an experimental murine tumor preparation, Ikekawa and coworkers[72] investigated the efficacy of cryochemotherapy and confirmed the phenomenon of entrapment of anticancer drugs after combined treatment. A prospective study at the Center Hospitalier Specialise en Pneumologie in Chevilly-Larue, France, was carried out on 12 patients to confirm these experimental data.[53] All patients were inoperable with endobronchial tumor obstructing one main bronchus. All received intravenous infusions of 15 mg of bleomycin labeled with cobalt.[57] Endoscopic treatment was performed using either a rigid or a flexible cryoprobe. Each patient was placed under a gamma camera, and a region of interest over the left ventricle was sampled to plot a time-activity curve corresponding to the disappearance of the radiolabeled bleomycin from the blood. The redistribution and elimination half-lives of the labeled bleomycin were calculated from this curve. Further regions of interest were studied to calculate uptake by both the tumor and normal tissue. A tumor-to-normal tissue ratio was then calculated. Since the washout time of radiolabeled bleomycin is 10 days, the same protocol was repeated 15 days later, 1 h after the cryotherapy procedure. A significant difference was found in the tumoral uptake of radiolabeled bleomycin before and after cryotherapy with a mean increase in the tumor-to-normal tissue ratio of 30 percent following cryotherapy. The pharmacokinetic parameters show that after cryotherapy there was accelerated plasma clearance. It can be postulated that bleomycin was trapped in the tumor because of the vascular disruption caused by freezing. As expected, the endoscopic findings after the initial 15 days, just before the cryotherapy, were not modified by the single injection of 15 mg of bleomycin, since the dose was clearly not high enough to have a therapeutic effect. This study thus confirms the experiments of Ikekawa and coworkers[72] in the mouse and offers an explanation for the initial clinical findings reported by Benson[71] in head and neck tumors treated with cryotherapy and chemotherapy. These results showed that the concentration of the chemotherapy drug was higher in the frozen zone and adjoining hypothermic areas. The tumor destruction was superior to that found with either chemotherapy or cryotherapy alone. The histology of the tumor did not influence the response. At this time too few patients have been treated with this combined approach to draw any meaningful conclusions. Nevertheless, when surgical resection of bronchial cancer is not feasible, cryochemotherapy might be a reasonable alternative treatment.

CRYOTHERAPY-RADIOTHERAPY

In localized inoperable bronchial cancers, radiotherapy is usually offered, but the mean survival of patients treated in this way is only 20 months,[51] and local eradication of tumor is obtained in only 35 percent of patients.[49] In obstructive tumors the regression of atelectasis after irradiation is achieved in only 21 percent of patients without local treatment.[50] Treatment of these obstructive tumors with neodymium: yttrium-aluminum-garnet (Nd:YAG) laser has been suggested before irradiation. This may result in a better survival and quality of life. Like laser therapy, cryotherapy will relieve bronchial obstruction and prevent local complications, which are often the cause of death. Studies have suggested a possible synergy between the effect of cryotherapy and that of external irradiation.[52,76] Using microangiography to study the cryolesion of a rabbit esophagus, Le Pivert and coworkers[76] showed marked neovascularization 15 days after cryotherapy. This hypervascularization may increase the radiosensitivity of tissues. In similar prospective studies, Vergnon and coworkers[52] and Homasson[43] have enrolled patients in a protocol using cryotherapy combined with radiotherapy. Satisfactory outcome was defined as >50 percent tumor destruction. Radiotherapy was performed two weeks after cryotherapy.

Our study group consisted of 29 patients. All presented with symptomatic obstructions and were considered unresectable either for local reasons (18 patients with tracheal or proximal main-stem neoplasm) or for functional reasons (11 patients). One or two sessions of cryotherapy were required; treatment was considered satisfactory in 16 patients and unsatisfactory in 13 due to persistent tumor. Twenty-one patients received 65 Gy and eight patients in poor general condition received 45 Gy of external radiation.

The results were evaluated with flexible bronchoscopy and biopsy 2 months following the completion of irradiation. All patients survived >3 months. In the unsatisfactory cryotherapy group, patients died sooner of local complications, with a median survival of 5 months. In the satisfactory cryotherapy group, the median survival was 11 months, indicating a significant improvement in survival. This study does not prove the potentiating effect of cryotherapy on the effect of radiotherapy. However, it confirms several significant points: Cryotherapy is a safe method that does not cause premature death and is successful in 70 to 80 percent of patients.[43] This study reinforces the earlier recommendations to eliminate an obstruction before irradiation to improve survival and avoid local complications. The survival curves obtained correspond closely to those obtained using laser resection of endobronchial lesions. For patients with inoperable lung cancer, the presence of local obstruction may be an important prognostic criterion, survival being more dependent on this factor than the TNM stage. This study also confirms the inadequacy of radiotherapy alone in relieving bronchial obstruction and achieving local eradication of obstructing tumors and emphasizes the possibility of increasing tumor radiosensitivity by new methods such as cryotherapy.

Equipment Needs

COOLING AGENTS

Several cooling agents can be used as cryogens. These are generally liquids so that on vaporization they remove heat at a constant temperature (heat of vaporization). The chlorofluorocarbons (CFCs) are commonly used in domestic and industrial refrigeration and have no clinical use. Carbon dioxide is attractive because it achieves a low temperature (−79° C). However, when it expands at atmospheric pressure, it produces snow. This is used for direct application to accessible lesions (as in dermatology). CO_2 cannot be used in fine-bore bronchial cryoprobes since the solid particles block the flow of liquid.

Several studies have shown that the core temperature needed for a lesion to be destroyed is between −20° and −40° C. Freezing to −40° C or below at the rapid rate of −100° C/min causes more than 90 percent cell death. The choice of an effective cryogen for cryodestruction is important, since the effect of treatment is directly related to the temperature achieved at the site. Therefore, a cooling agent should have the cooling power to produce a local temperature of −30° C or less. The two cryogens available to the pulmonologists are (1) liquid nitrogen and (2) nitrous oxide.

Liquid nitrogen (LN_2) is easily obtainable and is stored near its saturation temperature (−196° C) in a vacuum in insulated containers to reduce the loss of liquid by evaporation. Liquid nitrogen is nontoxic and not flammable. As LN_2 passes through the transfer line at room temperature, it evaporates and the gaseous nitrogen comes in contact with the metal tip of the cryoprobe. This results in relatively slow cooling of the tip. (With bronchial cryoprobes, the temperature of −196° C is reached in about 1 min for the first freeze-thaw cycle, and in 20 to 30 s for the other cycles.) When the temperature of the inner tube of the probe is sufficiently low to prevent evaporation of gas in transit, droplets of LN_2 bombard the inner wall of the tip of the probe. These evaporate, removing heat at a much faster rate and producing very low temperatures. When the flow is stopped, liquid remaining inside the transfer line is evacuated via the cryoprobe; thus thawing is delayed. Electrical heating of the bronchial cryoprobe tip cancels the well known adhesive effect of cold.

Nitrous oxide (N_2O) is the most common cooling agent used in tracheobronchial cryotherapy. It is stored at room temperature in the liquid state in high pressure bottles. The vapor phase of N_2O occurs at the metal tip of the cryoprobe, where it expands from a high pressure to atmospheric pressure (Joule-Thomson effect). This expansion lowers the temperature of the fluid and produces droplets of liquid reaching an equilibrium of −89° C at atmospheric pressure. These droplets strike the metal tip of the probe, removing heat from the wall of the probe as they evaporate. The heat exchanges between high-pressure fluid coming in and low-pressure gas exhausting occur only in the distal 1 or 2 cm from the expansion nozzle. Thus, the cooling occurs quickly just where it is needed since the metallic mass to be cooled is very small. The transfer line and the cryoprobe are small capillary tubes surrounded by sheaths of either metal or plastic, depending on whether the lines are rigid or flexible. Nitrous oxide produces an almost instant cooling effect, is readily available, and is slightly more expensive than LN_2.

CRYOTHERAPY EQUIPMENT

There are three parts to a cryomachine: the console, the cryoprobe, and the transfer line that connects the console and gas cylinder to the probe. Machines are made by several manufacturers (Table 6-1). The cryoprobes are rigid, semirigid, or flexible. Rigid and semirigid cryoprobes can be used only through a rigid bronchoscope, but flexible cryoprobes can be used either through the channel of a fiberoptic bronchoscope or through a rigid bronchoscope. The diameter of the flexible probes requires the use of a fiberoptic bronchoscope with the largest available (2.6 or 3.2 mm) working channels.

Monitoring of the freezing remains a problem,[77] and there is no ideal solution. The empirical method relies on the experience of the operator, who observes the change in color or consistency of the frozen tissue and the length of freezing. In clinical studies,[78] using rigid, semirigid, or flexible probes, each freeze-thaw cycle takes about 30 s. The thaw phase is almost immediate with rigid probes that have a reheating system, but spontaneous thawing with the flexible probes results in increased freeze-thaw cycle times.

A thermic method of freeze monitoring requires implantation of a thermocouple in the tumor and at the periphery and is not practical with a bronchoscope. With the S.M.T. cryoprobe the temperature reached inside the tip of the probe can be measured, and the time to obtain a temperature of −200° C is noted. In the Spembly model, a thermocouple is incorporated within the tip of the cryoprobe, allowing confirmation of correct functioning of the cryoprobe. However, even this does not show the temperature achieved in the frozen tissue, and the operator must rely on experience to estimate the length of time of freezing.

The only endoscopic method of monitoring freezing is the bioelectric method.[76] This method relies on the fact that complete extracellular crystallization is essential to produce tissue necrosis, and this change in the physical state of the extracellular milieu with freezing (crystallization) leads to a change in the impedance of the tissue. During cryotherapy, the cryoprobe represents one electrode. The other electrode is a metal plate placed in contact with the patient's body. The ice ball that is formed breaks the current between the two electrodes. A resistance attained between 200 and 500 kΩ indicates that the cryoprobe is working correctly.

ENDOSCOPE EQUIPMENT

The rigid and semirigid cryoprobes are used with rigid bronchoscopes and the flexible cryoprobes are used in the operative lumens of flexible bronchoscopes (2.6 or 3.2 mm). The choice of a particular rigid bronchoscope is not important; however, the lumen of the scope must have a diameter large enough to admit the cryoprobe and the rigid optic system. This usually requires an adult rigid bronchoscope with a minimum diameter of 8 mm.

The efficacy of a cryoprobe depends in part on its diameter; thus if a fiberoptic bronchoscope is used, the operative lumen must be as large as possible. The operative channel should be wide enough to allow smooth introduction of the cryoprobe. This means that the handle of the bronchoscope must be suitably angled, bearing in mind that the rigid metal tip of the cryoprobe is about 10 mm in length. There is no distortion of the optical equipment by cold, but during freezing the entire endoscope is cooled, and this effect may be magnified by retrofreezing if the cryoprobe becomes defective. This "retrofreezing" effect is caused by droplets of liquid gas within the return channel vaporizing against the metal shaft of the probe and further cooling it. When this happens, the cooling has to

Table 6-1
CRYOPROBES

Make	Country of Origin	Type	Length, cm	Diameter, mm	Length of Tip of Probe, mm	Coolant Source	Controls			Sterilization		
							P	Z	T	Autoclave	Gas	Soaking
Date[a]	France	Semirigid	60	3.0	10	N_2O cryo	✓	✓		✓	✓	✓
		Flexible	1300	2.0 B 2.3	10	N_2O cryo	✓	✓			✓	✓
				2.6 B 3.0								
Erbe[b]	Germany	Rigid	52	2.5	10	N_2O cryo	✓			✓	✓	✓
		Flexible	80	2.2 B 2.4	7	N_2O cryo	✓				✓	✓
				2.7 B								
Spembly[c]	United Kingdom	Rigid	45	2.0 B 3.0	10	N_2O cryo	✓		✓	✓	✓	✓
						N_2O						
						CO_2						

[a]Date, Quartier de la Condamine, BP 6, 38770 La Motte D'Aveillans, France.
[b]Erbe, 11 Chemin de l'Industrie, 69570 Dardilly, France.
[c]Spembly, Newsbury Road, Andover, Hampshire SP10, England.
NOTE: P, control of pressure at a bottle; Z, impedance; T, temperature.

be stopped to avoid damage to the cryoprobe and the endoscope. Cooling does no harm to a rigid bronchoscope. When a fiberoptic bronchoscope becomes frozen, it hardens and should not be manipulated.

No special accessories are needed beyond those normally used for tracheobronchial endoscopy. Photographic recording is essential. A video camera with recording facilities is always desirable.

HOW I DO IT

The key factor for successful tracheobronchial cryotherapy is not only the technique but more importantly the indications. All cryo units are equally satisfactory. The major difference is that the S.M.T. unit employs liquid nitrogen as a cooling agent. In the last 10 years the Date and the Erbe cryoprobes have been used in the United States. The Erbe cryoprobe is FDA approved. Following is a description of how we perform tracheobronchial cryotherapy using rigid or semirigid probes with a rigid bronchoscope and using the flexible probe with a flexible bronchoscope.

Patient Selection

Cryotherapy is indicated for tracheobronchial obstruction. The selection criteria are as follows:

1. Histologically proven carcinoma of the trachea or bronchi
2. Inoperability based on the location of the tumor
3. Unsuitability for lung resection because of poor respiratory function
4. Recurrence of tumor following other modes of treatment such as radiotherapy, chemotherapy, lung resection, or another endobronchial treatment (Nd:YAG laser, brachytherapy)
5. Intraluminal tumors with little external compression (Tumors with extraluminal pressure should not occlude the lumen by more than 75 percent.)
6. An inoperable microinvasive carcinoma
7. Hemotypsis caused by a visible benign or malignant lesion
8. Granulation tissue following lung transplantation
9. Foreign bodies

The palliative treatment of tracheobronchial carcinoma often requires the use of several complementary techniques. Studies have shown effectiveness of combined endobronchial and conventional cancer treatment, which improves quality of life and prolongs survival. These studies have been carried out with both Nd:YAG laser[79,80] and cryotherapy[52] with identical results. Patients should be treated at an early stage of illness. Previous studies seem to indicate a potentiating or synergistic effect with the combined treatment of cryotherapy and chemotherapy.[53] Further randomized studies are now necessary to confirm the benefit in quality of life and survival. Patients with extremely poor Karnofsky scores should not be considered for this type of therapy.

Preparation of the Patient

An initial endoscopy is performed along with other examinations such as chest roentsengraphy, CT scan, complete blood count, coagulation studies, blood gases, and respiratory function. Anticoagulant therapy is discontinued before the bronchoscopy. Reactive edema following cryotherapy is not severe, and corticosteroid is generally not indicated. As a precaution corticosteroids may be given for 24 h following cryotherapy for some tracheal or subglottic lesions.

Rigid bronchoscopy can be carried out under neuroleptic analgesia or general anesthesia. An intravenous access site is established. Local anesthesia is applied to the pharynx. Monitoring includes an electrocardiogram, noninvasive blood pressure recording, and arterial oxygen saturation. Rigid bronchoscopy under general anesthesia follows a period of preoxygenation. Anesthesia is induced with propofol, 0.70 to 1.5 mg/kg over a 30- to 120-s interval, depending on the condition of the patient. Further relaxation is provided with fentanyl, 1 to 1.2 g/kg. The procedure lasts between 20 and 30 min. Rigid bronchoscopy allows safe oxygenation and ventilation. Our anesthetists prefer manual ventilation, rather than jet ventilation. If jet ventilation is used, we recommend a frequency of 120 per minute, with an inspiratory ratio to total time (I/R) of 30 percent and FIO_2 of 50 percent. Naloxone (1 to 2 g/kg) is usually administered intravenously at the end of the procedure to reverse the effects of the drugs.

Technique

RIGID BRONCHOSCOPY

The patient is placed in the supine position, and the endoscope is introduced according to the classic method: the head is fully extended so the chin points vertically upward in the midline position (this can be achieved by using a pillow); the upper teeth must be protected with a swab or sponge. The rigid bronchoscope should be supported by the left forefinger (if right-handed) and a thumb. This protects the teeth and gums from trauma.

The operator inspects the lesions to be treated to determine their potential for hemorrhage, whether they are projecting into or infiltrating the airway, and to define their position and the extent of stenosis or extrinsic compression that may exist. If there is a high risk of bleeding, performing an initial freeze-thaw cycle is preferable prior to any biopsy that might be needed. In this way the hemostatic properties of cold are used to prevent bleeding, while adequate biopsy specimens are obtained for microscopic examination.

The freeze-thaw procedures are carried out under direct vision. The distal tip of the rigid bronchoscope should be placed about 0.5 to 1 cm above the lesion. The cryoprobe is introduced through the scope. Treatments may vary, depending on the appearance of the lesion to be treated.

The most suitable lesions are polypoid, either benign or malignant. The metallic tip of the cryoprobe is placed on the tumor or pushed into it, producing circumferential freezing of maximal volume. Three freeze-thaw cycles are carried out. The probe is then moved 5 to 6 mm and another three cycles carried out in the adjoining area. The points of impact are staggered with an overlap of the frozen zones. The procedure is continued until all the visible tumor has been frozen (Figs. 6-5 and 6-6).

The method is identical whether nitrous oxide or a liquid nitrogen is used to drive the cryoprobe. However, the larger ice ball and greater freezing power of the liquid nitrogen cryoprobe usually destroys the entire lesion with two to three cycles, resulting in a shortened duration of endoscopy time with this probe.

If the probe is equipped with a device for measuring impedance, reheating begins when a plateau between 250 and 500 kΩ is reached, depending on the tissue and the position of the cryoprobe. Subsequent cycles are begun when the impedance falls to 50 kΩ and before the probe becomes unstuck.

With the nitrous oxide-driven cryoprobes, the freezing time is around 30 s per cycle. There is no value in prolonging the freezing beyond this point. It has been shown that there is a greater cryodestructive effect when several freeze-thaw cycles are used.

With the liquid nitrogen device, freezing is continued until a temperature of −200° C is obtained (about 1 min for the first freeze cycle). Subsequent freeze procedures are shorter. With infiltrating lesions, cryotherapy can be used with lateral tangential contact (Figs. 6-7 and 6-8).

Eight to ten days after the first session, a repeat bronchoscopy is usually performed, most often with a flexible bronchoscope. This second examination enables assessment of cryodestruction, removal of any slough (Fig. 6-9), and repeat cryotherapy if required. A slough is generally present with large tumors and may be removed with forceps, by suction or by cryoadhesion with the cryoprobe.

FIBEROPTIC BRONCHOSCOPY

Patients undergo routine fiberoptic bronchoscopy with standard monitoring in a fully equipped bronchoscopy suite. Before the bronchoscopy, routine clinical data are obtained, including arterial blood gases, coagulation parameters, and chest radiography. An intravenous access site is established, and normal saline is infused during the procedure. Monitoring includes an electrocardiogram, noninvasive blood pressure recording,

Figure 6-5

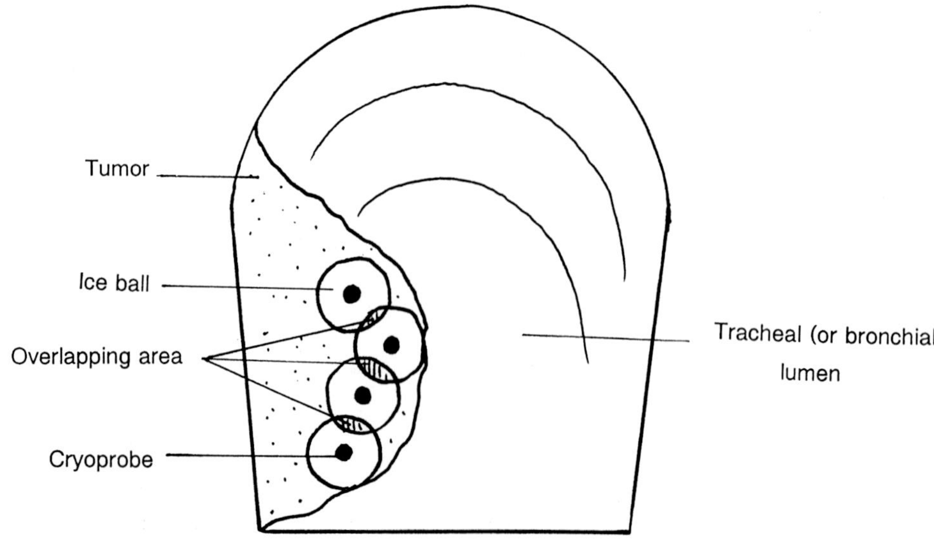

Freezing technique showing overlapping areas.

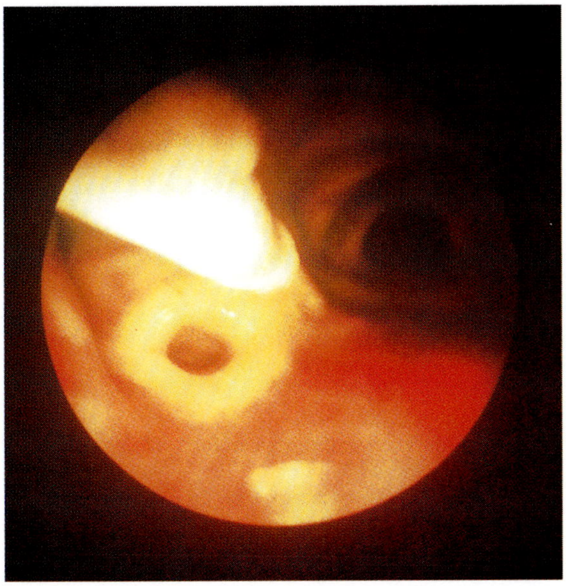

Figure 6-6

Freezing technique showing overlapping areas.

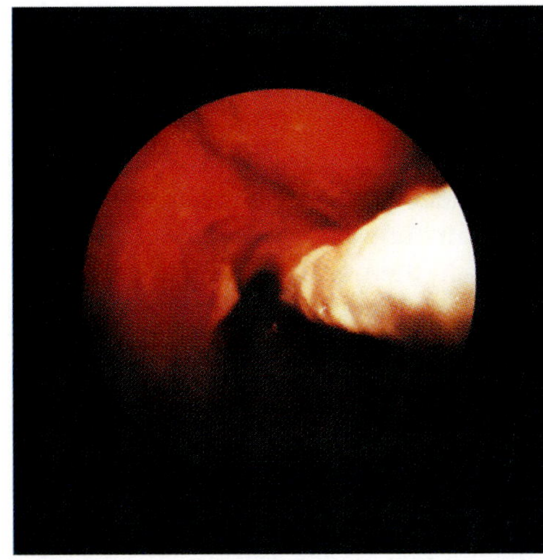

Figure 6-8

Tangential freezing.

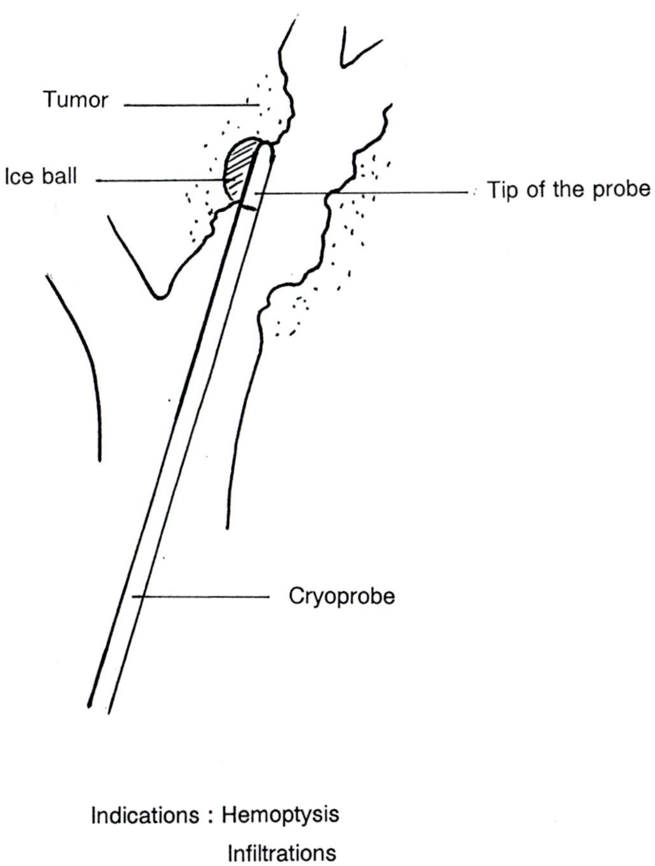

Figure 6-7

Tangential freezing.

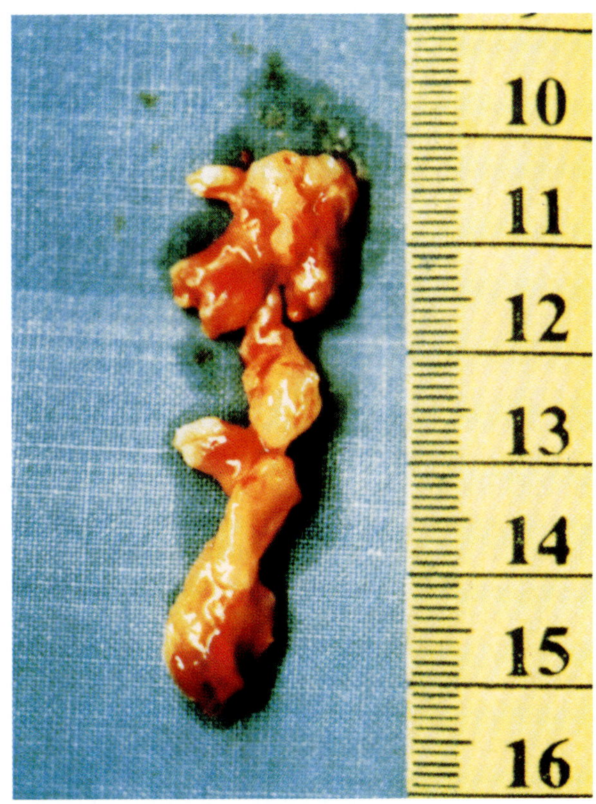

Figure 6-9

Slough removed.

and arterial oxygen saturation. Supplemental oxygen is given, and the bronchoscopy is carried out in a standard fashion with atropine premedication. Topical anesthesia of the oral-nasopharynx is achieved with 4% lidocaine. Conscious sedation is achieved with intravenous midazolam and meperidine or morphine.

The fiberoptic bronchoscope is passed through the nose or orally in the usual fashion, and a thorough inspection of the tracheobronchial tree is completed. Endoscopic therapy is then performed using a flexible cryoprobe (Erbe USA, Inc., Marietta, GA), which is passed through the working channel. The cryoprobe tip is visualized and directly applied to the tumor area. Once in the lumen of the airway, about 4 mm away from the tip of the bronchoscope, the cryoprobe is engaged with the foot pedal. Within 30 s an ice ball appears on the tip of the probe. One to three freeze-thaw cycles, each lasting 1 min, are applied to the same or immediate area. The tip of the probe can be applied perpendicularly or tangentially or driven into the tumor mass. The tissues are frozen at −30 to −40° C. The tissue destruction due to cryotherapy is readily visible. The cryoprobe is deactivated by removing the foot from the foot pedal. At the end of each freeze cycle, the ice ball is observed until thawing has been completed before the tip is removed from the airway lesion. It is occasionally necessary to suction some blood from the airway before each cycle.

Any devitalized or necrotic tissue can be removed with biopsy forceps during the bronchoscopy. Bronchoscopic examination is repeated in 1 to 2 weeks. During this procedure, more cryotherapy can be applied, and any slough can be removed. Other treatment modalities can be added any time after cryotherapy.

Postoperative Care

Cryotherapy does not require any particular immediate follow-up care. Keeping the patient under medical surveillance for 24 h after a general anesthetic is prudent. Patients treated under local anesthesia and conscious sedation have been sent home on the same day. Radiography of the chest immediately after therapy is not essential but is usually done. Occasionally rapid relief of bronchial obstruction may be accomplished by retraction of tumor tissue after freezing. Reventilation of the area can be confirmed with radiography. Nevertheless we recognize the delayed effect of cryonecrosis and generally do not expect a change in the chest film immediately after a cryotherapy procedure.

Corticosteroids are not routinely administered and are considered only following treatment of laryngeal and tracheal lesions, where the risk of an edematous reaction is greatest. The hemostatic effect of freezing is often sufficient to stop hemoptysis. Improvement may be delayed and occur only some hours to a day after cryotherapy. Occasionally trauma caused by the penetrating probe into an already hemorrhagic lesion may temporarily aggravate bleeding. Hemostatic drugs should then be prescribed. Minor hemoptysis immediately following therapy usually does not require treatment.

REFERENCES

1. Breasted JH: *The Edwin Smith Surgical Papyrus.* Chicago, University of Chicago Oriental Institute, 1930; 3:217.
2. Bartolini T: *De Nivis Usu Medico Observationes Variae.* Copenhagen, Haubold, 1991.
3. Larrey DJ: *Memoires de Chirurgie Militaire et Campagne.* In Buisson F (ed). Paris, 1812.
4. Arnott J: *On the Treatment of Cancer by Regulated Application of an Anaesthetic Temperature.* London, Churchill, 1851.
5. Arnott J: *On the Treatment of Cancer by Congelation and an Improved Mode of Pressure.* London, Churchill, 1855.
6. White AC: Liquid air; Its application in medicine and surgery. *Med Rec* 1899; 56:109.
7. White AC: Possibilities of liquid air to the physicians. *JAMA* 1901; 34:426.
8. Pusey WA: The use of carbon dioxide snow in the treatment of nevi and other lesions of the skin: A preliminary report. *JAMA* 1907; 49:1354.
9. Lortat-Jacob L, Solente G: *Cryotherapie.* Paris, Masson, 1930:6.
10. Fay T, Henny GC: Correlation of body segmental temperature and its relation to the location of carcinomatous metastasis: Clinical observations and response to methods of refrigeration. *Surg Gynecol Obstet* 1938; 66:512.
11. Fay T: Observations on prolonged human refrigeration. *NY State J Med* 1940; 40:1351.
12. Fay T: Early experiences with local and generalized refrigeration of the human brain. *J Neurosurg* 1959; 16:239.
13. Hass G, Taylor C: A quantitative hypothermal method for the production of local injury of tissue. *Arch Pathol* 1948; 45:563.
14. Rowbotham GF, et al: Cooling cannula for use in the treatment of cerebral neoplasms. *Lancet* 1959; 1:12.
15. Tytus J, Reis L: Further observations on rapid freezing and its possible application to neurosurgical techniques. *Bull Masson Clin* 1961; 15:51.
16. Tytus J: Cryosurgery, its history and development. In Rand R, et al (eds): *Cryosurgery.* Springfield, Ill., Charles C. Thomas, 1968: 3–18.
17. Cooper IS, Lee A: Cryostatic congelation: A system for producing a limited controlled region of cooling or freezing of biologic tissues. *J Nerv Ment Dis* 1961; 133:259.
18. Cooper IS: Cryogenic surgery: A new method of destruction or extirpation of benign or malignant tissues. *N Engl J Med* 1963; 268:743.
19. Cooper IS, Stellar S: Cryogenic freezing of brain tumors for excision or destruction in situ. *J Neurosurg* 1965; 24:237.
20. Cooper IS: Cryogenic surgery for cancer. *Fed Proc Suppl* 1965; 15:(24)237.
21. Cooper IS, Hirose J: Application of cryogenic surgery to resection of parenchymal organs. *N Engl J Med* 1966; 274:15.
22. Cahan WG, Brockmier G: Cryosurgery of the uterine cavity. *Am J Obstet Gynecol* 1967; 99:138.
23. Gonder MJ, et al: Experimental prostate cryosurgery. *Invest Urol* 1964; 1:610.
24. Rand RW, et al: Stereotactic cryohypophysectomy. *JAMA* 1964; 189:225.
25. Gage AA, et al: Cryotherapy for cancer of the lip and oral cavity. *Cancer* 1965; 18:1646.

26. Zacarian S, Adham M: Cryotherapy of cutaneous malignancy. *Cryobiology* 1966; 2:212.
27. Barton R: Cryosurgical treatment of nasopharyngeal neoplasms. *Am Surg* 1966; 32:744.
28. Lincoff H, et al: The cryosurgical treatment of intraocular tumors. *Am J Ophthalmol* 1967; 63:389.
29. Blackwood J, et al: Cryotherapy for malignant tumors. *Cryobiology* 1967; 4:33.
30. Ostergard D, Townsend DE: Malignant melanoma of the female urethra treated by cryotherapy with radical vulvectomy and anterior exenteration. *Obstet Gynecol* 1968; 31:75.
31. Gage AA: Cryotherapy for inoperable cancer. *Dis Colon Rectum* 1968; 2:36.
32. Marcove RC, Miller TR: Treatment of primary and metastatic bone tumors by cryosurgery. *JAMA* 1969; 207:1890.
33. Grana L, et al: Cryogenic techniques within tracheobronchial tree. *J Cryosurg* 1969; 2:62.
34. Thomford NR, et al: Morphological changes in canine trachea after freezing. *Cryobiology* 1970; 7:19.
35. Skivolocki WP, et al: Effect of cryotherapy on tracheal tumors in rats. *Arch Surg* 1971; 103:341.
36. Neel HB, et al: Cryosurgery of respiratory structures 1. Cryonecrosis of trachea and bronchus. *Laryngoscope* 1973; 83:1062.
37. Gorenstein A, et al: Transbronchoscopic cryosurgery of respiratory strictures. Experimental and clinical studies. *Ann Otol Rhinol Laryngol* 1976; 85:670.
38. Carpenter RJ, et al: Cryosurgery of bronchopulmonary structures. An approach to lesions inaccessible to the rigid bronchoscope. *Chest* 1977; 72:279.
39. Gage AA: Cryotherapy for cancer. In Rand R, et al (eds): *Cryosurgery*. Springfield, Ill., Charles C. Thomas 1968; 376–387.
40. Sanderson DR, et al: Cryotherapy of bronchogenic carcinoma. Report of a case. *Mayo Clin Proc* 1975; 50(8):435–437.
41. Rodgers BM, Talbert JL: Clinical application of endotracheal cryotherapy. *J Pediatr Surg* 1977; 13:662.
42. Rodgers BM, et al: Endotracheal cryotherapy in the treatment of refractory airway strictures. *Ann Thorac Surg* 1983; 35:52.
43. Homasson JP, et al: Bronchoscopic cryotherapy for airway strictures caused by tumors. *Chest* 1986; 90:159.
44. Maiwand MO: Cryotherapy for advanced carcinoma of the trachea and bronchi. *Br Med J* 1986; 293:181.
45. Astesiano A, et al: Distruzione crioterapica dei tumori invasivi tracheobronchiali. Casistica personale. *Min Med* 1986; 77:2159.
46. Homasson JP: Cryotherapy in pulmonary today and tomorrow. *Eur Resp J* 1989; 2:799.
47. Walsh DA, et al: Bronchoscopic cryotherapy for advanced bronchial carcinoma. *Thorax* 1990; 45:509.
48. Pesek M, et al: Kryokoagulation in der Behandhlung von Bronchialtumoren. *Z Erkrank Atm Org* 1990; 175:126.
49. Homasson JP, Bell NJ: *Cryotherapy in Chest Medicine*. Paris, Springer Verlag, 1992.
50. Maiwand MO, Homasson JP: Cryotherapy for tracheobronchial disorders. In Mathur PN, Beamis JF (eds): *Clinics in Chest Medicine*. Philadelphia, WB Saunders, 1995; 16:427–443.
51. Homasson JP: Bronchoscopic cryotherapy. *J Bronchology* 1995; 2:145.
52. Vergnon JM, et al: Initial combined cryotherapy and irradiation for unresectable non-small lung cancer *Chest* 1992; 102:1436.
53. Homasson JP, et al: Tumor fixation of bleomycin labeled with 57 cobalt before and after cryotherapy of bronchial carcinoma. *Cryobiology* 1992; 29:548.
54. Morasso A, et al: Cryosurgery in bronchoscopic treatment of tracheobronchial stenosis. *Chest* 1993; 103:472.
55. Fahy GM, et al: Physical problems with the vitrification of large biological systems. *Cryobiology* 1990; 27:492.
56. Gage AA, et al: Effect of varying freezing and thawing rates in experimental cryosurgery. *Cryobiology* 1985; 22:175.
57. Smith JJ, Fraser J: An estimation of tissue damage and thermal history in cryolesion. *Cryobiology* 1974; 11:139.
58. Miller RH, Mazur P: Survival of frozen-thawed human red cells as a function of cooling and warming velocities. *Cryobiology* 1976; 13:404.
59. Gage AA: Critical temperature for skin necrosis in experimental cryosurgery. *Cryobiology* 1982: 19:273.
60. Rand RW, et al: Cryolumpectomy for breast cancer: An experimental study. *Cryobiology* 1985; 22:307.
61. Rubinsky B, Ikeda M: A cryomicroscope using directional solidification for the controlled freeing of biological tissue. *Cryobiology* 1985; 22:55.
62. Mazur P: Kinetic of water loss from cells at sub zero temperatures and the likelihood of intracellular freezing. *J Gen Physiol* 1963; 47:347.
63. Mazur P: Cryobiology: The freezing of biological systems. *Science* 1970; 168:939.
64. Diller KR: Quantitative low temperature optical microscopy of biological systems. *J Microscopy* 1982; 126:9.
65. Chaw MW, Rubinsky B: Cryomicroscopical observations on directional solidification in onion cells. *Cryobiology* 1985; 22:392.
66. Mazur P: The role of intracellular freezing in the death of cells cooled at supra optimal rates. *Cryobiology* 1977; 14:251.
67. Forsyth M, Macfarlane DR: Recrystallisation revisited. *Cryo-letters* 1986; 7:367
68. Martino MN, Zariteky NE: Ice recrystallisation in a model system and in frozen muscle tissue. *Cryobiology* 1989; 26:138.
69. Beckman J, et al: Redefining cooling rate in terms of ice front velocity and thermal gradient: First evidence of relevance of freezing injury in lymphocytes. *Cryobiology* 1990; 27:279.
70. Gilbert JC, et al: Real time ultrasonic monitoring of hepatic cryosurgery. *Cryobiology* 1985; 22:319.
71. Benson JW: Combined chemotherapy and cryosurgery for oral cancer. *Am J Surg* 1975; 13:596.
72. Ikekawa S, et al: Basic studies of cryochemotherapy in a murine tumor system. *Cryobiology* 1985; 22:477.
73. Ablin RJ, et al: Prospects for cryo-immunotherapy in cases of metastasizing carcinoma of the prostate. *Cryobiology* 1971; 8:217.
74. Tanaka S: Immunological aspects of cryosurgery in general surgery. *Cryobiology* 1982; 19:247.
75. Ablin RJ: Cryoimmunology: A critique of the phenomenon and its future. *Cryosurgery. Mechanisms and Applications*. Intern Institute Refr 1995; 14:133–138.
76. Le Pivert P, et al: Measurement of intratissue bioelectrical low frequency impedance: A new method to predict perioperatively the destructive effect of cryosurgery. *Cryobiology* 1977; 14:245.
77. Gage AA, et al: A comparison of instrument methods of monitoring freezing in cryosurgery. *J Dermatol Surg Oncol* 1983; 9:209.
78. Homasson JP, et al: The operation and efficacy of cryosurgical, nitrous oxide-driven cryoprobe. Cryoprobe physical characteristics: Their effects on cell cryodestruction. *Cryobiology* 1994; 31:290.
79. Macha H, et al: Pattern of failure and survival in endobronchial laser resection. A matched pair study. *Chest* 1992; 145:967.
80. Eichenhorn MS, et al: Initial combination therapy with YAG laser photoresection and irradiation for inoperable non small cell carcinoma of the lung. A preliminary report. *Chest* 1986; 89:782.

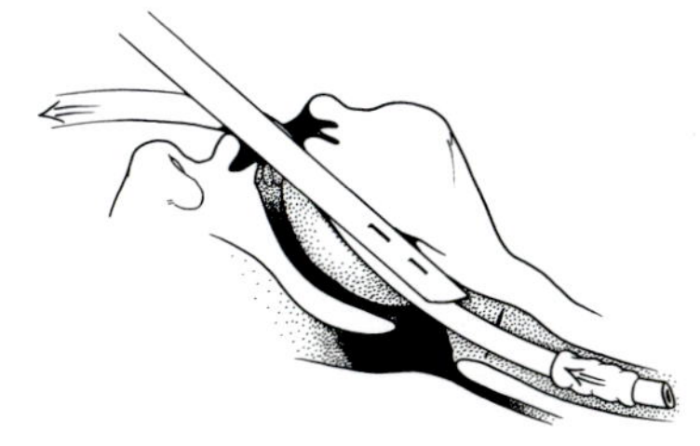

CHAPTER 7

ENDOBRONCHIAL ELECTROCAUTERY

Tom G. Sutedja and Pieter E. Postmus

Most lung cancers are inoperable because of locally advanced tumors, involvement of mediastinal lymph nodes, and/or distant metastases.[1] In recent years, there has been some improvement in the care of patients with advanced non-small cell lung cancer, in which combined modality treatment increasingly plays a role in management.[2–5] However, even after apparently curative surgery, a substantial risk of subsequent lung cancer, recurrent disease, and/or distant metastases still exists.[6–8]

In the majority of patients with locally advanced tumors, local control after conventional radiotherapy has been shown to be poor.[9–11] Local recurrence and distant metastases after radiotherapy are common. There is also a relatively high rate of second primary lung cancers after surgery. Close surveillance after surgery and early detection of a subsequent tumor followed by a second resection provide the best chance for survival.[6–8] Another category of patients, those who have received radical treatment for a head and neck tumor, is also at risk (10 to 40 percent) to develop a second or third primary pulmonary neoplasm.[12,13]

Survival after surgery in early stage squamous cell cancer detected by sputum cytology is close to 100 percent.[14–16] Surgery has been shown to improve survival in this group of patients. In these tumors, nodal metastasis has been shown to correlate with tumor size and was absent if tumor thickness was $\leq$ 3 mm and the longitudinal tumor axis was $<$ 2 cm.[6,17,18]

The main problems encountered in lung cancer management include: the relatively advanced stage at which patients present, the limited number of patients with stage $\leq$ IIIa disease in whom curative surgery is feasible (15 percent), the significant loss of healthy lung parenchyma after surgery or radiotherapy, the substantial risk of recurrent and metastatic disease after surgery (30 percent), and the high incidence (10 to 40 percent) of second primaries after initial treatment of respiratory tract malignancies. In the last decade, technical developments have facilitated the use of endoscopic instruments for diagnosis and therapy of pulmonary malignancies.[19–21] Improved imaging and the use of smaller and more practical equipment have allowed bronchoscopic treatment of tumors located proximal to the segmental bronchi. Palliation and curative treatment of patients with extra- and intraluminal tumors are now feasible.[19–22] The purpose of this chapter is to describe the background, technique, and clinical usefulness of endobronchial electrocautery in two situations. First, the treatment of patients with major airway obstruction after failure of, or prior to, other palliative treatments. For these patients, relief of symptoms by means of a simple technique is important to improve quality of life. The second group consists of patients in whom endobronchial electrocautery may provide substantial long-term benefit, especially if tumors are occult and completely intraluminal. In this particular group intraluminal bronchoscopic treatment with photodynamic therapy (PDT) has been shown to be effective.[19,20] Further investigations are needed, however, to develop simple, safe, and effective treatment alternatives, since cost effectiveness is becoming increasingly important.[23] A comparison of treatment efficacy, morbidity, and costs between electrocautery and other techniques such as neodymium: yttrium-aluminum-garnet (Nd:YAG) laser, brachytherapy, and photodynamic therapy is given.

Background and History

Endobronchial electrocautery is the application of heat, produced by electric current, via the bronchoscope to treat tumor tissue using a probe or a snare. Electrocautery itself has been applied in medicine for decades. Using high-frequency alternating current to avoid neural and muscular response, the electric current passes through living tissue and is converted to heat because tissue resistance is high.[24] Using a small probe which functions as an active electrode, the heat is concentrated in a tiny surface area to coagulate or vaporize tissue. The degree of tissue destruction depends on the power used, duration of contact, surface area, and density and water content of tissue treated. The monopolar technique is suitable for endoscopic application, that is, bronchoscopic intervention.[25]

There have been several published reports on the use of electrocautery to palliate patients with tumor obstruction in the major airways.[26–34] Both rigid and flexible instruments have been used effectively, under either general or local anesthesia.

Technique

The techniques of rigid and fiberoptic bronchoscopy are not reviewed here.[35] Endobronchial electrocautery can be applied either through a rigid or fiberoptic bronchoscope. The most frequently used technique is direct contact with (tumor) tissue. Deciding between rigid or flexible instruments for any kind of endobronchial therapy is dependent on the expertise of the bronchoscopist and risk assessment of the patient's condition.

The choice of anesthesia depends on the level of risk. Expertise and awareness of possible complications during and after treatment are essential.[36] Patients presenting with imminent respiratory failure, hemorrhage, and life-threatening airway obstruction are obviously at risk for any kind of bronchoscopic intervention. It is therefore more prudent to use general anesthesia under these circumstances.[36–39] If immediate tumor debulking is required, multiple techniques can be applied successfully. Treatment choice is academic whether it be electrocautery, Nd:YAG laser, mechanical tumor removal, or a combination of these.[19,20,26–34,36–41] Combined use of endoscopic techniques with stenting for extraluminal tumor is becoming a standard strategy.[22,28]

The rigid electrocautery technique is comparable to the transurethroscopic resection of prostatic tissue using a rigid loop. Gastroenterologists use a flexible endoscope and an electrosurgical loop to snare pedunculated polyps. The rigid bronchoscopic technique is more commonly used in Europe, and the fiberoptic bronchoscope is the most popular instrument in North America and the United Kingdom.[42–44] Endobronchial electrocautery is similar to electrocautery techniques that have been used to treat tumors in hollow organs using either a rigid or the fiberoptic method. An electrocautery unit is routinely used in every surgical suite.

A relatively new development is the noncontact technique of argon plasma coagulation (APC) to obtain superficial homogenous tissue necrosis. This may be attractive for the treatment of hemorrhagic tissue and superficial tumors.[45–47] Ionized argon gas functions as a conductor in the strong electrical field between the active electrode and tissue. APC has been reported to be effective in the treatment of small malignant gastrointestinal tumors.[47] Histologic studies have shown coagulative necrosis by the APC method to be similar to that of standard electrocautery.[45,46] However, APC causes more acute superficial tissue destruction and is efficient for obtaining hemostasis.

Palliative Treatment

Publications dealing with endobronchial electrocautery are shown in Tables 7-1 and 7-2.[26–34] Using either the rigid or flexible technique, initial success rates are good. Despite the unpredictable degree of necrosis and the danger of perforation, the complication rate of electrocautery in these studies was not excessive.

Treatment with Curative Intent

The number of patients with occult cancer treated with bronchoscopic therapy is small, and experience in using electrocautery is even more limited. Early stage cancer lesions are easily missed by conventional bronchoscopy. A high-risk population for subsequent primary lung cancer includes those patients who have had previous malignancies of the respiratory tract.[6–8,12,13] Occult cancers are often considered inoperable because of poor pulmonary function or because the patients have been previously treated with curative intent. Many were treated with photodynamic therapy. The choice of PDT was based on the theory of "selective" damage with relative sparing of normal tissue.[48,49] However, clinical data to support this selectivity, using hematoporphyrin derivatives as sensitizers, are lacking.[50–52] Cicatricial fibrosis, probably due to treatment-induced hyperthermia, may occur after PDT.[50,51]

Several bronchoscopic techniques seem to offer potential for cure of occult and intraluminal lung tumors[51–68] (See Table 7-3). This is possible because occult tumors are only several millimeters thick and early stage superficial tumors with ≤ 3 mm invasion of the

Table 7-1
PALLIATIVE RESULTS OF ENDOBRONCHIAL ELECTROCAUTERY USING THE RIGID BRONCHOSCOPE IN PATIENTS WITH LUNG TUMORS

Reference	*n*	*Technique*	*Response*	*Complications*
Ledingham and Goldstraw[26]	15	GA, rigid loop + radioactive grains	Successful palliation 11/15 alive > 1 month median 2.5 months	No
Pedersen et al.[27]	10	GA, jet ventilation and rigid loop	Palliative 3–14 months adenocystic 2–29 years	No
Petrou et al.[28]	29	GA and rigid loop (+ stents, + radioactive grains)	19/20 improved symptoms	No

NOTE: GA, general anesthesia.

bronchial mucosa, and a visible distal margin can be reached effectively with bronchoscopic therapy. Local therapy should not be performed, however, if tumors are extraluminal and if there is a chance of nodal metastasis.[6,17,18,53] The particular technique itself seems therefore less important. A small number of patients with more advanced tumors may also be treated prior to surgery to improve resectability by using PDT, Nd:YAG laser, and brachytherapy.[69–71] Low-grade malignant tumors such as typical carcinoids may also be treated with curative intent.[72,73]

Endobronchial Electrocautery and Other Treatment Modalities

How does endobronchial electrocautery compare to other bronchoscopic therapies such as mechanical re-

Table 7-2
PALLIATIVE RESULTS OF ENDOBRONCHIAL ELECTROCAUTERY USING THE FIBEROPTIC BRONCHOSCOPE IN PATIENTS WITH LUNG TUMORS

Reference	*n*	*Technique*	*Response*	*Complications*
Frizelly[29]	17	GA/LA, FB	Average palliation 4–5 months (9 months)	1 hemorrhage
Hooper and Jackson[30]	4	GA, FB + snare	All successful	1 fire/explosion + respiratory failure
Hooper and Jackson[31]	18	GA/LA FB + snare + bipolar probe	5 benign successful 13 palliation follow-up ≤ 3 years	1 bleeding and 1 fire
Gerasin and Shafirovsky[32]	14	GA, FB + snare	10/14 complete and 2/14 > 75% clearance	1 bleeding (100 ml 2 emergencies for bleeding/suffocation
Sutedja et al.[33]	17	LA and FB + probe	15/17 successful 2 extraluminal	1 minor bleeding 1 pneumonia
Homasson et al.[34]	32	LA; rigid + flexible probes	27/32 > 50% reduction 11/12 hemostasis	2 bleeding

NOTE: GA, general anesthesia; LA, local anesthesia; FB, flexible bronchoscope.

Table 7-3
RESULTS OF BRONCHOSCOPIC INTERVENTION FOR ROENTGENOLOGICALLY "OCCULT" LUNG CANCER

Photodynamic Therapy with Curative Intent

Reference	*n (lesions)*	*Response*	*Survival, months*
Edell and Cortese[55]	14	CR 10/14 (71%)	7–49 (10 patients)
Monnier et al.[51]	16	CR 11/16 (69%)	3–60
Furuse et al.[56]	59	CR 45/59 (83%)	14–32 (median 14)
Imamura et al.[57]	39	CR 25/39 (64%)	4–169 (17 patients)
Okunaka et al.[58]	10 synchronous	10/10 synchronous (100%)	Mean 38
	17 metachronous	16/17 metachronous (94%)	
Sutedja et al.[59]	39	CR 28/39 (72%)	2–95

Brachytherapy Treatment with Curative Intent

Reference	*n*	*Technique*	*Survival, months*
Macha and Wahlers[60]	9	15 Gy at 3 mm/4 × HDR	Up to 27
O'Driscoll et al.[61]	6	15–20 Gy/1 × HDR	12–21
Hernandez and Donath[62]	4	7.5 Gy/? HDR	8–24
Sutedja et al.[63]	2	10 Gy/2–3 × HDR	25,54
Ono et al.[64]	12	8–10 Gy/5–7 × HDR	2–8
Ono[65]	34	20–60 Gy	3–30

Endobronchial Electrocautery for Occult Cancer and Intraluminal Carcinoid

Sutedja et al.[66]	11 occult cancers 7 carcinoids	LA with flexible probe, carcinoid under GA	4–27 4–19

Nd-YAG Laser for Occult Cancer and Intraluminal Carcinoid

Cavaliere et al.[67]	19 in situ cancers	GA, rigid bronchoscope	Up to 12 years
Personne et al.[68]	3/30 carcinoids	GA, rigid bronchoscope	2–4 years

NOTE: CR, complete response with negative histology/cytology; HDR, high dose rate brachytherapy; GA, general anesthesia; LA, local anesthesia.

moval,[40] Nd:YAG laser,[22] cryosurgery,[74] brachytherapy,[60] and PDT?[48,54] Each technique has its own merits and limitations (Table 7-4). Treatment choice is usually based on several factors: clinical presentation, expertise of the bronchoscopist, anesthetic care, and technical facilities of each hospital. Financial aspects may further influence treatment choice, since every institution cannot offer every treatment modality[19] (Table 7-5).

Patients often present with imminent respiratory failure from bulky airway tumors with extraluminal components. Immediate tumor debulking is required using either Nd:YAG laser, electrocautery, or mechanical removal. A stent can also be inserted in cases of significant extraluminal compression.[22] In nonemergency cases, local anesthesia often suffices and brachytherapy may be the best alternative to obtain a durable response with minimal damage to normal tissue.[60,75] Comparison of various techniques and treatment costs is shown in Tables 7-4 and 7-5. A guideline for palliative treatment is given in Fig. 7-1. Cost considerations may become increasingly important.[19,23] It

Table 7-4
ADVANTAGES AND DISADVANTAGES OF VARIOUS BRONCHOSCOPIC INTERVENTION TECHNIQUES

Treatment	*Equipment/Technique*	*Result*	*Complication*
Mechanical removal	Standard, GA	Immediate and short-term	Bleeding
Cryotherapy	Special equipment, mostly GA	Late and superficial	Unpredictable necrosis (secondary)
Electrocautery	Standard, GA and LA, rigid and fiberscope	Immediate and superficial	Unpredictable necrosis (secondary)
Nd:YAG laser	Laser, mostly GA, or fiber through rigid	Immediate and in depth effect	Perforation
Brachytherapy	Afterloading, LA	Late and in depth effect	Late tissue damage
Photodynamic therapy	Dye laser, LA	Late and in depth effect	Late necrosis and skin photosensitivity

NOTE: GA, general anesthesia; LA, local anesthesia.

has been previously suggested that electrocautery may be a less costly alternative than Nd:YAG laser.[27] The cost effectiveness of any technique depends on equipment price, maintenance cost, and usefulness for various applications by different specialists. Electrocautery as a simple, standard instrument is therefore quite attractive. In our daily practice, most patients are treated for local palliation. Hence, treatment choice is more or less at the discretion of the operator.

Randomized studies in patients with occult lung tumors are difficult to perform, because of the small number of patients identified. Several techniques seem to be equally effective in treating tumor tissue several millimeters thick. Inaccurate assessment of tumor dimension is the real issue.[21,64] The limitations of our diagnostic accuracy in assessing peribronchial, nodal, and distant disease are well recognized.[6,17,18,53]

Table 7-5
TREATMENT COSTS OF BRONCHOSCOPIC INTERVENTIONS IN THE NETHERLANDS (CALCULATED IN U.S. DOLLARS)

	Price of Equipment	*Cost Reimbursement*[a]
Bronchoscopy		309
Anesthesia		318
Nd:YAG laser[b]	100,000	880
Photodynamic therapy[b]	200,000	3077
Brachytherapy (HDR)[b]	250,000	539
Electrocautery	20,000	309

[a]Based on tariffs of the COTG (Government Health Insurance Tariff).

[b]Diode lasers with similar wave length ≈ 40,000

NOTE: HDR, high dose rate.

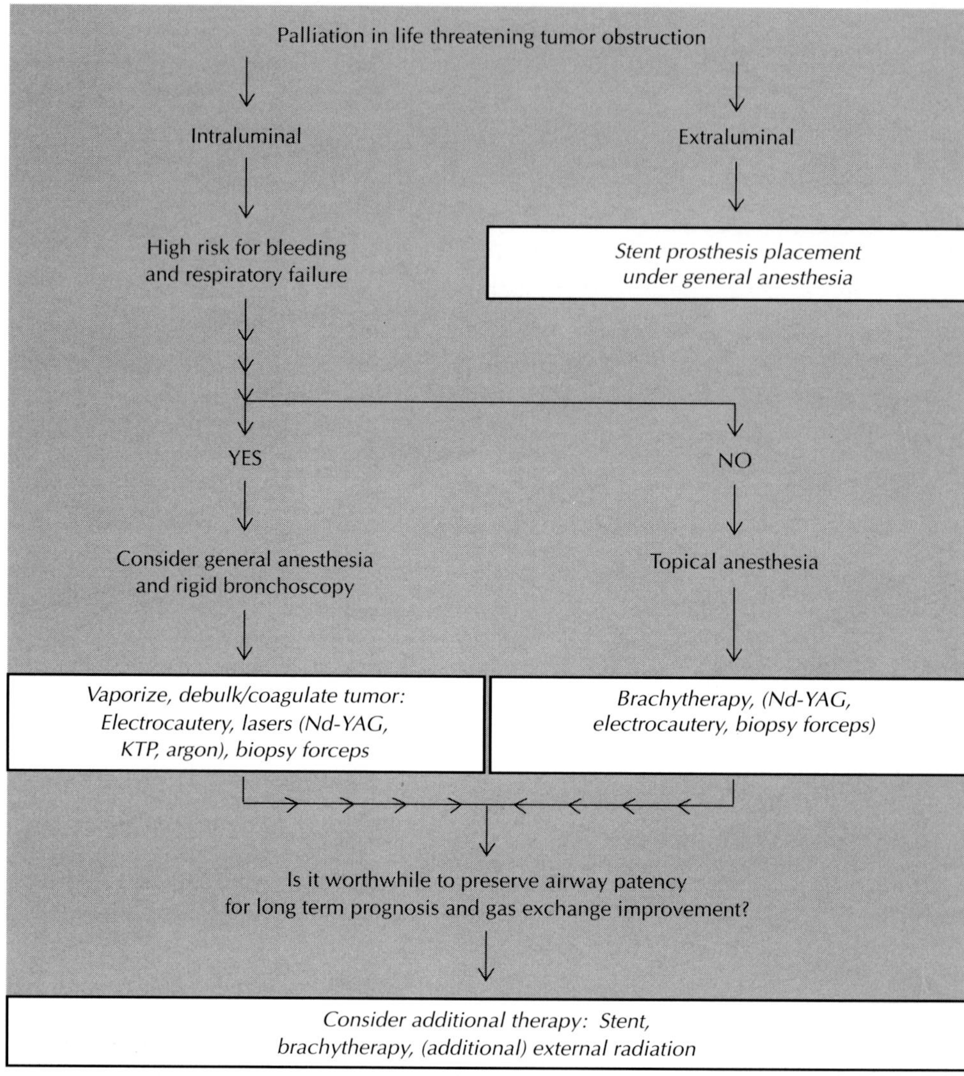

Figure 7-1

An algorithm for decision making in palliative treatment.

Conclusion

Tumors located in the central airways can be treated with various bronchoscopic techniques such as lasers [Nd:YAG, argon, potassium titanyl phosphate (KTP)], photodynamic therapy, brachytherapy, cryotherapy, and electrocautery. Extraluminal airway compression may be relieved by inserting a stent. Thus, multiple techniques are currently available to treat patients with major airway obstruction.

Bronchoscopists frequently deal with bulky tumors with extraluminal components in which the visible intraluminal tumor is only the tip of the iceberg. Bronchoscopic treatment may be indicated for immediate relief of obstruction. Improvement of gas exchange is the main goal of opening the airways, but some regions with poor gas exchange, for example, those that have been treated with external irradiation or those with significant extraluminal disease, may improve little with treatment. The patient's general, cardiac, and pulmonary condition; tumor dimension and stage; bronchoscopic findings; CT findings; and regional ventilation-perfusion are factors to be taken into account prior to any bronchoscopic intervention. Risk and potential benefit also depend on the expertise of the bronchoscopist and the facilities in each institution. Results are immediate with lasers (Nd:YAG, KTP, argon) and electrocautery, especially in combination with mechanical tumor removal using biopsy forceps. Techniques that induce late response or cause secondary necrosis, like brachytherapy, PDT, and cryotherapy, are less practical. The integrity of the tracheobronchial wall has to be respected to prevent airway perforation; therefore only intraluminal tumor can be removed. PDT and brachytherapy can result in a deep effect resulting in damage to normal tissue. This may lead to hemorrhage, fistula formation, and cicatricial fibrosis. Secondary necrosis and exudate may

Figure 7-2

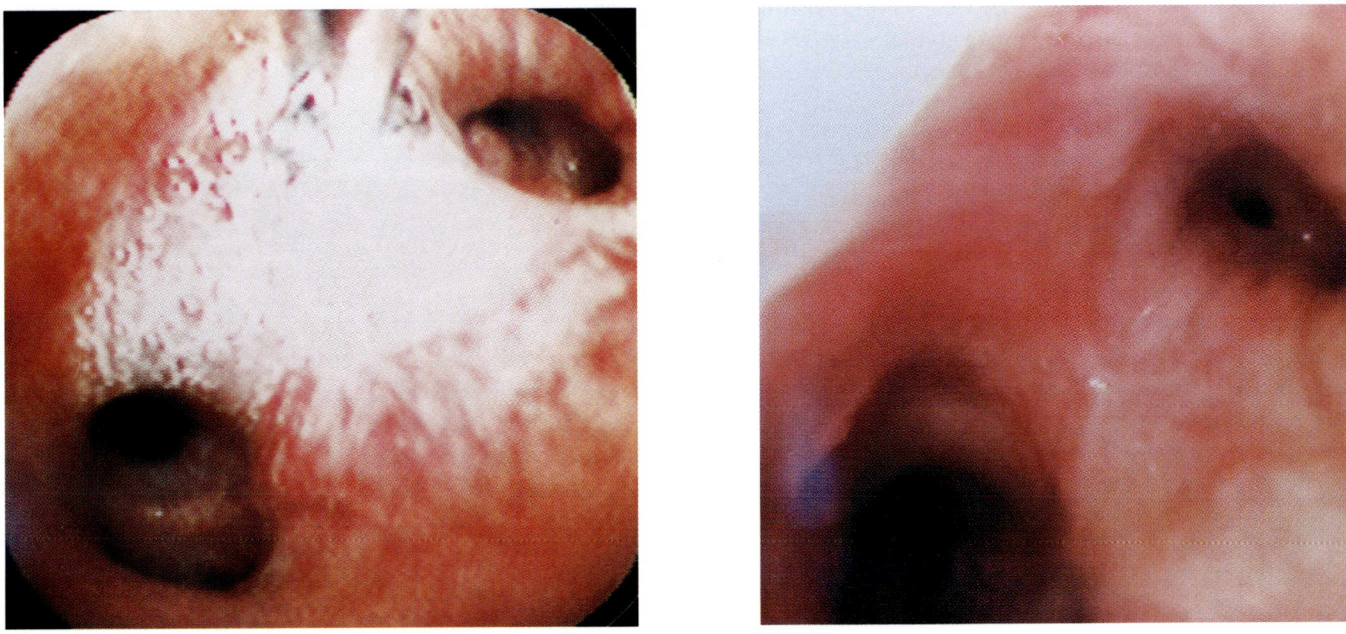

A B

A. Infiltrating squamous cell carcinoma of the carina of the left upper lobe before electrocautery treatment. This is a recurrence after photodynamic therapy. Patient could not have a surgical resection because of severe COPD. *B.* Carina left upper lobe after treatment. No tumor is seen and biopsy was negative for tumor. High-resolution CT scan images did not show any abnormality. Follow-up has been >4 years.

Figure 7-3

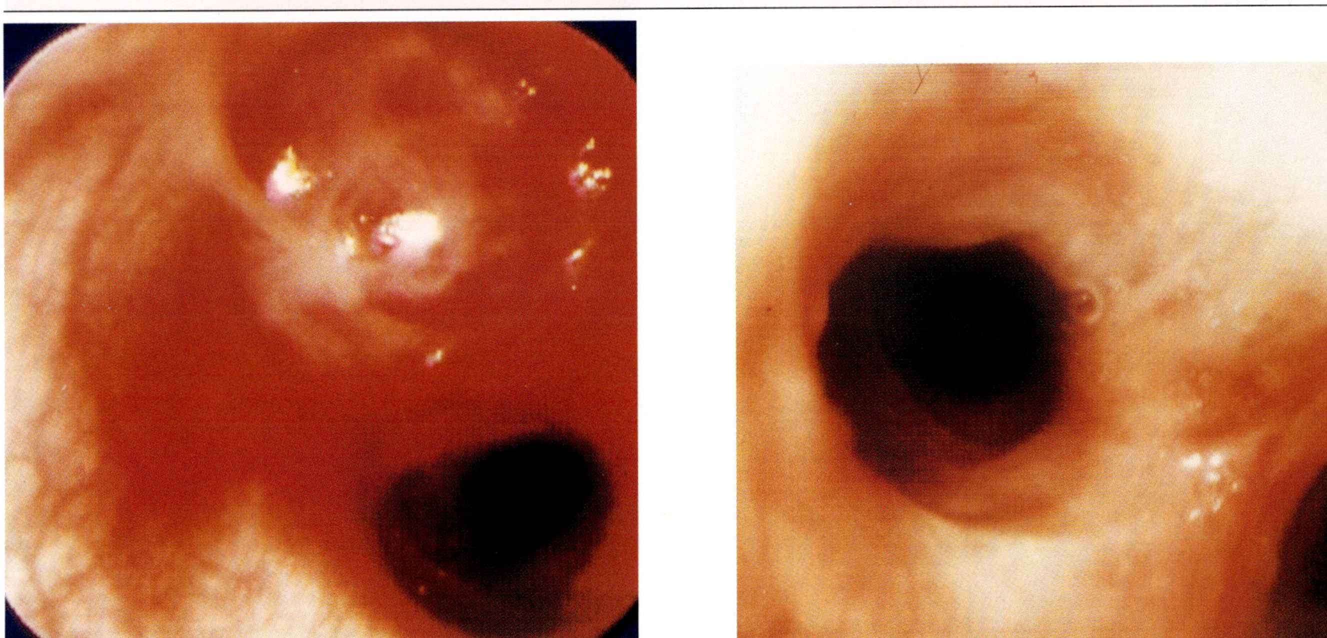

A B

A. Typical intraluminal bronchial carcinoid blocking the left upper lobe orifice. The left lower lobe bronchus is open. Treatment was with electrocautery with curative intent prior to surgical resection. *B.* Carina of the left upper lobe. The left upper lobe bronchus is completely open, with mild scarring of the orifice due to mucosal fibrosis after electrocautery. No tumor is seen; biopsy was negative for carcinoid. High-resolution CT showed no abnormality. An example of electrocautery as an alternative for surgical resection.

require additional bronchoscopy following cryosurgery and PDT. PDT skin photosensitivity also increases treatment morbidity. In case of significant extraluminal airway compression, a stent can be inserted.

The small number of patients with intraluminal occult lung cancer may benefit from bronchoscopic treatment with curative intent. Treatment may also be used to improve resectability. However, tumors ≥ 1 cm, with ≥ 3 mm invasion of the bronchial mucosa or with poorly visible distal tumor margins are unlikely to be cured by bronchoscopic treatment. Local therapy should not be performed if tumors are extraluminal or if there is a possibility of nodal or distant metastasis. A simple and inexpensive technique in the era of limited health care budgets is quite attractive, especially when more complicated and expensive techniques have not been shown to be superior. Endoscopic electrocautery has become more popular recently. High-frequency electric current is applied using a snare or a probe to generate heat in tissue. Clinical data so far have shown endobronchial electrocautery to be a simple and cost-effective palliative treatment modality. It may also be potentially curative for the treatment of superficial tumors, including benign, relatively benign, and low-grade malignant lesions such as typical bronchial carcinoids (Figs. 7-2 to 7-4).

HOW I DO IT

The clinical use of electrocautery as a therapeutic bronchoscopic technique assumes the need for immediate tumor debulking in patients with airway obstruction from intraluminal tumors. Heat is generated with standard equipment (Valleylab Force Generator with or without a Gas Surgical Unit/GSU, Erbe Beamer Two). Risk assessment should include factors previously mentioned following the guidelines shown in Fig. 7-1.

Figure 7-4

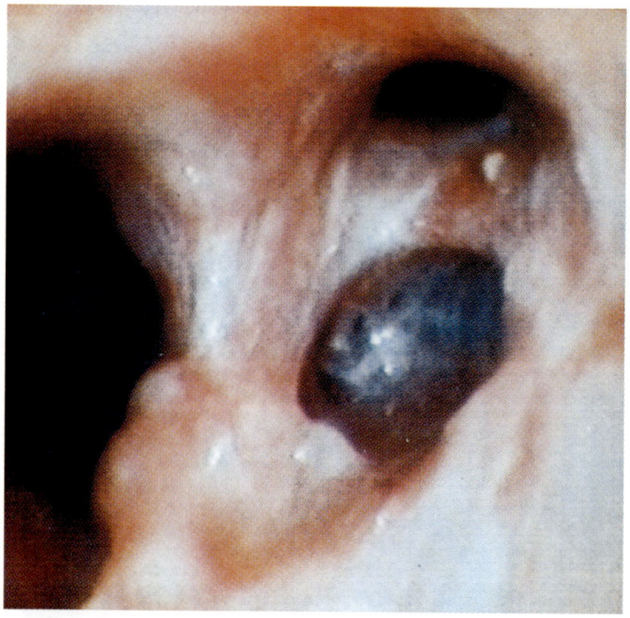

A

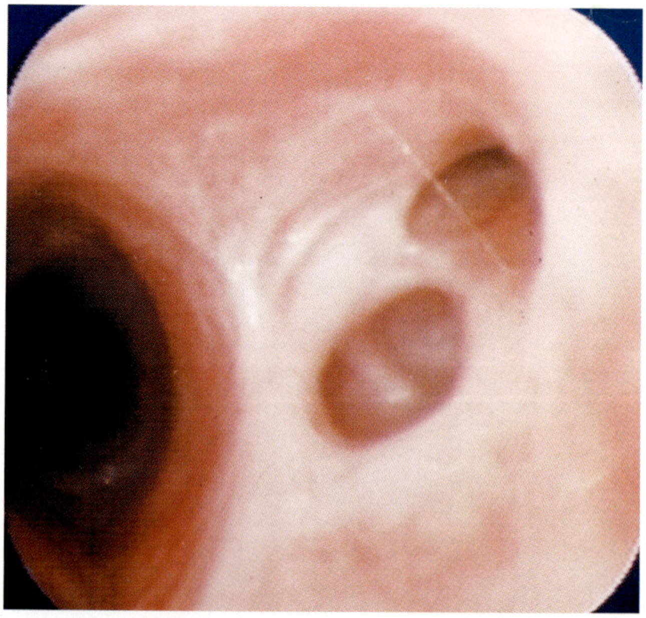

B

A. Infiltrating squamous cell carcinoma of the subcarina of the right upper lobe between the dorsal and anterior segmental bronchi (RB2 and RB3, respectively). Residual tumor or tumor recurrence 4 months after photodynamic therapy. Patient was not a surgical candidate because of left hemidiaphragm paralysis. Electrocautery with curative intent was an alternative treatment. *B.* Complete response after fiberoptic bronchoscopic electrocautery under local anesthesia. No tumor is seen, biopsy was negative for tumor. High-resolution CT did not show any abnormality in this area. The flexible monopolar probe enabled tumor coagulation of the segmental carina. This was easily achieved despite the fact that the tumor location required the extreme flexion of the distal tip of the flexible bronshoscope. Follow-up has been 4 years.

The Rigid Technique

Rigid bronchoscopy under general anesthesia must be considered if the bronchoscopist believes that maximal control is necessary during the treatment procedure in patients at high risk. The rigid scope may be safer and less time-consuming. It allows adequate ventilation and rapid tumor debulking in patients with imminent respiratory failure from bulky and hemorrhagic tumors. Tissue coagulation can be achieved by using the rigid probe or a flexible probe with the fiberoptic bronchoscope through the rigid scope. Electrocautery technique is quite similar to the contact mode of Nd:YAG laser therapy. Tissue blanching and charring is immediately apparent. The applied energy can be adjusted any time, based on tissue response. As with the Nd:YAG laser technique, coagulated tissue can be sheared off the wall using the tip of the rigid scope, a biopsy forceps, or the fiberscope shaft.[36] The process of coagulation or vaporization can be repeated until a sufficient airway lumen has been obtained.

The rigid technique of endobronchial electrocautery is usually performed under general anesthesia. After induction of anesthesia, the rigid scope is introduced

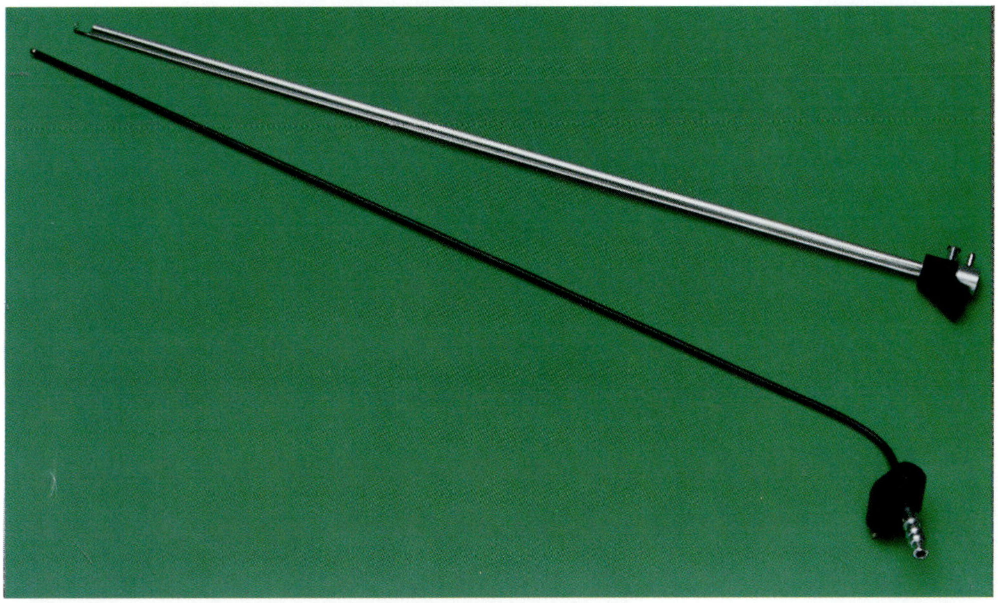

A

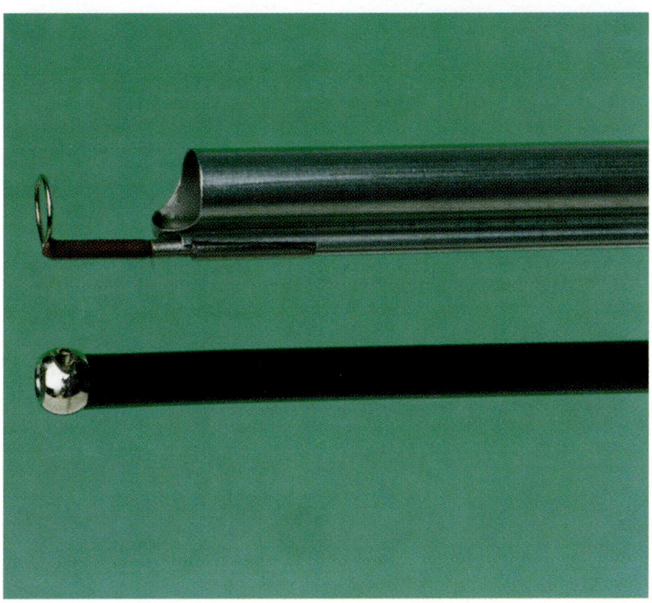

B

Figure 7-5

A. Rigid electrocautery instruments: the cutting loop without the rigid optic and the rigid coagulation suction probe. *B.* View of the distal tips of the rigid cutting loop and the rigid suction probe.

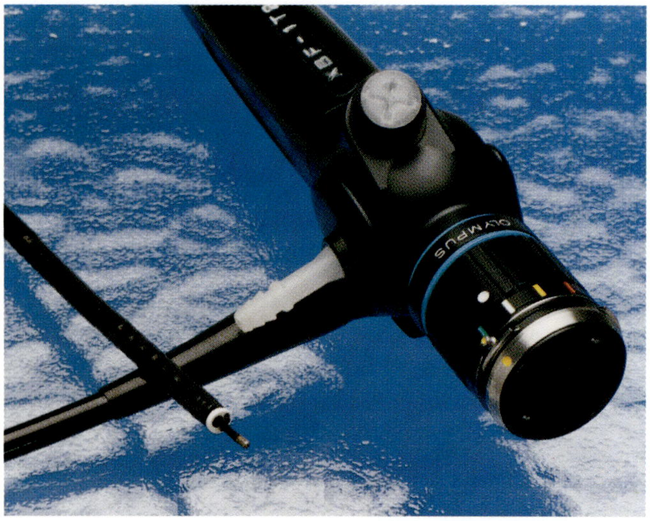

Figure 7-6

View of the fiberoptic electrocautery bronchoscope, showing the monopolar flexible probe protruding out of the insulated suction channel (white distal tip).

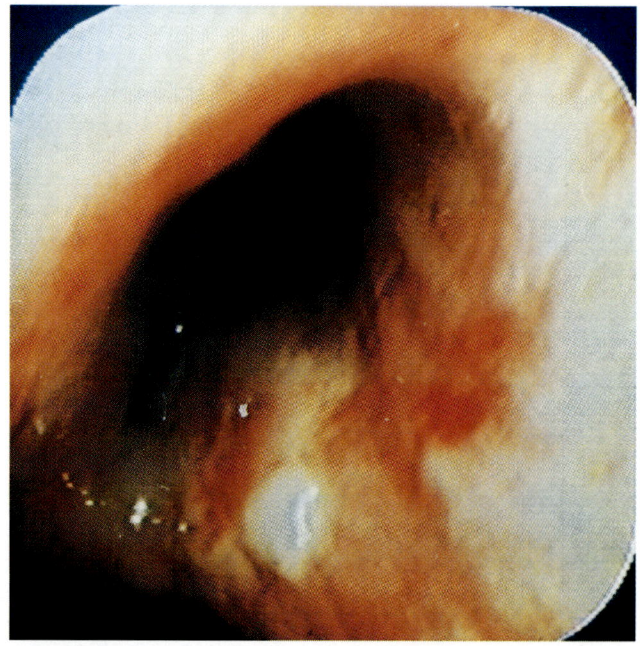

A

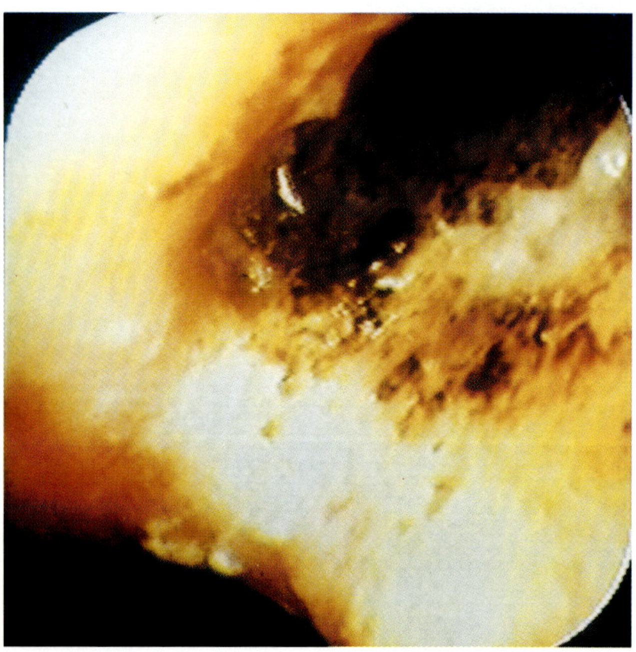

B

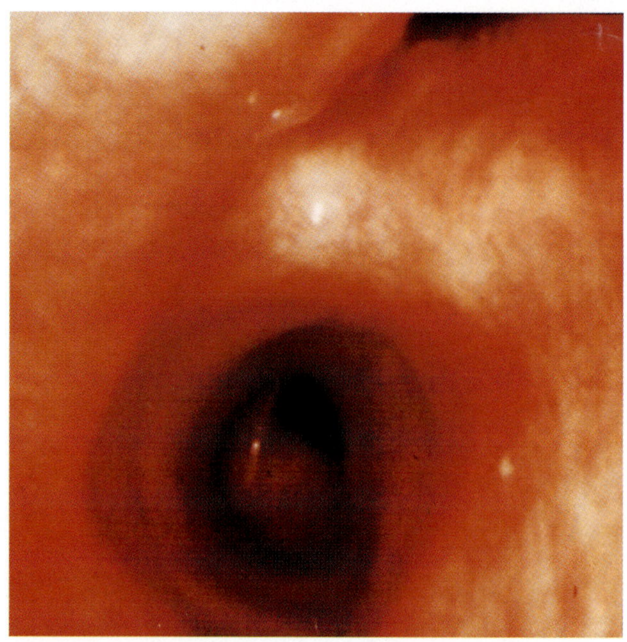

C

Figure 7-7

A. A patient with severe COPD and emphysema. A granulosa cell tumor of the carina of the right upper lobe. *B*. View immediately after argon plasma coagulation of the right upper lobe area showing coagulation necrosis. *C*. No recurrence of granulosa cell tumor is seen. Follow-up has been 3.5 years.

and ventilation maintained by jet ventilation. For rigid electrocautery probes, the Storz high-frequency loop electrode 10440 A or the rigid coagulation suction probe 10390 N can be used (Fig. 7-5). The intraluminal tumor mass is gently stripped or coagulated with the coagulation probe. Energy of ± 50 W is applied by activating the electric current using a foot pedal. Continuous suction of mucus, debris, and blood while performing coagulation can easily be carried out. Using the probe to palpate the tracheobronchial wall gives direct feedback about airway rigidity in assessing the significance of extraluminal compression.

The Flexible Technique

The flexible technique enables easier access to peripherally located tumors in the segmental bronchi. The use of an insulated fiberscope prototype (Olympus, Fig. 7-6) is theoretically safer in preventing electric current leak,[25] which may lead to uncontrolled coagulation or burns to the patient and the bronchoscopist. The tumor area should be kept free of blood or mucus by continuous suctioning. Coagulation can be achieved by gently touching the tumor base and applying 20 to 40 W of energy with the monopolar flexible probe.

With contact coagulation, the monopolar probe is pressed against the tumor base until sufficient blanching becomes apparent.[33] The noncontact method of argon plasma coagulation is another alternative. This is comparable to the noncontact mode of Nd:YAG laser or CO_2 laser therapy and can be used to superficially spray the tumor area. Tissue blanching is obtained in a matter of seconds[45–47] (Fig. 7-7). Treatment duration is very short if tumors are superficial and the surface area is limited to a few square centimeters. Therefore, treatment can be easily performed under local anesthesia. It is most important, however, to appreciate the indications and limitations of treatment with curative intent in patients with superficial cancers, as has been discussed.[6,17,18,53,55]

If local anesthesia is used, possible complications must be anticipated. An intravenous line is established for giving sedation.[76,77] Immediately before starting the bronchoscopic procedure, 2 mg of midazolam is injected as a bolus via the intravenous line. Additional midazolam can be titrated during the session. The procedure is done under continuous monitoring by pulse oximetry. Supplemental oxygen is given.[78–80] The bronchoscopist should possess the skills to intubate the patient or insert a rigid scope in case of emergency. We always keep the rigid scope ready for use. The rigid scope can be mounted with two cuffs, similar to a double-lumen endotrochael tube,[80] enabling simultaneous ventilation and treatment to continue.

The depth of tissue necrosis with electrocautery has been shown to be 2 to 3 mm, which is shallower than that of Nd:YAG laser necrosis.[46,81] Fibrin plugs and exudate may require a cleanup bronchoscopy in the post-treatment days. Treatment efficacy should be evaluated by bronchoscopy at 4 to 6 weeks to consider the need for additional treatment to maintain airway patency[19,20] (Fig. 7-1).

REFERENCES

1. Benfield JR: The lung cancer dilemma. *Chest* 1991; 100:510–511.
2. Ruckdeschel JC: Future directions in non-small cell lung cancer. A personal view. *Lung Cancer* 1995; 12(2):S147–152.
3. Souhami RL, et al: A data-based meta-analysis of randomised trials of chemotherapy versus best supportive care (BSC) in advanced non-small cell lung cancer (NSCLC). *Lung Cancer* 1994; 11(2):24–25.
4. Bonomi P: Combined modality treatment for stage III non-small cell lung cancer. *Lung Cancer* 1995; 12(2):S41-S52.
5. Ginsberg RJ: Neoadjuvant (induction) treatment for non-small cell lung cancer. *Lung Cancer* 1995; 12(2):S33–S40.
6. Woolner LB, et al: Roentgenographically occult lung cancer: Pathologic findings and frequency of multicentricity during a 10-year period. *Mayo Clinic Proc* 1984; 59:453–466.
7. Thomas PA, Rubinstein L: Malignant disease appearing late after operation for T1NO non-small-cell lung cancer. *J Thorac Cardiovasc Surg* 1993; 106:1053–1058.
8. Martini N, et al: Incidence of local recurrence and second primary tumors in resected stage I lung cancer. *J Thorac Cardiovasc Surg* 1995; 109:120–129.
9. Chetty KG, et al: Effect of radiation therapy on bronchial obstruction due to bronchogenic carcinoma. *Chest* 1989; 95:582–584.
10. Majid DA, et al: The response of atelectasis from lung cancer to radiation therapy. *Int J Rad Oncol Biol Phys* 1986; 12:231–232.
11. LeChevalier M, et al: Radiotherapy alone versus combined chemotherapy and radiotherapy in nonresectable non-small cell lung cancer—First analysis of a randomized trial in 353 patients. *J Natl Cancer Inst* 1991; 83:417–423.
12. Slaughter DP, et al: Field cancerization in oral stratified squamous epithelium. *Cancer* 1953; 6:963–968.
13. Lippman SM, Hong WK: Second malignant tumors in head and neck squamous cell carcinoma: The overshadowing threat for patients with early-stage disease. *Int J Rad Oncol Biol Phys* 1989; 17:691–694.
14. Watanabe Y, et al: Early hilar lung cancer: Its clinical aspect. *J Surg Oncol* 1991; 48:75–80.
15. Strauss GM, et al: Chest x-ray screening improves outcome in lung cancer. A reappraisal of randomized trials on lung cancer screening. *Chest* 1995; 107:270S–279S.
16. Flehinger BJ, et al: The effect of surgical treatment on survival from early lung cancer. Implications for screening. *Chest* 1992; 101:1013–18.
17. Nagamoto N, et al: Relationship of lymph node metastasis to primary tumor size and microscopic appearance of roentgenographically occult lung cancer. *Am J Surg Pathol* 1989; 13(12):1009–1013.
18. Usuda K, et al: Relation between bronchoscopic findings and tumor size of roentgenologically occult bronchogenic squamous cell carcinoma. *J Thorac Cardiovasc Surg* 1993; 106: 1098–1103.
19. Sutedja G, Postmus PE: Bronchoscopic treatment of lung tumors. Review article. *Lung Cancer* 1994; 11:1–17.
20. Edell ES, et al: Ancillary therapies in the management of lung cancer: Photodynamic therapy, laser therapy and endobronchial prosthetic devices. *Mayo Clin Proc* 1993; 68:685–690.

21. Lam S, et al: Detection of dysplasia and carcinoma in situ with a lung imaging fluorescence endoscope device. *J Thorac Cardiovasc Surg* 1993; 105:1035–1040.
22. Dumon JF: A dedicated tracheobronchial stent. *Chest* 1990; 97:328–332.
23. Sutedja G, Postmus PE: The cost-effectiveness of intraluminal bronchoscopic treatment. *Am Rev Resp Dis* 1995; 151(2):A850 (abstr).
24. Jackson R: Basic principles of electrosurgery: A review. *Can J Surg* 1970; 13:354–361.
25. Barlow DR: Endoscopic applications of electrosurgery: A review of basic principles. *Gastrointestinal Endoscopy* 1982; 28:73–76.
26. Ledingham SJ, Goldstraw P: Diathermy resection and radioactive gold grains for palliation of obstruction due to recurrence of bronchial carcinoma after external irradiation. *Thorax* 1989; 44:48–51.
27. Pedersen U, et al: Palliative resection with high-frequency cutting loop in malignant tracheobronchial diseases. *J Bronchol* 1994; 1:23–25.
28. Petrou M, Kaplan D, Goldstraw P: Bronchoscopic diathermy resection and stent insertion: A cost effective treatment for tracheobronchial obstruction. *Thorax* 1993; 48:1156–1159.
29. Frizelly R: Le traitement par électrocoagulation en pathologie maligne trachéo-bronchique. *Rev Pneumol Clin* 1986, 42:235–237.
30. Hooper RG, Jackson FN: Endobronchial electrocautery. *Chest* 1985; 87:712–714.
31. Hooper RG, Jackson FN: Endobronchial electrocautery. *Chest* 1988; 94:595–598.
32. Gerasin VA, Shafirovsky BB: Endobronchial electrosurgery. *Chest* 1988; 93:270–274.
33. Sutedja G, et al: Fiberoptic bronchoscopic electrosurgery under local anesthesia for rapid palliation in patients with central airway malignancies. A preliminary report. *Thorax* 1994; 49:1243–1246.
34. Homasson JP, et al: Traitement des tumeurs bronchiques par thermocoagulation haute fréquence. Etude préliminaire. *Rev Pneumol Clin* 1885; 51:77–81.
35. Prakash UBS: *Bronchoscopy.* New York, Raven, 1992.
36. Dumon JF, et al: Principles for safety in application of neodymium-YAG laser in bronchology. *Chest* 1984; 86:163–168.
37. George PJ, et al: Laser treatment for tracheobronchial tumours: Local or general anaesthesia? *Thorax* 1987; 42:656–660.
38. Hanowell LH, et al: Complications of general anesthesia for Nd:YAG laser resection of endobronchial tumors. *Chest* 1991; 99:72–76.
39. McCaughan JS, et al: Management of endobronchial tumors: A comparative study. *Sem Surg Oncol* 1989; 5:38–47.
40. Mathissen DJ, Grillo HC: Endoscopic relief of malignant airway obstruction. *Ann Thorac Surg* 1989; 48:469–475.
41. Macha HN, et al: New technique for treating occlusive and stenosing tumours of the trachea and main bronchi: Endobronchial irradiation by high dose iridium-192 combined with laser canalization. *Thorax* 1987; 42:511–515.
42. Simpson FG, et al: Postal survey of bronchoscopic practice by physicians in the United Kingdom. *Thorax* 1986; 41:311–317.
43. Prakash UBS, et al: Bronchoscopy in North America: The ACCP survey. *Chest* 1991; 100:1668–1675.
44. Sutedja G, et al: A postal survey of bronchoscopic practice in the Netherlands. *J Bronchology* 1996; 3:17–21.
45. Go PM, et al: The argon beam coagulator provides rapid hemostasis of experimental hepatic and splenic hemorrhage in anticoagulated dogs. *J Trauma* 1991; 31:1294–1300.
46. Rusch V, et al: Use of the argon beam electrocoagulator for performing pulmonary wedge resections. *Ann Thorac Surg* 1990; 49:287–291.
47. Sessler MJ, et al: Therapeutic effect of argon plasma coagulation on small malignant gastrointestinal tumors. *J Cancer Res Clin Oncol* 1995; 121:235–238.
48. Dougherty TJ: Photodynamic therapy for early stage lung cancer. Preferable to resection? *Chest* 1992; 102:1314.
49. Smith SGT, et al: Experimental studies to assess the potential of photodynamic therapy for the treatment of bronchial carcinomas. *Thorax* 1993; 48:474–480.
50. Sutedja G, et al: Photodynamic therapy for treatment of bronchial carcinomas. *Thorax* 1994; 49:289–290.
51. Monnier Ph, et al: Photodetection and photodynamic therapy of 'early' squamous cell carcinomas of the pharynx, oesophagus and tracheobronchial tree. *Lasers Med Sci* 1990; 5:149–169.
52. Braichotte DR, et al: Clinical pharmacokinetic studies of Photofrin by fluorescence spectroscopy in the oral cavity, the esophagus and the bronchi. *Cancer* 1995; 75:2768–2778.
53. Sutedja G, et al: Bronchoscopic treatment modalities in lung cancer, indications and limitations. *Ann Oncol* 1995; 6:951–952.
54. Hayata Y, et al: Photodynamic therapy (PDT) in early stage lung cancer. *Lung Cancer* 1993; 9:287–294.
55. Edell ES, Cortese DA: Photodynamic therapy in the management of early superficial squamous cell carcinoma as an alternative to surgical resection. *Chest* 1992; 102:1319–1322.
56. Furuse K, et al: A prospective phase II study on photodynamic therapy with photofrin II for centrally located early-stage lung cancer. *J Clin Oncol* 1993; 11:1852–1857.
57. Imamura S, et al: Photodynamic therapy and/or external beam radiation therapy for roentgenologically occult lung cancer. *Cancer* 1994; 73:1608–1614.
58. Okunaka T, et al: Photodynamic therapy for multiple primary bronchogenic carcinoma. *Cancer* 1991; 68:253–258.
59. Sutedja G, et al: Response and pattern of failure after photodynamic therapy for intraluminal stage I lung cancer. *J Bronchol* 1994; 1:295–298.
60. Macha HN, Wahlers B: Endobronchiale Brachytherapie: Die endoluminale Kleinraumbestrahlung von Bronchialtumoren mit dem Afterloading HDR-Verfahren. *Pneumonologie* 1991; 45:95–99.
61. O'Driscoll BR, et al: Radical treatment of lung cancer by high dose rate intraluminal radiotherapy. *Am Rev Resp Dis* 1991; 143:A60.
62. Hernandez P, Donath D: High dose rate endobronchial brachytherapy in the treatment of bronchogenic carcinoma. *Chest* 1993; 104:989–990.
63. Sutedja G, et al: High dose rate brachytherapy has a curative potential in patients with intraluminal squamous cell lung cancer. *Respiration* 1993; 61:167–168.
64. Ono R, et al: Bronchoscopic ultrasonography and brachytherapy in roentgenologically occult bronchogenic carcinoma. *J Bronchol* 1994; 1:281–287.
65. Ono R: *Brachytherapy.* Tokyo, Nakayama-Schoten, 1995.
66. Van Boxem T, et al: Radiographically occult lung cancer treated with fiberoptic bronchoscopic electrocautery: A pilot study of a simple and inexpensive technique. *ERJ* 1998; 11:169–172.
67. Cavaliere S, et al: Nd:YAG laser therapy in lung cancer: An 11-year experience with 2,253 applications in 1,585 patients. *J Bronchol* 1994; 1:105–111.
68. Personne C, et al: Indications and technique for endoscopic laser resections in bronchology. *J Thorac Cardiovasc Surg* 1986; 91:710–715.
69. Kato H, et al: Preoperative laser photodynamic therapy in combination with operation in lung cancer. *J Thorac Cardiovasc Surg* 1985; 90:420–429.
70. Shankar S, et al: Elective resection of tumours of the trachea and main carina after endoscopic laser therapy. *Thorax* 1990; 45:493–495.

71. Sutedja G, et al: High dose rate brachytherapy improves resectability in squamous cell lung cancer. *Chest* 1992; 102:308–309.
72. Shah H, et al: Benign tumors of the tracheobronchial tree. Endoscopic characteristics and role of laser resection. *Chest* 1995; 107: 1744–1751.
73. Sutedja G, et al: Bronchoscopic therapy in patients with intraluminal typical bronchial carcinoid. *Chest* 1995; 107:556–558.
74. Homasson JP: Bronchoscopic cryotherapy: A review. *J Bronchol* 1995; 2:145–153.
75. Speiser BL, Spratling L: Radiation bronchitis and stenosis secondary to high dose rate endobronchial irradiation. *Int J Rad Oncol Biol Phys* 1993; 25:580–597.
76. Midazolam—Is antagonism justified? *Lancet* 1988; II:140–142.
77. Rees PJ, et al: Premedication for fibreoptic bronchoscopy. *Thorax* 1983; 38:624–627.
78. Ovassapian A: Hemoglobin saturation monitoring; Should its use be mandated? *J Bronchol* 1995; 2:2–4 (edit).
79. Schiffman P, et al: Arterial oxygen saturation during Nd:YAG laser photoresection of endobronchial tumours under local anaesthesia. Use of intermittent supplemental oxygen with pulse oximetry guidance. *Chest* 1988; 94:1300–1301.
80. Sutedja G, et al: Nd-YAG laser under local anesthesia in obstructive endobronchial tumors. *Respiration* 1991; 58:238–240.
81. Lanzafame RJ, et al: Comparison of local tumor recurrence following excision with the CO_2 laser, Nd:YAG laser and argon beam coagulator. *Lasers Surg Med* 1988; 8:515–520.

C H A P T E R 8

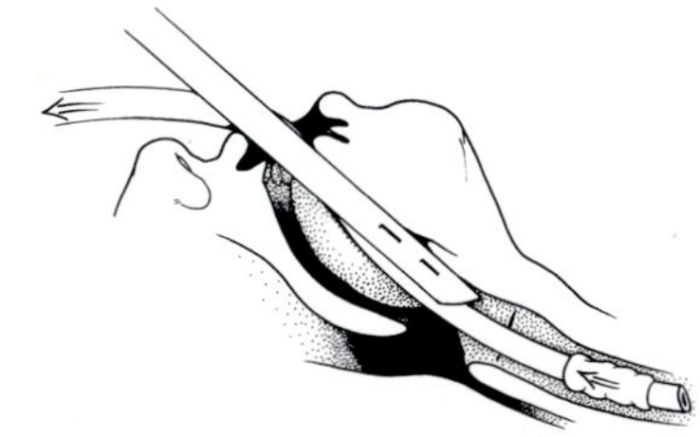

SILICONE AIRWAY STENTS

Henri G. Colt

The Random House Dictionary of the English Language defines prosthesis as "a device, either external or implanted, that substitutes for or supplements a missing or defective part of the body."[1] Referred to as *stents,* tracheobronchial prostheses have become essential to the interventional pulmonologist. Substantial anecdotal evidence suggests that airway stent insertion results in resolution of symptoms, prolonged symptom-free survival, and improved quality of life in selected patients with obstructed central airways.

Stents are temporarily inserted for palliation in patients with benign strictures or used permanently in nonsurgical candidates and in patients with evidence of stricture recurrence despite surgical or bronchoscopic treatment. Strictures resulting from intubation or inhalation injury, inflammatory processes, and systemic diseases are readily treated. Often, long-term palliation or cure is possible without resorting to open-surgical techniques.

Central airways obstruction is most commonly caused by intraluminal growth or extrinsic compression from malignant disease. Airway narrowing is also caused by a combination of exophytic growth and extrinsic compression or cartilaginous wall collapse. Many patients have exhausted or failed attempts at rigid bronchoscopic debulking, radiation or chemotherapy, bronchoscopic laser resection, or cryotherapy. In some patients, intraluminal lesions are not amenable to laser resection.[2,3] Symptomatic patients with any of the above airway abnormalities may be eligible for airway stents. Indeed, stenting may be the only therapeutic alternative available to satisfactorily preserve airway patency, improve quality of life, and prevent death from suffocation.

History of Silicone Airway Stents

Silicone rubber is a synthetic rubber made from silicone elastomeres, introduced originally in the 1940s. Silicone contains polymers with alternate silicon and oxygen atoms. Silicone's properties (resinous, rubbery, stable at high temperatures, and water-repellent) are determined primarily by organic groups attached to these atoms. Silicone has been employed successfully as an adhesive, a lubricant, and a sealant. It is used in insulation, cosmetics, and many other industries. The word *silicone* should not be confused with the word *Silastic,* which is a trademark name for any group of substances containing polymeric silicone and is the trademark substance used most commonly in the manufacture of medical prosthetic devices.

Prosthetic replacement of the obstructed airway with a silicone graft was described by Graciano and associates in 1967.[4] Previously, metal tubes were used by Harkins in the 1950s to relieve benign tracheal stenosis.[5] Silicone prostheses were further introduced by Neville and coworkers,[6] who sutured them into place during open thoracotomy and tracheal resection. Although bronchoscopic stent implantation was considered by Chevalier Jackson[7] early in the 20th century, stenting had not become an accepted therapeutic alternative until this decade. Indeed, recently, some interventional pulmonologists have increasingly recognized the limitations of bronchoscopic laser resection, and explored other means of restoring central airway patency.[8,9]

The majority of silicone stents used today derive from the Montgomery silicone tracheal T tube introduced in the 1960s.[10] Originally, the Montgomery T tube was designed to maintain a satisfactory airway and to provide support in the reconstructed trachea. It is, therefore, both a stent and a tracheotomy tube. An external side limb protrudes through the tracheostomy orifice, allowing ventilation or aspiration as necessary. When the side limb is occluded, patients are able to breath and speak without difficulty. During the past 25 years, several modifications were made to the T-tube design. Duvall and Bower demonstrated stent insertion through the larynx over a rigid bronchoscope.[11] Modified T tubes were used in patients with endobronchial disease. Westaby designed a T tube in which the distal branch was lengthened and bifurcated to saddle the carina.[12] Other modifications included removal of the external side limb or extending the length of the distal limb to stent the lower trachea and right or left main bronchi. Stents were inserted into the airways during laryngoscopy or rigid bronchoscopy or over bronchial boogies. Clark modified Sutar's esophageal stent for airway lesions.[13] Cooper and colleagues removed the side limb altogether, and introduced a smooth-walled silicone stent into the airway by placing it onto a rigid bronchoscope and pushing it into place with an endotracheal tube or chest tube.[14] In 1987, Orlowski designed a modified tracheoflex tracheostomy tube with a side hole cut into it. The stent was inserted into the trachea through the rigid bronchoscope using a polyethylene tube as a pusher.[15] In the late 1980s, Dumon experimented with modified Montgomery T tubes, finally publishing preliminary results of his Endoxane stent in 1990.[16,17] Today, the patented Dumon stent is probably the most commonly used tracheobronchial prosthesis in the world. This silicone stent introduced the concept of small studs placed on the external surface of the stent to increase adherence to airway-wall mucosa. In addition, a specially designed stent introducer system was conceived to facilitate stent insertion through, rather than over, the rigid bronchoscope. This also facilitates preliminary dilatation and allows deployment of a stent with maximal outer diameter.[18]

Because of concerns regarding impaired mucociliary clearance through the silicone protheses, stent migration, and the need for multiple stents in certain patients with extensive tracheobronchial disease, "hybrid" stents have become commercially available recently.

Figure 8-1

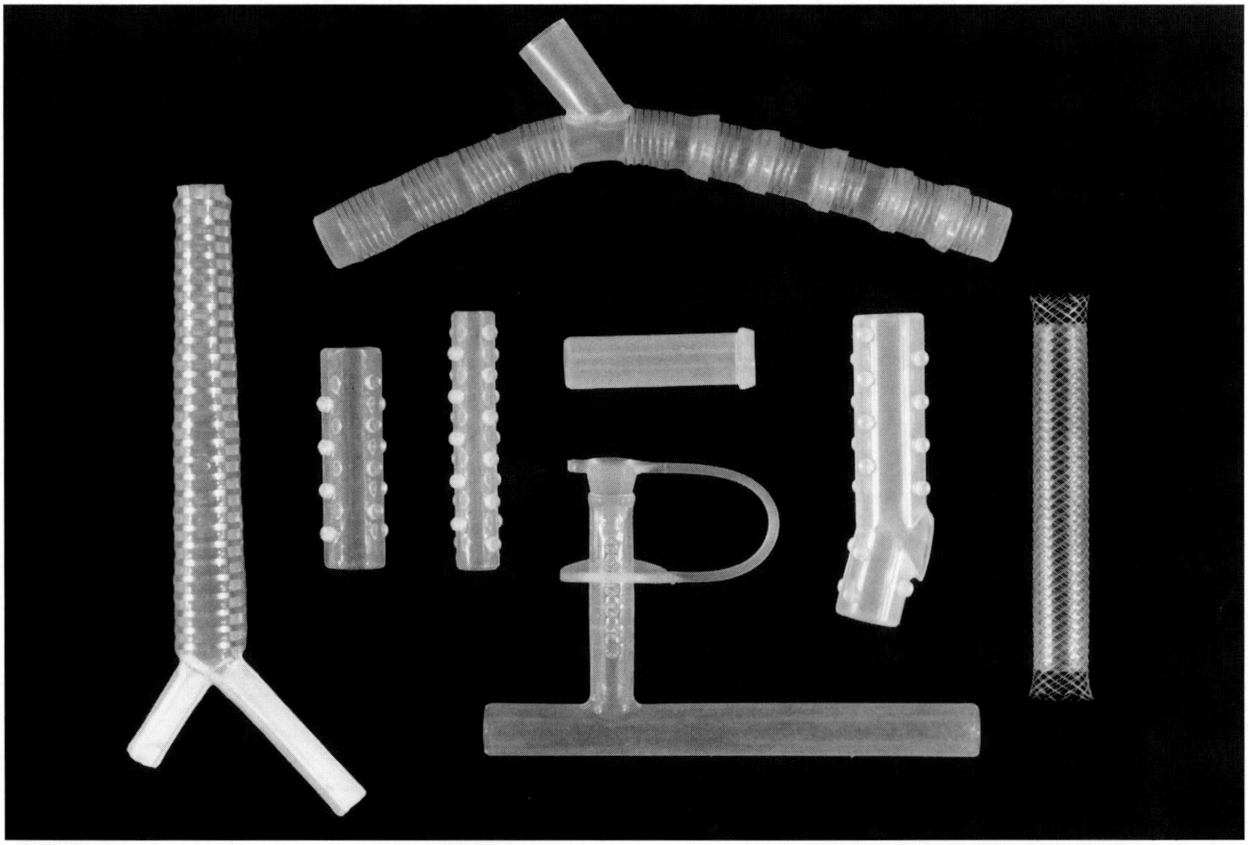

Commercially available models of silicone and hybrid stents. From *left* to *right:* Rusch stent, Dumon tracheal stent, Dumon bronchial stent, Montgomery T-tube (*bottom*), Hood bronchial stent (*middle*), Orlowski stent (*top*), Hood custom tracheobronchial stent, covered Schneider Wallstent.

These stents are made of silicone rubber, stainless steel, or nitinol wire mesh.[19–22] Future research devoted to finding an ideal stent for selected patients, as well as a way to facilitate flexible bronchoscopic stent insertion, will probably result in the design of additional models of tracheobronchial prostheses.

Commercially Available Silicone Stents (Fig. 8-1, Table 8-1)

MONTGOMERY T TUBE (Boston Medical Products, Inc., Waltham, MA)

As mentioned earlier, the Montgomery T tube rapidly became a popular method of palliation in patients with subglottic tracheal stenosis.[23,24] Originally introduced in the 1960s, this silicone tube requires a permanent tracheotomy. Subglottic tracheal dilatation is achieved prior to or at the time of stent insertion. The intratracheal limbs of the T tube are smooth-walled with tapered distal extremities. The recently designed Safe-T-tube includes some modifications that make it easier and safer to use.[25] Ridges and grooves along the extraluminal limb of the tube allow a ring washer to be attached to it to prevent posterior displacement. The proximal portion of the T tube extends above the tracheostomy, lying directly within the subglottic stricture and below the vocal cords. The distal limb of the T tube extends below the tracheostomy and lies within the lumen of the upper and middle third of the trachea. The external side limb protrudes through the tracheostomy maintaining its patency and allowing suctioning as needed (Fig. 8-2). The external side limb must be plugged to avoid drying of secretions. Should the patient be unable to breathe through the mouth at any time, this external side limb may be unplugged, providing immediate access to the inside of the stent and to the airways. T tubes come in multiple sizes ranging from 10- to 16-mm outside diameter. An extralong intraluminal portion is available. T tubes also come in pediatric sizes ranging from 6- to 9-mm outside diameter. If necessary, the internal limbs of the T tube may be shortened, although care must be taken to smooth any of the cut edges with fine sandpaper and hand filing. Customizing kits are available from the manufacturer.

THE HOOD STENT (Hood Laboratories, Pembrook, MA)

Short silicone stents were also manufactured for use within the tracheobronchial tree without requiring a tracheostomy. In 1989, Cooper and colleagues de-

Table 8-1
DESCRIPTION OF CURRENTLY AVAILABLE SILICONE STENTS

Stent	*Description*
	Simple
Montgomery T-tube	Requires tracheotomy. Suctioning and cleaning are possible through external limb. Palliation of subglottic stenosis and midtracheal strictures.
Dumon	Studs on external surface prevent migration. Easily removed.
Reynders-Noppen	Self-expanding, fine wire mesh stent of different lengths and diameters. Insertion using loading catheter. Prior dilatation of strictures unnecessary.
Hood	Smooth walled, can be custom-designed in various lengths, shapes, and diameters.
	Hybrid
Rusch Y stent	Silicone with stainless-steel struts offered in 3 sizes (11, 13, and 15 mm). Special forceps facilitates placement.
Schneider covered Wallstent	Silicone-wrapped braided wire mesh. Insertion using loading catheter. Prior dilatation of strictures necessary.
Gianturco/Rusch covered esophageal design	Polyethylene covered metal Z stent. Lengths: 10, 12, 14 cm. Outer diameter 18 mm. Used in esophagus but can be deployed in trachea.
Rusch-Orlowski	Silicone with circular metal armor interior.

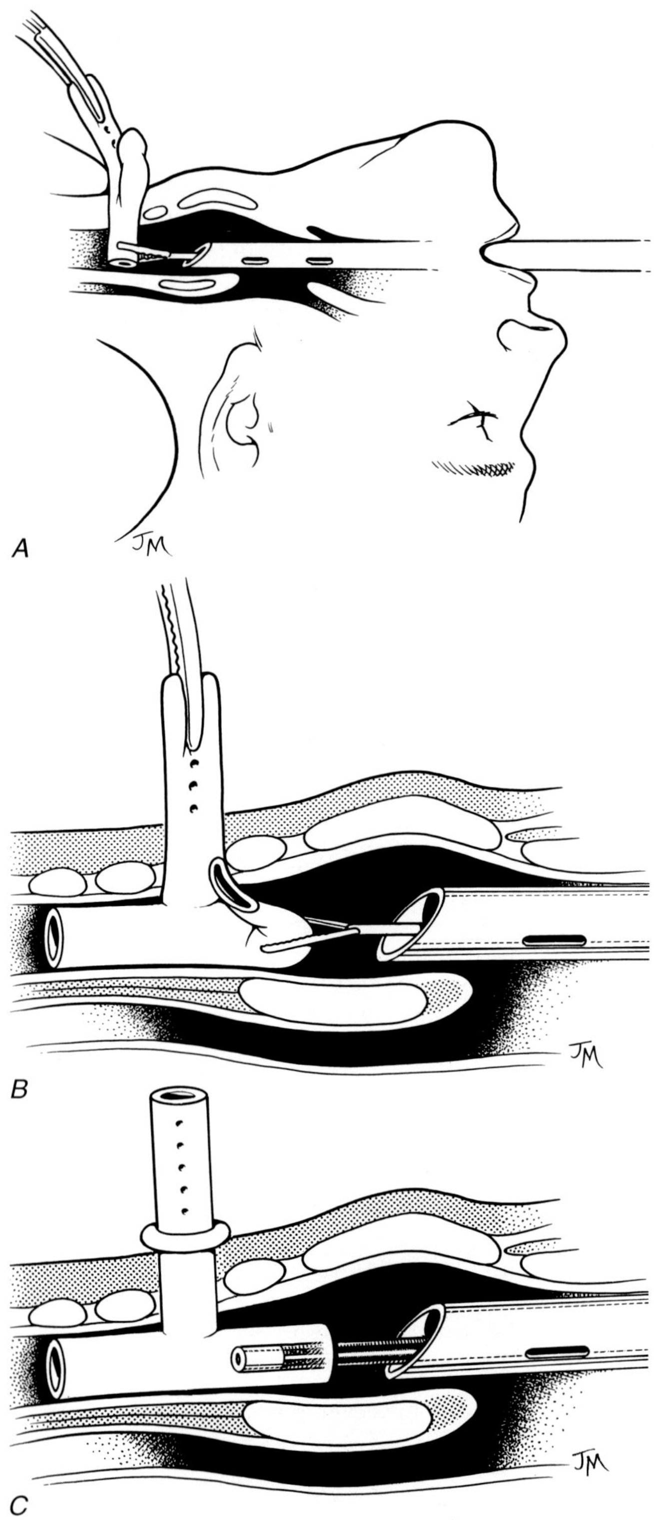

Figure 8-2

The Montgomery T tube. *A*. Introduction of Montgomery T tube through tracheostomy assisted with Kelly clamp and rigid forceps pushing distal limb downward. *B*. Once the distal limb is in place, forceps are used to pull the proximal limb upward while firmly maintaining the rigid bronchoscope in place within immediate subglottis. *C*. Once unfolded, bronchial toilet is performed using the flexible bronchoscope through the external limb of the T tube. The rigid bronchoscope is gently withdrawn to assess distance between the proximal limb and the vocal cords. The patient is extubated and the external limb is capped.

scribed endoscopic insertion of a short segment of silicone tubing in patients with benign bronchial strictures.[14] These stents were well tolerated, although one patient coughed up a stent several days after its placement. A bronchial stent was fashioned from the horizontal limb of a silicone T tube. A flared end was made from the junction of the horizontal and vertical limbs of the T tube at the distal aspect of the stent. A smaller flare or circle of silicone rubber was placed as a flange at the proximal end to help prevent migration. Eventually, the manufacturer produced stents with flanges on one or both ends. These are available commercially in multiple lengths and diameters. Custom-designed Y stents for use in the trachea and bronchial tree were also designed. Studded silicone stents similar to the Dumon stent, have also become available recently from this manufacturer. Both the Y stent and straight silicone stents can be inserted through or over the rigid bronchoscope using a pushing device. It is noteworthy that in Cooper's report of tracheobronchial stenting, tenacious secretions caused obstruction of the stent lumen in some patients, prompting bronchoscopy for aspiration, and resulting in the author's recommendation for twice daily inhalation therapy using acetylcysteine (Mucomist).

THE DUMON STENT (Novatech, Aubagne, France, distributed by Bryan Corporation, Woburn, MA)

Following a vast experience with Montgomery T tubes and smooth-walled indwelling tracheobronchial stents, Dumon designed an indwelling stent made of molded silicone with regularly placed studs on its external surface to help prevent dislodgement.[16] These studs imbed themselves slightly into the airway mucosa, yet do not cause ischemia, necrosis, infection, or perforation. In addition, the studs allow collateral ventilation between the prosthesis wall and the airway wall. This is particularly beneficial if the stent partially occludes the entrance of an upper lobe bronchus. Stents come in 30- to 60-mm lengths, and 10- to 16-mm diameters. The original insertion technique using an external pusher over the rigid bronchoscope raised concerns about possible damage to the larynx during stent insertion. Also, maximally sized stents could not be inserted using this technique. A specially designed Stent Introducer System (EFER, La Ciotat, France, distributed in the United States by Bryan Corporation, Woburn, MA) is now commercially available so that stents can be inserted through, rather than over, the rigid bronchoscope.[26–28] This stent can be inserted using bronchoscopes made by any manufacturer, but is particularly destined for use with the EFER-Dumon rigid bronchoscope, with its tubes of various lengths and diameters and universal rotating swivel base (EFER, La Ciotat, France, distributed in the United States by Bryan Corporation, Woburn, MA). Today, the

Dumon stent is probably the most widely used indwelling silicone stent in the world. There is no doubt that its design, distribution, and demonstrated efficacy have been catalysts responsible for promoting interventional pulmonology. Like the Hood stents, these prostheses can be custom-designed as step-down stents (a proximal portion of larger diameter than its distal portion), as stents with tapered extremities, and as stents with bifurcations using angles of various degrees or side holes providing ventilation of an upper-lobe, middle-lobe, or lower-lobe segmental bronchus. In these particular cases, stent insertion may be difficult, and rotation of the side port away from the take-off of the segmental bronchus can be problematic. At the time of this writing, many of the custom-designed stents and stents with side holes are not approved by the U.S. Food and Drug Administration (FDA).

THE REYNDERS STENT (Reynders Medical Supply, Lennik, Belgium)

Another interesting stent design was described by Noppen and coworkers in 1996.[29] A specially manufactured Tygon synthetic cylindric tube is thermetically molded to a screw-thread prosthesis, making this stent far more rigid than those made of silicone rubber. Only a single diameter (17 mm), however, is available. The stent is inserted into the airway stricture using an external pusher device. The external screw threads are designed to maintain stent stability within the airway. Only 10 patients, however, were described in the author's initial report, and conclusions regarding efficacy and ease of use are probably premature. Further studies are needed to demonstrate long-term effectiveness and safety of this prosthesis.

THE RUSCH STENT (Rusch AG, Deluth, GA)

This stent was introduced in the early 1990s in Germany and has been recently approved by the FDA in the United States. This Y-shaped stent is made of silicone with horseshoe-shaped steel struts incorporated into the anterior and lateral walls of the stent. The shapes of the steel struts change from longitudinally oval at the level of the cricoid cartilage, to transversely oval at the level of the main carina. A flexible, somewhat thinner posterior silicone membrane presumably facilitates dynamic compression during cough. The stent is Y shaped with long tracheal and left main bronchial limbs and a shorter right main bronchial limb.[30–32] The stent comes in only three sizes (three stents, each with a different length and diameter). The bronchial limbs are not reinforced with metal and have smaller diameters than the tracheal limb. The stent's design potentially avoids secretion accumulation and facilitates expectoration, but there is no doubt that if obstruction occurs from thick mucous plugging, emergent intervention is necessary to avoid respiratory compromise. This is particularly the case if the tracheal limb of the stent becomes obstructed. An additional purpose of the stent's design was to prevent migration, but several cases of stent displacement and even expectoration with forceful cough have been reported (verbal communications). The stent is usually inserted during rigid laryngoscopy under general anesthesia, and after preliminary tracheobronchial dilatation or bronchoscopic laser resection.

THE COVERED WALLSTENT (Schneider Inc., Minneapolis, MN)

Another example of a hybrid stent is the thin, silicone-membrane-covered wall stent manufactured by Schneider. This stent comes in sizes ranging from 20 to 90 mm in length, and 5 to 24 mm in width. Although it appears that the silicone membrane covering the wire metal mesh prevents granulation tissue formation or growth of tumor through the metal struts in the mid-portion of the stent, both the distal and proximal aspects of the stent are uncovered.[33] At these levels, therefore, stents may become obstructed, prompting either insertion of another stent within the first or a long procedure to entirely remove the stent that has been epithelialized into the airway mucosa. The covered wall stent can be inserted using rigid or flexible bronchoscopy, fluoroscopy, and a loaded catheter introducer system. Techniques are similar to those used for insertion of metal stents described in Chap. 9.

As manufacturers strive to develop the ideal stent for all circumstances, it is likely that additional hybrid stents using a variety of different alloys will become available.

Indications for Silicone Stent Insertion (Table 8-2)

Stenting is indicated when central airway patency cannot be preserved using other bronchoscopic or adjuvant therapeutic techniques, and if patients have respiratory symptoms, impaired functional status, or diminished quality of life. These occur with malignancies, benign strictures, and malacia, and after lung transplantation. Stents are used alone or in addition to other bronchoscopic techniques to restore airway patency in patients with intraluminal disease, as well as in patients with extrinsic compression of the airways without exophytic disease. In experienced hands, stent insertion is safe and effective and provides excellent palliation of the symptoms and effects of central-airway obstruction.[18,34–39]

Patients with central-airway obstruction often present with cough, stridor, wheezing, hemoptysis, or dyspnea. Others have postobstructive pneumonia or respiratory failure, often requiring endotracheal intubation and mechanical ventilation. Many patients,

Table 8-2
POTENTIAL INDICATIONS FOR TRACHEOBRONCHIAL STENT INSERTION

Malignant tracheobronchial obstruction with extrinsic compression of large airways in patients who have exhausted curative therapeutic options
Malignant tracheobronchial obstruction despite laser resection and dilatation
Malignant tracheobronchial obstruction in patients undergoing external beam radiation
Postintubation subglottic stenosis after failure of laser resection or dilatation
Benign, complex tracheal stenosis in patients who are not surgical candidates
Benign tracheal stenosis after failure of laser resection or dilatation
Benign tracheal or bronchial stenosis from inflammatory or infectious processes while waiting for response to systemic therapy or pending open surgical resection
Localized or extensive tracheobronchomalacia regardless of cause
Anastomotic strictures after lung and heart-lung transplantation
Tracheal or broncheal-esophageal fistula

however, are asymptomatic until critical narrowing of the airway occurs. Pulmonary function tests and flow-volume curves are infrequently sensitive, but may be helpful when grossly abnormal. Often, patients have failed treatment with oral or inhaled corticosteroids and β agonists for presumed asthma, or have received courses of antitussives, mucolytics, and even racemic epinephrine prior to referral. Consequently, although central-airway obstruction is a relatively infrequent finding in the absence of known underlying pulmonary neoplasm, many interventional pulmonologists have a tendency to perform flexible fiberoptic bronchoscopy early on in the course of their evaluation of patients with chronic cough, adult-onset asthma, a history of airway intervention, tracheal intubation, mechanical ventilation, or smoke inhalation.

The indication for stent insertion is usually made during diagnostic flexible bronchoscopy, although most operators will make final determinations and "tactical decisions" during therapeutic bronchoscopy when resection of an obstructing lesion or dilatation of an airway stricture fails to reestablish patency. Once inserted, tracheobronchial stents are usually well tolerated and will not adversely effect external beam radiation therapy, brachytherapy, or subsequent bronchoscopic laser resection.[40–44] If recurrent granulation tissue or tumor growth requires resection, however, it is wise to remove the silicone stent prior to laser firing. This prevents intraluminal airway burns and facilitates complete debulking of remaining exophytic disease.

Malignancies also cause airway narrowing because of significant extrinsic compression from bronchogenic tumors or lymphadenopathy, or because of extensive submucosal infiltration. Such abnormalities may or may not be accompanied by exophytic tumor growth in patients with primary lung cancer, endobronchial metastases, or neoplasms metastatic to the lung. Bronchoscopic debulking is often necessary prior to stent insertion. In patients with lung, thyroid, or esophageal cancer, dyspnea should prompt flexible bronchoscopy, which can reveal extrinsic compression of the trachea or main bronchus from the adjacent tumor. Silicone stent insertion can be safely followed by surgical resection, or external beam irradiation therapy. In many cases, patients are better able to tolerate adjuvant therapies (which require multiple outpatient visits) once airway patency has been restored by stenting, than if they were referred for therapy without prior establishment of a satisfactory tracheobronchial lumen. Once patients respond to therapy, stents are easily removed. In patients with esophageal cancer, infiltration of the posterior and left-lateral tracheal wall may be noted during bronchoscopy, and sometimes, patients present with tracheobronchial-esophageal fistulas at the level of the carina and left main bronchus.[45] Simultaneous or sequential insertion of an esophageal and airway stent often prevents complications resulting from the fistulous track. Bronchoscopy is warranted in any patient with an indwelling esophageal stent complaining of dyspnea because the stent itself can cause extrinsic compression of the airway which can be palliated using a tracheobronchial stent.[46]

Benign tracheobronchial strictures may result from prolonged intubation, previous airway interventions, or systemic illnesses such as amyloidosis, relapsing polychondritis, *Klebsiella rhinoscleromata,* fibrosing mediastinitis, tuberculosis, and Wegener's granulomatosis. Other indications include fixed obstruction from scarring due to radiation therapy and intermittent central-airway obstruction from localized or extensive tracheobronchial malacia. In these patients, stents are occasionally used pending surgical intervention or when patients are ineligible for curative surgical repair. Individuals with stricture recurrence despite open surgery may be candidates for long-term stent placement. Patients with localized and extensive tracheobronchial malacia, however, present a particularly difficult problem. In this setting, stents often migrate, and multiple bronchoscopic interventions may be necessary before a properly fitting stent is found. Some operators may choose to perform a tracheostomy with insertion of a modified T tube. Others attempt Y or custom stent insertion, select a Rusch stent, or insert multiple straight-silicone stents to impede dynamic airway wall collapse. Tracheobronchomalacia usually results from recurrent infection and prolonged mechanical ventilation, but can also be discovered in some patients with severe chronic obstructive pulmonary disease. Patients and physicians must be made aware that multiple procedures are often necessary in these instances. They should not become discouraged if initial bronchoscopic therapy fails to provide long-term relief of dyspnea or cough.

Airway strictures, usually at the level of, or just beyond, the site of tracheal or bronchial anastomosis, are occasionally found in lung transplant recipients. Therefore, most transplant surgeons and interventional pulmonologists agree that flexible bronchoscopic examination of the airway anastomoses is indicated in lung transplant recipients with abnormal spirometry, cough, or dyspnea. Care must be taken, however, not to misjudge airway caliber during flexible bronchoscopic examination nor to misinterpret a telescoping anastomosis and recipient-to-donor step-down as an airway stricture.

Strictures occur probably as part of the healing process after airway dehiscence, granulation, necrosis, or infection. Although it appears that airway strictures occur in up to 15 percent of all lung transplant recipients, not all require stent placement.[38,47] Granulation tissue or circumferential fibrous scarring, for example, is easily resected, but stenting is necessary when the airway lumen is reduced by 60 percent of more, especially if respiratory symptoms are manifested or ventilatory function declines. Some patients have only malacia of airways distal to the anastomotic site. This is not identical with the perianastomotic bronchomalacia seen in association with obliterative bronchiolitis. A thorough analysis of the incidence of posttransplantation airway complications is difficult, in part because of the absence of a universally accepted classification of airway abnormalities.

The etiology of posttransplantation airway strictures is probably multifactorial. Bronchial ischemia appears to be central to the development of anastomotic complications. Surgical technique, perioperative use of corticosteroids, acute allograft rejection, prolonged postoperative ventilation, and concomitant infections such as aspergillosis are also believed to influence airway healing.[48–50] Younger patients undergoing lung transplantation for cystic fibrosis may have an increased propensity for granulation tissue formation and bronchial stenosis. It is unclear whether neovascularization, different mechanisms of organ preservation, pathologic changes in airway cartilage, retained secretions, or multiple bronchoscopic examinations and bronchoscopic lung biopsies performed as part of routine surveillance affect airway healing.[38,51]

In summary, many benign strictures are initially amenable to rigid bronchoscopic laser resection and dilatation. Stenting is necessary, however, in the case of recurrence or inability to satisfactorily achieve a patent airway. Increased experience with silicone stents suggests that stents should be left in place for 12 months or more. Stent tolerance is usually excellent in the abscence of complications such as migration, obstruction by secretions, or granulation tissue formation. Many patients have had indwelling stents for several years. After a period of time, a circumferential band of tissue usually forms around the stent, firmly holding it place, but also maintaining adequate tracheobronchial patency after stent removal. By initially leaving stents in position for at least 1 year, airway strictures, particularly from lung transplantation, may not recur as often as when stents are removed after 1 or 2 months. Operators must resist the temptation to remove stents too soon just to "see what happens" or at the urging of patients who may not fully understand the necessity for leaving stents in place for longer periods. Because many silicone stents can eventually be removed without stricture recurrence, particularly in patients with stenoses after lung transplantation, most operators avoid using permanent metal stents in these instances. The silicone stent is easily inserted and easily replaced or removed, and there is no risk of airway wall perforation.

Setting Up for Stent Insertion

BRONCHOSCOPIC ASSESSMENT

The tracheobronchial tree is a complex organ that is ever-changing in shape. Length and diameter may vary as the structure is exposed to large pressure variations during breathing and coughing. Factors for consideration during stent design and development of insertion techniques include (1) the relatively rigid cartilaginous structure, (2) the relatively dynamic and malleable membranous structure, (3) close proximity of hollow organs and great vessels, (4) the need to maintain adequate mucocilliary clearance and expectoration of secretions, (5) potential reactions to chronic inflammation and foreign bodies, and (6) the focal or circumferential effects of tumor compression, fibrous strictures, and stent expansion.

In many cases, bronchoscopic airway dilatation and debulking is necessary prior to stent insertion. In some cases, however, it is better to maintain a somewhat narrowed airway that will help stabilize the stent and maintain its position. Debulking, laser resection, and tracheal dilatation can be performed at the time of stent insertion. For this reason, most experienced operators agree that silicone stents be placed by bronchoscopists familiar with all techniques of interventional pulmonology. If a stent is placed for temporary palliation of airway obstruction in a patient destined to undergo surgical resection, the precise location of the airway stricture, its length, and its distance from the vocal cords and carina need to be noted. The presence of airway inflammation, necrosis, or purulent secretions is also important. The stent's precise length, diameter, and location should be noted in the procedure note. Informed consent should be obtained so patients and their families are aware of the potential complications of stent insertion as well as the need for routine surveillance. Either may lead to increased utilization of health care resources; repeated chest radiographs or bronchoscopic examinations may be necessary. At the University of California at San Diego Medical Center, patients are instructed to call in cases of increasing dyspnea, cough, or hemoptysis. Patients are also provided with a wallet-size medical alert document describing the indication for stent placement, location of the stent, and emergency procedures to follow in case of complications.

ANESTHESIA TECHNIQUES AND PRECAUTIONS

Stent insertion is usually performed under general anesthesia. Because the airway may be lost or complete obstruction may occur during stent placement, satisfactory ventilation and oxygenation must be provided during the entire procedure. Rigid bronchoscopy is safely performed using spontaneous assisted ventilation techniques or jet ventilation.[52–56] Paralysis and muscle relaxation are occasionally necessary. Particular care is taken if stents are placed during rigid laryngoscopy. Restenosis from malacia, unsatisfactory tumor debulking, or laryngospasm can lead to loss of the airway. The rigid bronchoscope should be readily available, and a physician expert at airway intubation must be present. Ideally, stent insertion should be performed only by a bronchoscopist expert at interventional pulmonary techniques and supported by a well-trained team of nurses and technicians. Close collaboration with an experienced anesthesiologist is essential. When dealing with a severe subglottic stenosis, it may be desirable to have an emergency tracheotomy tray available.

BRONCHOSCOPIC SILICONE STENT INSERTION (BEFORE STENTING)

During bronchoscopic examination, the type and extent of airway stricture should be noted. If the length and diameter of the stenosis must be assessed, the stricture must be first passed with either the rigid or flexible bronchoscope. Preliminary dilatation is performed carefully to avoid substantial mechanical or thermal damage to bronchial epithelium. The diameter of the stenosis is measured using the rigid bronchoscope or open-flexible biopsy forceps. The length of the stricture can be precisely measured using the flexible bronchoscope by placing the scope at the distal aspect of the stricture and withdrawing the scope slowly to the proximal aspect. By measuring the length of the part of the withdrawn endoscope, the extent of the stricture can be determined accurately. This is also possible during rigid bronchoscopy using either a suction catheter or the rigid telescope. Only direct visualization results in perfect measurements of stricture length and diameter. Fluoroscopic examination without bronchoscopic control provides estimations of these measurements. A miscalculation can result in improper stent placement and the need for additional therapeutic intervention.

Immediately prior to stent insertion, depth of general anesthesia and preoxygenation with 100% oxygen are assured. These are important because complete airway obstruction or even loss of the airway may occur at the time of stent insertion. It is noteworthy that stent insertion under local anesthesia should be performed only in rare cases of distal tracheal or bronchial stenosis and if the residual airway lumen allows safe ventilation during insertion. Silicone stent insertion under local anesthesia, although possible, is generally not advocated.[31,57,58]

BRONCHOSCOPIC SILICONE STENT INSERTION (DURING STENTING)

Regardless of stent implantation technique, the largest possible diameter prosthesis should be selected to prevent stent migration. In addition, silicone stents should extend 1 cm beyond the proximal and distal margins of the stricture to assure airway patency and prevent recurrent obstruction by tumor overgrowth or granulation tissue. Preliminary bronchial toilet should always be performed with a flexible bronchoscope to remove secretions, blood, or necrotic debris within the airways.

Once the stent is inserted, distal or proximal malposition is corrected by pulling or pushing the stent with the beveled tip of the bronchoscope or using grasping forceps. Insufficient stent expansion may require additional dilatation with smaller-caliber rigid bronchoscopes or a balloon catheter. Occasionally, the stent may be left in place partially expanded since it will gradually expand on its own during the subsequent 24 to 48 h. If, however, the stent is too small and does not appear firmly fixed within the airway stricture, a larger stent should be immediately placed since there is little doubt that stent migration will occur. Because straight silicone stents do not adapt well to the bends and curves of the tracheobronchial tree, these stents lean into the airway wall, facilitating secretion accumulation and obstruction. In certain cases, however, the stent is sufficiently rigid to straighten the airway and maintain patency. If the proximal or distal aspect of the stent rubs against the wall, however, cough and granulation tissue formation may result. This will eventually require repeat bronchoscopy, laser resection, or stent removal.

BRONCHOSCOPIC SILICONE STENT INSERTION (AFTER STENTING)

After stent insertion, flexible bronchoscopy should again be performed to ensure complete airway patency and to remove any additional secretions or blood resulting from the insertion technique itself. Because oxygen saturation usually falls during stent insertion, 100% oxygen and assisted ventilation should be delivered immediately following placement. Patients are extubated when hemodynamically stable. After a short time in the postanesthesia care unit, and usually after obtaining a radiograph of the chest to document stent position, patients can be discharged. Thus, many procedures are performed on a same-day-admission basis, although patients with subglottic strictures may warrant overnight observation and corticosteroids because of the greater risks and consequences of laryngospasm and complete upper tracheal obstruction.

Results

There is no doubt that stent insertion is safe and effective when performed by experienced bronchoscopists who are knowledgeable of the indications and limitations of this procedure. In patients with malignancy, stent placement is justifiable for palliation of dyspnea and to improve quality of life. Although randomized, prospective controlled studies are not available and are probably ethically unjustifiable at this point, several studies have demonstrated the effectiveness of stents in this patient population (Table 8-3). Few studies have been designed to assess the stent's effect on outcome, quality of life, or survival. Obviously, it is difficult to control for many confounding factors such as extent of disease, type of underlying malignancy, and effects of previous or subsequent adjuvant therapy when evaluating the therapeutic utility of this procedure. Effect on pulmonary function is also difficult to assess because so many stents are inserted under emergency conditions in suffocating patients. In cases where pulmonary function studies have been obtained prior to stent insertion, it appears that restored large airway patency leads to improvement of flow-volume curves and expiratory flows.[59–61]

The majority of authors, therefore, provide a descriptive, often experiential analysis of retrospective case studies. The majority report substantial clinical improvement, relief of dyspnea, and subjectively

Table 8-3
LARGER STUDIES OF SILICONE TRACHEOBRONCHIAL STENTS

Author	*No. of patients*	*Outcome*
Colt et al., 1993[18]	206	Complications usually minor (migration 15%, granulation 20%, and obstruction by secretions or tumor 3%). Follow-up to 3 years.
Bolliger et al., 1993[34]	31	90% had lasting improvement. Complications in 30%. Median survival 2.5 months in case of malignancy.
Sonett et al., 1995[38]	57	Stent adjustment frequently required. All patients had symptomatic relief. Median survival in cancer 3–10 months, migration most frequent in transplant patients.
Martinez-Ballarin et al., 1996[41]	63	Migration 17%, granuloma 6%, obstruction 6%. Follow up to 18 months.
Strausz et al., 1994[58]	38	Migration in 28%. Follow up to 5 months.
Dumon et al., 1996[37]	1058	Multi-institutional study, 7-year experience. Migration 10%, secretion 4%, granulation 8%. Mean duration (benign disease) 14 months, (malignancy) 4 months.

demonstrated improved quality of life. Stents efficiently restore airway patency. It also appears that time to tumor recurrence and central-airway obstruction is less than after laser resection alone. Because stents are often inserted as part of a life-saving intervention in terminally ill patients, survival is understandably limited. In several studies, patients lived only 3 to 10 months after stent insertion for malignant-airway disease.

Patients with benign central-airway obstruction also benefit from airway stenting. It appears, however, that stents must be left in position for a minimum of 12 months to prevent stricture recurrence. Controlled studies comparing stenting to open-surgical procedures or to other bronchoscopic interventions alone are not available. There is no doubt, however, that stents are particularly beneficial in patients with severe, recurrent, central airway obstruction due to systemic illnesses such as amyloidosis or Wegener's granulomatosis, or as a result of scarring after infection with tuberculosis or fungi. In these patients, mucosal changes are often extensive enough to preclude any form of open-surgical intervention.

Figure 8-3

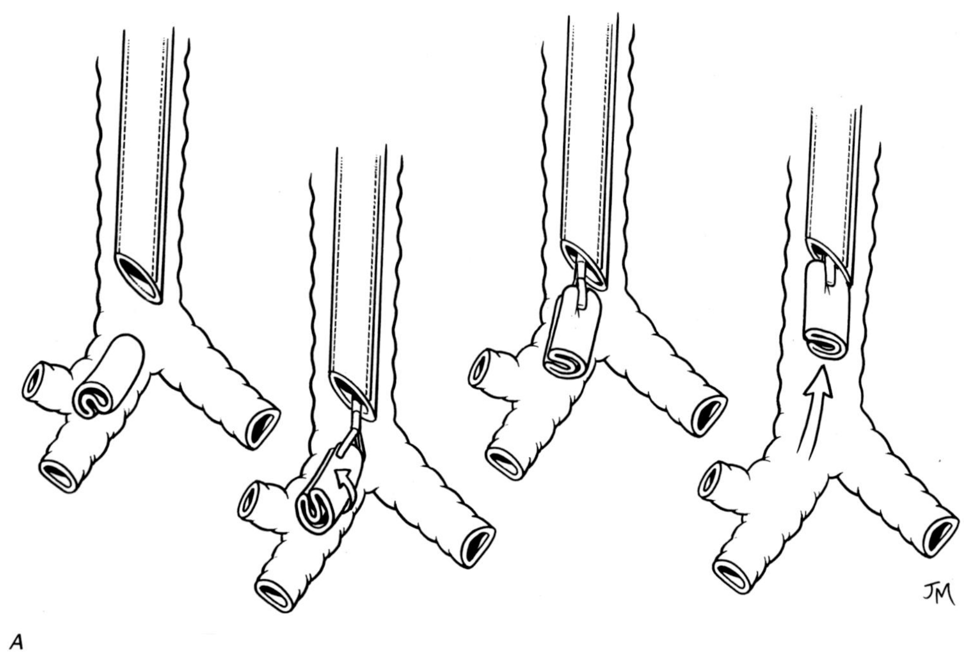

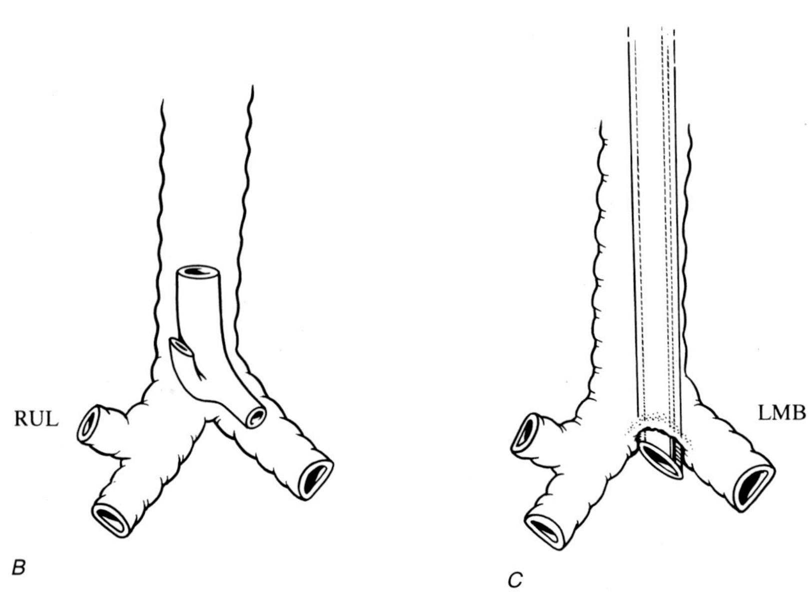

Potential problems. *A*. Straight silicone stent does not unfold. If stent expansion does not occur (*far left*) despite using forceps, balloons, or rigid tubes of smaller diameter, the stent must be grasped with forceps (*second from left*), twisted and pulled up into the rigid bronchoscope (*third from left*). The bronchoscope-stent-forceps ensemble is removed (*far right*). *B*. Malpositioned Y stent with folding of the short limb at or above the carina. This can often be avoided by using the Fogarty catheter guide technique. *C*. Unsatisfactory positioning of the bronchoscope into the left or right main bronchus. Forceful ejection of the stent can result in laceration of the posteromedial wall of the bronchus and stent ejection into the mediastinum.

Complications

The complications of stent insertion are related primarily to malposition (Fig. 8-3), obstruction by granulation tissue or tumor, stent migration, or infection (MOMI). Physicians working with stented patients should be aware of these potential problems because careful clinical, radiographic, or bronchoscopic surveillance is warranted.

Malposition results from unsatisfactory rigid bronchoscopic technique, altered tracheobronchial anatomy due to the underlying disease, and errors in stent selection. A stent too large or too long may fully obstruct a lateral segmental bronchus. During insertion, stents may not unfold longitudinally, or, as in the case of Y stents, a distal bronchial limb may get "caught" at the carina. A stent too small will likely migrate later, or may even be dislodged shortly after insertion. A stent too short may not span the stricture and result in fibrous tissue formation or granulation tissue formation. Tumor may also cause obstruction of the proximal or distal openings of the stent. Stent malposition may result in complete lobar atelectasis, postobstructive pneumonia, cough, fever, or dyspnea. In selected instances, however, there may be no choice but to partially or totally obstruct a segmental bronchus.

Migration occurs more frequently in patients requiring stent insertion for benign disease than in patients with airway neoplasms. This is probably because substantial extrinsic compression by a growing neoplasm wedges the stent in place. In patients with cancer, migration may occur because of resolving extrinsic compression after systemic therapy. Although troublesome, migration is very rarely life-threatening. In patients with either benign or malignant stenosis, migration may occur during a powerful or persistent cough, or because recurrent stricture formation at the distal or proximal margin of the stent pushes the prosthesis out of position. Distal stent migration results in recurrent stricture with its subsequent symptoms. Proximal stent migration may result in cough, hoarseness, or loss of voice. Sometimes stents are expectorated, accidently ingested, or caught between the vocal cords. Rigid or flexible bronchoscopy is immediately warranted[62] to determine need for stent removal or repositioning.

In carefully selected cases of subglottic stenosis, percutaneous stent fixation, either internal or external, may be desirable[63,64] (Fig. 8-4). In these cases, malposition is primarily a result of technical error. Either inaccurate measurements of the stricture's diameter and length were made, or the general relationship of the stricture to surrounding tracheobronchial anatomy (especially distance from the vocal cords) was misjudged.

Cough or hemoptysis may be caused by rubbing of the distal or proximal aspect of the stent against bronchial mucosa. Friction promotes granulation tissue formation. The impact of underlying inflammatory airway disease on granulation tissue formation, however, is unknown. As the stent moves during inspiration and expiration, further friction occurs. Abundant granulation tissue may require stent removal and laser resection for tissue ablation. Similarly, extensive tumor growth at the proximal or distal aspects of the stent may also cause stent obstruction. In selected cases, se-

Figure 8-4

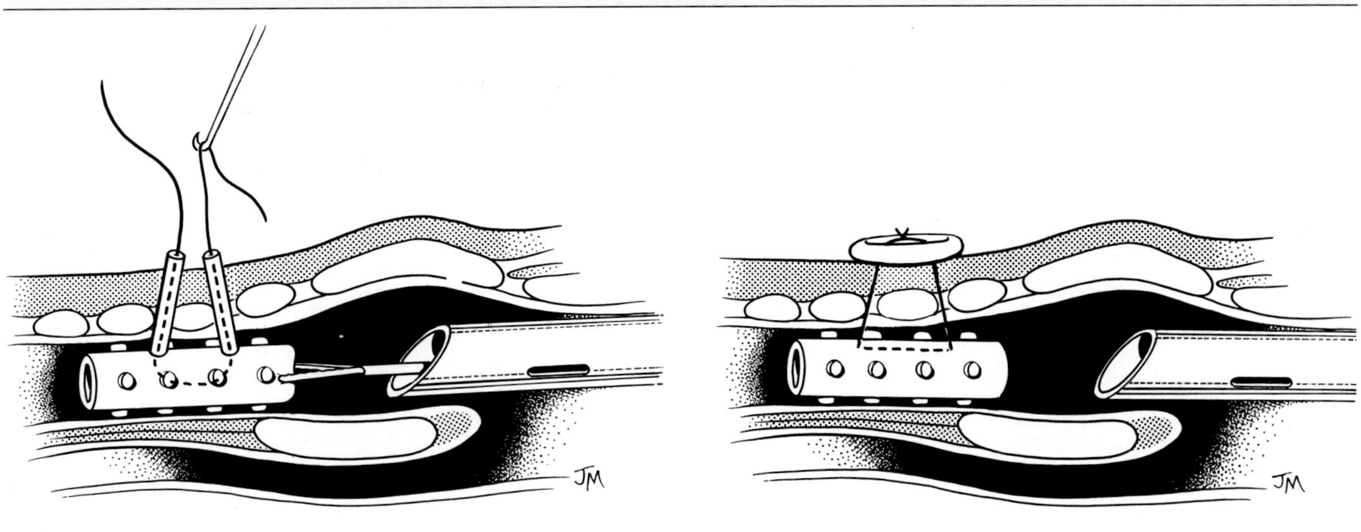

A B

Stent fixation technique. *A*. With the stent in position and held in place with forceps through the rigid scope, two angiocatheters are inserted through the anterior neck and trachea into the stent. Needles are withdrawn, leaving the catheters in place. The suture is inserted through one of the catheters and withdrawn using a Bodkin threader through the other. *B*. The suture is secured over a silicone button fixing the stent externally, or knotted and buried within subcutaneous tissues (internal fixation).

quential insertion of stents of increasing length and diameter may become necessary.

Overall, silicone stents are extremely well tolerated, and infection is very rare. Flexible bronchoscopy, however, should probably be performed if patients present with productive cough. The stent may be partially obstructed from tenacious mucoid or purulent secretions, or there may be evidence of substantial airway inflammation distal to the stent. Aspiration of secretions is usually performed by flexible bronchoscopy alone. Antibiotics may also be warranted. To prevent obstruction by tenacious secretions and enhance mucocillary clearance expectoration, humidification of the airways using large drop or ultrasound saline nebulization is advocated.

Surveillance after Stent Insertion

There are few rules regarding clinical, radiographic, or bronchoscopic surveillance. Most silicone stents are visible on chest radiographs and present as straight edges within the tracheobronchial tree. For this reason, many operators routinely obtain postinsertion radiographs for use as baseline controls. When patients are seen many months later, stent migration, atelectasis, or pneumonia can be readily diagnosed by viewing a repeat chest film, even in asymptomatic patients. The clinical examination is suggestive of stent obstruction if breath sounds are decreased or absent. Repeat bronchoscopic evaluation every 2 to 3 months may also be necessary if sequential stenting with increasing larger or longer stents is warranted, or if migration is suspected, as in patients undergoing adjuvant therapy for cancer. It is unclear whether surveillance bronchoscopy performed in the absence of symptoms suggestive of a complication is either warranted or cost-effective.

Training, Competence, and Maintenance of Proficiency

In the ideal setting, physicians performing stent procedures should be trained in both flexible and rigid bronchoscopy and be familiar with most, if not all, techniques of interventional pulmonology. The most efficient way of managing patients with benign and malignant central airway obstruction is to have a complete arsenal of therapeutic modalities available. This includes rigid bronchoscopic debulking, laser resection, stent insertion, brachytherapy, and of course potential for close collaboration with otolaryngologists, thoracic surgeons, radiation oncologists, and anesthesiologists. Training, competence, and maintenance of proficiency have not yet been addressed by the pulmonary societies. As interest in interventional pulmonology grows, however, these delicate issues need to be faced. Nationally and internationally sponsored training seminars with hands-on workshops are increasingly offered to provide interested physicians and surgeons with a basic understanding of the indications and techniques of stent insertion and introduce them to commercially available equipment. Credentialing, of course, is always determined within individual institutions.

Conclusion

The rigid bronchoscope is the workhorse of the interventional pulmonologist. Silicone stents are almost always inserted during rigid bronchoscopy under general anesthesia. In experienced hands, stent insertion is safe and effective, providing excellent palliation against the dreadful, life-threatening effects of central airway obstruction. Although migration, obstruction, or infection may occur, complications are usually managed easily. Unlike metal stents, silcone stents can be easily removed or replaced. Properly designed clinical studies are necessary, however, to assess the effect of silicone stents on pulmonary function, quality of life, survival, and utilization of health care resources.[65] Of course, the indications for silicone stent insertion are limited to symptomatic central-airway obstruction despite other bronchoscopic or adjuvant therapies in patients with malignant or benign airway disease. Whether stenting should be performed exclusively in centers of excellence where operators have a complete arsenal of therapeutic intervention and clinical research available is a controversial issue that health care reorganization may force us to address in the future.

HOW I DO IT

Using the Rigid Bronchoscope to Insert the Stent

Straight silicone stents are inserted through the rigid bronchoscope, using a specially designed stent introducer system, or over the rigid bronchoscope, using either an endotracheal tube or a chest tube as a stent pusher. A third technique is to load the stent onto the beveled aspect of the rigid bronchoscope with the telescope inside, exerting pressure onto the stent with the telescope from the inside while exerting pressure from the opposite end of the bronchoscope. In general, however, direct visualization of the stent insertion process is not necessary if the bronchoscope has been satisfactorily placed through the stricture prior to stent ejection and the bronchoscopist has sufficient experience with the techniques and "feel" of rigid bronchoscopy. The stent may be folded in half longitudinally and inserted either into the distal end of the rigid bronchoscope or ideally into the hollow stent introducer tube. Inserting the stent into the rigid bronchoscope only (without using an introducer tube) is dangerous because the stent will completely obstruct the distal aspect of the bronchoscope and visualization cannot be assured during intubation. Using the stent introducer system, the rigid bronchoscope is left in place within the stricture, the telescope is removed, and the "loaded" introducer tube is inserted into the rigid bronchoscope. The stent is ejected using a pusher while the rigid bronchoscope is pulled proximally. If the stent does not unfold completely or is not entirely ejected from the rigid bronchoscope, it may be pushed into place with a rigid telescope that is reintroduced into the rigid tube once the introducer and pusher are withdrawn. The stent can also be manipulated with grasping forceps (Fig. 8-5). When a stent is loaded onto the outer aspect of the rigid bronchoscope, the rigid bronchoscope, stent, and rigid telescope are inserted together into position within the stricture. Prior to intubation, an uncuffed endotracheal tube or cut chest tube is placed over the rigid bronchoscope. This tube is used to push the stent into position as the rigid bronchoscope is withdrawn. Satisfactory preliminary airway dilatation is essential. Y-shaped stents can also be loaded into the specially designed introducer and pushed out into the stricture through the rigid bronchoscope. Several other techniques are also possible. Stents may be loaded onto the outside of the rigid bronchoscope and pushed into place using a 36 Fr straight silicone chest tube; the proximal aspect of the stent may be sutured to decrease its overall lumen, facilitating insertion and preventing intussusception of

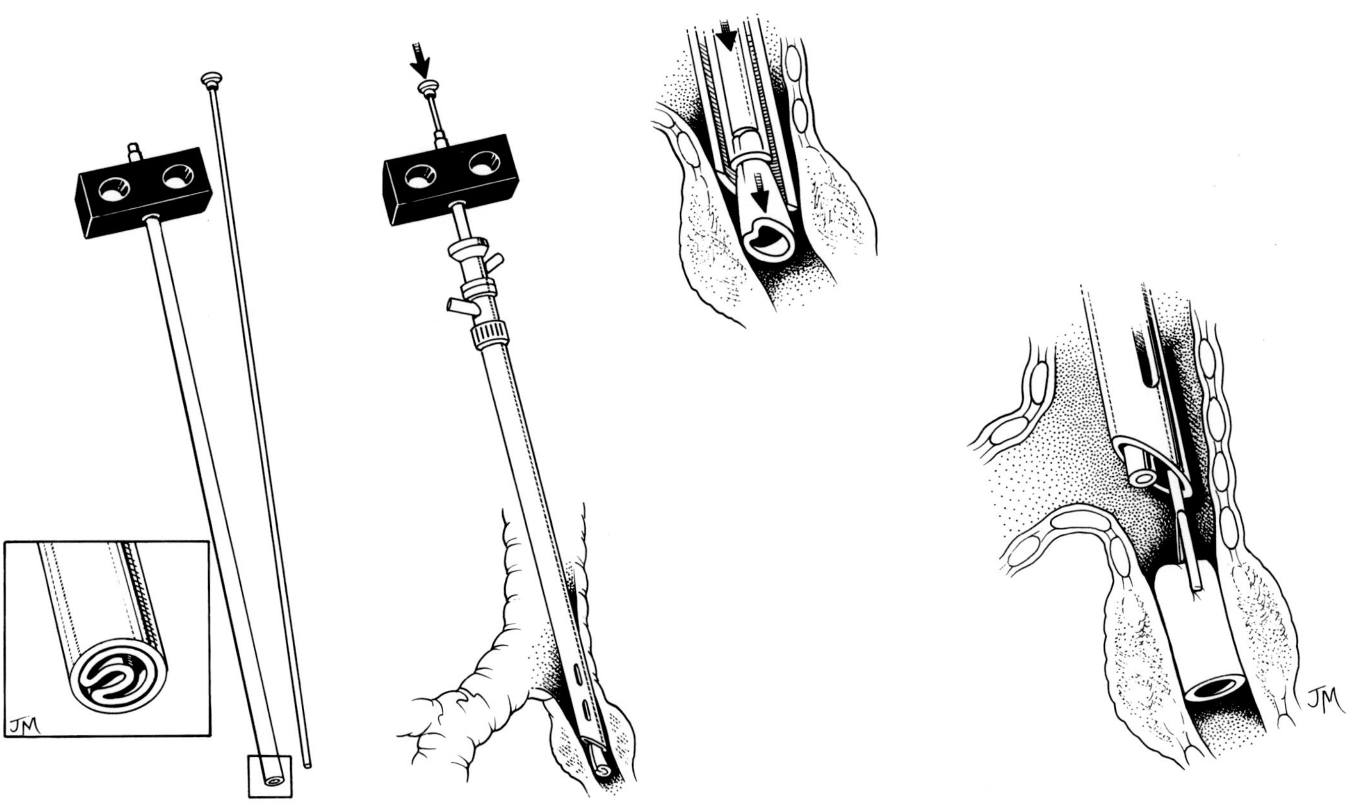

A B C

Figure 8-5

The stent introducer system. *A*. The rigid bronchoscope is in position with its beveled tip at the distal aspect of the stricture. The telescope has been removed, and the stent, loaded into the introducer, is placed into the rigid scope. *B*. The pusher is used to eject the stent as the rigid scope is pulled proximally. As the stent is gradually ejected, the scope is pulled back through the stricture. If necessary, the telescope can be inserted to push the stent out of the scope into position. *C*. The stent can be unfolded using forceps through the rigid tube. The stent is grasped and rotated 180 to 360 degrees. The stent is easily pulled or pushed into place within the stricture.

the chest tube into the stent; or a guide wire or Fogarty balloon catheter may be inserted adjacent to the rigid bronchoscope and through the right bronchial limb of the stent to prevent folding of the shorter limb of the Y stent at the level of the carina (Fig. 8-6).

Using the Flexible Bronchoscope to Insert the Stent

This technique has been described by Strausz and coworkers.[58] It may be helpful on rare occasions if stent insertion is necessary and patients cannot tolerate general anesthesia. A chest tube or endotracheal tube is placed over the flexible fiberoptic bronchoscope. A 100-cm-long silk or polypropylene suture is then placed through the distal aspect of the silicone stent to help secure its position at the distal aspect of the flexible fiberoptic bronchoscope adjacent to the chest tube pusher. The flexible bronchoscope with the stent and pusher on it is inserted through the mouth and past the vocal cords. Substantial preliminary dilatation of the airway stricture is essential. As the flexible bronchoscope is introduced through the stricture, the scope is held at the mouth and the stent is pushed into position through the stricture. The stent is held firmly in place using the sutures, and the flexible bronchoscope is gently withdrawn. The endotracheal tube or chest tube can be left in place in case further adjustments are necessary. If the stent is distal to the stricture, it can be pulled back into position using the sutures. Flexible bronchoscopy then ensures that the stent is in its appropriate position, the threads are withdrawn, the pusher is pulled back over the flexible bronchoscope, and the flexible bronchoscope is removed.

Using the Rigid Laryngoscope to Insert the Stent

This technique can be used to insert the Rusch Y stent or other silicone Y stents. Such bifurcated stents can be placed using an operating laryngoscope, or during

Figure 8-6

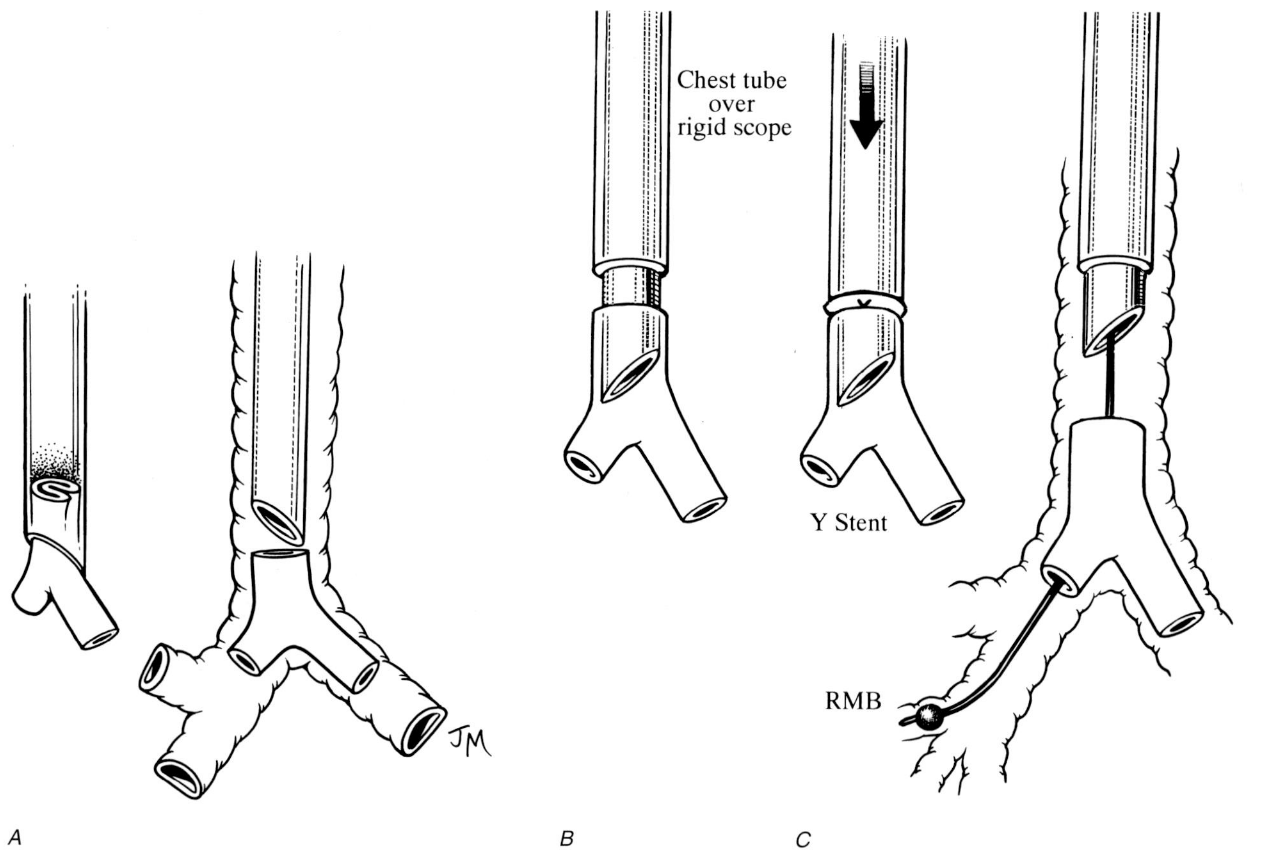

Y stent insertion. *A*. Sometimes the Y stent is loaded into the introducer, carefully preserving left and right direction (*left*). The stent is ejected at the carina so each limb slips naturally into the appropriate bronchus (*right*). *B*. Y stents can be loaded onto the rigid bronchoscope and pushed into place using a chest tube pusher. *C*. Alternative techniques include using (*left*) a suture to narrow the proximal limb of the stent to prevent intussusception of the chest tube into the stent and (*right*) a Fogarty catheter used as a guide through the distal right bronchial limb of the stent. The balloon is inflated to fix the catheter into position, and the right or left bronchial limb of the stent is loaded onto the bronchoscope, then pushed into place using the chest tube pusher.

Figure 8-7

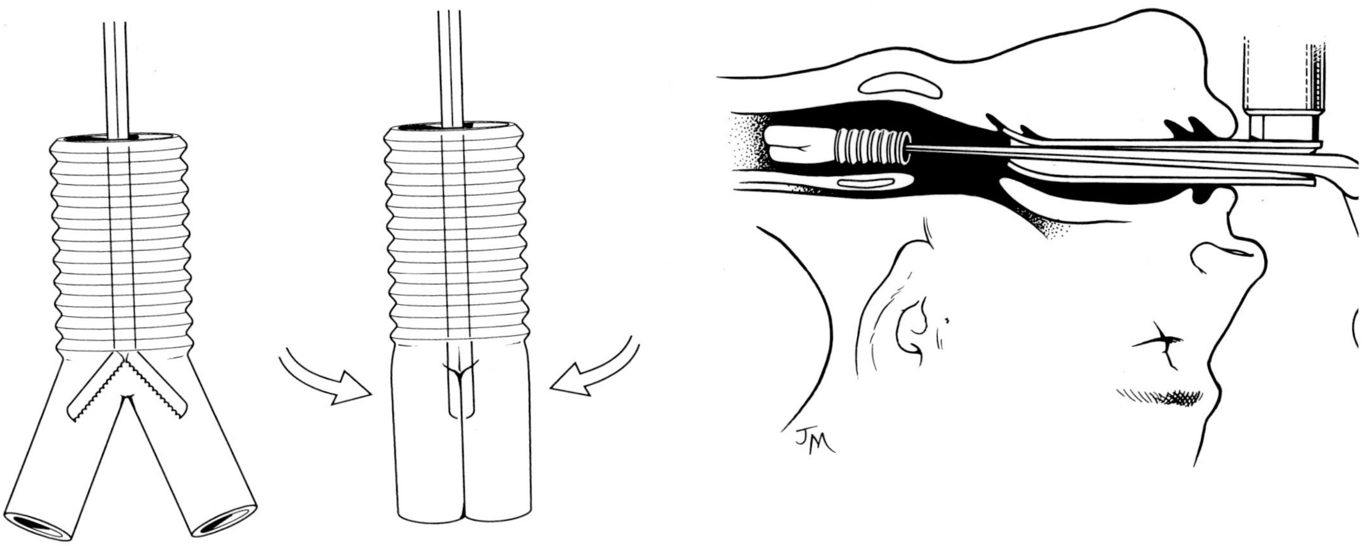

A *B*

The Rusch stent. *A*. The stent is grasped at its bifurcation using a specially designed forceps with built-in pusher. *B*. Rigid laryngoscopy exposes the vocal cords. The stent is then inserted into the airways.

rigid laryngoscopy with or without the help of fluoroscopy and guide catheters. More recently, the Storz Manufacturing Company has marketed a special stent forceps which both grasps and pushes the stent into place. The bifurcated stent is grabbed from the inside with the stent forceps. Rigid laryngoscopy is performed, and the stent is inserted past the vocal cords on the rigid forceps (Fig. 8-7). Once past the larynx and the tracheal stricture, the forceps are carefully opened, and the bronchial limbs can be felt extending into their respective main bronchi. The adjustable pusher mounted on the forceps can be used to anchor the stent in place while the grasping component of the forceps is withdrawn. With the stent in place, the forceps are withdrawn, and the patient is intubated with the rigid bronchoscope to verify stent position and patency. To ensure complete expansion and proper positioning of the bronchial limbs, several techniques are advocated. The stent may be pushed into the left main bronchus and gradually withdrawn allowing the bronchial limbs to open; the stent may be placed at the level of the carina as the bronchial limbs snap open into their appropriate positions; or skin markers and fluoroscopy, as well as a guide wire or Fogarty balloon catheter, can be used to ensure proper stent placement and complete unfolding of the bronchial limbs.

REFERENCES

1. Flexner SB (ed): *The Random House Dictionary of the English Language.* New York, Random House, 1987:1553.
2. Colt HG, Dumon JF: Airway obstruction in cancer: Pros and cons of stents. *J Respir Dis* 1991; 12:741–749.
3. Becker HD: Stenting of the central airways. *J Bronchol* 1995; 2:98–106.
4. Graziano J, et al: Prosthetic replacement of the tracheal carina. *Ann Thorac Surg* 1967; 4:1–11.
5. Harkins WB: An endobronchial metallic prosthesis in the treatment of stenosis of the trachea. *Ann Otol Rhinol Laryngol* 1952; 61:663–675.
6. Neville WE, et al: Replacement of the intrathoracic trachea and both stem bronchi with a molded silastic prosthesis. *J Thorac Cardiovasc Surg* 1972; 63:569–576.
7. Jackson C: Bronchoscopy and esophagoscopy: *A Manual of Peroral Endoscopy and Laryngeal Surgery.* Philadelphia, Saunders, 1927.
8. Colt HG, Dumon JF: Airway stents: Present and future. *Clin Chest Med* 1995; 16:465–478.
9. Edell ES, et al: The use of prosthetic stents in tracheobronchial, gastrointestinal, and genitourinary diseases. *Diag Therap Endosc* 1994; 1:1–8.
10. Montgomery WW: T-tube tracheal stent. *Arch Otolaryngol* 1965; 82:320–321.
11. Duvall AJ, Bauer W: An endoscopically introducible T-tube for tracheal stenosis. *Laryngoscope* 1977; 87:2031–2037.
12. Westaby S, et al: A bifurcated silicone rubber stent for relief of tracheobronchial obstruction. *J Thorac Cardiovasc Surg* 1982; 83:414–417.
13. Clarke DB: Palliative intubation of the trachea and main bronchi. *J Thorac Cardiovasc Surg* 1980; 80:736–741.
14. Cooper JD, et al: Use of silicone stents in the management of airway problems. *Ann Thorac Surg* 1989; 47:371–378.
15. Orlowski TM: Palliative intubation of the tracheobronchial tree. *J Thorac Cardiovasc Surg* 1987; 94:343–348.
16. Dumon JF: A dedicated tracheobronchial stent. *Chest* 1990; 97:328–332.
17. Shapshay SM, et al: Total cervical tracheal stenosis: treatment by laser, dilatation, and stenting. *Ann Otol Rhinol Laryngol* 1989; 98:890–895.
18. Colt HG, Dumon JF: Tracheobronchial stents: Indications and applications. *Lung Cancer* 1993; 9:301–306.
19. Domscke W, et al: Self-expanding mesh stent for esophageal cancer stenosis. *Endoscopy* 1990; 22:134–136.

20. George PJ, et al: Covered expandable metal stent for recurrent tracheal obstruction. *Lancet* 335:582–584, 1990.
21. Schaer J, et al: Treatment of malignant esophageal obstruction with silicone-coated metallic self-expanding stents. *Gastrointest Endosc* 1992; 38:7–11.
22. Wong K, Goldstraw P: Role of covered eosphageal stents in malignant esophagorespiratory fistula. *Ann Thorac Surg* 1995; 60:199–200.
23. Cooper JD, et al: Use of the silicone tracheal T-tube for the management of complex tracheal injuries. *J Thorac Cardiovasc Surv* 1981; 82:559–568.
24. Insall RL, Morritt GN: Palliation of malignant tracheal strictures using silicone T tubes. *Thorax* 1991; 46:168–171.
25. Montgomery WW, Montgomery SK: Manual for use of Montgomery layrngeal, tracheal, and esophageal prostheses: Update 1990. *Ann Otol Rhinol Laryngol* 1990; 99(suppl):1–28.
26. Acuff TE, et al: Simplified placement of a silicone tracheal Y stent. *Ann Thorac Surg* 1994; 57:496–497.
27. Gaer JAR, et al: Use of endotracheal silicone stents for relief of tracheobronchial obstruction. *Ann Thorac Surg* 1992; 54:512–516.
28. Noppen M, et al: A simplified insertion technique for tracheobronchial stents. *Chest* 1994; 106:520–523.
29. Noppen M, et al: A new screw thread tracheal endoprosthesis. *J Bronchol* 1996; 3:22–26.
30. Freitag L, et al: Theoretical and experimental basis for the development of a dynamic airway stent. *Eur Respir J* 1994; 7:2038–2045.
31. Freitag L, et al: Bifurcated dynamic airway stent insertion using flexible bronchoscopy. *J Bronchol* 1995; 2:130–134.
32. Freitag L, et al: Mechanical properties of airway stents. *J Bronchol* 1995; 2:270–278.
33. Bolliger CT, et al: Covered Wallstent insertion in a patient with conical tracheobronchial stenosis. *J Bronchol* 1996; 2:215–218.
34. Bolliger CT, et al: Silicone stents in the management of inoperable tracheobronchial stenoses; Indications and limitations. *Chest* 1993; 104:1653–1659.
35. Cortese DA, Edell ES: Role of phototherapy, laser therapy, brachytherapy, and prosthetic stents in the management of lung cancer. *Clin Chest Med* 1993; 1:149–159.
36. Diaz-Jimenez JP, et al: Silicone stents in the management of obstructive tracheobronchial lesions: 2 year experience. *J Bronchol* 1994; 1:15–18.
37. Dumon JF, et al: Seven year experience with the Dumon prosthesis. *J Bronchol* 1996; 3:6–10.
38. Sonett JR, et al: Endobronchial management of benign, malignant, and lung transplantation airway stenoses. *Ann Thorac Surg* 1995; 59:1417–1422.
39. Tsang V, Williams AM, Goldstraw P: Sequential silastic and expandable metal stenting for tracheobronchial strictures. *Ann Thorac Surg* 1992; 53:856–860.
40. Cavaliere S, et al: Nd:YAG laser therapy in lung cancer: An 11 year experience with 2,253 applications in 1,585 patients. *J Bronchol* 1994; 1:105–111.
41. Martinez-Ballarin JI, et al: Silicone stents in the management of benign tracheobronchial stenoses: Tolerance and early results in 63 patients. Chest 1996; 109:626–629.
42. Petrou M, et al: Bronchoscopic diathermy resection and stent insertion: A cost effective treatment for tracheobronchial obstruction. *Thorax* 1993; 48:1156–1159.
43. Sutedja G, et al: Stent placement is justifiable in end stage patients with malignant airway tumors. *Respiration* 1995; 62: 148–150.
44. Witt C, et al: Flexible bronchoscopic stenting followed by radiation in malignant obstruction of central airways. *J Bronchol* 1995; 2:118–122.
45. Albes JM, et al: Tracheal stenting for malignant tracheoesophageal fistula. *Ann Thorac Surg* 1994; 57:1263–1266.
46. Colt HG, et al: Double stents for carcinoma of the esophagus invading the tracheobronchial tree. *Gastrointest Endosc* 1992; 38:485–489.
47. Shennib H, Massard G: Airway complications in lung transplantation. *Ann Thorac Surg* 1994; 57:506–511.
48. Colt HG, et al: Endoscopic management of bronchial stenosis after double lung transplantation. *Chest* 1992; 102:10–16.
49. Schafers HJ, et al: Decreased incidence of bronchial complications following lung transplantation. *Eur J Cardio-thorac Surg* 1992; 6:174–179.
50. Haydock DA, et al: Lung transplantation. Analysis of thirty-six consecutive procedures performed over a twelve month period. *J Thorac Cardiovasc Surg* 1992; 103:329–340.
51. Yousem SA, et al: Bronchial cartilage alterations in lung transplantation. *Chest* 1990; 98:1121–1124.
52. Duckett JE, et al: General anesthesia for Nd;YAG laser resection of obstructing endobronchial tumors using the rigid bronchoscope. *Can Anesth Soc* 1985; 32:67–72.
53. Hermens JM, et al: Anesthesia for laser surgery. *Anesth Analg* 1983; 62:218–229.
54. Lennon RL, et al: Monitoring and analysis of oxygenation and ventilation during rigid bronchoscopic neodymium-YAG laser resection of airway tumors. *Mayo Clin Proc* 1987; 62:584–588.
55. Perrin G, et al: Safety of interventional rigid bronchoscopy using intravenous anesthesia and spontaneous assisted ventilation: A prospective study. *Chest* 1992; 102:1526–1530.
56. Vourc'h G, et al: Anesthetic management during Nd:YAG laser resection for major tracheobronchial obstructing tumors. *Anesthesiology* 1984; 61:636–637.
57. deCastro FR, et al: Tracheobronchial stents and fiberoptic bronchoscopy *Chest* 1991; 99:792 (letter).
58. Strausz J, et al: Tracheobronchial silicone stent implantation with the flexible bronchoscope. *J Bronchol* 1994; 1:123–125.
59. Gelb AF, et al: Physiologic studies of tracheobronchial stents in airway obstruction. *Am Rev Respir Dis* 1992; 146:1088–1090.
60. Edell ES, et al: Ancillary therapies in the management of lung cancer: Photodynamic therapy, laser therapy, and endobronchial prosthetic devices. *Mayo Clin Proc* 1993; 68:685–690.
61. Vergnon JM, et al: Efficacy of tracheal and bronchial stent placement on respiratory functional tests. *Chest* 1995; 107:741–746.
62. Wassermann K, et al: Emergency removal of a dislodged endobronchial silicone prosthesis using a valvuloplasty catheter through a flexible bronchoscope. *J Bronchol* 1994; 1:304–306.
63. Colt HG, et al: External fixation of tracheal stents. *Chest* 1994; 105:1653–1657.
64. Temes RT, et al: Internal fixation of high tracheal stents. *Ann Thorac Surg* 1995; 59:1023–1024.
65. Colt HG: The art and science of airway stenting. *J Bronchol* 2:263–266, 1995.

CHAPTER 9

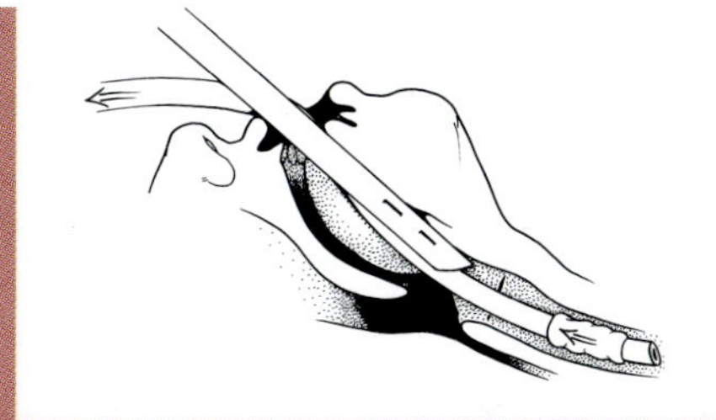

EXPANDABLE ENDOBRONCHIAL STENTS

Chris T. Bolliger and Praveen N. Mathur

Obstructing lesions of the central airways, usually defined as the trachea, both main bronchi, and the lobar orifices, are difficult to treat. In industrialized countries these obstructions are mainly caused by malignancies, whereas in developing countries they are frequently caused by benign disorders, such as tuberculosis. In addition to conventional therapy such as surgery, chemotherapy, and radiotherapy in malignancies, and antibiotic or anti-inflammatory treatment in benign disorders, local endoscopic treatment modalities are being used increasingly to treat these disorders. Endoluminal lesions (Fig. 9-1) can be treated by coring out with the rigid bronchoscope and a forceps, resection with heat (laser, high-frequency electrocautery), application of cold (cryotherapy), endoluminal irradiation (brachytherapy), or laser irradiation of previously sensitized cells (photodynamic therapy). For endoluminal lesions the choice of a specific endobronchial treatment or the combination of such modalities often depends on the preference of the interventional endoscopist and the available equipment. Obstructions caused by extraluminal or mixed lesions with an important extraluminal component (Fig. 9-1), however, are not amenable to local treatment other than by endoprostheses or stents. This chapter discusses the role of such stents in the treatment of central-airway stenoses caused by malignant and benign diseases with the focus on expandable stents. An in-depth description of silicone stents is discussed elsewhere in this book (Chap. 8).

Etiology of Central-Airway Obstruction

MALIGNANCIES

The majority of patients who present with central-airway obstruction suffer from malignancies, which include primary bronchogenic carcinoma, metastatic lesions, and direct invasion by esophageal or thyroid cancers. Most of these tumors are inoperable because of their advanced stage.[1] A minority of patients are deemed functionally inoperable because of poor cardiopulmonary reserve. Thus, the main therapeutic aim is palliation. Stent placement in malignant central-airway obstructions is indicated when a stenotic airway is either compressed from outside or in mixed stenoses if the resection of the endoluminal component is insufficient to relieve the obstruction (Fig. 9-2). In our institutions we consider stent insertion whenever the diameter of the affected airway remains below 50 percent of normal after endoscopic therapy with laser and/or dilatation.[2] Further indications are loss of cartilaginous support by tumor destruction of the airway wall, exhaustion of therapeutic options such as external beam irradiation and brachytherapy, and fast endoluminal tumor recurrence despite repetitive sessions of endoscopic tumor resection.

BENIGN DISORDERS

Benign disorders that lead to central airway obstruction are primarily postintubation stenoses with or with-

Figure 9-1

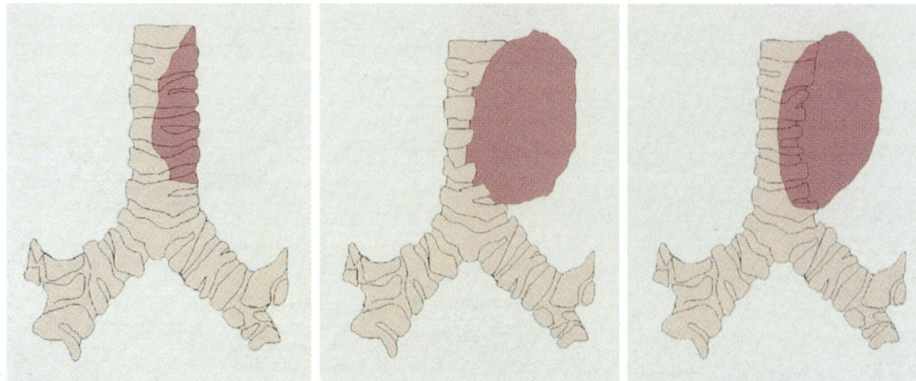

Schematic illustration of the three most important types of central airway obstruction, shown at the tracheal level with identical degree of obstruction. *A*, Endoluminal; *B*, extraluminal; and *C*, mixed.

out tracheomalacia after prolonged intubation. With the use of endotracheal tubes (ET) with low-pressure cuffs, these stenoses have become rare in industrialized countries, but they are still encountered quite frequently in areas where there is a lack of adequate finances to cover the cost of modern intensive care units with necessary equipment such as disposable ET tubes. Other etiologies are infectious diseases such as tuberculosis with enlarged lymph nodes, which can compress airways from outside or penetrate through the airway wall leading to endoluminal obstruction by

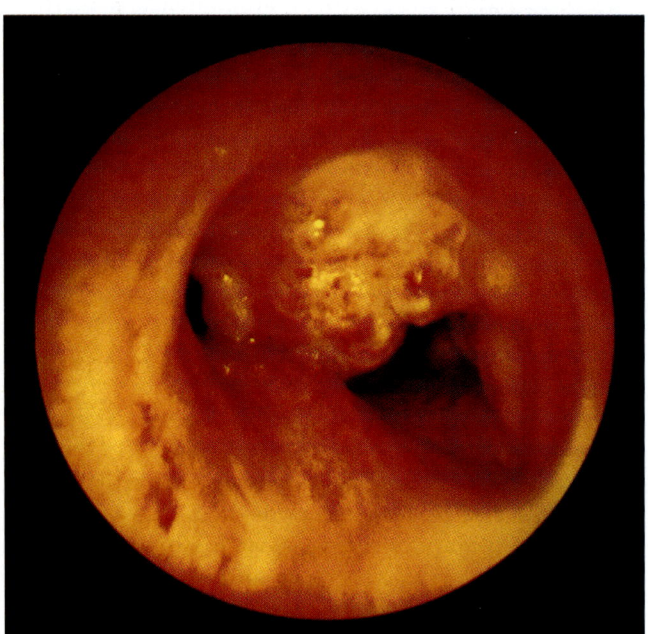

Figure 9-2

Mixed obstruction at the level of the main carina, laser resection alone is possible for the right main bronchus, whereas the left main bronchus will need a stent due to a large extraluminal component of the obstruction.

caseating material. Rarer conditions are Wegener's disease with endobronchial involvement,[3] relapsing polychondritis, tracheopathia osteoplastica, fibrosing mediastinitis, or endobronchial papillomatosis. Anastomotic stenoses after pulmonary sleeve resection[4] or stenoses after lung transplantation can lead to stenoses which can be dealt with endoscopically.[5–7] The basic principle for the treatment of benign disorders leading to obstruction of the central airways is that curative surgery should be attempted whenever feasible. The best treatment option should therefore be discussed between the specialists who are usually involved in the care of such patients, namely, interventional pulmonologists, otolaryngologists, and thoracic surgeons. Thanks to pioneering work by surgeons such as Grillo[8] and Pearson,[9] even extensive resections of the major airways have become feasible in specialized centers. There are, however, quite a few reasons for benign disorders to become unresectable: the length of the lesions may exceed resectability; the disease tends to recur after resection such as in bronchial papillomatosis, or the patient is debilitated and will or cannot undergo surgery, for example, for a goiter obstructing the trachea. Whenever stents are used in benign disorders, models should be chosen which can be removed if necessary, especially in younger patients with a long life expectancy.

Diagnosis of Central Airway Obstruction

In patients with pronounced stridor and dyspnea, obstruction of the central airways is usually easily diagnosed. If a stenosis at the tracheal, and sometimes also bronchial, level develops insidiously and the patient gets used to slowly increasing dyspnea, even advanced obstructions are misdiagnosed as asthma, emphysema, or dyspnea due to heart failure. The physician has therefore to think of the possibility of central airway obstruction and investigate patients promptly. Unexplained dyspnea should lead to a careful clinical evaluation, which might show diminished motion of half of the chest during respiration or localized wheezing on auscultation. The chest roentgenogram can indicate a central tumor or atelectasis of a lobar segment or a whole lung; CT scanning adds further information, especially about the mediastinum, and possibly vascular tumor invasion, especially of the pulmonary artery. An invaluable tool is the flow-volume loop, which is a fine diagnostic tool for the evaluation of airflow obstructions at different levels of the tracheobronchial tree.[10,11] However, obstruction of less than 50 percent of a given airway diameter is often not detected. The most important investigation is bronchoscopy with the flexible bronchoscope. This allows assessment of the type of obstruction and its extent.

Endobronchial Stents

Various stent models or endoprostheses are used for the endoscopic treatment of inoperable stenoses of the central airways, Historically the silicone T tubes by Montgomery[12] were the best known types. Anchorage of these tubes was guaranteed by the external limb which passed through a tracheostomy opening. This allowed suctioning of the trachea as through any conventional tracheostomy tube but had the same disadvantages: cosmetic problems and excessive drying of the inspired air when the T limb was not closed, leading to encrustation of dried secretions within or below the tube. For these reasons, Dumon[13,14] further developed the concept of the silicone tube by eliminating the T limb of the Montgomery tube. This resulted in a cylindrical tube with regularly placed studs on the outer surface to provide anchorage of the stent in the airway mucosa. Currently this stent (Endoxane, Novatech, Aubagne, France and Bryan Corp., Woburn, MA), available in different lengths and diameters, is the most widely used type. It is usually inserted with a special rigid delivery device without direct visual control, but its final position can be adjusted with a forceps. Its advantages are good tissue tolerance, elasticity with good clearance of secretions, and removability even after years. The disadvantages are a relatively unfavorable wall/inner-diameter ratio, especially in tight stenoses where the studs on the outside of the stent can impair full deployment. This is the case in any stenosis where the diameter remains less than 10 mm after dilation and does not allow passage of the smallest Dumon stent. Further, because of its cylindrical nature, this stent may migrate when used in conical stenoses, especially if they are less than 2.5 cm in length.[2]

In addition to various silicone stents,[15–17] expandable metal stents have also been widely used.[18–22] Although originally developed for vascular use, insertion in the tracheobronchial tree proved to be quite successful.[23,24] These stents consist of various forms of woven wire struts or meshes and are usually inserted under fluoroscopic control. Although they provide excellent initial palliation, their long-term results are often disappointing.

Theoretically these stents become epithelialized and should be well tolerated. In reality they often lead to complications. In malignant disease, tumor ingrowth through the wire mesh often occludes the stent within 2 to 3 months after placement.[25] In benign disease, the same problem arises through excessive granuloma formation.[5] Further, all these stents are more difficult to remove than the Dumon stent. Many institutions have therefore abandoned the use of uncovered metal stents. However, their very favorable wall/inner-diameter ratio, the excellent adaptability to varying airway wall diameters, and the near absence of kinking are clear advantages of metal stents. The current trend in metal stent development is therefore to cover the wire mesh with a thin layer of synthetic material to prevent stent reocclusion. So far the Gianturco[26] and the Wallstent[27] have been used in a covered version in malignant stenoses of the esophagus. Recently a new covered Wallstent called Airway Wallstent has been developed and commercialized in Europe.[28] This chapter focuses on the different types of expandable endobronchial stents. The silicone stents are discussed separately in Chap. 8.

EXPANDABLE ENDOBRONCHIAL STENTS

In the early 1980s various expandable vascular stents were developed. The different devices all follow the same technical principle. Metal wires are assembled in different ways to form a highly compressible tube, which can be inserted into a vascular stenosis and opened up after delivery from the introducer set either by spontaneous expansion (Gianturco, Wallstent) or after balloon dilatation (Palmaz, Strecker). Once the stent is open and the stenosed vessel has become patent, the stent becomes covered by vascular epithelium and can be left in place indefinitely. These stents are introduced under fluoroscopic control by radiologists and cardiologists. Currently vascular and coronary artery stenting are firmly established therapies.[21,29–31] In addition to vessels, the esophagus[32] and the biliary tract[33] are increasingly being stented with similar stents with very good results. Most of these stents can be used in the tracheobronchial tree as well, mainly because of their ease of insertion and the lack of other available devices designed for the lung. Unlike the vascular bed, however, the airways are not round muscular tubes but more complex structures with a horseshoe-shaped cartilaginous part and a soft collapsible posterior membrane. Further, the vessel lumens are kept patent by a more or less constant blood flow, whereas the airways are kept open by the cartilaginous support. On coughing, their anterior-posterior diameter narrows considerably by the inward bulging of the posterior membrane which enhances expectoration of secretions or of aspirated material. Thus, the shape of the ideal tracheobronchial stent would have to imitate the cross section of the natural airways. All the available expandable stents are cylindrical tubes and clearly do not fulfill these requirements. Fortunately, central airway obstruction requiring stent insertion has often altered the anatomy and the function of the stenotic segment to such an extent that insertion of a round stent leads to dramatic functional improvement despite the conceptual shortcomings of the stent design.

TYPES OF EXPANDABLE STENTS

The Gianturco stent consists of a continuous loop of stainless steel zigzag wire (William Cook Europe, Bjaeverskov, Denmark) and is available for tracheobronchial use in either single units of 2.5 cm in length or a double length with two units welded together resulting in a 5-cm length.[18] The unconstrained stent diameters are 15, 20, and 30 mm. Small metal hooks near the stent ends guarantee firm hold in the mucosa (Fig. 9-3). These stents can be inserted in highly compressed form through a long introducer sheath that contains the stent at its distal end. Deployment takes place under fluoroscopy. The stent is pushed out of the sheath by a stent positioner and expands immediately. Although deployment of this stent is very simple, the single stent of 2.5-cm length has a tendency to jump forward if released too quickly, which can result in too distal placement. The Gianturco stents rarely ever migrate but are almost impossible to remove. The reports on the long-term outcome vary greatly from center to center. Some authors report good results with epithelialization of the stent and uneventful follow-up over years in malignant[23,34] and benign airway strictures.[7,35–37] The majority of specialists using different stent types find the Gianturco stent prone to cause unacceptable complications. In malignant disease, the wire zigzag offers virtually no protection from tumor ingrowth,[38] and very often the airway is completely reoccluded by recurrent tumor growth after 1 to 2 months. In benign disorders, the stent may become imbedded in columnar epithelium and give satisfactory long-term results. However, the mucosa often reacts with granuloma formation, leading to the same reocclusion of the airway as in malignant disease.[5] Other serious complications are stent fractures[39] and penetration through the airway wall, which can occasionally lead to fatal erosion of major vessels[35] or to tracheoesophageal fistulas.[40] Penetration through the airway wall is most likely at the tracheal level when stents with an oversize unconstrained diameter of 30 mm are used. In light of the emerging number of complications, many institutions have abandoned the use of the Gianturco stent. Recently a covered version of the Gianturco stent has been introduced for esophageal use[26]; a covered version for the tracheobronchial tree has been described,[41] but has not been commercialized.

The Strecker Stent (Boston Scientific International, Natack, MA) is a balloon-expandable vascular prosthesis which consists of a flexible, knitted tantalum wire mesh tube.[20,42] It is available for bronchial use in 2- and 4-cm lengths with an expanded lumen of 8 and 11 mm. It is mounted in compressed form on a balloon catheter and deployed under fluoroscopy (Figs. 9-4 and 9-5). The stent is knitted from a single filament resulting in a series of loosely connected loops which make the stent elastic and very flexible. The endless wire makes removal in one piece possible as long as the stent has not been overgrown by mucosa. Although the Strecker stent represents much more of a

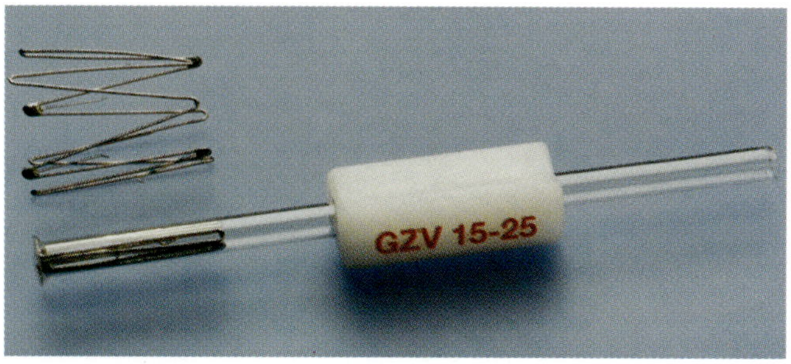

Figure 9-3

The Gianturco z-stent, shown compressed in the cartridge and fully expanded.

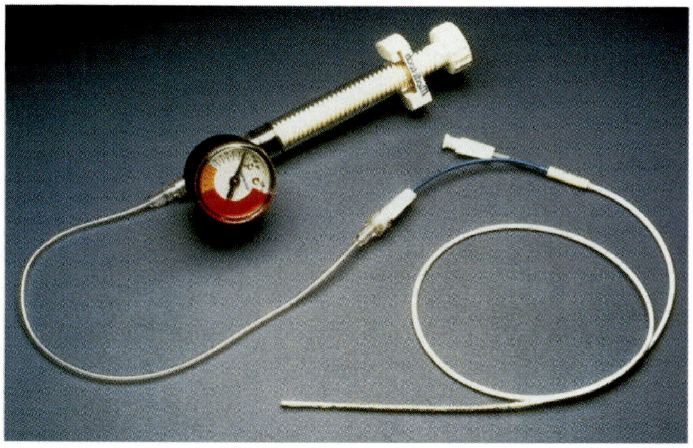

Figure 9-4

The Strecker stent: shown is the balloon-catheter with the stent mounted near its tip, the manometer for the generation of the necessary pressure to inflate the balloon is attached.

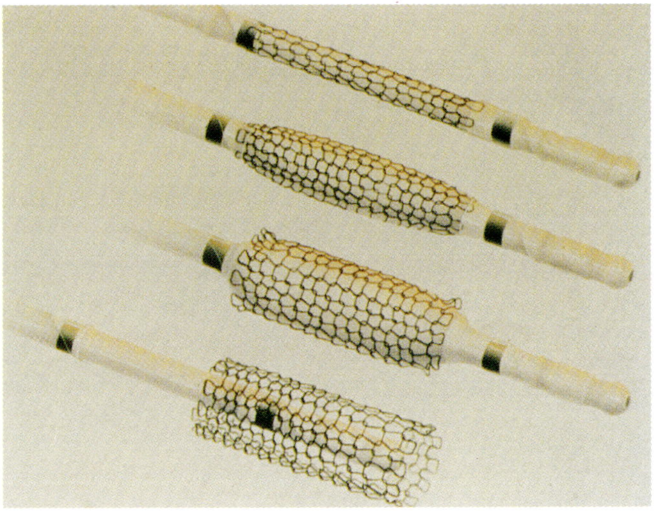

Figure 9-5

The Strecker stent: the different phases of deployment shown from *top* to *bottom*.

mesh than the zigzag struts of the Gianturco stent, tumor ingrowth or granuloma formation often lead to reocclusion similar to that seen with the Gianturco stent. On the other hand, airway wall perforation does not occur because the stents cannot be expanded beyond the preset diameters of 8 and 11 mm, respectively. Reocclusion and lack of diameters greater than 11 mm have prevented the wide use of the Strecker stent. It is, however, quite easily inserted since the very thin catheter carrying the stent can be passed through the working channel of a therapeutic fiberscope into very narrow airways.[43] So far no covered versions of the Strecker stent have been commercialized.

The Palmaz stent (Johnson and Johnson Interventional Systems Co., Warren, NJ) is another balloon-inflatable wire stent which deploys similarly to the Strecker stent.[19,44] Analyses of the mechanical properties have shown that the Palmaz stent exhibits plastic rather than elastic behavior.[45] Once deployed it can be recompressed by external compression such as vigorous coughing, and its plastic behavior will keep it from reexpanding afterward, thus partially obstructing the lumen of the airway. The Palmaz stent is therefore not suitable for the tracheobronchial tree.

A new exciting material is nitinol, a nickel titanium alloy with shape memory, that is, the alloy deforms plastically at low temperatures (martensitic state) and regains its original shape at higher temperatures (austenitic state) in the body.[46–48] Stents made from nitinol wires will therefore shrink at low temperatures and expand at body temperature. The biocompatibility of nitinol is very good,[49] and analyses of the mechanical properties of stents made from this alloy have shown them to exert almost equal pressure on the mucosa independent of the airway diameter. In an hourglass-type stenosis for instance, the pressure exerted at the narrowest part is not much greater than on either side.[45] Currently, uncoated and coated nitinol stents are available for the tracheobronchial tree (Ultraflex stent, Boston Scientific, Natack, MA).[40]

A well-known stent is the Wallstent [Schneider (Europe) AG, Buelach, Switzerland], which is a self-expandable wire mesh made of woven cobalt-based alloy filaments. It is widely used in the vascular system.[22,50,51] When used in the tracheobronchial tree, the uncovered version of the Wallstent is fraught with the same problems of reocclusion as all other uncovered metal stents and should therefore not be used. A new fully covered version called the Airway Wallstent has recently been commercialized in Europe after extensive testing in a prospective multicenter study.[28] The stents have a full polyurethane covering on the outside of the filaments, which does not interfere with the high flexibility of the stent (Fig. 9-6). The unconstrained stent dimensions designed for the airways are combinations of various diameters (12, 14, 16, and 18 mm) and lengths (25, 30, 35, 45, and 60 mm) (Fig. 9-7). There are two different delivery devices: a flexible device (Telestep) on which the stent is mounted in a compressed and elongated shape (Fig. 9-8) and a specially designed rigid bronchoscope (Rigidstep) (Fig. 9-9). With the Telestep the radiopaque stent is usually deployed under fluoroscopic control. The airway segment to be stented is determined endoscopically, and under fluoroscopy the distal and proximal ends of the stenosis are marked on the skin of the patient with the aid of metal clips (Fig. 9-10*A*). Under fluoroscopic con-

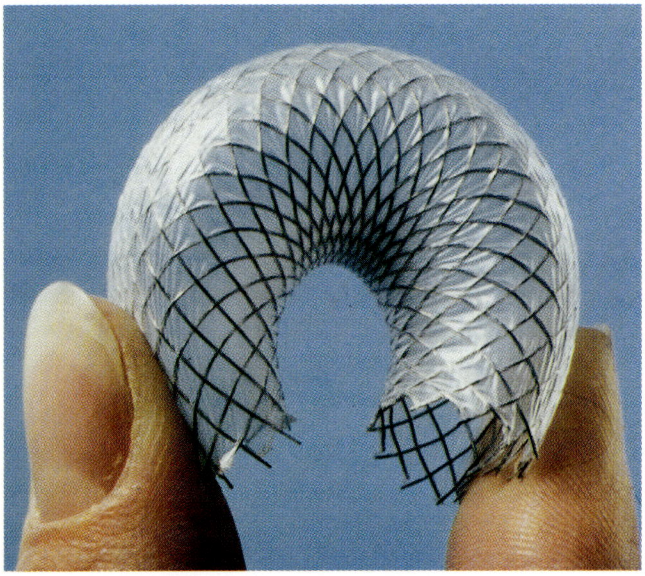

Figure 9-6

The Airway Wallstent: illustration of the high flexibility despite the polyurethane covering.

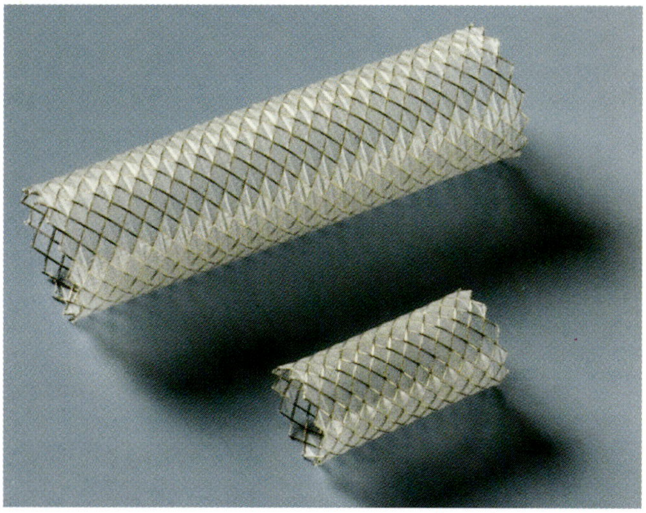

Figure 9-7

The Airway Wallstent: two different sizes, unconstrained diameters are shown.

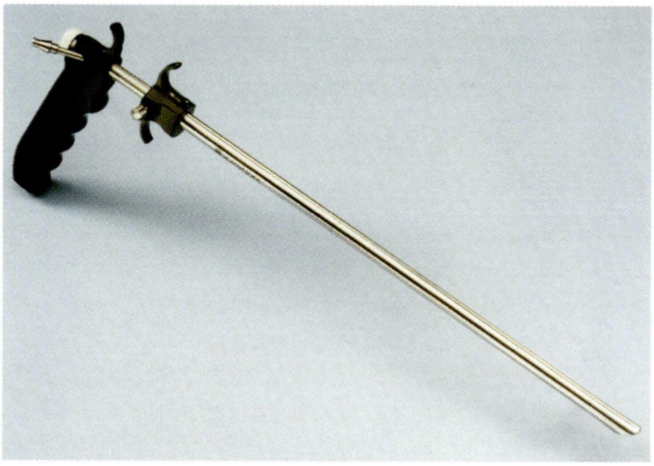

Figure 9-9

The Airway Wallstent: the rigid delivery device (Rigidstep); a specially designed bronchoscope: the hand grip is on the inner barrel, over which the outer barrel with the grip for two fingers is retracted to deploy the stent (invisible inside the tip of the scope).

trol the distal tip of the device is placed at the distal skin marker and the outer sheath slowly pulled back revealing the distal end of the stent (Fig. 9-10*B*). In the early deployment phase, the stent can be fine adjusted by moving the whole device proximally or distally, or the stent can be completely reintroduced into the device by advancing the outer sheath over it. Once the stent is fully released, it opens quickly and becomes firmly lodged in the mucosa by the sharp ends of the filaments (Fig. 9-10*C*). Inherent to its design, the stent shortens considerably with expansion. This shortening of the stent on expansion is of minor importance in vessels or in the esophagus. In the tracheobronchial tree with its many bifurcations, however, the choice of the adequate stent dimensions requires some experience to estimate the final length of the stent. For example, to treat a stenotic segment of diameter 10 mm and length 25 mm, the ideal unconstrained stent dimensions would be 12 mm in diameter and 30 mm in length. With the Rigidstep, the stent is loaded in only a slightly compressed form and therefore shortens less on deployment. The tip of the scope is passed just beyond the lesion to be stented, and the stent is deployed by retraction of the outer barrel of the scope while the stent is being held in position by an inner barrel. The procedure is controlled endoscopically using a rigid lens passed down the middle of the scope to visualize the stent as it is deployed. The Rigidstep can be used only if the lesion can be dilated enough for the scope to pass through. In stenoses narrower than 12 mm after dilatation the Telestep must be used. In comparison with silicone stents, the Airway Wallstent has the disadvantage of causing more granuloma formation at the ends of the stents and more retention of secretions,[28] but compared with the other uncovered metal stents, these complications occur much less often. A major advantage of the Airway Wallstent is its feasibility for the treatment of narrow, short and conical stenoses. For these situations it is currently the only stent available that can be placed securely and will not become reoccluded.

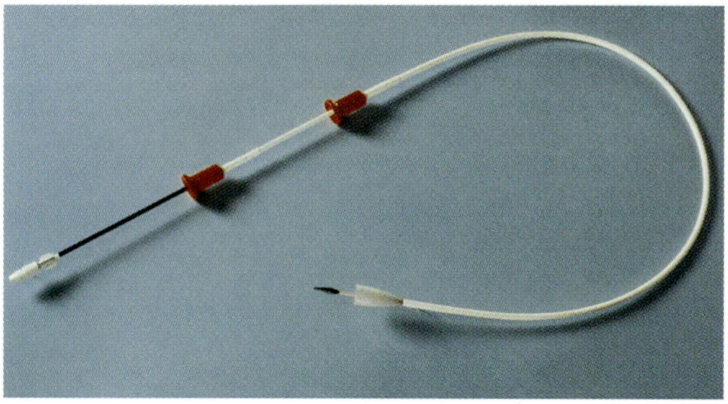

Figure 9-8

The Airway Wallstent: the flexible delivery device (Telestep) is shown with a stent half deployed at the tip.

A hybrid between a silicone and metal stent is the new Novastent (Novadis, Saint-Victoret, France), which consists of a thin silicone sheet containing small metallic hoops of a nitinol alloy (Fig. 9-11). For insertion the stent is rolled up like a cigarette paper and introduced through a rigid bronchoscope using a special forceps. Placement can be controlled fluoroscopically or endoscopically. After placement the metal hoops expand the stent to its full preset diameter. Silicone bands are mounted on the outside at both ends of the stent to prevent migration. Data on its performance are not available yet, but different sizes of the Novastent are

Figure 9-10

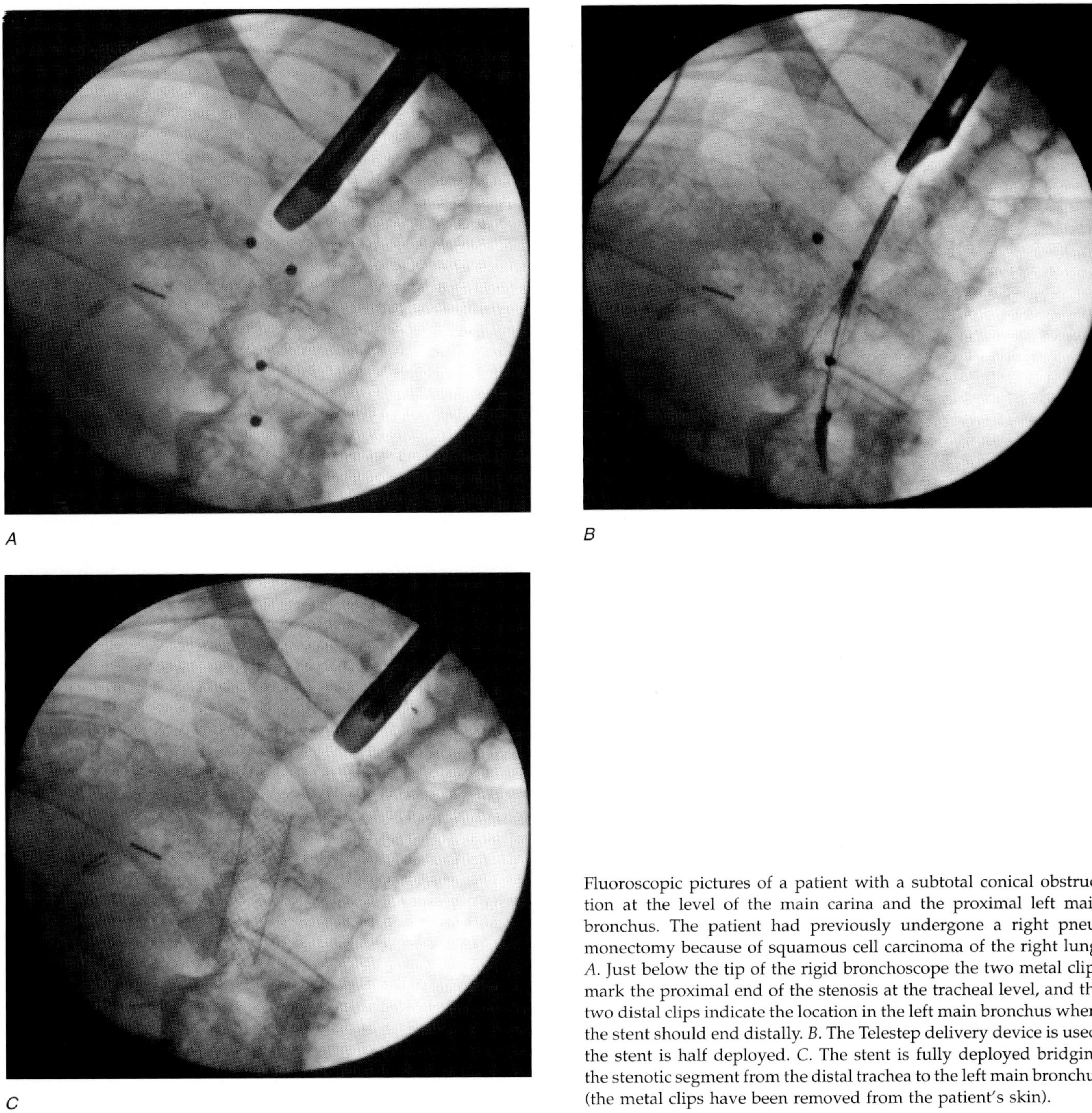

Fluoroscopic pictures of a patient with a subtotal conical obstruction at the level of the main carina and the proximal left main bronchus. The patient had previously undergone a right pneumonectomy because of squamous cell carcinoma of the right lung. *A*. Just below the tip of the rigid bronchoscope the two metal clips mark the proximal end of the stenosis at the tracheal level, and the two distal clips indicate the location in the left main bronchus where the stent should end distally. *B*. The Telestep delivery device is used; the stent is half deployed. *C*. The stent is fully deployed bridging the stenotic segment from the distal trachea to the left main bronchus (the metal clips have been removed from the patient's skin).

currently being tested prospectively in patients with malignant airway obstruction in a multicenter study in France and Switzerland.

Table 9-1 contains a summary of the advantages, disadvantages, and feasibility for the treatment of central airway obstructions for all expandable stents. The prices of all stents are currently in flux and therefore not indicated in this chapter; as a general rule the Dumon stent is still the least expensive, and most expandable stents cost at least twice as much. Ultimately only reasonably priced stents with excellent technical properties will remain competitive in a medical climate of increasing financial constraints.

Tracheobronchial Fistulas

Tracheobronchial fistulas can be caused by malignant and benign disorders and communicate with the esophagus, the mediastinum, or the pleura. The cause

Figure 9-11

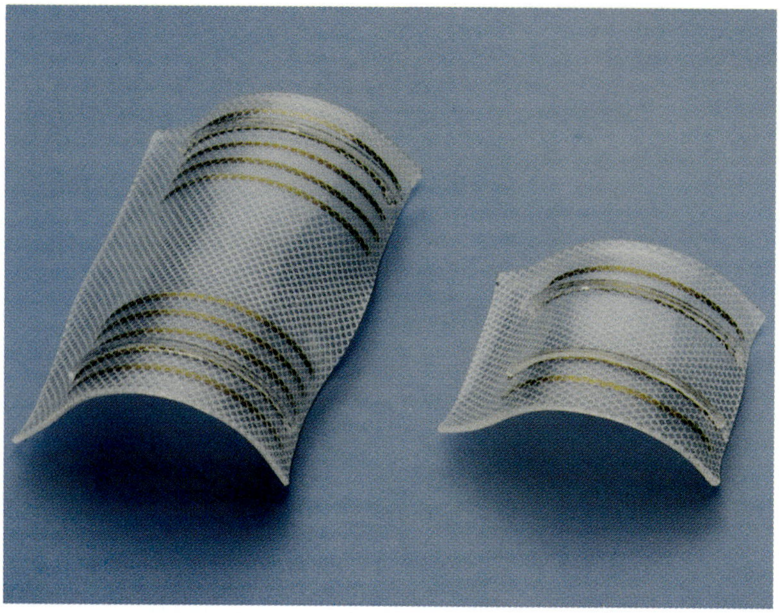

A

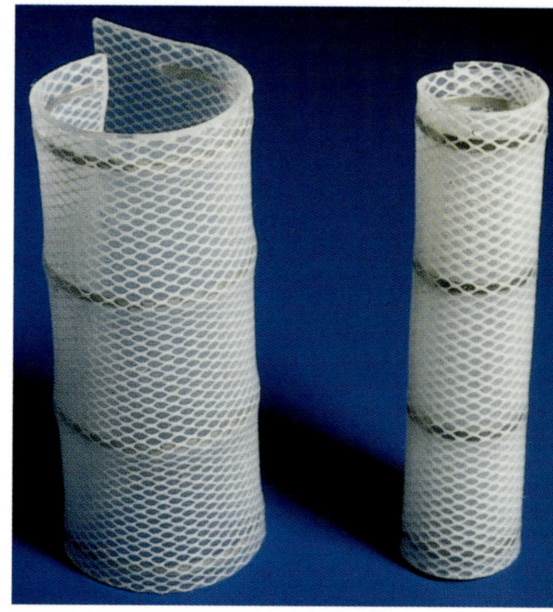

B

The Novastent: *A*. Two sizes are shown unconstrained. Nitinol hoops act as expansion force; on the outside two silicone bands prevent stent migration. For insertion the stent is rolled up like a cigarette and introduced with a special forceps or through the delivery device used with the Dumon silicon stents. *B*. The Novastent shown rolled up as it will look inside the airway (the picture shows the first models of the Novastent without the silicone bands on the outside).

of benign fistulas can be trauma to the airways. This may heal spontaneously or must be repaired surgically.[52] Postoperative bronchopleural fistulas after pulmonary resections have become rare and can be dealt with endoscopically if the diameter of the fistula does not exceed a few millimeters.[53] Fistulas caused by malignant disease are more difficult to manage. If the fistula develops in a tumor which also produces airway obstruction, various stents may be used successfully to seal it.[54,55] A malignant fistula in an airway without concomitant tumor stenosis, however, represents a real challenge for endoscopic treatment. The most frequent sites are between the esophagus and the tracheobronchial tree or bronchopleural fistulas due to tumor recurrence after pneumonectomy. Techniques such as sealing with glue,[56] laser application,[53] or closure with spongiosa graft,[57] used successfully in small postoperative fistulas after lung resections, seldom lead to closure of malignant fistulas, which invariably increase in size as the disease progresses. The optimal solution in these patients who usually have advanced disease and thus a short life expectancy, is the sealing of the fistula by a tightly fitting stent, rather than surgical closure by thoracotomy. In our experience, the available silicone stents, such as the Dumon[13] or the dynamic Y stent,[55] do not seal off fistulas in airways of normal diameter, whereas the Airway Wallstent seems to be effective in these situations[58] (Fig. 9-12). Effective sealing at the tracheal level requires large stent diameters of 18 or even 20 mm. Covered versions of a nitinol stent based on the Strecker design have also been reported to seal tracheobronchial fistulas.[40]

Assessment of Treatment Outcome

Early reports on treatment efficacy of the various expandable stents were mainly descriptive case series. Now, more than a decade into the use of such devices, analyses of treatment results should be reported with measurable parameters making terms such as "stent placement was easy" and patients had "good symptomatic relief" a thing of the past. Three main aspects of treatment outcome should always be reported: (1) technique of insertion and removal of stents, (2) efficacy of palliation, and (3) complications.

TECHNIQUE OF STENT INSERTION AND REMOVAL

All expandable stents have the advantage of an excellent wall/inner-diameter ratio; they can usually be compressed and mounted onto a thin balloon-catheter (Palmaz, Strecker) or loaded into an introducer sheath (Gianturco, Airway Wallstent). The entire procedure of deployment can either be controlled under fluoroscopy since the metal stents are all radiopaque or endoscopically with either a rigid lens or a flexible bron-

Table 9-1
ADVANTAGES AND DISADVANTAGES OF EXPANDABLE ENDOBRONCHIAL STENTS

Stent	*Advantages*	*Disadvantages*	*Feasibility*
Gianturco (Cook)	Simple insertion Several stents can be overlapped No migration	Removal extremely difficult Granulation tissue Tumor ingrowth Stent fracture Penetration through airway wall: Fatal erosion of vessels Tracheoesophageal fistula	Should not be used
Strecker (Boston Scientific)	Simple insertion Excellent flexibility Good in narrow stenoses Several stents can be overlapped	Late removal very difficult Granulation tissue Tumor ingrowth	Use in narrow stenoses, only if no covered stent available
Palmaz (Johnson, Johnson)	Simple insertion Good in narrow stenoses Several stents can be overlapped	Late removal very difficult Granulation tissue Tumor ingrowth Permanent deformation of stent (not elastic)	Should not be used
Nitinol (Boston Scientific)	Excellent flexibility Good biocompatibility Seals fistulas (if covered)	Late removal ? Granulation tissue ? Tumor ingrowth ? Longevity of covering ? Insufficient data	Promising stent Insufficient data
Airway Wallstent stent (Schneider)	Simple insertion Excellent flexibility Good in narrow stenoses Several stents can be overlapped Seals fistulas	Removal somewhat difficult Some granulation at stent ends Some retention of secretions Shortening requires experience	Only covered expandable Currently available Best for: fistulas and narrow stenoses
Novastent (Novadis)	Simple insertion Good biocompatibility Easy early and late removal Seals fistulas ?	Migration ? Granulation tissue ? Insufficient data	Promising stent More data needed

choscope. Most endoscopists prefer the rigid bronchoscope[59] for safe ventilation during the procedure. On the other hand, very thin introducer sheaths can be passed down the working channel of a flexible bronchoscope, making stent placement under local anesthesia feasible.[43] Deployment of all the expandable stents discussed above is quick and very accurate. The accuracy is very important because, with the exception of the Novastent, fine adjustment is almost impossible once the stents are fully deployed. Well-placed metal stents migrate very seldom, but they are usually more difficult to remove than silicone stents. The Gianturco stent with its sharp metal hooks is extremely difficult to remove, and extraction is often piecemeal, requiring several fractures of the stent.[35] The other uncovered metal stents can be removed during the first few days after placement; later the wire mesh will be overgrown by tumor, granulomata, or a layer of mucosa. At this stage any attempt at removal is a tedious and messy affair. Covered expandable stents such as the Airway Wallstent still cause some granuloma formation at the stent ends, but once the proximal end of the stent is loosened, it can be removed in one piece through the rigid bronchoscope like a silicone stent.

EFFICACY OF PALLIATION

All expandable stents have been shown to be very efficacious at relieving symptoms of dyspnea, cough, retention of secretions, and postobstructive pneumonia. The efficacy of symptom relief should be measured with objective parameters such as pulmonary function tests,[60–63] radiologic appearance of lung parenchyma, and endoscopic assessment of the stented airways. Also, and just as important, subjective parameters such as degree of dyspnea, and Karnofsky or WHO activ-

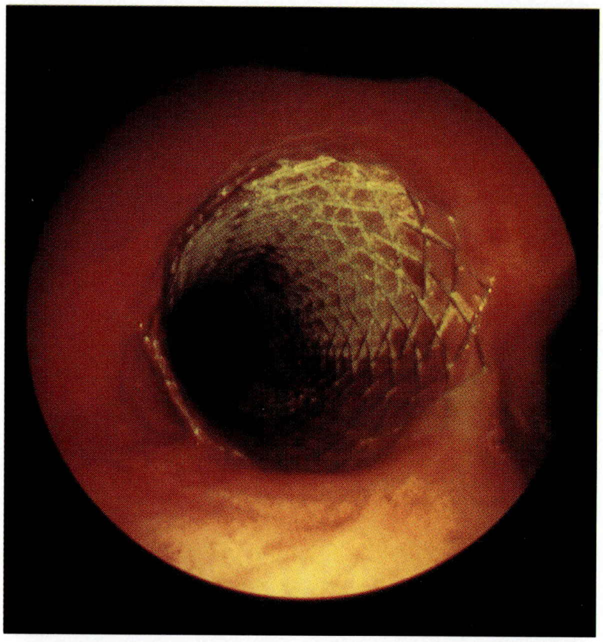

A

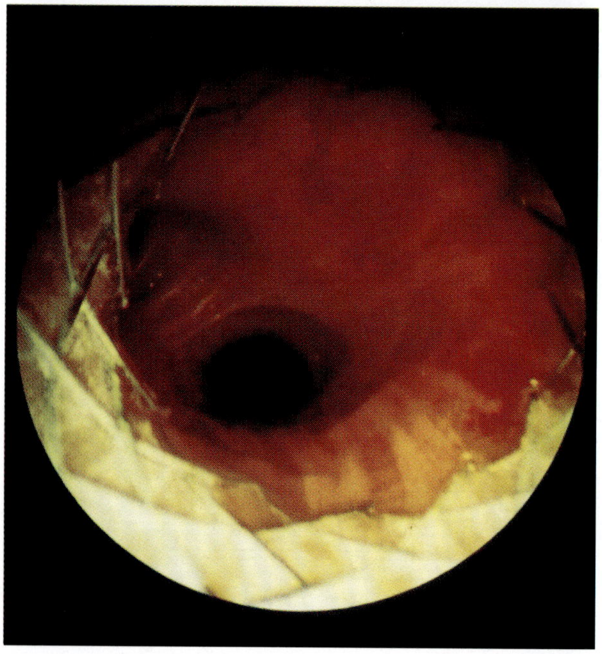

B

Figure 9-12

Patient with a malignant fistula between the esophagus and the left main bronchus: an Airway Wallstent sealed the fistula perfectly. *A.* Proximal end of stent seen at the level of the main carina. *B.* Distal end of stent in the left main bronchus, the openings of the left upper and lower lobes are visible.

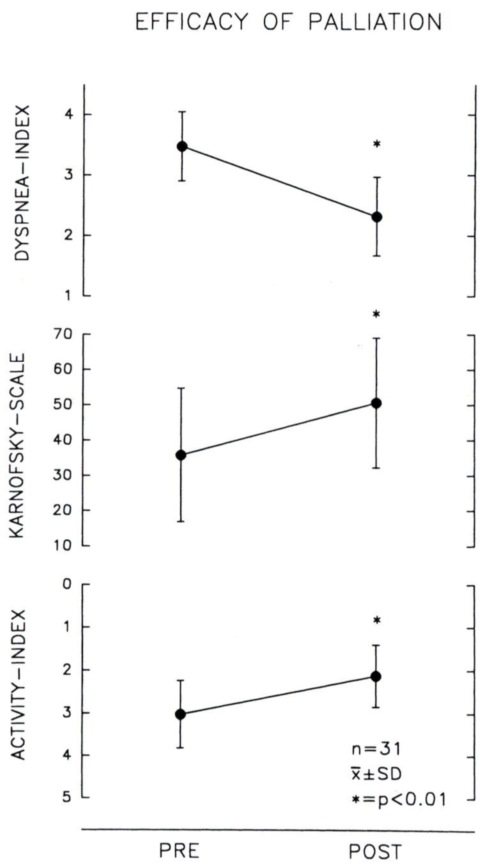

Figure 9-13

Highly significant improvement in the degree of dyspnea, Karnofsky and WHO-activity indices in 31 patients after endobronchial treatment with laser and stent placement (measurements are 1 day before and 1 week after treatment) (according to Bolliger, et al.[2]).

ity indexes[2] (Fig. 9-13) should be reported. Although in patients with malignant disease the emphasis is on palliation or quality of life, recent reports have shown that good palliation also increases survival.[64–66] Any new stent should be tested prospectively with subjective and objective parameters, allowing direct comparison between different stent models. In our institution we have found serial flow-volume loops to be the single best follow-up parameter after endobronchial treatment; an unchanged loop over time usually obviates the need for repetitive routine bronchoscopies or chest roentgenograms.

COMPLICATIONS

Expandable stents very rarely lead to complications initially. They fit varying airway diameters snugly and provide excellent initial palliation. After some months, however, uncovered stents are often obstructed by tumor ingrowth when used in malignant disease, even if the initial stenosis had been purely extraluminal and the stenosed airway had exhibited a normal mucosa. The experience with silicone stents has shown that once a stent is open, tumor will not recompress the stent but grow where it meets least resistance, namely, above and below the stent. Therefore in the future most expandable stents will be covered stents, the Airway Wallstent and the Novastent being the first models commercially available. Granuloma formation at the stent ends and retention of secretions are generally more frequent with metal stents than with silicone stents. Although most metal stents are elastic, they loose this property once they are epithelialized and integrated into the airway wall. This leads to impaired mucus clearance at the level of the stent. All patients with indwelling stents should therefore be encouraged to inhale saline solution at least once daily to humidify the internal surface of their prosthesis, which helps to prevent mucous impaction within and around the stent. Another important complication is migration of the stent proximally or distally to its original site. This is usually noted by the patient as sudden onset or worsening of cough and dyspnea. In general, expandable stents migrate less than silicone stents; if they do, the event is fortunately rarely ever life-threatening since the stent is a hollow tube moving within a tube.[67] Any symptom of displacement should, however, lead to prompt investigation with a chest roentgenogram and flexible bronchoscopy, and removal of the stent if necessary. Longevity of expandable stents, especially of new covered models will have to be assessed carefully and must withstand comparison with the durable silicone stents. In this respect the Palmaz stent with its lack of elasticity and the Gianturco stent with its severe complications are not suited for the endobronchial use. In our opinion these two stent types should be replaced with the newer covered, expandable stents now available.

HOW I DO IT (BOLLIGER)

In our institution stent placement is considered in patients with central-airway stenosis of more than 50 percent of the normal diameter after therapeutic endoscopy or with highly collapsible airway walls due to loss of the cartilaginous support. In all but life-threatening situations, the nature and extent of the stenosis is first determined by flexible bronchoscopy. In subtotal to total obstruction of the airway lumen, in which the anatomy distal to the stenosis cannot be inspected, we instill some saline into the occluded airway with the patient in a sitting position. Disappearance of the liquid and/or slight bubbling of the air-fluid level indicates minimal patency. We further try to pass a small brush catheter or closed forceps past the tumor. If the probe can be advanced relatively easily into the periphery, the presence of anatomically normal airways distal to the tumor is highly likely. When in doubt, we perform a chest CT scan with thin sections at and especially distal to the level of the stenosed airway. With the advent of helical CT, three-dimensional reconstructions of the area of interest have become quite helpful.

Almost all our therapeutic procedures are performed under general anesthesia. For narrow (<10 mm in diameter after dilation) and conical stenoses and for the sealing of malignant fistulas without concomitant stenosis, we use expandable stents. Of the available expandable types, the Airway Wallstent is the one we currently use most. For stent placement we mainly use the rigid bronchoscope in combination with the Telestep delivery device. Stent delivery is performed as described above (Fig. 9-10*A* to *C*). For straight stenoses with a diameter of >12 mm, we use the second delivery device (Rigidstep) (Fig. 9-9) for which fluoroscopy is not necessary. The choice of the stent depends on the diameter and length of the stenosis; the diameter is estimated by the diameter of the bronchoscope used to pass the stenosis or by the balloon diameter used for its dilatation. In fistulas without concomitant airway stenosis, the best estimate is obtained by CT measurement. The length of the stenosis is determined endoscopically. One caveat must be mentioned: the considerable shortening of the Wallstent, which is more pronounced when using the Telestep, makes the choice of the dimensions of the stent more difficult than with stents that do not shorten on placement. This problem is overcome with increasing experience with the device. We find it useful to choose an unconstrained diameter of about 2 mm larger than the lumen to be stented, which, depending on the size of the stent, results in a final length of about 2 to 5 mm longer than the unconstrained length. For bronchial stents, when in doubt, we choose a slightly shorter stent to prevent occlusion of bronchial side branches or protrusion of the proximal stent end into the trachea, thereby partially obstructing the entrance to the contralateral main bronchus. At the tracheal level, this effect of shortening is less important.

With the Telestep, placement of the Airway Wallstent can also be performed under local anesthesia with the patient lightly sedated. Because the outer diameter of the Telestep measures 5.3 mm, it cannot be passed through the working channel of a flexible bronchoscope. A guide wire must first be placed by flexible bronchoscopy. After removal of the bronchoscope, the Telestep is then advanced over the wire under fluoroscopic control—similar to the technique used for vascular stenting. This maneuver is somewhat cumbersome and does not guarantee adequate control of the ventilation. We therefore prefer to place Airway Wallstents with the rigid bronchoscope. Covered expandable stents that could be mounted on a catheter thin enough to pass through a working channel of a flexible bronchoscope are currently not available.

One day after stent placement, we routinely obtain the following for all our patients: (1) a chest roentgenogram, (2) a flow-volume loop, and (3) a repeat flexible bronchoscopy. This guarantees a thorough assessment of position and patency of the stent. Even if the chest film shows good stent patency, we perform the bronchoscopy, because quite often some degree of obstruction within the stent lumen by fibrin, mucus, or old blood will have occurred, especially if laser resection had preceded stent placement during the therapeutic endoscopy session. Every patient is instructed to inhale a normal saline solution one to three times daily to humidify the inner stent surface and prevent subsequent mucous impaction within the stent. The average hospital stay including diagnostic, therapeutic, and control endoscopy rarely exceeds 48 h, after which the patient is discharged home. Regular clinical follow-up evaluations are done by the referring pulmonologist or the patient's primary doctor.

HOW I DO IT (MATHUR)

The European version of the Airway Wallstent differs from the ones available in the United States. See Table 9-2.

The Unistep and Classic delivery systems are positioned and deployed under fluoroscopy. A rigid bronchoscope could also be used to visualize the proximal end of the stent during deployment. The bronchoscopic delivery system can be deployed through the working channel of the flexible bronchoscope, allowing for direct visualization during deployment (minimum 2.6 mm working channel). The Rigidstep and Telestep are not available in the United States.

In our institution also stent placement is considered in patients with central airway stenosis of more than 50 percent of the normal diameter after therapeutic endoscopy or with highly collapsible airway walls due to loss of the cartilaginous support. In all but life-threatening situations, the nature and extent of the stenosis is first determined by flexible bronchoscopy. In cases of subtotal to total obstruction of the airway lumen, in which the anatomy distal to the stenosis cannot be inspected, we instill some saline into the occluded airway. Disappearance of the liquid and/or bubbling of the fluid indicates some degree of patency. We then try to pass a closed forceps past the tumor under fluoroscopic guidance. If this is possible with the forceps advancing relatively easily into the periphery, the presence of anatomically normal airways distal to the tumor is highly likely. We perform a helical CT and three-dimensional reconstructions of the area of interest. The stent size is determined with the help of the helical CT scan and the reconstruction of the airway. If stent placement is considered, almost all our therapeutic procedures are performed under local anesthesia and conscious sedation. For narrow (<10 mm in diameter after dilation) and conical stenoses and for the sealing of malignant fistulas without concomitant stenosis, we use expandable stents. Of the available expandable types, the Airway Wallstent is the one we currently use most. For stent placement, we use the flexible bronchoscope in combination with the Unistep or Classic delivery device. The patient is prepared in the routine manner for a flexible bronchoscopy with local anesthesia and conscious sedation. The Unistep stent is first prepared for delivery by removing the stylet and inspecting for any defects. The delivery system is attached to a 10-ml syringe, saline is flushed, and the stopcock is closed. A soft J wire is placed through the flexible bronchoscope, and the bronchoscope is then removed. The Unistep catheter is passed over the J wire. To deploy the prosthesis the stainless steel tube remains stationary and the valve body is pulled toward the hub. Once 50 percent of the stent is deployed, we assess the location. To reposition we wedgelock the stent and pull the stainless steel tube back into the unopened stent. The stent is moved to the final position by holding the valve body and pulling entire catheter back. Once the desired location is confirmed, the rest of the Wallstent is deployed by pulling the valve body toward the hub.

The Classic delivery system also has to be prepared. The Permalume (covered Wallstent) has a rolling membrane which has to be purged. A 20-ml syringe is attached and the plunger pulled back to create a negative pressure, which is maintained for several seconds until the maximal amount of air has been aspirated. The stopcock is closed, maintaining a negative pressure. This process is repeated several times. The aspiration syringe is replaced with an inflation syringe equipped with a pressure gauge and filled with saline. The stopcock is opened and the inflation syringe is pressurized to 4.0 atm. The pressure is maintained until the saline solution has advanced to the stent. The pressure is monitored for 1 min. If the pressure drops below 3.0 atm or perforation of the rolling membrane is seen, the delivery system should not be used. It is important to ensure that the rolling membrane completely covers the constrained stent and does not overlap the enlarged portion of the distal tip and that none of the wires have perforated the rolling membrane. If the rolling membrane does not cover the stent, the system should not be used. The inflation syringe is then pulled to create a negative pressure, and the stopcock is closed. The delivery system is now ready for deployment. Once again we place a soft J wire through the stricture using the flexible bronchoscope. Using flu-

Table 9-2
DIFFERENCES BETWEEN THE U.S. AND EUROPEAN WALLSTENT TRACHEOBRONCHIAL ENDOPROSTHESES

	United States	*European*
Stent	Bare metal or Partially covered (5 mm bare wire on each end of stent)	Fully covered
Stent covering	*Silicone*	*Polyurethane*

Delivery systems	Bare stent
	  Unistep
	    Working length 75 cm
	    Flexible delivery system
	    Single-use delivery system
	  Bronchoscopic Unistep
	    Working length 135 cm
	    Flexible delivery system
	    Single-use delivery system for use through flexible bronchoscope
	Covered stents
	  Classic
	    Working length 75 cm
	    Flexible delivery system
	    Single-use delivery system to deploy stent-catheter pressurized to 4 atm with saline
		Covered stents
		  Rigidstep
		    Working length 350 mm
		    Rigid delivery system
		    Reusable delivery system
		  Telestep
		    Working length 90 cm
		    Flexible delivery system
		    Single-use delivery system

oroscopy, the stent is placed across the site of the stricture, the leading markers positioned a minimum of 2 cm beyond the distal area of the dilated segment. As the stent shortens upon deployment, these markers are used as approximate markers for the final stent position. The stopcock is opened and the rolling membrane inflated with saline to 4.0 atm of pressure, which is maintained for 1 min to allow for adequate perfusion of the delivery system. Then we immobilize the stainless steel tube with one hand and grasp the valve body with the other hand, and gently slide the valve body along the stainless steel tube toward the hub until the stent is approximately 50 percent deployed. Pressure within the rolling membrane will fall as the stent is deployed. It is imperative that the pressure is maintained at 4.0 atm. If the stent is deployed too far distally, it can be pulled back by aspirating the inflation syringe and pulling the delivery system to the desired location. The membrane is then reinflated to 4.0 atm, and the deployment continued. A partially deployed stent can be pulled back, *but* a stent deployed too far proximally cannot be advanced distally. In summary, a guide wire must first be placed by flexible bronchoscopy. After removal of the bronchoscope, the delivery system is then advanced over the wire under fluoroscopic control—similar to the technique used for vascular stenting. The choice of adequate stent depends on the diameter and length of the stenosis; the diameter is estimated by the diameter of the bronchoscope used to pass the stenosis or by the balloon diameter used for its dilatation. In fistulas without concomitant airway stenosis, the best estimate is obtained by CT measurement. The length of the stenosis is determined endoscopically. One must appreciate the considerable shortening potential of the Wallstent. However, this problem is overcome with increasing experience with the device.

One day after stent placement, we routinely obtain chest radiography for all patients. This guarantees a thorough assessment of position and patency of the stent. Even if the chest film shows good stent patency, we perform bronchoscopy at 2 weeks because quite often some degree of obstruction within the stent lumen by fibrin, mucus, or old blood will have occurred. Every patient is instructed to inhale albuterol and normal saline solution three to four times daily to humidify the inner stent surface and prevent subsequent mucous impaction within the stent.

Summary

The use of stents to treat central airway obstruction is firmly established. In experienced hands, the short- and long-term results are excellent (Fig. 9-13). Of all the various stents on the market, the cylindrical silicone stent designed by Dumon is the one most widely used and represents the standard against which all other models have to compete. Expandable stents have advantages over silicone stents because of their thin walls and their excellent adaptability to greatly varying airway diameters. The current development of covered expandable stents should make it possible to combine the excellent biocompatibility of silicone stents with the increased flexibility and favorable wall/inner-diameter ratio of the metal stents. This development will make expandable stents much more versatile for the treatment of malignant and benign obstructions of the central airways.[68] Effective sealing of fistulas in airways without a concomitant obstructive component is another most welcome indication for these stents. The future might well belong to hybrid stents with metallic components and a smooth synthetic covering of silicone or polyurethane. The Novastent and the Airway Wallstent are the first examples of this generation. Nitinol with its shape memory effect might well become an important alloy for stents in the near future.[40] The ongoing development clearly shows that the ideal stent has not been found and will almost certainly never exist. Quite often the specific stent type needed can be identified only during a therapeutic endoscopy. Every specialist practicing in the area of stenting should therefore have an armamentarium of several different types of stents available and use the one best indicated in a specific situation.

REFERENCES

1. Belani CP: Multimodality management of regionally advanced non-small-cell lung cancer. *Sem Oncol* 1993; 20:302.
2. Bolliger CT, et al: Silicone stents in the management of inoperable tracheobronchial stenoses. Indications and limitations. *Chest* 1993; 104:1653.
3. Daum TE, et al: Tracheobronchial involvement in Wegener's granulomatosis. *Am J Respir Crit Care Med* 1995; 151:522.
4. Tsang V, Goldstraw P: Endobronchial stenting for anastomotic stenosis after sleeve resection. *Ann Thorac Surg* 1989; 48:568.
5. Colt HG, et al: Endoscopic management of bronchial stenosis after double lung transplantation. *Chest* 1992; 102:10.
6. Gaer JAR, et al: Use of endotracheal silicone stents for relief of tracheobronchial obstruction. *Ann Thorac Surg* 1992; 54:512.
7. Carré P, et al, and the Toulouse lung transplantation group: Balloon dilatation and self-expanding metal wallstent insertion for management of bronchostenosis following lung transplantation. *Chest* 1994; 105:343.
8. Grillo HC: Notes on the windpipe. *Ann Thorac Surg* 1989; 47:9.
9. Pearson FG: *Surgery of the Trachea. Coventry Conference.* London, Butterworth, 1973.
10. Miller RD, Hyatt RE: Evaluation of obstructing lesions of the trachea and larynx by flow-volume loops. *Am Rev Respir Dis* 1973; 108:475.
11. Bolliger CT, et al: The flow-volume loop in bilateral vocal cord paralysis. *Chest* 1993; 104:1302.
12. Montgomery WW: The surgical management of supraglottic and subglottic stenosis. *Ann Otol Rhinol Laryngol* 1968; 77:534.
13. Dumon JF: A dedicated tracheobronchial stent. *Chest* 1990; 97:328.
14. Colt HG, Dumon JF: Airway stents. Present and future. In Mathur PN, Beamis JF (eds): *Clinics in Chest Medicine, Interventional Pulmonology.* Philadelphia, WB Saunders, 1995, 16: 465–478.
15. Westaby S, et al: A bifurcated silicone rubber stent for relief of tracheobronchial obstruction. *J Thorac Cardiovasc Surg* 1982; 83:414.
16. Cooper JD, et al: Use of silicone stents in the management of airway problems. *Ann Thorac Surg* 1989; 47:371.
17. Neville WE, et al: Clinical experience with the silicone tracheal prosthesis. *J Thorac Cardiovasc Surg* 1990; 99:604.
18. Wallace MJ, et al: Tracheobronchial tree: Expandable metallic stents used in experimental and clinical applications. *Radiology* 1986; 158:309.
19. Palmaz JC, et al: Intraluminal stents in atherosclerotic iliac artery stenosis: Preliminary report of a multicenter study. *Radiology* 1977; 168:727.
20. Strecker E-P, et al: Expandable tubular stents for the treatment of arterial occlusive diseases. Experimental and clinical results. *Radiology* 1990; 175:97.
21. Sigwart U, et al: Intravascular stents to prevent occlusion and restenosis after transluminal angioplasty. *N Engl J Med* 1987; 316:701.
22. Zollikofer CL, et al: Endovascular stenting of veins and grafts: Preliminary clinical experience. *Radiology* 1988; 167:707.
23. Rousseau H, et al: Self-expandable prostheses in the tracheobronchial tree. *Radiology* 1993; 188:199.
24. Varela A, et al: Use of Gianturco self-expandable stents in the tracheobronchial tree. *Ann Thorac Surg* 1990; 49:806.
25. Hürter T, et al: Bronchiale Endoprothesen (Stents) beim inoperablen Bronchuskarzinom. *Pneumologie* 1991; 45:19.
26. Schaer J, et al: Treatment of malignant esophageal obstruction with silicone-coated metallic self-expanding stents. *Gastrointest Endosc* 1992; 38:7.
27. Fleischer DE, Bull-Henry K: A new coated self-expanding metal stent for malignant esophageal strictures. *Gastrointest Endosc* 1992; 38:494.
28. Bolliger CT, et al: A covered Airway Wallstent for the treatment of malignant tracheobronchial stenoses. *Thorax* 1996; 51:1127.
29. Serruys PW, et al: Angiographic follow-up after placement of a self-expanding coronary-artery stent. *N Engl J Med* 1991; 324:13.
30. Serruys PW, et al: A comparison of balloon-expandable-stent implantation with balloon angioplasty in patients with coronary artery disease. *N Engl J Med* 1994; 331:489.
31. Fischman DL, et al: A randomized comparison of coronary-stent placement and balloon angioplasty in the treatment of coronary artery disease. *N Engl J Med* 1994; 331:496.
32. Neuhaus H, et al: Implantation of self-expanding esophageal metal stents for palliation of malignant dysphagia. *Endoscopy* 1992; 24:405.
33. Lammer J, et al: Obstructive jaundice: Use of expandable metal endoprosthesis for biliary drainage. *Radiology* 1990; 177:789.
34. Sawada S, et al: Malignant tracheobronchial obstructive lesions: Treatment with Gianturco expandable metallic stents. *Radiology* 1993; 188:205.

35. Nashef SAM, et al: Expanding wire stents in benign tracheobronchial disease: Indications and complications. *Ann Thorac Surg* 1992; 54:937.
36. Spatenka J, et al: Gianturco self-expanding metallic stents in treatment of tracheobronchial stenosis after single lung and heart and lung transplantation. *Eur J Cardiothorac Surg* 1991; 5:648.
37. Tsang V, Williams AM, Goldstraw P: Sequential silastic and expandable metal stenting for tracheobronchial strictures. *Ann Thorac Surg* 1992; 53:856.
38. Bolliger CT, et al: Covered Wallstent insertion in a patient with conical tracheobronchial stenosis. *J Bronchol* 1995; 2:215.
39. Schäfers H-J: Gianturco self-expanding metallic stents. *Eur J Cardiothorac Surg* 1992; 6:278.
40. Becker HD: Stenting of central airways. *J Bronchol* 1995; 2:98.
41. George PJM, et al: Covered expandable metal stent for recurrent tracheal obstruction. *Lancet* 1990; 335:582.
42. Breyer G, Häussinger K: Tracheobronchiale Stents - Indikationen und Möglichkeiten. *Pneumologie* 1991; 45:997.
43. Becker H: Flexible versus rigid bronchoscopic placement of tracheobronchial prostheses (stents). Pro flexible bronchoscopy. *J Bronchol* 1995; 2:252.
44. Palmaz J: Intravascular stents. In Kollath J, Liermann D (eds): *Stents II*. Konstanz, Schnetztor-Verlag, 1992:162–173.
45. Freitag L, et al: Mechanical properties of airway stents. *J Bronchol* 1995; 2:270.
46. Dotter CT, et al: Transluminally expandable nitinol coil stent grafting: Preliminary report. *Radiology* 1983; 147:259.
47. Cragg A, et al: Nonsurgical placement of arterial endoprostheses. A new technique using nitinol wire. *Radiology* 1983; 147:261.
48. Vinograd I, et al: A new intratracheal stent made from nitinol, an alloy with "shape memory effect." *J Thorac Cardiovasc Surg* 1994; 107:1255.
49. Castelman LS, et al: Biocompatibility of nitinol as an implant material. *J Biomed Mater Res* 1976; 10:695.
50. Zollikofer CL, et al: Perkutane transluminale Behandlung von Stenosen und Verschlüssen im venösen System mittels Gefässendoprothesen (Stents). *Schweiz Med Wochenschr* 1994; 124:995.
51. Stock KW, et al: Treatment of malignant obstruction of the superior vena cava with the self-expanding Wallstent. *Thorax* 1995; 50:1151.
52. Lin M-C, et al: Emergent flexible bronchoscopy for the evaluation of acute chest trauma. *J Bronchol* 1995; 2:188.
53. Wang K-P, et al: Closure of bronchopleural fistula by Nd-YAG Laser. *Am J Respir Crit Care Med* 1995; 151:A847.
54. Colt HG, et al: Double stents for carcinoma of the esophagus invading the tracheobronchial tree. *Gastrointest Endosc* 1992; 38:485.
55. Freitag L, et al: Theoretical and experimental basis for the development of a dynamic airway stent. *Eur Respir J* 1994; 7:2038.
56. Scappaticci E, et al: Postoperative bronchopleural fistula: Endoscopic closure in 12 patients. *Ann Thorac Surg* 1994; 57:119.
57. Stamatis G, et al: Autologous spongiosa graft and fibrin sealant for endoscopical treatment of bronchopleural stump fistulas. Update and future trends in fibrin sealing in surgical and nonsurgical fields. November 1992, Vienna A 175.
58. Bolliger CT, et al: Use of the covered Airway Wallstent in tracheobronchial malignancies. *Eur Respir J* 1995; 8:458s.
59. Freitag L: Flexible versus rigid bronchoscopic placement of tracheobronchial prostheses (stents). Pro rigid bronchoscopy. *J Bronchol* 1995; 2:248.
60. Moshenifar Z, et al: Physiologic assessment of lung function in patients undergoing laser photoresection of tracheobronchial tumors. *Chest* 1988; 93:65.
61. Desai SJ, et al: Survival experience following Nd:YAG laser photoresection for primary bronchogenic carcinoma. *Chest* 1988; 94:939.
62. Gelb AF, et al: Physiologic studies of tracheobronchial stents in airway obstruction. *Am Rev Respir Dis* 1992; 146:1088.
63. Vergnon J-M, et al: Efficacy of tracheal and bronchial stent placement on respiratory functional tests. *Chest* 1995; 107:741.
64. Ross DJ, et al: Survival characteristics after neodymium: YAG laser photoresection in advanced stage lung cancer. *Chest* 1990; 98:581.
65. Vergnon JM, et al: Initial combined cryotherapy and irradiation for unresectable non-small cell lung cancer. *Chest* 1992; 102: 1436.
66. Macha HN, et al: Pattern of failure and survival in endobronchial laser resection. A matched pair study. *Chest* 1994; 105:1668.
67. Edell ES, et al: Tracheobronchial prostheses. In Prakash UBS (ed): *Bronchoscopy*. New York, Raven, 1994: 301–311.
68. Goldstraw P: Endobronchial stents. In Hetzel MR (ed): *Minimally Invasive Techniques in Thoracic Medicine and Surgery*. London, Chapman and Hall, 1995: 233–246.

CHAPTER 10

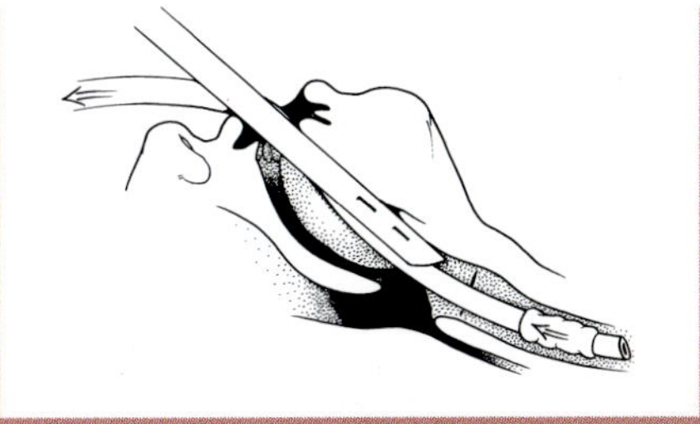

BALLOON DILATION OF BENIGN TRACHEOBRONCHIAL STENOSIS

Francis D. Sheski and Praveen N. Mathur

Benign tracheobronchial stenosis of the proximal airway has various medical and/or surgical etiologies. The result is dyspnea or recurrent pulmonary infections. Some of the etiologies of stenosis are lung transplantation, bronchial reimplantation after lobectomy for bronchial carcinoma, tuberculosis, long-term endotracheal or tracheostomy tube placement, Wegener's granulomatosis, trauma, berylliosis, smoke inhalation, foreign body reaction, and sarcoidosis (Table 10-1).

In infants, prior use of endotracheal and tracheostomy tubes or congenital lesions are the primary reasons for such stenoses. Thus subglottic or tracheal sites are common.[1] In adults, the etiologies are variable with the mainstem or lobar bronchi commonly involved.[2] In patients with tuberculosis, despite adequate antitubercular therapy, progression of tracheobronchial stenosis may occur. Similarly, when systemic therapy fails to relieve stenosis owing to endobronchial sarcoidosis, local treatment of the narrowed airway may be required.

Bronchial stenosis may produce symptoms, such as dyspnea, cough, wheeze, stridor, or recurrent lower respiratory tract infections. Local treatment of stenosis has included surgical resection, laser resection, and bougie dilation during rigid bronchoscopy. Balloon bronchial dilation has been used in combination with other modalities such as laser resection, cryotherapy, and electrocautery (Table 10-2).

Under laminar flow conditions in a tubular system, flow is proportional to the tube radius raised to the fourth power (Poiseuille's law), and under turbulent conditions flow is proportional to the radius raised to the fifth power.[3] Since the respiratory tract is modeled as a system of branching tubes with laminar and turbulent flow, increasing the tube radius slightly can increase flow significantly. Thus the purpose of bronchoscopic balloon dilation is to establish an adequate bronchial lumen by a simple, nontraumatic, rapid method enlarging the stenosis and restoring airflow.

In 1984, Cohen and colleagues reported the successful balloon dilation of a surgical anastomosis in a 4-1/2-month-old infant.[4] Similarly, 1 year later, Groff and Allen reported successful balloon dilation of a stenosis thought to be related to prolonged intubation and frequent suctioning in a 5-month-old infant.[5] In 1987, Fowler and colleagues described bronchoscopic balloon dilation in an adult who had had a sleeve resection for an endobronchial squamous cell carcinoma of the right mainstem bronchus some 2 years earlier.[6] The following year Carlin and associates reported two cases of bronchoscopic balloon dilation in conjunction with Nd:YAG laser therapy.[2] The first patient had a stenosed bronchus intermedius due to granulation tissue caused by an aspirated pill fragment; the second patient had undergone a right pneumonectomy for squamous cell carcinoma 13 years earlier and external beam irradiation for recurrence 1 year prior, and presented with tumor growth at the stump, compromising the left mainstem bronchus. Not until 1991 was balloon dilation with flexible bronchoscopy (FB) described.[7] Since then, several reports have been published.[8–13]

Table 10-1
ETIOLOGIES OF STENOSIS

Lung transplant or sleeve resection anastomosis	Tuberculosis
Endotracheal or tracheostomy tube	Wegener's granulomatosis
Trauma	Berylliosis
Smoke inhalation	Bronchial artery embolization
Caustic chemical inhalation	Foreign body reaction
Carcinoma	Congenital lesions
Sarcoidosis	Idiopathic

This chapter describes flexible bronchoscopic balloon dilation in adults, including indications and contraindications, technique, complications, and outcome.

Indications and Contraindications

To date there are no prospective controlled studies comparing the various modalities of treatment for tracheobronchial stenosis; therefore, the physician's experience in a particular modality has been the guide. In selecting bronchoscopic balloon dilation, several factors should be considered.

First, the patient should be medically able to undergo FB.[14] Second, a bronchoscopist familiar with the technique should be available. The bronchoscopist should also be capable of using other modalities if needed. Third, the patient should have a clinical picture consistent with airway stenosis. Last, the stenosis should be amendable to balloon dilation. Several factors discussed below will help in making this decision.

Although balloon dilatations of tracheal lesions in adults have been reported, the most common sites involve either the mainstem or lobar bronchi.[13,15] Most tracheal stenoses are treated by alternative means or by combination therapy which may involve balloon dilation. Narrowed segmental bronchi are considered for dilation if thought to contribute to the patient's symptoms. Since the balloon catheter must extend beyond the lesion, it is desirable to visualize the airway distal to the stenosis even if the bronchoscope cannot be passed completely through the opening. Visualizing the stenosis and analyzing radiographic studies allows for the approximation of the length and diameter of the stenosis and the choice of an appropriate balloon size. Several authors have suggested that the process causing the stenosis, such as fibrosis, malacia, inflammation, calcification, carcinoma, and compression, may effect the outcome. Fibrotic stenosis is said to lend itself to a better result. Visual characteristics, such as pale, nonedematous mucosa, may suggest a lesion with little inflammation and a greater likelihood of successful opening.[1,13]

Contraindications to FB balloon dilation are similar to those for FB.[14] In addition, balloon dilation is contraindicated if there is nonvisualization of the distal orifice or lack of a channel through the obstruction.

Table 10-2
LOCAL TREATMENT MODALITIES

Surgery
Laser
Biopsy forceps
Cryotherapy
Electrocautery
Rigid or flexible bronchoscopic dilation
Angioplasty, valvuloplasty, or embolectomy catheter balloon dilation with or without bronchoscopy

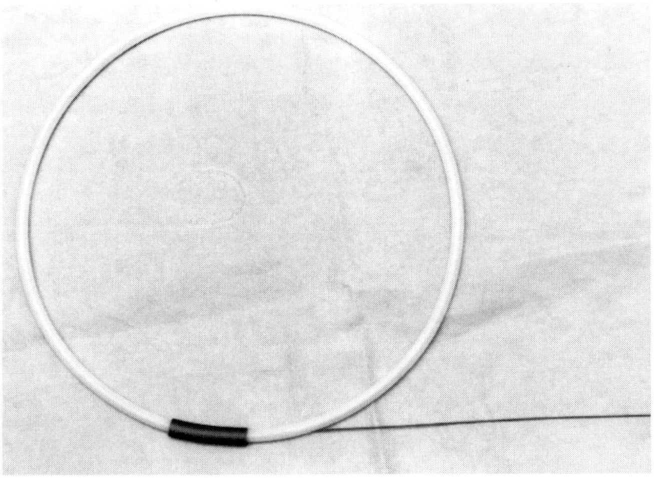

Figure 10-1

The guide wire in the protective plastic casing.

Technique

Balloon dilation is performed using FB with topical anesthesia and conscious sedation. Thus the preoperative patient evaluation and patient monitoring during the procedure are the same as that for standard FB using conscious sedation.[14]

Since bleeding may be a complication, assessment of the patient's coagulation status and withholding any anticoagulant or antiplatelet medication seems prudent. After topical anesthesia is applied and the patient sedated (usually with a benzodiazipine and a narcotic), the bronchoscope is inserted either nasally or orally. The airways are then inspected and the stenosis identified. Since this procedure involves placing a balloon catheter over a guide wire and not through the working channel of the bronchoscope, a bronchoscope with a 2.0 mm or larger working channel can be used.

When the stenosis has been identified and deemed treatable by balloon dilation, a guide wire (0.89 mm diameter, Cook Incorporated, Bloomington, IN) is passed through the working channel and advanced beyond the stenosis (Fig. 10-1). This is performed under fluoroscopy to avoid extending the wire to the lung periphery (Fig. 10-2). The bronchoscope is then removed, leaving the guide wire in place. Next, a balloon catheter (Olbert Catheter System, Meadox Surimed, Oakland, NJ, and Rigiflex OTW, Boston Scientific Corporation, Watertown, MA) is selected, based on balloon length and diameter in relation to the stenosis dimensions (Fig. 10-3). The choice of a balloon diameter is based primarily on the estimated stenosis diameter and on the diameter to be achieved. The

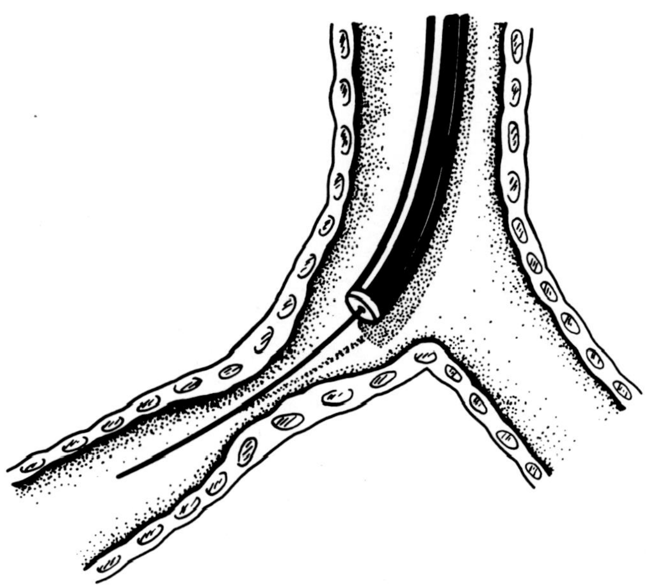

Figure 10-2

A guide wire is passed beyond the stenosis, using bronchoscopy and fluoroscopy.

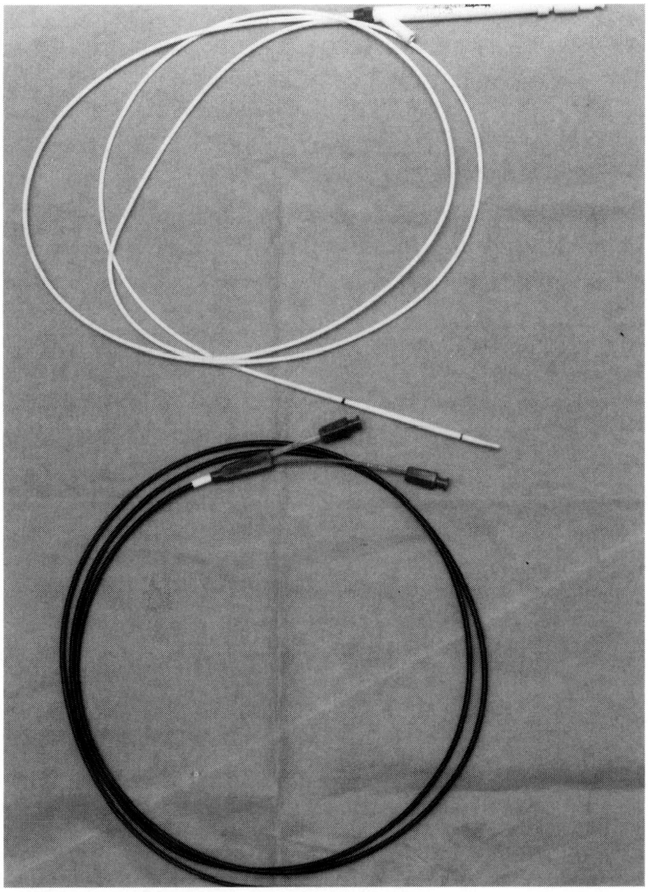

Figure 10-3

Balloon catheters from Olbert Catheter Systems (*top*) and Rigiflex OTW (*bottom*.)

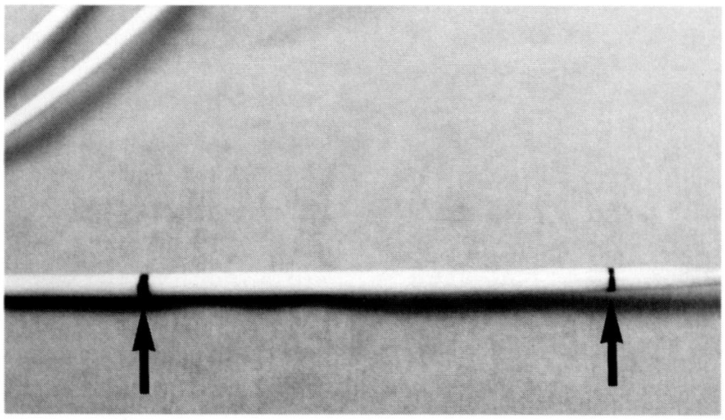

A

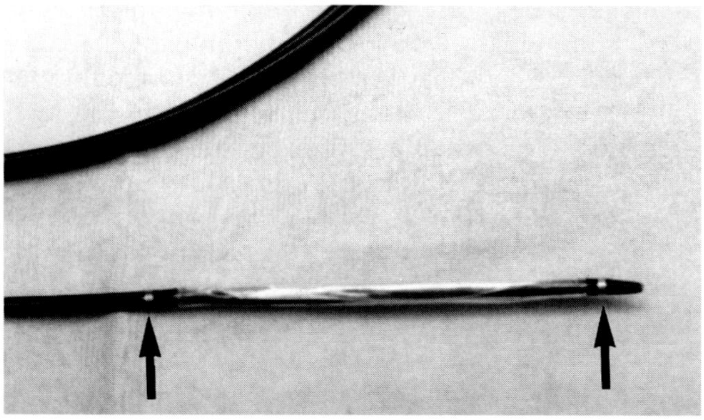

B

Figure 10-4

Radiopaque markers (*arrows*) delineate the proximal and distal ends of the balloon. *A*. Olbert catheter. *B*. Rigiflex catheter.

catheter has radiopaque markers at the proximal and distal ends of the balloon (Fig. 10-4*A* and *B*).

With fluoroscopic guidance the catheter is passed over the guide wire and the balloon markers properly located with respect to the stenosis (Fig. 10-5). The bronchoscope is again inserted to visualize the stenosis and catheter (Fig. 10-6). This allows direct monitoring of the balloon during inflation (Figs. 10-7 and 10-8). Some authors use a dilute contrast medium to inflate the balloon, allowing for better fluoroscopic imaging.[1,4,12] Repeat inflations can be made if needed, based on the stenosis diameter after deflating the balloon. Success is based on a stable increase in airway diameter after balloon deflation (Fig. 10-9). Adjunctive treatments such as laser vaporization or stent placement may precede or follow balloon dilation. This procedure may be performed on intubated mechanically ventilated patients as well.[1,10,16]

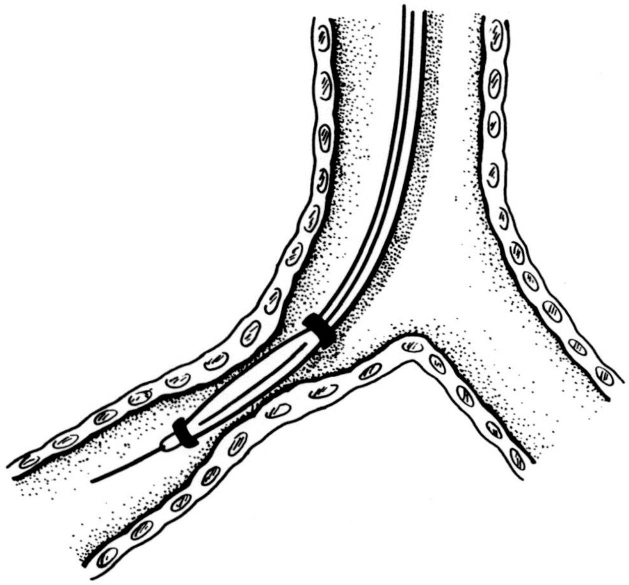

Figure 10-5

The balloon is advanced over a guide wire and positioned under fluoroscopy.

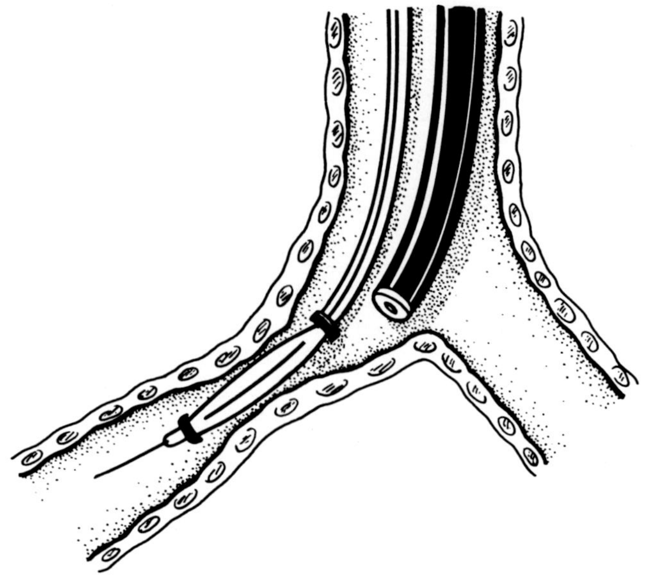

Figure 10-6

Proper positioning of the proximal end of the balloon is confirmed with visualization through the bronchoscope.

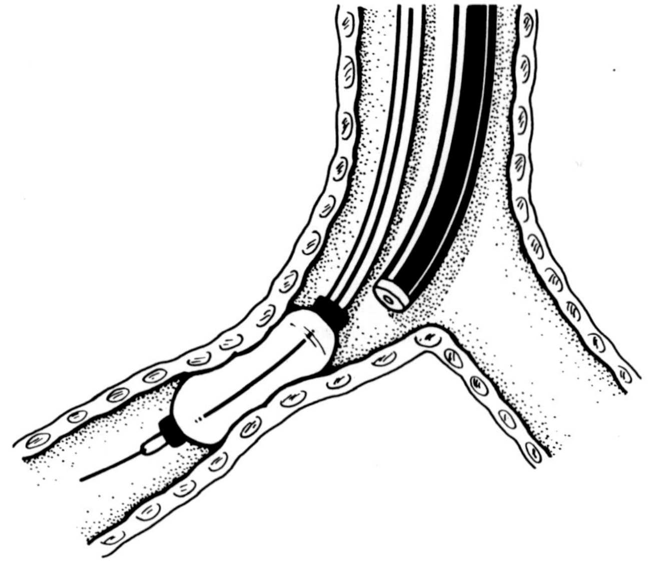

Figure 10-7

Bronchoscopy allows visualization of balloon inflation and deflation.

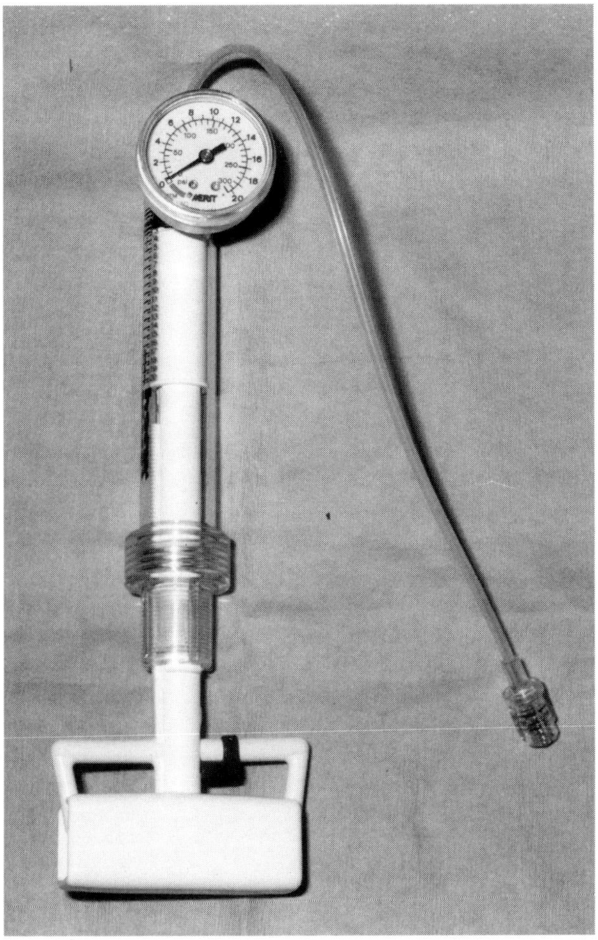

Figure 10-8

The basic inflation syringe is used to inflate the balloon and monitor the inflation pressure.

Complications

Complications associated with FB are detailed elsewhere.[14] Chest pain has been reported during balloon inflation. Bronchospasm and atelectasis have been described by several authors.[1,16,17] Excessive balloon inflation may lacerate or rupture the airway, causing hemorrhage, pneumothorax, pneumomediastinum, or mediastinitis. However, no reports of these potential complications have been documented in the literature. Similarly, no deaths have been attributed to balloon dilation.

Results

A number of reports of bronchoscopic balloon dilation in adults are available.[2,6–8,10–13] The number of patients in these studies has varied from 1 to 16. Follow-up has ranged from 1 to 36 months. Most patients have required more than one dilation. Several patients had balloon dilation in conjunction with other therapies.

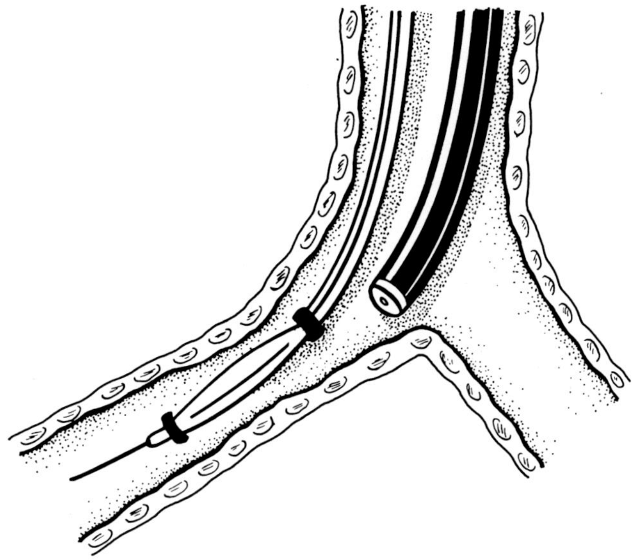

Figure 10-9

The immediate result is assessed through the bronchoscope.

Short-term success was defined as an immediate increase in postdilation airway diameter. Long-term success was based on the patient remaining asymptomatic. Some patients have undergone radiologic evaluation with chest roentgenography or CT scan, pulmonary function testing, or FB as part of follow-up care. If symptoms or signs suggested that tracheobronchial stenosis had recurred, the patient usually was bronchoscoped. Ferreti and colleagues[13] described the largest series of patients (16). The etiology of the stenosis varied: 10 patients had undergone lung transplant, four had bronchial reimplant, one followed radiation therapy, and one had Wegener's granulomatosis. Nine of the stenosis patients required only one modality of therapy. Table 10-3 summarizes detailed data reported in the literature.

At Indiana University Medical Center we have performed 55 FB balloon dilations on 14 patients, nine male and five female. The patients ranged in age from 35 to 72 years. Seven patients had a main-stem bronchial stenosis after either single-lung or bilateral sequential lung transplants for chronic obstructive pulmonary disease (COPD) (4), α_1-antitrypsin deficiency (1), pulmonary fibrosis (2), or pulmonary hypertension (1). Of the remaining seven patients, all with a main-stem bronchial stenosis, three had a sleeve resection pneumonectomy for non-small cell lung cancer (NSCLC), two had irradiation for NSCLC, and two had fibrosing mediastinitis, presumably caused by histoplasmosis. The time since the last dilation varied between 3 months and 5 years. All attempted dilations but one were judged an immediate success. The one unsuccessful attempt was on a stenosis in a lung transplant patient who also had bronchiolitis obliterans.

Table 10-3
DATA SUMMARY

Study (number of patients)	*Age*	*Etiology*	*BD*	*Other Therapy*	*Time from last BD, mo*
Fowler et al., 1987[6] (1)	58 y	Sleeve resection	2	None	1.5 mo
Carlin et al., 1988[2] (2)	52 y	Pill fragment	1	Laser	14 mo
	71 y	NSCLC	2	Laser	4 mo
Girard et al., 1990[8] (1)	34 y	Bronchial artery embolization	1	Pneumonectomy	1 mo
Nakamura et al., 1991[7](2)	58 y	Tuberculosis	1	None	8 mo
	46 y	Tuberculosis	1	NA	NA
Keller and Frost, 1992[10](3)	42 y	DLT	11	Left SLT	NA
	43 y	D-SLT	3	None	NA
	42 y	SLT	1	Stent	NA
Carre et al., 1994[11](8)	47 y	DLT	6	Stent	11 mo
	50 yr[a]	SLT	1	None	10 mo
	43 yr	DLT	1	Stent	NA
	57 yr	SLT	2	Stent/laser	NA
	57 yr	SLT	2	None	10 mo
	57 yr	SLT	2	Stent/Laser	6 mo
	40 yr	DLT	1	None	1 mo
	56 yr[b]	SLT	1	None	12 mo
Fouty et al., 1994[12](6)	40 yr	sarcoid	1	None	6 mo
	31 yr	sarcoid	3	None	12 mo
	36 yr[c]	sarcoid	2	None	36 mo
	40 yr	sarcoid	2	None	6 mo
	36 yr	sarcoid	2	None	9 mo
	32 yr	sarcoid	2	None	NA

NOTE: BD, balloon dilations; DLT, double-lung transplant; SLT, single-lung transplant; D-SLT, double-single-lung transplant; XRT, irradiation therapy; NA, not available; NSCLC, non-small cell lung cancer.

[a]This patient had one stenosis treated with a stent and one with dilation.

[b]This patient had one stenosis treated with dilation and stent (not included in table) and one with dilation.

[c]This patient required dilation every 9 months.

One lung transplant patient died during an attempted Y-stent placement. No other complications occurred. Table 10-4 summarizes our experience at Indiana University Medical Center. Figures 10-10 to 10-14 show a stenosis before balloon dilation, after guide-wire balloon placement, during balloon inflation, and after balloon deflation. This result would be considered an immediate success. This patient did well for several months before symptoms suggesting restenosis occurred and repeat balloon dilation was accomplished.

Table 10-4

SUMMARY OF FLEXIBLE BRONCHOSCOPIC BALLOON DILATION AT INDIANA UNIVERSITY MEDICAL CENTER

Patient age, gender	*Etiology*	*Number of BDs*	*Other Therapy*	*Time from Last BD, months*	*Current Status*
38 yr, male	SLT	3	Stent	22	Dead
56 yr, male[a]	B-SLT	2	None	60	Alive
35 yr, female	B-SLT	5	Cryotherapy	36	Alive
52 yr, male[b]	B-SLT	6	Stent	6	Dead
42 yr, male	B-SLT	2	Cryotherapy	12	Alive
53 yr, male[c]	SLT	30 plus	Stent	6	Died during Y-stent placement
60 yr, female	B-SLT	1	None	36	Alive
53 yr, male	Sleeve resection NSCLC	1	None	24	Dead
68 yr, female	Sleeve resection NSCLC	1	None	12	Dead
54 yr, male	Sleeve resection NSCLC	1	None	18	Dead
69 yr, male	XRT NSCLC	1	None	6	Dead
72 yr, female	XRT NSCLC	1	None	3	Dead
62 yr, female	Fibrosing mediastinitis	1	None	36	Alive
65 yr, male	Fibrosing mediastinitis	1	None	12	Dead

NOTE: BD, balloon dilations; SLT, single-lung transplant; B-SLT, bilateral sequential lung transplant; XRT, irradiation therapy; NSCLC, non-small cell lung cancer.

[a]This patient had left and right main-stem bronchial stenoses, dilated one time each.

[b]This patient had left and right main-stem bronchial stenoses, dilated three times each.

[c]All deaths except one occurred from causes unrelated to the procedure.

Discussion

Benign tracheobronchial stenosis of the proximal airway is a complication of several medical conditions, as outlined above. The pathogenesis of the bronchial stenosis caused by tuberculosis has been well described. Pathologically, it progresses through three stages: a submucosal infiltration by tubercles and lymphocytes, followed by ulceration and growth of granulation tissue. Finally a fibrous scar characteristic of the healed stage develops.[18-23] Stenosis from other medical causes may also finally result in a fibrous scar. In single- or double-lung transplantation, this endobronchial stenosis may be a result of airway rejection

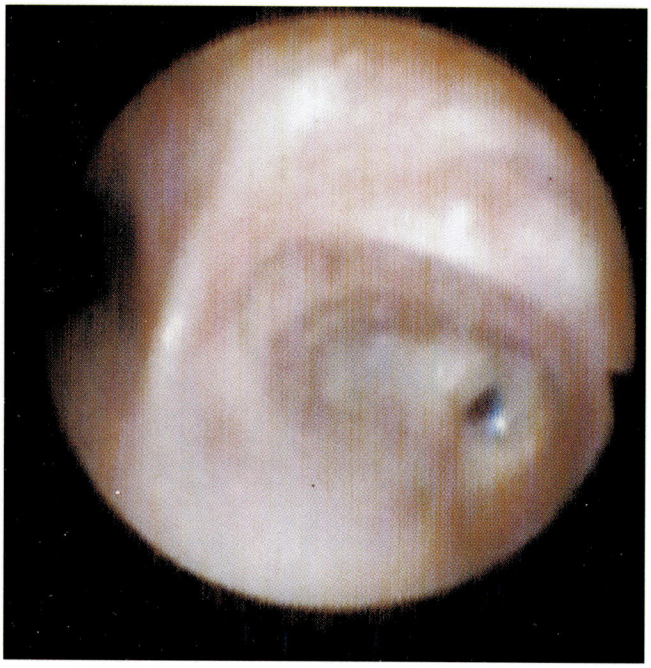

Figure 10-10

This lung transplant patient had a right main-stem bronchial stenosis at the anastomotic site.

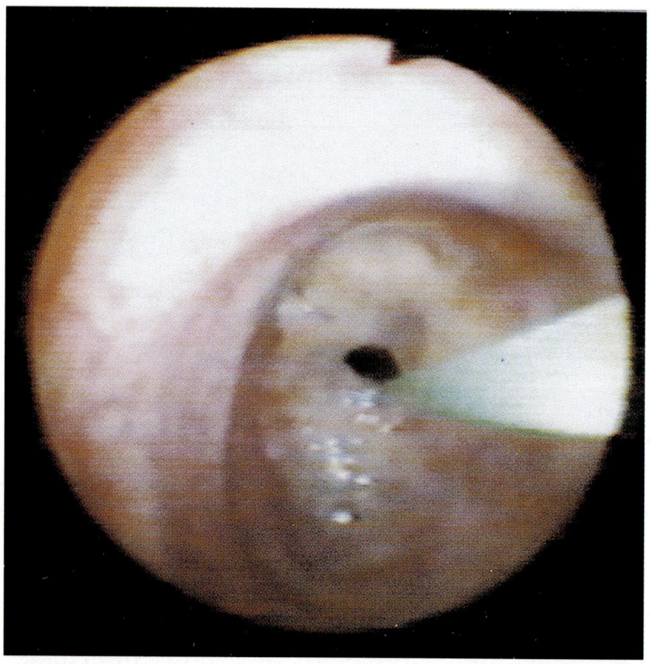

Figure 10-11

The guide wire is placed through the stenosis.

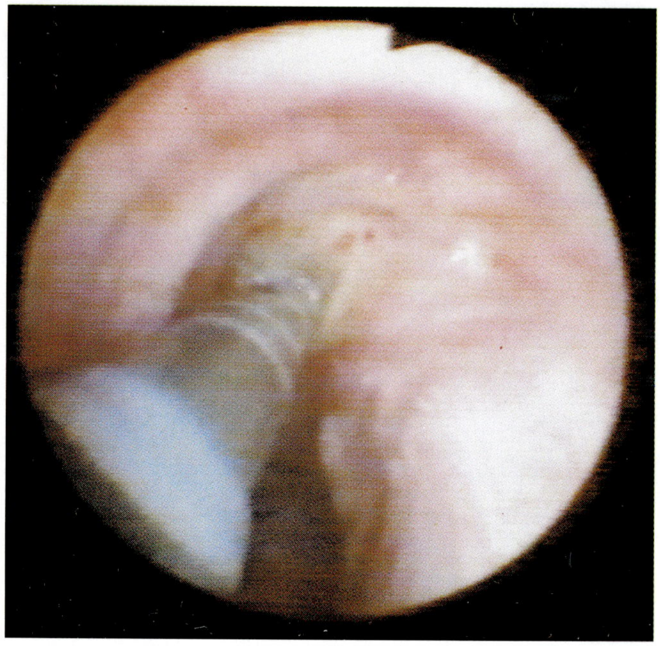

Figure 10-12

The balloon catheter is placed over the guide wire through the lesion so the radiopaque marker is visible (*light band in lower left corner*).

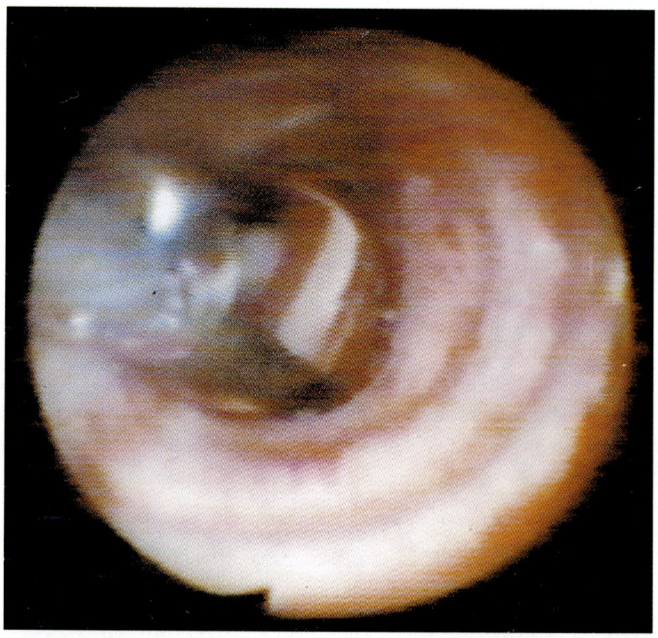

Figure 10-13

The balloon is inflated.

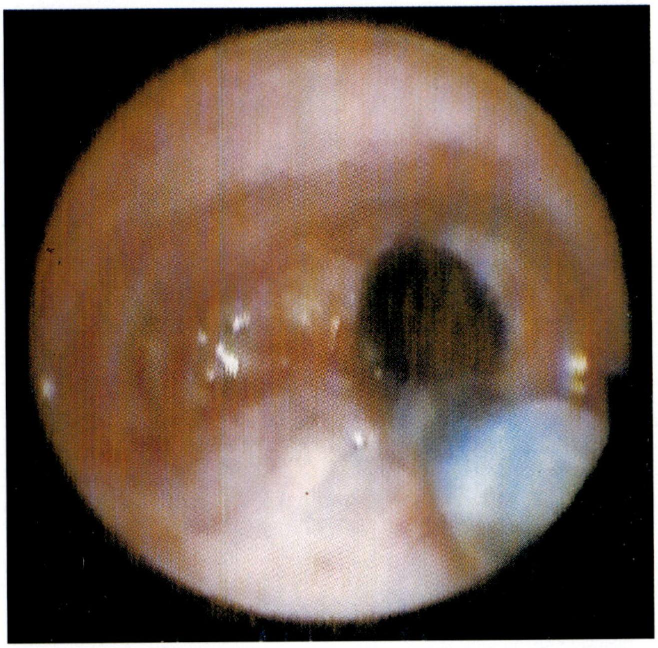

Figure 10-14

After balloon deflation the airway is significantly wider than before dilation. This was judged an immediate success.

or due to ischemic changes at the site of the bronchial implantation. This bronchial stenosis at the anastomotic site could develop with or without previous bronchial dehiscence.[10] Since repeated balloon dilation is often required in this group of patients, there must be an ongoing process such as airway rejection or ischemia that contributes to the recurrence and results in the poor success rates of balloon dilation in this condition. Dumon[24] classified acquired benign tracheal stenosis into two types: concentric and bottleneck, which is accompanied by collapse of the wall due to the loss of cartilage. Either type may be treated by balloon dilation; however, the bottleneck type often requires subsequent stenting.

Various procedures have been used to improve the airway caliber. Surgical resection remains controversial owing to the associated high risk with this option and the high rate of recurrence.[25] Mechanical dilation of the stenosis can be performed using rigid bronchoscopy. This requires general anesthesia and passage of a series of metal bougies through the rigid bronchoscope.[26] Nd:YAG laser photocoagulation has been used alone or with balloon dilation. Laser resections are technically difficult and in this particular situation may present a risk of bronchial perforation and/or bleeding.[2,27] Endobronchial cryotherapy in conjunction with balloon dilation has been used in two cases with success.[28] Regardless of the method of dilation, if there is cartilage damage in the trachea or bronchi resulting in bronchomalacia, an airway stent is usually needed to support the airway.[11] To prevent complications of overdistention, balloon size must be carefully chosen, according to the location of the stenosis and the diameter of the bronchus.

HOW I DO IT

The procedure outlined below is similar to that described by Ferretti.[13] Both the nasal and oral intubation routes may be utilized. We anesthetize both areas with topical agents. Atropine (0.4 to 0.8 mg) is given intravenously to block parasympathetic responses. After sedating the patient, usually with a benzodiazepine (midazolam) and a narcotic (morphine), the bronchoscope is inserted either nasally or orally. A thorough inspection on the airways is done, and the stenosis is identified. Since this procedure will take longer than a routine diagnostic bronchoscopy, it is necessary to titrate the sedation accordingly. Because this procedure involves placing a balloon catheter over a guide wire and not through the working channel of the bronchoscope, a bronchoscope with a 2.0-mm greater working channel can be used.

Once the stenosis has been identified and deemed amendable to balloon dilation, a guide wire (0.89 mm diameter, Cook Incorporated, Bloomington, IN) is advanced through the working channel, placing the tip beyond the stenosis (Fig. 10-1). This is performed under fluoroscopy to avoid creating a coil or extending the wire to the lung periphery (Fig. 10-2). The bronchoscope is then removed, leaving the guide wire in place. The placement of the guide wire should be confirmed with fluoroscopy after the bronchoscope has been removed.

Next, a balloon catheter (Olbert Catheter System, Meadox Surimed, Oakland, NJ, or Rigiflex OTW, Boston Scientific Corporation, Natick, MA) is selected based on balloon length and diameter and on the stenosis dimensions (Fig. 10-3). The balloon should protrude from each end of the stenosis so that the entire stenosis will be dilated when the balloon is inflated. If the balloon extends too far distally there is a potential for airway damage. Similarly, if the balloon does not extend sufficiently through the stenosis, it tends to slip out of the stenosis on inflation. Balloons from 2.5 to 4.0 cm long are usually adequate. The choice of a balloon diameter is based primarily on the estimated stenosis diameter. The inflated balloon needs to be larger than the lesion for dilation to occur, but should not be so large that excessive airway injury results. A 1.0- to 1.5-cm-diameter balloon is usually sufficient. The initial balloon catheter can always be replaced should it be too narrow. The balloon catheter has radiopaque markers at the proximal and distal ends of the balloon, allowing the balloon location to be assessed with fluoroscopy. (Fig. 10-4*A* and *B*).

While using fluoroscopy, the catheter is passed over the guide wire so the balloon markers are properly located with respect to the stenosis (Fig. 10-5). The bronchoscope is then reinserted through another intubation route, e.g., the other nostril or mouth, to visualize the stenosis and the balloon catheter (Fig. 10-6). This allows the operator to directly monitor the balloon during inflation (Fig. 10-7). The balloon is inflated with water to pressures between 45 and 131 lb/in^2 based on that particular balloon catheter's characteristic. The inflation is achieved with a basic inflation syringe (Merit Medical Systems, Inc., Salt Lake City, UT) (Fig. 10-8). Some authors have used a dilute contrast agent to inflate the balloon, allowing for better fluoroscopic imaging.[1,4,12] The balloon is kept inflated for approximately for 1 to 2 min, depending on how the patient tolerates complete occlusion of a main bronchus or lobar bronchus. Occasionally the initial inflation times must be very short, but they can be increased as the dilation occurs. Based on the stenosis diameter after deflation, repeated inflations can be performed if needed. A longer or wider balloon may be used by exchanging the balloon catheter for another over the guide wire. Since the catheter is not placed through the working channel of the bronchoscope, the balloon catheter size is not limited. Immediate success is based on an increased airway diameter after balloon deflation (Fig. 10-9). Figures 10-10 to 10-14 show a stenosis before balloon dilation, after guide-wire and balloon placement, during balloon inflation, and after balloon deflation. We routinely perform a flexible bronchoscopy about 2 weeks after the procedure. Other follow-up bronchoscopies are based on the patient's signs and symptoms. More than one stenosis may be dilated at a session. Likewise, adjunctive treatment such as laser therapy, cryotherapy, or stent placement may follow balloon dilation. This procedure may be performed on intubated, mechanically ventilated patients as well.[1,10,16]

Summary

Flexible bronchoscopic balloon dilation is effective therapy for benign tracheobronchial stenosis. The advantage of this procedure in comparison with other procedures is that it is minimally invasive, safe, and rapid. It avoids general anesthesia. Using fluoroscopy, balloon placement and inflation-deflation are monitored. A guide wire permits easy exchange of the balloon catheter. Complications are infrequent and minor, and no deaths have been attributed directly to balloon dilation. Only fibrous stenosis responds to balloon dilation alone. Bronchial stenosis with coexisting bronchomalacia usually requires combination therapy with another therapeutic modality such as stent placement. The procedure often must be repeated to achieve a satisfactory result.

REFERENCES

1. Brown SB, et al: Tracheobronchial stenosis in infants: Successful balloon dilation therapy. *Pediatr Radiol* 1987; 164:475.
2. Carlin BW, et al: The treatment of endobronchial stenosis using balloon catheter dilation. *Chest* 1988; 93:1148.
3. West JB: Mechanics of breathing. In West JB (ed): *Respiratory Physiology—The Essentials*, 4th ed. Baltimore, Williams & Wilkins, 1990.
4. Cohen MD, et al: Balloon dilation of tracheal and bronchial stenosis. *AJR* 1984; 142:477.
5. Groff DB, Allen JK: Gruentzig balloon catheter dilation for acquired bronchial stenosis in an infant. *Ann Thorac Surg* 1985; 93:379.
6. Fowler CL, et al: Dilation of bronchial stenosis with Gruentzig balloon. *J Thorac Cardiovasc Surg* 1987; 93:308.
7. Nakamura K,et al: Tuberculous bronchial stenosis: Treatment with balloon bronchoplasty. *AJR* 1991; 157:1187.
8. Girard P, et al: Left mainstem bronchial stenosis complicating bronchial artery embolization. *Chest* 1990; 97:1246.
9. Ball JB, et al: Endoscopic bougie and balloon dilation of multiple bronchial stenoses: 10 year follow up. *Thorax* 1991; 46:933.
10. Keller C, Frost A: Fiber optic bronchoplasty: Description of a simple adjunct technique for the management of bronchial stenosis following lung transplantation. *Chest* 1992; 102:995.
11. Carre P, et al, and the Toulouse Lung Transplantation Group: Balloon dilation and self-expanding metal wallstent insertion for management of bronchostenosis following lung transplantation. *Chest* 1994; 105:343.
12. Fouty BW, et al: Dilation of bronchial stenoses due to sarcoidosis using a flexible fiber optic bronchoscope. *Chest* 1994; 106:677.
13. Ferretti G, et al: Benign noninflammatory bronchial stenosis: Treatment with balloon dilation. *Radiology* 1995; 196:831.
14. Golden JA, et al: Bronchoscopy, lung biopsy, and other diagnostic procedures. In Murray JF, Nadel JA (eds): *Textbook of Respiratory Medicine* 2d ed. Philadelphia, Saunders, 1994.
15. Van Steenkiste JF, Lacquet LM: Possibilities and Indications for Nd-YAG Laser and Dilation Therapy in the Management of Tracheal Stenosis. *Acta Oto-rhino-laryngol Belg* 1995; 49:359.
16. Elkerbout SC, et al: Endoscopic balloon dilation of acquired airway stenosis in newborn infants: A promising treatment. *Arch Disease Childhood* 1993; 68:37.
17. Hebra A, et al: Balloon tracheoplasty in children: Results of a 15 year experience. *Pediatr Surg* 1991; 26:957.
18. Wilson NJ: Bronchoscopic observations in tuberculous tracheobronchitis: Clinical pathological correlation. *Dis Chest* 1945; 11:36.
19. Bugher JC, et al: Tuberculous tracheobronchitis: Its pathogenseisis. *Am J Med Sci* 1937; 193:515.
20. Auerbach O: Tuberculosis of the trachea and major bronchi. *Am Rev Tuberc* 1949; 60:604
21. Eloesser L: Bronchial stenosis in pulmonary tuberculosis with some notes on tuberculous stenosis of the trachea and the bronchioles. *Am Rev Tuberc* 1934; 30:123.
22. Salkin D, et al: The natural history of tuberculous tracheobronchitis. *Am Rev Tuberc* 1943; 47:351.

23. Judd AR: Tuberculous tracheobronchitis: A study of 500 consecutive cases. *J Thorac Surg* 1947; 16:512.
24. Dumon JF: Yag laser bronchoscopy. New York, Praeger, 1985:117.
25. Grillo HC, Mathisen DJ: Surgical management of tracheal strictures. *Surg Clin North Am* 1988; 68:511.
26. Iles PB: Multiple bronchial stenoses: Treatment by mechanical dilation. *Thorax* 1981; 36:784.
27. Dumon JF, et al: Treatment of tracheobronchial lesions by laser photoresection. *Chest* 1982; 81:278.
28. Mathur PN, et al: Fiberoptic bronchoscopic cryotherapy in the management of tracheobronchial obstruction. *Chest* 1996; 110:718.

CHAPTER 11

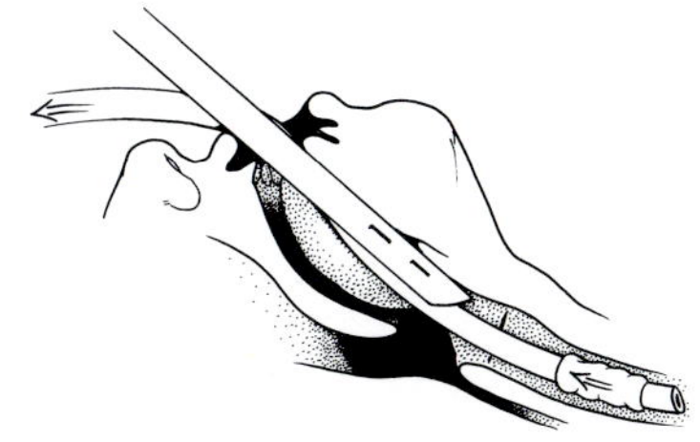

ENDOBRONCHIAL BRACHYTHERAPY

Andrew G. Villanueva, Anthony W. Gray, Jr., and Theodore C. M. Lo

Description of Endobronchial Brachytherapy

Brachytherapy (a term derived from the Greek *brachys*, meaning "short") is a form of radiation treatment in which encapsulated radioactive sources are placed within or near a tumor. Endobronchial brachytherapy has been used to treat patients with many types of tumors involving the tracheobronchial tree, but it has been used most frequently for the treatment of bronchogenic carcinoma. Lung cancer has become the leading cause of cancer deaths in both men and women in the United States; of the greater than 170,000 patients diagnosed each year, more than 80 percent will die of this disease.[1] Fewer than 25 percent of patients with bronchogenic carcinoma have a tumor that is surgically resectable at the time of diagnosis,[2] and 75 percent have non-small cell lung cancer (NSCLC), which responds poorly to chemotherapy. Radiation therapy, therefore, is an important treatment modality for many patients with lung cancer.

In the majority of patients with NSCLC, the tumor will be located in the central part of the tracheobronchial tree,[3] often causing atelectasis, hemoptysis, or postobstructive pneumonia. External beam irradiation is considered standard therapy for such patients, but it is effective in reversing atelectasis in only about 21 percent of patients.[4,5] Moreover, recurrence of tumor after external beam irradiation is common, occurring in up to 50 percent of patients,[6] for which additional external beam irradiation is rarely possible because of the limited radiation tolerance of normal tissue.[7] Several methods are now available that can be used singly or in combination, with or without external beam irradiation, to treat endobronchial tumors.[8] These methods include biopsy recanalization, electrocoagulation (see Chap. 7), cryosurgery (see Chap. 6), laser therapy (see Chap. 5), endobronchial prosthesis (see Chaps. 8 and 9), and endobronchial brachytherapy.

HISTORY

Yankauer[9] reported the first successful case of endobronchial brachytherapy for the relief of bronchial obstruction from lung cancer 75 years ago. He introduced encapsulated "radium emanations" (radon) attached to a cord into the bronchus with a rigid bronchoscope and left the capsule in for 4 to 6 h. In 1929, Kernan and Cracovaner[10] reported the insertion of radium needles and the use of electrocoagulation through a bronchoscope to remove a malignant tumor in a patient's left main bronchus that had caused atelectasis of the lung. In his classic paper on superior pulmonary sulcus tumors, Pancoast[11] reported using brachytherapy in three patients to treat apical carcinoma by implanting radium in tubes or needles directly into the tumor during thoracotomy. In 1933, Kernan[12] summarized eight cases of lung cancer successfully treated with "radon seeds" implanted by means of rigid bronchoscopy. By 1939, Ormerod[13] had collected 100 patients with bronchogenic carcinoma treated with endobronchial brachytherapy, of whom 21 survived for more than 1 year. He either put radon into a "container" and left it in situ for 5 to 7 days or directly inserted radon seeds into the tumor mass. Pool[14] later reviewed his successful experience using a similar technique in 42 patients. In the 1960s, cobalt-60 beads, which have more than two times the specific activity of radon, were used and permitted shorter treatment times.[15] This technique, however, was abandoned because of the considerable personnel exposure to radiation. Indeed, because of the lack of a satisfactory radiation source, the need for rigid bronchoscopy or thoracotomy and general anesthesia for radiation source implantation, and the risk of radiation exposure for medical personnel, endobronchial brachytherapy was not widely used for several years.

Technical developments that led to the resurgence of endobronchial brachytherapy in the 1980s included flexible bronchoscopy, endobronchial laser therapy, the introduction of the radioactive source iridium-192, and the invention of the remote afterloader. The advent of flexible bronchoscopy permitted the insertion of small-caliber afterloading catheters in every major branch of the tracheobronchial tree using only intravenous sedation and local anesthesia.[15] The development of laser bronchoscopy with the neodymium: yttrium-aluminum-garnet (Nd:YAG) laser made possible rapid recanalization of an airway totally or nearly totally occluded by tumor to create a channel through which an afterloading catheter could be inserted. Other techniques have been used for rapid recanalization of airways, such as cryotherapy, balloon dilation, and electrocautery, but the Nd:YAG laser has become the most widely used.[16]

A variety of radionuclides have been used for endobronchial brachytherapy, including cobalt-60, radon-222, cesium-137, gold-198, iodine-125, and palladium-103, but iridium-192 has become the radionuclide of choice since the 1980s because of its high potency and ease of handling. It became available as multiple end-to-end seeds simulating a line source[17] or as a high-activity seed driven by a remote afterloader. The prototype of the modern afterloader was introduced by Henschke and coworkers[18] in 1964 when they described a hand-cranked, remote afterloading device with a cobalt-60 source for use in cervical carcinoma. The hand crank was later replaced by a motor, and the stepwise motion of the source permitted the delivery of tailored brachytherapy. In 1979, a remote afterloader with microprocessor controls, named GAMMAMED I, became available for endobronchial treatment. The development of remote afterloaders and the availability of high-activity radiation sources, such as iridium-192, made endobronchial brachytherapy easier, more convenient, and safer for medical personnel. Brachytherapy for patients no longer needed to be performed using a rigid bronchoscopy, thoracotomy, or general anesthesia, but it could be performed using flexible bronchoscopy and local anesthesia in an outpatient facility. These developments may explain the resurgence of endobronchial brachytherapy and its increasing popularity in the 1980s and 1990s.

In 1983, Mendiondo and associates[19] first reported endobronchial brachytherapy using fiberoptic endoscopy to insert polyethylene tubes loaded with iridium-192 filaments. When remote afterloading equipment and computerized treatment planning programs became commercially available, numerous investigators[20–40] reported on the therapeutic value of endobronchial brachytherapy using primarily radioactive iridium seeds in various doses. Doses for brachytherapy, which depend on the radioactivity of the source, have been described as low dose rate (LDR), intermediate dose rate (IDR), and high dose rate (HDR). Low dose rate is arbitrarily defined as a dose rate up to 1 Gy/h at the point of reference, IDR is defined as a dose rate of 2 to 10 Gy/h, and HDR is defined as a dose rate greater than 10 Gy/h. All dose rates have been described as effective in inducing substantial regression of tumor in the tracheobronchial tree, but relative advantages and disadvantages have been described with each of the dose rates.

BENEFITS AND COMPLICATIONS

Data from several studies, all retrospective, that examined the efficacy of endobronchial brachytherapy are summarized in Table 11-1. All of these studies looked at patients undergoing palliative treatment for malignant tumor involving the tracheobronchial tree, the most common indication for endobronchial brachytherapy. In most of these studies, the response to brachytherapy was assessed both subjectively and objectively. Subjective improvement meant symptomatic palliation, such as cessation of hemoptysis, relief of cough, and improvement of dyspnea. Objective improvement meant the resolution of obstructive pneumonitis or atelectasis as seen on radiography of the chest or the demonstration of increased bronchial patency as seen on follow-up bronchoscopy. No standardized methods were reported to assess palliation in any of these studies.

Low dose rate was the modality most commonly used during the early years of endobronchial brachytherapy. In studies using LDR brachytherapy, the total dose ranged from 20 to 40 Gy calculated at a 0.5 to 2 cm radius.[20,27,30,32,34,35,44] Effective palliation ranged from 60 to 100 percent of patients. Speiser and Spratling[38] reported their experience using IDR brachytherapy (2 to 10 Gy/h for 1 to 4 h) and obtained a response rate, 69 percent, comparable to their results using the LDR.

In 1985, Seagren and associates[41] published the first paper on HDR brachytherapy using the isotope cobalt-60. Apparatus designed to deliver HDR subsequently became commercially available, and iridium-192 be-

Table 11-1
SUMMARY OF RESULTS OF STUDIES ON HIGH DOSE RATE, INTERMEDIATE DOSE RATE, AND LOW DOSE RATE BRACHYTHERAPY

Study	*Year*	*No. of Patients*	*Dose Range*	*Palliation (% Patients)*	*Severe Complications (% Patients)*
Seagren et al[41]	1985	20	HDR	100	0
Allen et al[20]	1985	15	LDR	100	0
Macha et al[29]	1987	56	HDR	74	0
Schray et al[35]	1988	65	LDR	83	11
Mehta et al[30]	1990	38	LDR	70	10
Speiser and Spratling[38]	1990	45	IDR	69	0
Roach et al[34]	1990	17	LDR	60	0
Bedwinek et al[22]	1991	38	HDR	76	32
Speiser[37]	1991	342	HDR	80	7
Lo et al[27]	1992	110	LDR	63	4
Sutedja et al[42]	1992	31	HDR	71	42
Paradelo et al[32]	1992	32	LDR	83	0
Nori et al[43]	1993	32	HDR	91	0
Pisch et al[33]	1993	39	HDR	93	3
Zajac et al[40]	1993	82	HDR	74	2
Chang et al[24]	1994	76	HDR	87	4
Suh et al[44]	1994	37	LDR	75	30
Lo et al[28]	1995	59	HDR	71	0

NOTE: HDR, high dose rate; IDR, intermediate-dose rate; LDR, low dose rate.

came the radionuclide of choice. High dose rate was at least as effective as LDR,[22,24,28,29,33,37,40–43] with response rates ranging from 71 to 100 percent. The variability of results reflects the variability of the methodology among the studies.[15] Included were inhomogeneous groups of patients and tumor; variable additional treatments, such as laser and external radiation; and different treatment schema. The exact contribution of each of these variables was impossible to determine. Some authors[45] suggested that the addition of the laser improved response, but this theory was not corroborated by other larger studies.[39] It was also unclear whether there was a dose-response relationship with HDR, so that the optimal dose and dosage fractionation scheme were unknown. None of the studies directly compared LDR with HDR in a prospective, randomized fashion. Furthermore, none of the studies, regardless of the dose rate used, demonstrated an improvement in survival rates.

The two most serious reported complications from endobronchial brachytherapy were massive hemoptysis and fistula formation to the mediastinum. The incidence of these serious complications ranged from 0 to 42 percent in several large series.[20,22,27,31,35,41,42,46] The incidence of severe complications with LDR brachytherapy ranged from 0 to 11 percent in most studies,[20,27,30,32,34,35,44] although one group[44] reported a 30 percent incidence of exsanguination. In most studies,[24, 29, 33, 37, 40, 41, 43] HDR brachytherapy also appeared relatively safe, with an incidence of severe complications no higher than that associated with LDR brachytherapy. Bedwinek and coworkers[22] and Sutedja and colleagues,[42] however, found higher rates up to 32 and 42 percent, respectively. Although it is possible that the risk of massive pulmonary hemorrhage is related to higher dose rates, it is also likely related to the proximity of the pulmonary arteries to the main stem and upper lobe bronchi. Indeed, Bedwinek and associates[22] found that massive hemoptysis occurred only in patients with recurrent tumor in the right upper lobe, right main stem, or left upper lobe bronchi, and Suh and coworkers[44] found that 6 of their 11 patients who had exsanguination had lesions in the right or left upper lobes.

Other complications include pneumothorax, bronchospasm, bronchial stenosis, and radiation bronchitis.[20,22,27,31,35,39,41,46] These complications are uncommon, and although the rates of some of these complications are related to the dose of brachytherapy, they may also be related to other factors, such as previous external beam irradiation. For example, Speiser and Spratling[39] found that variables associated with an increased incidence of radiation bronchitis and stenosis included large cell carcinoma histology, curative intent, prior laser photoresection, and concurrent external radiation. To summarize, in retrospective, nonrandomized studies of palliative endobronchial brachytherapy for malignant tumors of the tracheobronchial tree, both LDR and HDR provided effective palliation in 70 to 100 percent of patients. Neither dose rate was shown to improve survival rates. The incidence of serious complications appeared similar for both dose rates, although results from some investigators[35,47] suggest that the risk may be higher with HDR. Other factors, such as location of the tumor, may also affect the risk of serious complications.

The decision to use LDR or HDR endobronchial brachytherapy may rest more with cost considerations and an institution's resources since the effectiveness of the two dose rates is similar. Low dose rate requires no expensive equipment and is relatively simple to perform. The major disadvantages include the need for inpatient treatment for 30 to 72 h, catheter intolerance, and potential radiation exposure to hospital personnel. High dose rate can be performed on an outpatient basis and reduces the risk of radiation exposure to medical personnel. Disadvantages include the high initial costs for equipment and setup and the requirement for multiple bronchoscopies. Moreover, although the consensus is that the effective total radiation dose with LDR brachytherapy should be about 30 Gy delivered at 1 cm from the radioactive source in the trachea and at 0.5 cm from the radioactive source in the bronchi,[35] much speculation remains on the optimal dose fractionation schemes with HDR. There is a lack of standard dosage schedules and uncertainty about the optimal fractionation schedule or time period between treatments.[48]

Indications and Contraindications

Endobronchial brachytherapy has been used almost exclusively to treat patients with malignant endobronchial tumors. Although specific indications may vary among institutions, the general criteria for treatment[49] include the following:

1. Non-small cell carcinoma of the lung or metastatic carcinoma
2. Biopsy-proved disease
3. Patient not eligible for or whose disease fails to respond to potentially curative therapies
4. Patient with symptoms caused by a malignant endobronchial lesion or lesions: dyspnea, pneumonitis from obstruction of an airway; hemoptysis; or intractable cough
5. After Nd:YAG laser debulking of tumor
6. Site of lesion suitable for placement of the brachytherapy catheter for delivery of the radiation source

Patients with unresectable primary carcinoma of the lung, recurrent carcinoma of the lung, or cancers metastatic to the airway are potential candidates for endobronchial brachytherapy. The lesions to be treated should be visible by bronchoscopy and located in the trachea, main stem bronchi, or lobar bronchi. Tumors can be either intrinsic or extrinsic to the airway.[20] When the catheter for delivery of the radiation source can be passed beyond an extrinsic or intrinsic airway lesion, brachytherapy can be given. The usual goal for brachytherapy is palliation of symptoms caused by airway obstruction from tumor. Brachytherapy, however, has also been used as an adjunct to external beam radiotherapy for the curative treatment of primary non-small cell carcinoma of the lung.[47] Other investigators[50,51] have used it in patients who have undergone surgical resection of bronchogenic carcinoma but who have histologically positive or suspicious margins after resection. Brachytherapy may thereby offer the potential for cure to patients who have residual tumor after operation.

A few absolute contraindications to endobronchial brachytherapy are known. Contraindications include known fistulas to nonbronchial tissue areas, patients in whom the malignancy has not been proved pathologically or cytologically, and patients who are not symptomatic from the tumor (unless the intent for treatment is curative).[49] Patients with endotracheal carcinoma causing high-grade obstruction should be treated with the Nd:YAG laser and possibly placement of a stent before brachytherapy because of the potential for postradiation edema and total airway obstruction. Brachytherapy should be avoided in patients who cannot safely undergo bronchoscopy or who are moribund.

Required Equipment

To perform modern endobronchial brachytherapy, afterloading catheters can be placed in the tracheobronchial tree using flexible bronchoscopy. To perform LDR brachytherapy, a strand of iridium-192 seeds with 1-cm spacing can be loaded into the catheter. The number of seeds to be used is based on the length of the

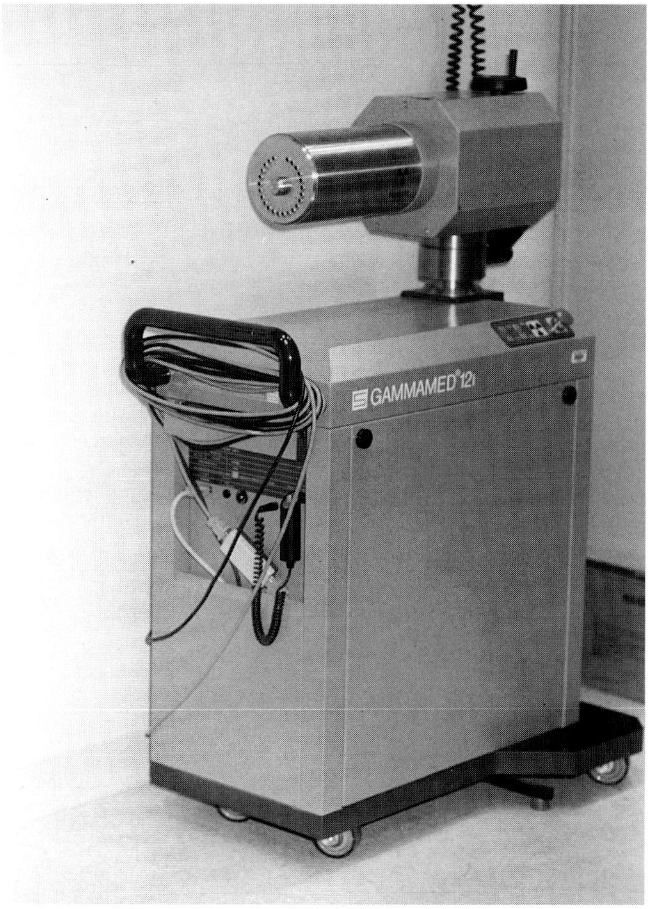

Figure 11-1

The GAMMAMED 12i afterloader used at the Lahey Clinic Medical Center for high dose rate endobronchial brachytherapy.

segment to be treated. For example, if the treatment length is to be 9 cm, 10 iridium-192 seeds can be loaded. The dose of radioactivity ranges from 250 to 470 MBq per seed. The median activity of iridium-192 seeds used for LDR was 330 MBq in our experience, which yielded a dose rate of 45 to 60 cGy per hour at a 2 cm radius from the radioactive source, similar to that reported by Mehta and coworkers.[31]

More sophisticated and expensive equipment is necessary to perform HDR brachytherapy. An HDR remote afterloading brachytherapy system consists of a housing unit for a source with high radioactivity, a source-drive mechanism with operating control, a safeguard system, and a treatment planning computer system (Fig. 11-1). Iridium-192 is the most commonly used radionuclide source today in HDR brachytherapy. The activity of the source is usually in the range of 370 GBq (10 Curie). The average gamma-ray energy is 380 KeV. The radioactive material is sealed inside a metal capsule, which is welded to the end of a cable. Source capsule length varies between 5 and 15 mm, and the source-drive cable length varies from 90 to 150 cm. The cables are generally made of stainless steel, with a diameter of less than 1.2 mm. In the housing unit for the apparatus is a simulated (dummy) source of cable. This serves as an important safeguard since the simulated source must succeed a "dry run" to ensure that the channel, connector, catheter, and applicator are patent through the entire path and without significant curvature to interfere with the travel of the radioactive source. If the test fails, the real source will not be permitted to leave the unit for treatment. Other safety features include a backup battery for the unit, an emergency source retraction system, and a radiation detector and alarm system. In the event of power failure, the emergency system is activated, either to complete the treatment or terminate the treatment by retracting the radioactive source and returning it to the shielded housing in the unit. With HDR treatment, it is necessary that treatment be given in a room heavily shielded and the operation be controlled with a remote unit outside the room. Video and audio communication between the operator and the patient needs to be established for the safety of the operation.

The faceplate of the unit can provide multichannel connection, depending on the applicator used and the specific application. An indexer motor moves the indexer to prescribed channels for proper treatment. Either the actual intraluminal catheters can be connected to the channel outlets of the unit or source-guide tubes can be used to connect the unit to the applicator in the patient.

The source-drive mechanism moves the radioactive source or the simulated dummy source from the HDR unit to the catheter or applicator in the patient in a matter of seconds. Source movement can be a "step-forward" or a "step-backward" design. The source will stop at "dwell points" for a designated time to deliver the prescribed dose. The interval between dwell points is usually prescribed for 0.5 or 1.0 cm, and the number of dwell points is determined by the computer to deliver the optimal dose to the tumor volume. The plan can be complicated when multiple channels are used in the same treatment.

The remote control unit is located outside the treatment room and is a dedicated microprocessor that operates the HDR unit and the source movement. It may be connected to the treatment planning computer through a serial port. The two can be integrated so that treatment can be delivered as prescribed and calculated. For permanent records, all treatment data are printed out on the printer and also stored in the computer. At the time of this writing, three commercial HDR units are available on the market worldwide: GAMMAMED (Isotopen-Technik Dr. Sauerwein GmbH, Haan, Germany), MicroSelectron (Nucletron Corporation, Columbia, MD), and VariSource (Varian, Marietta, GA). All use a radioactive iridium-192 source with a normal activity of 370 GBq (10 Curie) requiring a source change every 3 to 4 months. The manufacturers also produce appropriate catheters and applicators according to the customers' needs (Fig. 11-2).

Figure 11-2

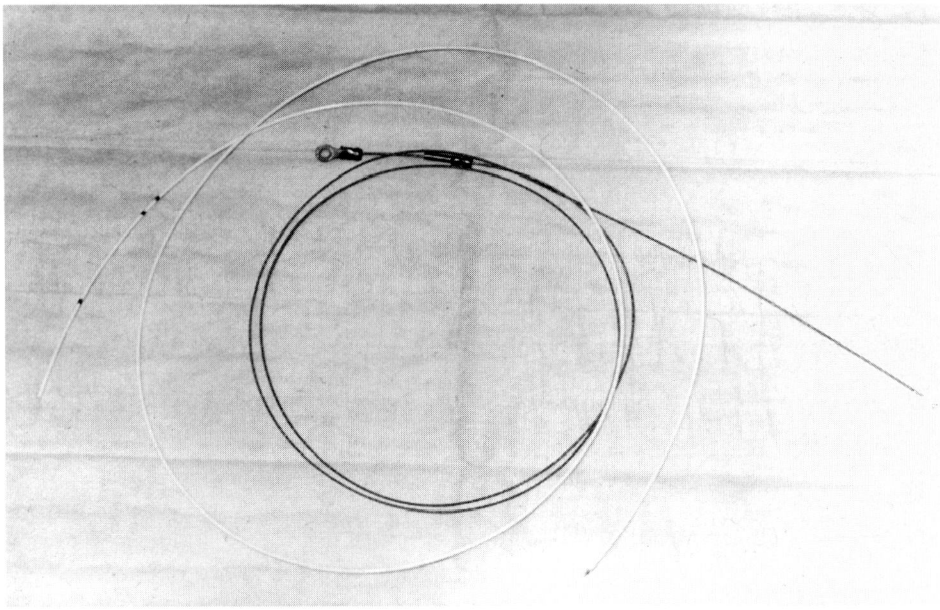

Hollow, plastic afterloading brachytherapy (*white*) catheter with marks 5, 10, and 11 cm from the distal end. The "dummy" source (*dark colored*) is a nonradioactive radiopaque wire that can be inserted into the afterloading brachytherapy catheter to check for patency and position of the catheter. It is removed just before loading of the radioactive source by a remote afterloader.

Figure 11-3

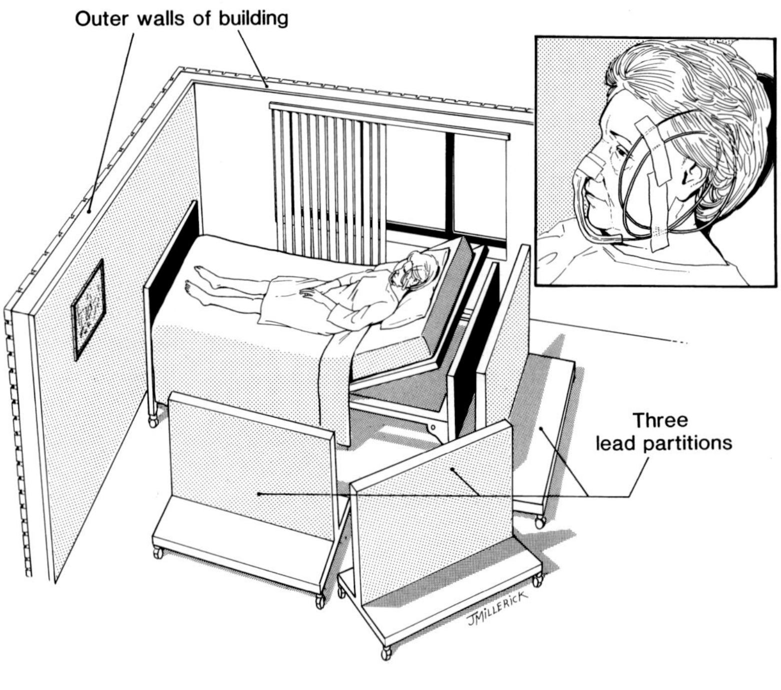

Patient undergoing low dose rate endobronchial brachytherapy in a lead-lined room and surrounded with portable lead shields. The iridium seeds are placed manually into the brachytherapy catheter (*inset*) and left in place for 48 to 72 h.

HOW I DO IT

Technique of Endobronchial Brachytherapy

The instillation of a radioactive source in close proximity to a region affected by the tumor was originally performed by rigid bronchoscopy using direct interstitial implantation. This technique is rarely used today because this procedure can be performed with the less invasive flexible bronchoscope without difficulty by most practicing pulmonologists. Endobronchial brachytherapy was first performed by means of the flexible bronchoscope in 1983 by Mendiondo and colleagues.[19] The technique has undergone further refinement and today is perhaps safer to perform with less risk of accidental radiation exposure to medical personnel.

The procedure, using a standard transnasal approach, is performed by introducing the bronchoscope into the airway to inspect the endobronchial tumor directly and to plan the course of the brachytherapy catheter. The special hollow catheter is then used to provide access for a radioactive source to be placed in

Figure 11-4

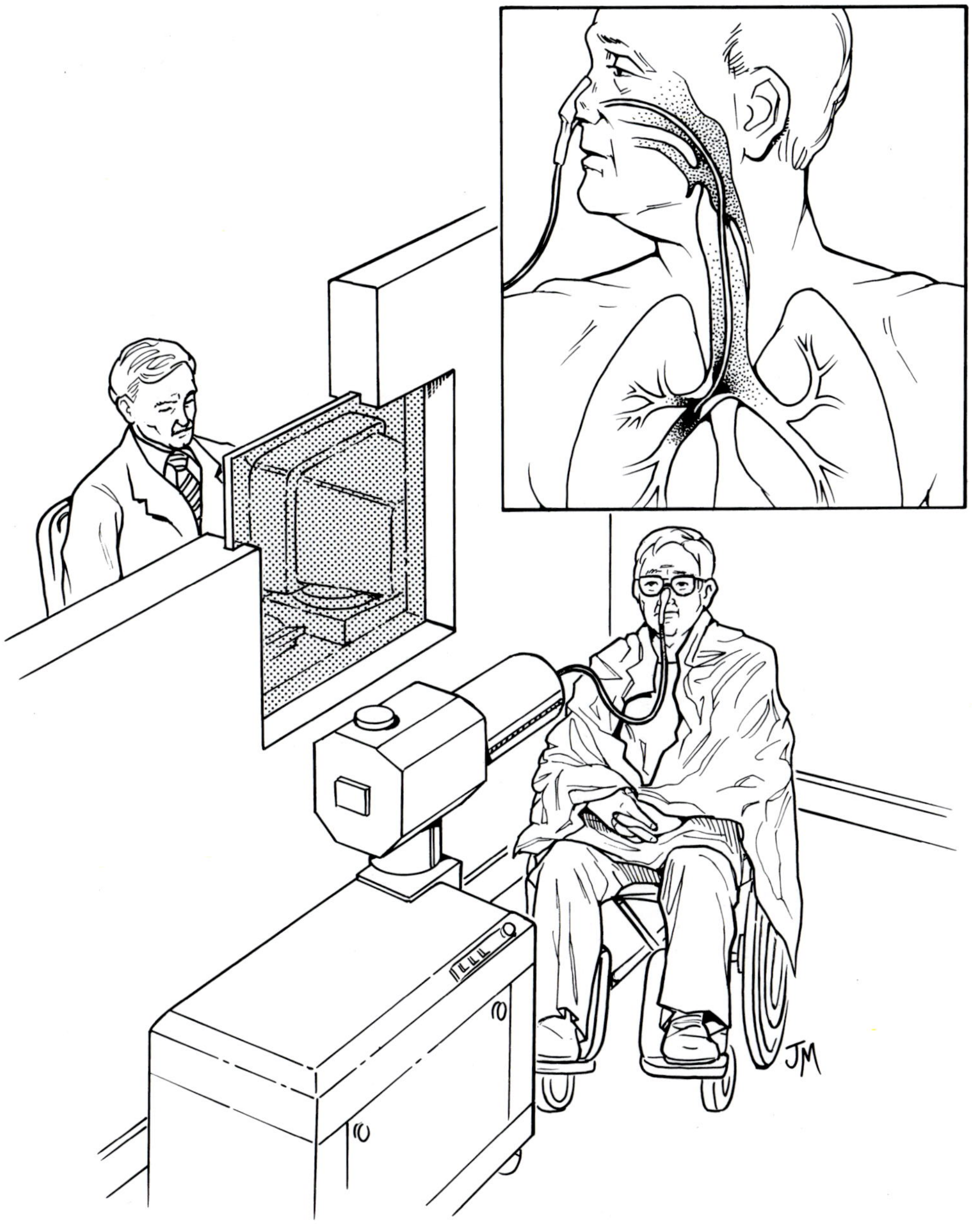

Patient undergoing high dose rate brachytherapy in our Department of Radiation Oncology, where our afterloader is located. A computerized treatment plan is generated and verified. The *inset* shows a patient undergoing treatment of a tumor in the right main stem bronchus. The catheter is positioned so that the 5-cm mark is at the approximate midpoint of the tumor.

close proximity to the diseased region. This catheter is designed to accept a radioactive source through its open proximal end while being capped at its distal end to prevent both contamination of the radioactive source from secretions and accidental passage of the radioactive pellet(s) beyond the distal end of the catheter into the lower airways. Before the catheter is advanced into the bronchoscope, it is marked in several places along its external surface to aid in a more exact radiation prescription. We have found that marks at 5, 10, and 11 cm from the distal end provide sufficient accuracy in estimating the location of the catheter in relation to the proximal and distal extents of the endobronchial tumor. The catheter is advanced through the working channel of the bronchoscope and passed beyond the area of endobronchial disease where special note is made of the exact location of the catheter. The bronchoscope is then slowly withdrawn, and the catheter is advanced at an equal pace by the bronchoscopy assistant. The catheter is held in position at the nose while the bronchoscope is reintroduced alongside the catheter into the airway to ensure that the catheter had not become dislodged while the bronchoscope was removed. Once again, careful note is made of the exact position of the catheter, often placed several centimeters beyond the midpoint of the tumor. After the operator confirms direct visual inspection, the catheter is secured to the nose, and a radiopaque guidewire is inserted. Chest radiography or fluoroscopy is used to ensure maintenance of proper catheter position after transport of the patient to the radiation oncology department where the endobronchial radiation is delivered by an afterloading technique.

Before 1991, we used LDR brachytherapy. After the brachytherapy catheter was placed using bronchoscopy, the patient was admitted to the hospital and placed in a lead-lined room and surrounded with portable lead shields (Fig. 11-3). The iridium seeds were placed manually by one of our radiation oncologists and left in place for 48 to 72 h. A strand of iridium-192 seed with 1 cm spacing (Best Industries, Springfield, VA) was inserted into the distal end of the brachytherapy catheter. The number of seeds used was based on the length of the segment treated. For most applications, 10 iridium-192 seeds were used, resulting in a treatment length of 9 cm at the distal end of the catheter. The dose of radioactivity ranged from 250 to 470 MBq per seed, and the medium activity was 330 MBq, which yielded a dose rate of 45 to 60 cGy/h at a 2 cm radius from the radioactive source.

Since 1991, we have been using HDR brachytherapy. After the brachytherapy catheter is placed, we now perform brachytherapy on an outpatient basis in our Department of Radiation Oncology, where our afterloader is located (Fig. 11-4). We use a remote afterloading unit (GAMMAMED 12i) to load the iridium-192 source with a nominal activity of 370 GBq per seed. After the endobronchial catheters are placed, dummy seeds are inserted, and radiography of the chest is obtained to verify the position of the catheter. The stopping points of the source and the number of stops are determined to ensure coverage of the segment of endobronchial tumor with adequate margins. The separation between stopping points is 1 cm. Computerized treatment planning is performed and verified. Our protocol aims for a dose of 7 Gy calculated at a 1 cm radius, and the treatment time is usually less than 15 min. After each session, the catheters are removed manually, and the patient is discharged to home. The patient typically undergoes 3 or 4 weekly treatments.

REFERENCES

1. Ries LAG, Kosary CL, Hankey BF, et al (eds): *SEER Cancer Statistics Review, 1973–1994, National Cancer Institute.* NIH Publication No. 97-2789: Bethesda, MD; 1997.
2. Shields TW: Surgical therapy for carcinoma of the lung. *Clin Chest Med* 1982; 3:369–387.
3. Gelb AF, Epstein JD: Laser in treatment of lung cancer. *Chest* 1984; 86:662–666.
4. Slawson RG, Scott RM: Radiation therapy in bronchogenic carcinoma. *Radiology* 1979; 132:175–176.
5. Chetty KG, Moran EM, Sassoon CSH, Viravathana T, Light RW: Effect of radiation therapy on bronchial obstruction due to bronchogenic carcinoma. *Chest* 1988; 95:582–584.
6. Perez CA, Stanley K, Grundy G, Hanson W, Rubin P, Kramer S, Brady LW, Marks JE, Perez-Tamayo R, Brown GS, Concannon JP, Rotman M: Impact of irradiation technique and tumor extent in tumor control and survival of patients with unresectable non-oat cell carcinoma of the lung: Report by the Radiation Therapy Oncology Group. *Cancer* 1982; 50:1091–1098.
7. Sullivan FJ: Radiation biology of lung cancer. In Pass HI, Mitchell JB, Johnson DH, et al (eds): *Lung Cancer: Principles and Practice.* Philadelphia: Lippincott-Raven; 1996:219–249.
8. Mehta MP: Endobronchial radiotherapy for lung cancer. In Pass HI, Mitchell JB, Johnson DH, et al (eds): *Lung Cancer: Principles and Practice.* Philadelphia: Lippincott-Raven; 1996:741–750.
9. Yankauer S: Lung tumor treated bronchoscopically. *NY Med J* 1922; 115:741–742.
10. Kernan JD, Cracovaner AJ: Carcinoma of the lung. *Arch Surg* 1929; 18:315–321.
11. Pancoast HK: Superior pulmonary sulcus tumor: Tumor characterized by pain, Horner's syndrome, destruction of bone and atrophy of hand muscles. *JAMA* 1932; 99:1391–1396.
12. Kernan JD: Carcinoma of the lung and bronchus: Treatment with radon implantations and diathermy. *Arch Otolaryngol* 1933; 17:457–475.
13. Ormerod FC: Some notes on the treatment of carcinoma of the bronchus. *J Laryngol Otol* 1941; 56:1–10.
14. Pool JL: Bronchoscopy in the treatment of lung cancer. *Ann Otol Rhinol Laryngol* 1961; 70:1172–1178.
15. Mehta MP, Speiser BL, Macha HN: High dose rate brachytherapy for lung cancer. In Nag S (ed): *High Dose Rate Brachytherapy: A Textbook.* Armonk, NY: Futura Publishing: 1994; 295–319.
16. Ramser ER, Beamis JF Jr: Laser bronchoscopy. *Clin Chest Med* 1995; 16:415–426.
17. Shahabi S, Mehta MP, Wiley AL, et al: The role of computed tomography in dosimetric evaluation of endobronchial implants. *Endocurie/Hypertherm Oncol* 1988; 4:187.
18. Henschke UK, Hilaris BS, Mahan GD: Remote afterloading with intracavitary applicators. *Radiology* 1964; 83:344–345.

19. Mendiondo OA, Dillon M, Beach JL: Endobronchial irradiation in the treatment of recurrent non-oat cell bronchogenic carcinoma. *J Ky Med Assoc* 1983; 81:287–290.
20. Allen MD, Baldwin JC, Fish VJ, Goffinet DR, Cannon WB, Mark JB: Combined laser therapy and endobronchial radiotherapy for resectable lung carcinoma with bronchial obstruction. *Am J Surg* 1985; 150:71–77.
21. Aygun C, Weiner S, Scariato A, Spearman D, Stark L: Treatment of non-small cell lung cancer with external beam radiotherapy and high dose rate brachytherapy. *Int J Radiat Oncol Biol Phys* 1992; 23:127–132.
22. Bedwinek J, Petty A, Bruton C, Sofield J, Lee L: The use of high dose rate endobronchial brachytherapy to palliate symptomatic endobronchial recurrence of previously irradiated bronchogenic carcinoma. *Int J Radiat Oncol Biol Phys* 1992; 22:23–30.
23. Burt PA, O'Driscoll BR, Notley HM, Barber PV, Stout R: Intraluminal irradiation for the palliation of lung cancer with high dose rate micro-Selectron. *Thorax* 1990; 45:765–768.
24. Chang LF, Horvath J, Peyton W, Ling SS: High dose rate afterloading intraluminal brachytherapy in malignant airway obstruction of lung cancer. *Int J Radiat Oncol Biol Phys* 1994; 28:589–596.
25. Fritz P, Schraube P, Becker HD, Loffler E, Wannenmacher M, Pastyr O: A new applicator, positionable to the center of tracheobronchial lumen for HDR-IR-192-afterloading of tracheobronchial tumors. *Int J Radiat Oncol Biol Phys* 1991; 20:1061–1066.
26. Lang N, Maners A, Broadwater J, Shewmake K, Chu D, Westbrook K: Management of airway problems in lung cancer patients using the neodymium-yttrium-aluminum-garnet (Nd:YAG) laser and endobronchial radiotherapy. *Am J Surg* 1988; 156:463–465.
27. Lo TCM, Beamis JF Jr, Weinstein RS, Costey GE, Andrews CF, Webb-Johnson DC, Girshovich L, Leibenhaut MH: Intraluminal low-dose rate brachytherapy for malignant endobronchial obstruction. *Radiother Oncol* 1992; 23:16–20.
28. Lo TCM, Girshovich L, Healey GA, Beamis JF Jr, Webb-Johnson DC, Villanueva AG, Gray AW Jr, Wu TR: Low dose rate versus high dose rate intraluminal brachytherapy for malignant endobronchial tumors. *Radiother Oncol* 1995; 35:193–197.
29. Macha HN, Koch K, Stadler M, Schumacher W, Krumhaar D: New technique for treating occlusive and stenosing tumours of the trachea and main bronchi: Endobronchial irradiation by high dose iridium-192 combined with laser canalisation. *Thorax* 1987; 42:511–515.
30. Mehta M, Shahabi S, Jarjour N, Seinmetz M, Kubsad S: Effect of endobronchial radiation therapy on malignant bronchial obstruction. *Chest* 1990; 97:662–665.
31. Mehta MP, Shahabi S, Jarjour NN, Kinsella TJ: Endobronchial irradiation for malignant airway obstruction. *Int J Radiat Oncol Biol Phys* 1989; 17:847–851.
32. Paradelo JC, Waxman MJ, Throne BJ, Beller TA, Kopecky WJ: Endobronchial irradiation with 192 Ir in the treatment of malignant endobronchial obstruction. *Chest* 1992; 102:1072–1074.
33. Pisch J, Villamena PC, Harvey JC, Rosenblatt E, Mishra S, Beattie EJ: High dose-rate endobronchial irradiation in malignant airway obstruction. *Chest* 1993; 104:721–725.
34. Roach M 3d, Leidholdt EM Jr, Tatera BS, Joseph J: Endobronchial radiation therapy (EBRT) in the management of lung cancer. *Int J Radiat Oncol Biol Phys* 1990; 18:1449–1454.
35. Schray MF, McDougall JC, Martinez A, Cortese DA, Brutinel WM: Management of malignant airway compromise with laser and low dose rate brachytherapy: The Mayo Clinic experience. *Chest* 1988; 93:264–269.
36. Schray MF, McDougall JC, Martinez A, Edmundson GK, Cortese DA: Management of malignant airway obstruction: Clinical and dosimetric considerations using an iridium-192 afterloading technique in conjunction with theneodymium-YAG laser. *Int J Radiat Oncol Biol Phys* 1985; 11:403–409.
37. Speiser B: Advantages of high dose rate remote afterloading systems: Physics or biology (editorial). *Int J Radiat Oncol Biol Phys* 1991; 20:1133–1135.
38. Speiser B, Spratling L: Intermediate dose rate remote afterloading brachytherapy for intraluminal control of bronchogenic carcinoma. *Int J Radiat Oncol Biol Phys* 1990; 18: 1443–1448.
39. Speiser BL, Spratling L: Remote afterloading brachytherapy for the local control of endobronchial carcinoma. *Int J Radiat Oncol Biol Phys* 1993; 25:579–587.
40. Zajac AJ, Kohn ML, Heiser D, Peters JW: High-dose-rate intraluminal brachytherapy in the treatment of endobronchial malignancy: Work in progress. *Radiology* 1993; 187:571–575.
41. Seagren SL, Harrell JH, Horn RA: High dose rate intraluminal irradiation in recurrent endobronchial carcinoma. *Chest* 1985; 88:810–814.
42. Sutedja G, Baris G, Schaake-Koning C, van Zandwijk N: High-dose rate brachytherapy in patients with local recurrences after radiotherapy of non-small cell lung cancer. *Int J Radiat Oncol Biol Phys* 1992; 24:551–553.
43. Nori D, Allison R, Kaplan B, Samala E, Osian A, Karbowitz S: High dose-rate intraluminal irradiation in bronchogenic carcinoma: Technique and results. *Chest* 1993; 104:1006–1011.
44. Suh JH, Dass KK, Pagliaccio L, Taylor ME, Saxton JP, Tan M, Mehta AC: Endobronchial radiation therapy with or without neodymium yttrium aluminum garnet laser resection for managing malignant airway obstruction. *Cancer* 1994: 73: 2583–2588.
45. Miller JI Jr, Phillips TW: Neodymium: YAG laser and brachytherapy in the management of inoperable bronchogenic carcinoma. *Ann Thorac Surg* 1990; 50:190–195.
46. Speiser B, Spratling L: High dose rate remote afterloading brachytherapy in the control of endobronchial carcinoma. In Martinez AA, Orton CG, Mould RF (eds): *Brachytherapy: HDR and LDR.* Columbia, MD: Nucletron Corp; 1990: 10–23.
47. Sutedja G, Baris G, van Zandwijk N, Postmus PE: High-dose rate brachytherapy has a curative potential in patients with intraluminal squamous cell lung cancer. *Respiration* 1994; 61:167–168.
48. Villanueva AG, Lo TCM, Beamis JF Jr: Endobronchial brachytherapy. *Clin Chest Med* 1995; 16:445–454.
49. Kress WS: Overview of endobronchial brachytherapy. In Martinez AA, Orton CG, Mould RF (eds): *Brachytherapy: HDR and LDR.* Columbia, MD: Nucletron Corp; 1990:3–9.
50. Aye RW, Mate TP, Anderson HN, Johnson LP, Hill L: Extending the limits of lung cancer resection. *Am J Surg* 1993; 165:572–576.
51. Sutedja G, Baris G, Zoetmulder F, van Zandwijk N: High dose rate brachytherapy improves resectability in squamous cell lung cancer. *Chest* 1992; 102:308–398.

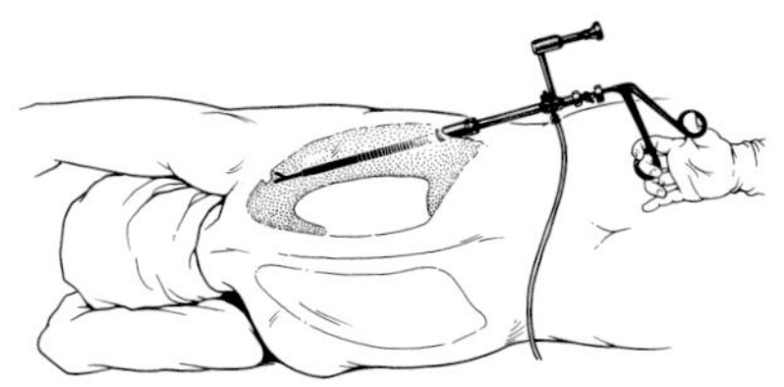

MEDICAL THORACOSCOPY

C H A P T E R 1 2

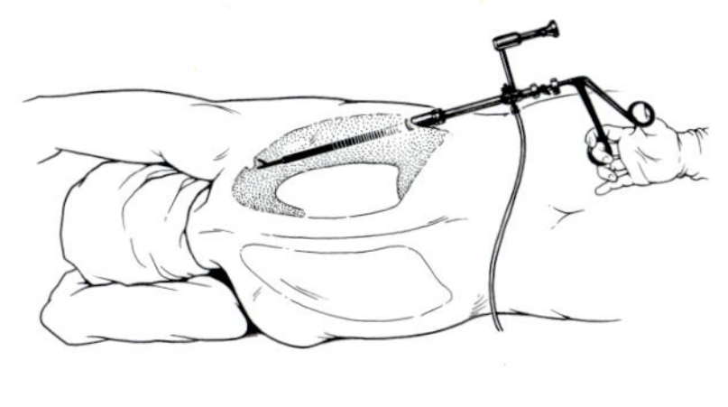

CHEST TUBE PLACEMENT

Karen M. Wolf, David C. Mares, and Praveen N. Mathur

Variations of chest tube placement have been used as a complement to patient care through the entire history of modern medicine. The initial description of the use of a metal tube inserted into the pleural space to drain the "bad humors" is credited to Hippocrates.[1] Playfair described the treatment of an empyema with closed chest drainage and underwater seal in 1872. The procedure was, however, not used routinely until 1917 when postinfluenza empyema became a common therapeutic dilemma.[2] Finally, during World War II intercostal drains were widely used for traumatic hemothoraces and pneumothoraces and eventually led to the dramatic decline in mortality from thoracic trauma.[3] In modern medicine, a chest tube is used to drain abnormal collections of fluid and/or air from the pleural space, causing expansion of the lung and restoration of pulmonary physiology.

Chest tube placement is a commonly performed procedure and an essential part of the procedural knowledge base of all pulmonary and critical care physicians. The American Board of Internal Medicine has required competency in chest tube placement for Critical Care Board Certification, yet in a recent survey of pulmonary physicians, only 60 percent reported chest tube placement as a procedure which they perform in their clinical practice. The survey suggested that the median number of thoracostomy placements was ten per year with a 25 to 75 percent median range of 4 to 20 procedures per year.[4] Because the routine function of pulmonary and critical care physicians includes: care for critically ill patients, frequent placement of central venous accesses, care for patients with pneumonia complicated by effusions, and care for patients with spontaneous pneumothoraces, it is essential that these physicians obtain and maintain competency in thoracostomy tube placement.

Who should place chest tubes? The technique of chest tube placement for emergent evacuation of a tension pneumothorax should be well known to pulmonologists, surgeons, anesthesiologists, radiologists, and all physicians engaged in emergency care practices, placing central lines or managing ventilator patients. Physicians caring for patients with complex pleural diseases, e.g., patients with parapneumonic effusions, malignant effusions, or with chest trauma, should be adept in lateral chest wall large caliber tube thoracostomy. Basic operational skills include: the ability to recognize pneumothoraces or effusions by physical examination and chest radiograph, an understanding of thoracoabdominal anatomy, competence in basic surgical procedures such as sterile technique, blunt dissection and suturing, the ability to administer local anesthesia and intravenous analgesia, and access to appropriate equipment, supplies, and assistance.[5]

The purpose of this chapter is to describe the indications and a variety of techniques for pleural space drainage by means of tube thoracostomy. Contraindications and complications are discussed. Care for the drainage system is addressed as is the technique for chest tube removal.

Indications for Chest Tube Placement

The pleural space is defined by the reflection of the visceral and parietal pleura at the hilum onto the mediastinal, chest wall, and lung surfaces. In health, the pleural surfaces are moistened by scant fluid, maintained by a balance of oncotic and hydrostatic pressures in the subpleural vessels and lymphatics. Intrapleural pressure is negative to that of atmospheric pressure. Processes that disrupt the integrity of the pleural lining or the balance of oncotic and hydrostatic pressures, cause air or fluid to accumulate in the space between the visceral and parietal pleura. Air or fluid compresses the lung causing partial or complete collapse. If the process which caused air or fluid accumulation ceases through medical management, the pleural surface and contents may revert to normal without longstanding sequelae. Should the insult prove irreversible or cause overwhelming symptoms, invasive intervention is required. Air or fluid can be removed from the pleural space by simple aspiration or chest tube drainage.

PNEUMOTHORAX

A pneumothorax is the presence of air between the visceral and parietal pleura. Air enters into the pleural space either from the alveoli through the visceral pleural surface or by transthoracic perforation of the parietal pleura. Pneumothoraces are categorized into two subsets, traumatic and spontaneous. Spontaneous pneumothoraces are further divided into primary and secondary subcategories.[5] Spontaneous primary pneumothoraces are those which occur in otherwise healthy adults. Spontaneous secondary pneumothoraces are those associated with underlying lung disease such as bullous emphysema. A tension pneumothorax is air under positive pressure in the pleural space causing compression and shift of the mediastinum and impeding cardiac output. Pneumothoraces may resolve without intervention.[6,7] Pneumothoraces require evacuation if persistent or if cardiopulmonary function is significantly impaired.

A pneumothorax without concomitant fluid accumulation can be treated with needle or catheter aspiration rather than chest tube insertion.[8–11] This procedure is suitable for mildly to moderately symptomatic patients with no significant underlying pulmonary disease. The needle or catheter aspiration technique is also appropriate for emergent treatment of a tension pneumothorax until trained personnel can place a chest tube. Pneumothoraces that recollect following simple aspiration, or occur in patients with underlying lung disease and moderate to severe symptoms, are best treated with a chest tube.

PLEURAL FLUID

Infected pleural effusions, parapneumonic effusions at high risk for complication, and hemothoraces should be tapped dry by aspiration or chest tube drainage.[12] Tube or catheter drainage followed by chemical pleurodesis has been recommended for symptomatic recurrent pleural effusions if refractory to medical management.[13,14]

Chest tube placement is indicated postoperatively following cardiopulmonary surgery and for bronchopleural fistula. Although only 5 percent of mechanically ventilated patients develop pneumothorax, barotrauma occurs in 30 to 50 percent of ventilated patients with acute, diffuse parenchymal injury.[15–17] Prophylactic chest tube placement has been suggested for patients at high risk of pneumothorax, for example, patients with high inspiratory pressures and the adult respiratory distress syndrome (ARDS). The only support of this practice is the finding that the diagnosis of ventilator-associated pneumothorax is delayed in as many as 30 percent of mechanically ventilated patients, one-third of whom can be expected to develop tension pneumothorax.[18]

Contraindications to Chest Tube Placement

Chest tube placement is not recommended for small, asymptomatic pneumothoraces or effusions occurring in competent, compliant patients. These can be observed for spontaneous remission, or, in the case of small effusions, for response to noninvasive therapies.[19,20] Coagulopathies should be corrected prior to chest tube placement. Chest tubes should not be placed through infected tissue or next to abraded tissue to which dressings and tape would cause further irritation.

Complications and Outcomes

Complications of chest tube placement are listed in Table 12-1.[12,21–32] These reflect experiences with large caliber (24 French and greater) chest tubes. Large caliber tubes are most commonly placed by means of blunt dissection through the lateral thoracic wall into the pleural space. This technique causes less trauma to the lung and adjacent tissues compared to sharp penetration techniques.[33] In a retrospective review by Millikan, empyema and penetration of adjacent organs were the two most frequent complications, 2 and 1 percent, respectively.[23] Similarly, Etoch evaluated complications in 379 trauma patients who underwent 599 tube thoracostomies.[24] The overall complication rate was 21 percent. Complications noted by Etoch's group were: inadequate drainage of the effusion or pneumothorax, recurrent pneumothorax after chest tube removal, inadequate positioning requiring replacement, empyema, patient removal of the chest tube and lung laceration. The complications which most frequently led to repeat chest tube placement were: postremoval pneumothorax, improper placement, and undrained pneumothorax or hemothorax.

Heffner and coworkers recently described the incidence of recurrent pneumothorax in a retrospective review of a mechanically ventilated population from whom trauma cases were excluded. Staff surgeons placed the initial chest tubes using the lateral thoracic approach. Thirty-four percent of pneumothoraces recurred with an ipsilateral chest tube in place. Recurrence was most common for patients with ARDS. Fifty-six percent of recurrent pneumothoraces had tension physiology.[26]

Laceration of an intercostal vessel or inadvertent penetration of an adjacent organ or tissue can cause

Table 12-1
COMPLICATIONS OF CHEST TUBE PLACEMENT

Malpositioning into interlobar fissures, lung, adjacent organs (e.g., esophagus), central vasculature, subcutaneous tissue
Recurrent ipsilateral pneumothorax or fluid collection
Contralateral pneumothorax
Cardiogenic shock from compression of right ventricle
Nerve damage, e.g., intercostal nerve, phrenic nerve
Unilateral noncardiogenic pulmonary edema (Reexpansion pulmonary edema)
Bronchopleural fistula
Adhesions with lung entrapment
Pain
Bleeding
Infection

significant bleeding. The intercostal neurovascular bundle is usually adjacent to the inferior border of the rib but can be found above and below the rib anteriorly, or near the superior surface of the adjacent rib in geriatric patients.[34] Hemostasis might be achieved by local pressure and correction of any coagulopathy. Picone and colleagues reported tamponade of a brisk intercostal vessel bleed by covering the wound site with a pressure dressing after replacing the chest tube with a balloon-tipped Foley catheter attached to 20 cm water suction and a 1-lb weight for traction.[35] Urschel reported success by anchoring the Foley balloon, pulled tight against the chest wall, with a catheter clamp at the surface of the skin.[36] Bleeding refractory to these measures requires surgical intervention.

While the complications noted above pertain to large caliber tubes used predominantly in surgical settings, small caliber tubes are frequently employed in both surgical and nonsurgical situations. Sargent and Turner described a small bore catheter over sharp trocar technique for emergent drainage of pneumothorax in 1970.[37] The safety and efficacy of this technique and its modifications for the treatment of pneumothorax, empyema, and pleurodesis are reported in a number of publications.[37–51] Quinn and Demlow also described the placement of large caliber (24 to 28 French) catheters using a guide wire and dilator technique instead of blunt dissection for pneumothoraces or empyemas.[52]

Small caliber chest tubes should successfully treat 70 to 100 percent of pneumothoraces, 50 to 100 percent of effusions and many complicated parapneumonic effusions which initially fail traditional chest tube drainage.[53–55] Key to the success of these catheters is placement under radiologic guidance, patient selection and timing.[56,57] The types of complications attributable to small bore catheter placement are similar to large caliber chest tube, though the rate of complications is lower. For the 538 small gauge catheters detailed in Table 12-2, the complication rate was 5 percent. The majority of these complications were incompletely drained or recurrent pneumothoraces or catheter occlusion. Recent series have been less troubled by catheter occlusion, likely due to improved equipment and techniques.

What are the outcomes and costs for simple aspiration or chest tube placement? Little data specifically address these issues. Delius and coworkers successfully treated 90 percent of 131 simple pneumothoraces with catheter aspiration.[45] In this study, emergency room patients were discharged to home if the 6-h follow-up chest radiograph showed complete resolution. Patients with residual pneumothoraces were treated with either chest tube or application of suction to the aspiration catheter. The average length of stay was 11 days for the former and less than 5 days for the latter. Ninety-one percent of LeMense's empyema patients were discharged from the hospital after an average stay of 20 hospital days.[57] This group had a 56 percent success rate with image directed catheter drainage of empyema. Surgical intervention, such as thoracotomy with decortication, Eloesser flap, or empyema tube (Chamberlain procedure), was successful for 93 percent. The surgical cases were hospitalized approximately 10 days longer than the nonsurgical in part due to failed attempts at nonsurgical interventions. These two reports suggest that prompt, staged invasive management of pneumothoraces and parapneumonic effusions is effective.

Table 12-2
USE OF AND RESULTS AND COMPLICATIONS FROM SMALL-BORE (8–16 FRENCH) PERCUTANEOUS CHEST TUBE PLACEMENT

Author (Year)	*Patients/Catheters*	*Problems*	*Success Rate, %*	*Complications Rate*
Peters[38] (1984)	25/27	Pneumothorax, I9	95	Occluded, 15
		Effusion, 6	100	Dislodged, 7
		Lung abscess, 1	100	Malpositioned, 4
Crouch[39] (1987)	44/53	Empyema, 20	70	Pneumothorax, 9
		Pneumothorax, 10	90	Occlusion, 6
		Effusion, 9	56	Catheter fracture, 2
		Lung Abscess, 4	100	Infection, 2
		Mediastinal, cyst 1	100	SQ emphysema, 2
Conces[40] (1988)	79/84	Pneumothorax	87	None
Guyton[43] (1988)	13/13	Pneumothroax, 10	80	Pneumothorax, 8
		Effusion, 3	100	
Parker[44] (1989)	13/13	Effusion	62	Pneumothroax, 15
Delius[45] (1989)	114/131	Pneumothorax	69	Hemothorax, 1 Catheter fracture, 2
Molina[46] (1990)	10/11	Pneumothorax	90	Malpositioned, 10
Samelson[47] (1991)	16/16	Pneumothorax	100	Patient removed, 13 Hematoma, 6
Kerr[48] (1991)	12/17	Empyema	83	None
Pollak[49] (1994)	8/9 (8 pigtail catheters)	Loculated effusion	50	None
Seaton[50] (1995)	47	Malignant effusion	81 (of evaluable patients)	N/A
Moulton[51] (1995)	118/NA	Empyema, 79 Loculated effusion, 27 Hemothorax, 10 Exudative effusion, 2	94 overall	None

HOW I DO IT

The proper placement and management of intercostal drains requires knowledge of thoracic anatomy, sterile techniques, a procedure for tube placement, the contraindications to tube placement, and possible complications of thoracostomy.

ANATOMY

Thoracic and specifically intercostal anatomy is depicted on many of the included figures. The skin overlies subcutaneous adipose tissue which is superficial to the fascial lining of the intercostal muscles. The three layers of intercostal muscles lie over and between the ribs. Lining the inside of the thoracic cavity is the parietal pleura. The intercostal neurovascular bundle traverses the chest wall from the vertebral body around the circumference of the chest and to the midline anteriorly in a depression on the inferior aspect of each rib, the intercostal groove. In certain areas other muscle groups may be present between the skin and thoracic cage, such as the pectoralis group anteriorly and the latissimus dorsi posteriorly. Also it must be remembered that the internal mammary artery and vein travel parasternally at a distance of approximately 20 mm from each edge of the sternum.[58] Surgically placed structures, such as mammary implants must also be observed and avoided.[59]

INDICATIONS FOR CHEST TUBE PLACEMENT

Of the many clinical situations in which chest tube placement is indicated, all involve drainage of an abnormal collection of air or fluid. The indications include: pneumothorax, pleural effusion, hemothorax, chylothorax, or any combination of the above.[5] Specific indications are listed in Table 12-3. Fluid drainage usually requires a large bore tube, 28 French to 32 French for uncomplicated effusions, while more viscous fluids, hemothorax, and complicated or infected effusions require at least 36 French and possibly as large as 42 French tubes to prevent occlusion of the tube by the viscous fluid. In many situations drainage of a pneumothorax can be accomplished by a smaller bore tube, 8 to 20 French.

Table 12-3
INDICATIONS FOR CHEST TUBE PLACEMENT

Pneumothorax
Infected pleural effusion (empyema)
Complicated parapneumonic effusion
Recurrent pleural effusion
Hemothorax
Postthoracotomy chest drainage
Pleurodesis
Bronchopleural fistula

CONTRAINDICATIONS

Often, indications for thoracostomy occur in a tenuous and relatively ill population of patients. As with any procedure, the risks must be weighed against the benefits in determination of the necessity for and timing of thoracostomy (Table 12-4). Major concerns include: coagulopathies, multiple pleural adhesions, ability to lay in the proper position without moving, allergies or hypersensitivities to medications used, and massive hemothorax without adequate fluid resuscitation.[60] Treatment of correctable coagulopathies ideally would occur prior to chest tube placement if the patient will tolerate a delay. If possible the platelet count should exceed 50,000. Unfortunately there is little data regarding the safety of thoracostomy placement in patients with coagulopathies. In thoracentesis, however, McVay and coworkers demonstrated that there was no increased risk when prothrombin and activated partial thromboplastin times were below twice control values.[61] In addition, increased risk of bleeding was not noted for platelet counts exceeding 25,000, however, there was a significant increase in bleeding complications if the serum creatinine was above 6 mg/dl. The level of invasiveness of the two procedures must be contemplated when interpreting this data. Obviously if a patient has an immediate need for open thoracotomy and such therapy is available, thoracostomy may be an unneeded delay in definitive therapy and a compromise in surgical sterility. In all situations, the relative risks and benefits must be weighed in making decisions regarding thoracostomy placement.

CHOOSING A SITE

The two most common sites for chest tube placement are the lateral and anterior sites, but nearly any site may be used if radiographic guidance is utilized. The anterior site lies along the midclavicular line at the second or third intercostal space and is specifically used for drainage of small pneumothoraces (Fig. 12-1). This site is limited to small tubes 8 to 18 French because the intercostal space is at its smallest anteriorly. The lateral site has a wider intercostal space allowing tubes as large as 42 French. The typical location for lateral thoracostomy is along the anterior or mid-axillary line at the fifth or sixth intercostal space (Fig. 12-2). Tube placement at this location allows the operator to either direct the tube anteriorly to drain air or posteriorly to drain fluid. Any anatomically possible site may be used, however, if appropriate radiographic guidance

Table 12-4
CONTRAINDICATIONS FOR CHEST TUBE PLACEMENT

Small, asymptomatic pneumothorax or effusion
Uncorrected coagulopathy
Transudative effusions for which adequate medical therapy has not been attained

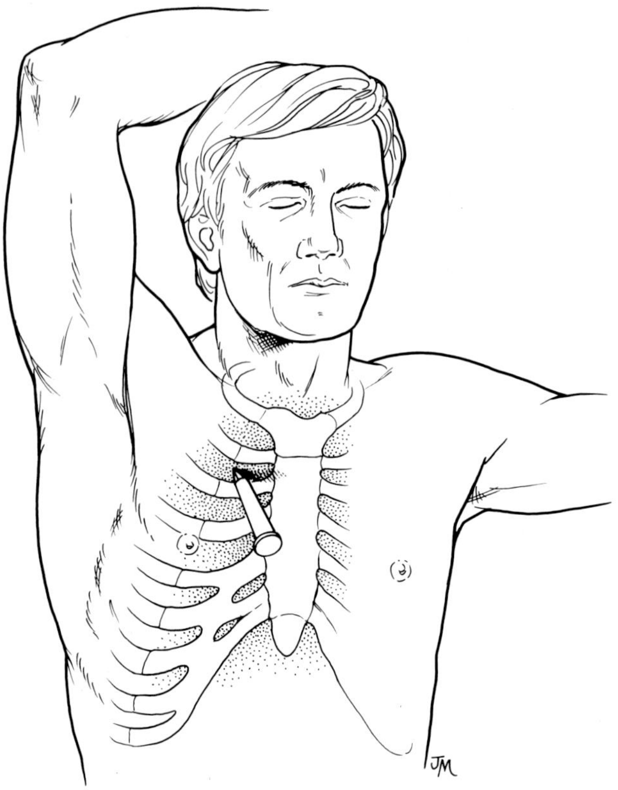

Figure 12-1

The anterior site lies along the midclavicular line at the second or third intercostal space.

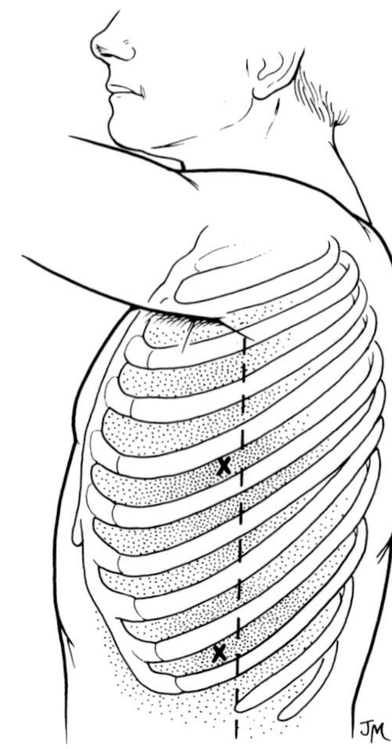

Figure 12-2

Location for lateral chest tube placement.

is used to minimize risk and optimize drainage of the desired fluid collection. Techniques have also been described for blind placement of apical tubes posteriorly.[62] Chest tubes should always be placed over the superior costal margin to avoid the damage to the intercostal nerves and vessels coursing along the inferior rib border. Intercostal vessels may be injured more readily in geriatric patients since the vessels can sag onto the superior costal margin of the adjacent rib.

PATIENT PREPARATION

Adequate positioning of the patient aids in maintenance of sterility and ease of the thoracostomy tube insertion. Position depends on the chosen site of tube placement. Ideally the best position would be one where the underlying lung is protected from the procedural instruments by a layer of intervening air or fluid, but ideal positioning is not always possible. For the lateral tube site, the best position is with the patient lying in the lateral decubitus position with a pillow under the flank on the side opposite the intended site. This causes the spine to flex laterally, widening the intercostal spaces on the procedural side. The ipsilateral arm is then placed over the head. It may be helpful to restrain the arm above the head depending on the patient's level of cooperativeness. For anterior chest tube placement a supine position with slight elevation of the head is adequate.

A sterile field is established. The intended thoracostomy site is prepared with surgical cleansing agent in a wide area. Sterile towels are then placed around the site to establish an area large enough for the intended procedure. The sterile field must be slightly larger in the case of the modified Seldinger (guide wire) technique, as the sterility of the lengthy guide wire must be maintained.

Cardiopulmonary monitoring usually is not needed, but may be warranted depending on the degree of the patient's illness or intentions to proceed with conscious sedation. Atropine, 0.4 to 0.8 mg given either intravenously or intramuscularly prior to the procedure, may be used to prevent vasovagal reactions, a common result of invasion of the pleural space.

EQUIPMENT PREPARATION

The various techniques of thoracostomy placement require differing equipment. For the standard blunt dissection technique, a sterilized surgical instrument tray is the most efficient way to gather the necessary equipment. For either the catheter over needle approach or the Seldinger approach, packaged disposable kits are commercially available. Further details regarding the necessary equipment will be discussed in the following sections. A Mayo stand or other mobile table is used to hold the instruments as the procedure is being completed. A commercial multi-chamber chest drainage system (Fig. 12-3) may be chosen for drainage of fluid or air contents or a Heimlich valve may be used

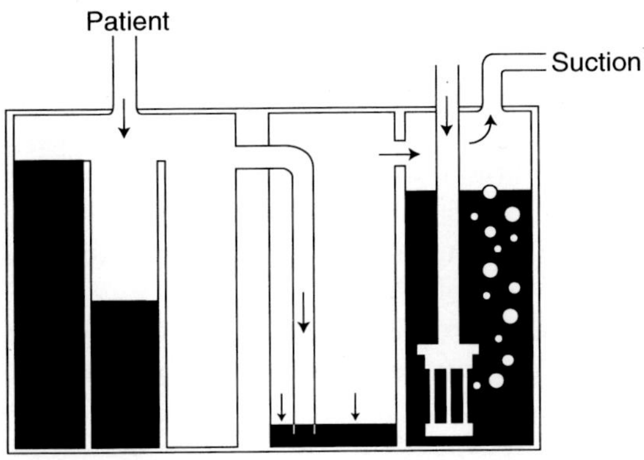

Figure 12-3

A commercial multi-chamber chest drainage system.

in the case of simple pneumothorax. In the specific case of drainage of a loculated empyema cavity, a simple plastic drainage collection bag is all that is necessary. Should the commercial vacuum system be chosen, a small setup procedure to add fluids to the vacuum and water seal chambers should be completed prior to placement of the thoracostomy. Supplies for the sterile preparation of the skin and operator are also essential, including a surgical scrub solution, sterile towels, gowns, and gloves (Table 12-5). The readers should refer to the product package insert for specific descriptive information.

ANESTHESIA

Adequate anesthesia and analgesia are essential to the success of the procedure regardless of site chosen or technique used. Before the procedure, narcotic analgesics (morphine, fentanyl, etc.) and benzodiazapines (midazolam, lorazapam, etc.) may allay the patient's anxiety about the procedure, provide analgesia for areas not anesthetized with the local anesthetic, and provide amnesia. In general though, careful local anesthesia is sufficient alone. Choice of the specific local anesthetic is a matter of personal preference. As long as sufficient quantities are used, adequate local block of pain sensory fibers will be attained.

The chosen local anesthetic (lidocaine 2% approximately 20 cc) is then injected immediately subcutaneously with a small gauge needle (25 or 27 gauge 1/2 in.) to form a local wheal. A larger needle (21 or 22 gauge 1-1/4 in.) is then used to anesthetize the deeper structures. This deeper anesthesia should only be in-

Table 12-5
SUPPLIES FOR A CHEST TUBE TRAY

Povidine-iodine solution
Gauze pads, 4 in. × 4 in.
Sterile towels and drapes
Lidocaine HCl (1 to 2%) with or without epinephrine (1:2000,000)
Syringes
Needles, 25 and 22 gauge
Scalpel
Kelly clamps (medium and large)
Chest tube
Trocar (optional)
1-0 or 2-0 silk suture with needle
Suture scissors
Bactericidal ointment
Sterile dressing
Tape
Flutter valve or chest drain and suction system
Wall suction regulator (if suction system is used)

jected after the plunger is withdrawn partially to ensure that the needle has not penetrated a vascular structure. The deep anesthesia should include several passes in multiple directions and angles to adequately block the procedural area. Deep anesthesia should include anesthesia of the periosteum of the rib. The needle is then walked superiorly up the surface of the rib until it passes over the top of the rib. The final step in adequate anesthesia is to advance the needle into the pleural space while withdrawing the plunger just until a flow of air or pleural fluid is obtained. The needle is then again withdrawn with suction on the plunger until the flow stops. The tip of the needle is then assumed to be just outside the parietal pleura. Injection of 8 to 10 cc of the anesthetic agent in this location will then anesthetize the parietal pleura. Careful attention to this particular step is essential to minimize the sensation of puncturing the pleura.

Intercostal nerve block can be an effective technique for anesthesia of a specific dermatomal area in anticipation of thoracostomy. The technique is relatively uncomplicated and easily performed during placement of a chest tube. Again a wheal is placed subcutaneously, followed by exchange to a larger needle and anesthesia of the subcutaneous tissues and the periosteum of the desired rib. The needle is then walked inferiorly off of the bottom of the rib and advanced approximately 2 mm. This places the tip of the needle in the area of the intercostal neurovascular bundle. After aspiration to ensure that the needle is not within a vascular structure, approximately 2 cc of the desired local anesthetic is instilled. The skin surface is then tested for adequate anesthesia.[63]

CATHETER OVER NEEDLE TECHNIQUE

This technique is used in a limited number of conditions, including nonventilator associated spontaneous or iatrogenic pneumothoraces. It is not indicated for traumatic pneumothoraces, hydropneumothoraces, or other pleural effusions. Some controversy exists regarding the use of this system in iatrogenic pneumothoraces in patients on mechanical ventilation. A commercial kit (Arrow Pneumothorax Kit, Arrow International, Inc. Reading, PA) is packaged with a Heimlich valve and contains all that is necessary for the placement of this type of thoracostomy tube (Fig. 12-4). Also because of the size of the included catheter, the kit is ideal for placement of anterior chest tubes. Other small bore catheter over needle kits are available for the drainage of fluid collections and are very successfully when used with radiologic guidance into small loculated collections.

The catheter over needle approach is the easiest and quickest of chest tube placements. The first step is to examine the contents of the kit and ensure that all are present and in proper functional state; specifically verifying that the catheter will pass freely off of the needle and is not stuck due to the sterilization procedure. After sterilely preparing the patient and anesthetizing as above, a small skin nick is made with the scalpel superficial to the rib below the intended intercostal space. The syringe is placed on the needle with the catheter in place and the apparatus is oriented perpendicularly with the skin. The needle catheter assembly is advanced into the skin and soft tissues while maintaining vacuum in the syringe and inserted until contact is made with the rib. The needle catheter apparatus is then removed a fraction of a millimeter and moved superiorly and then readvanced. This movement is repeated and the apparatus is "walked" up the rib until the needle passes over the rib. As soon as a flow of air or fluid is felt or visualized in the syringe, the catheter is advanced off the needle without moving the needle. After the catheter is placed to the desired depth, the needle is withdrawn and either the collection system or Heimlich valve is attached with use of the enclosed adapter.[64] The tube is then sutured in place and dressed as below.

GUIDE WIRE TECHNIQUE

The guide wire technique is the most recently introduced technique for placement of a thoracostomy tube.[65] With this technique also, commercially prepared kits are available in multiple sizes (Percutaneous Thal-Quick Chest Tube Set, Cook Critical Care, Bloomington, IN). Based on the Seldinger technique for vascular catheter placement, a needle is first used to enter the pleural space in a similar fashion to the needle

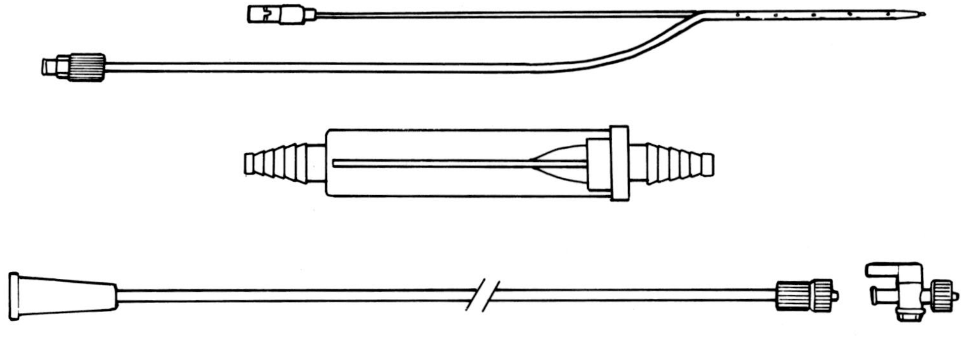

Figure 12-4

A generic pneumothorax kit containing an 8 F catheter over needle device, connecting tubes, and Heimlich valve.

over catheter technique (Fig. 12-5*A*). The needle is oriented in the desired direction and the guide wire is advanced through the needle to a depth of several centimeters deeper than the needle tip (Fig. 12-5*B*). The needle is removed by retracting along the length of the wire. Each dilator is serially placed over the guide wire to a depth to ensure dilatation of the full thickness of the chest wall (Fig. 12-5*C*). Several dilators may be necessary to progressively enlarge the thoracostomy site to allow passage of the desired size of tube. The tube is finally advanced over the guide wire in the desired direction (Fig. 12-5*D*). The guide wire is removed and the tube is connected to the desired drainage system and sutured in place as below (Fig. 12-5*E*).

Overall, this technique provides a rapid and minimally traumatic way to place thoracostomy tubes, however there are some potential concerns. This technique is a relatively blind access to the pleural space,

Figure 12-5

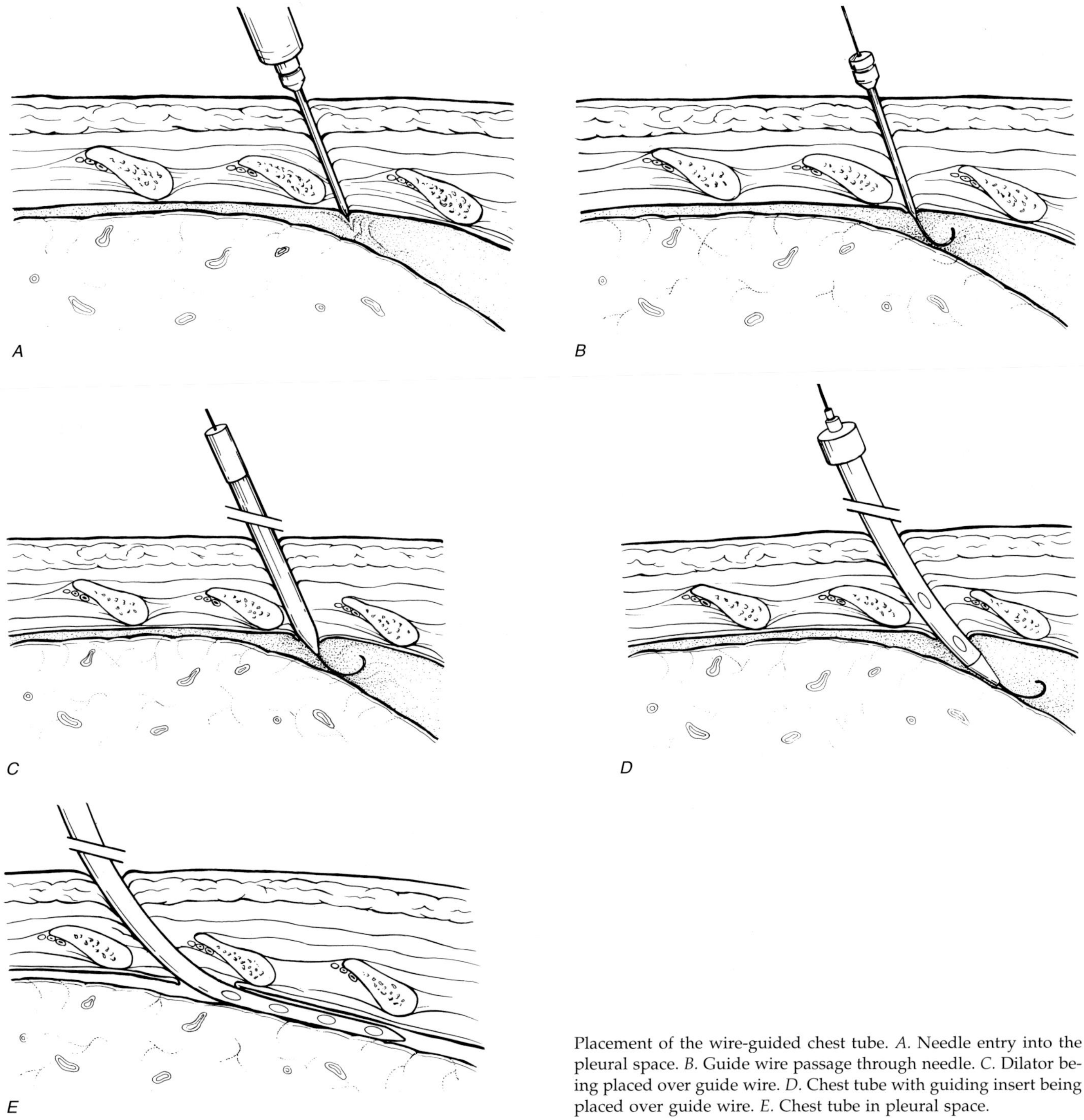

Placement of the wire-guided chest tube. *A*. Needle entry into the pleural space. *B*. Guide wire passage through needle. *C*. Dilator being placed over guide wire. *D*. Chest tube with guiding insert being placed over guide wire. *E*. Chest tube in pleural space.

and as a result, the chance to manually palpate the pleura and break down adhesions or verify their absence is lost. For this reason this technique is not advocated in the placement of drains into loculated fluid collections. In addition, the thoracostomy site is relatively tight around the tube itself and may limit the operator's ability to determine the direction of catheter advancement. A possible concern also is that the guide wire is relatively long and the free end of the wire may easily contact objects outside of the sterile field and potentially compromise the sterility of the procedure.

BLUNT DISSECTION TECHNIQUE

The most commonly used technique for chest tube placement involves blunt dissection of the subcutaneous tissues and intercostal muscles. Any indication for tube placement can be appropriately managed with this procedure. For this method, a sterilely prepared instrument pack is necessary; see Table 12-5 for a suggested list of contents. The setup and sterile preparation are similar to that used in the other techniques. The skin, subcutaneous tissues, periosteum, and pleura are anesthetized as for the other techniques. The skin is incised superficial to the rib below the desired interspace. A Kelly forceps is used for blunt dissection through the subcutaneous tissues, intercostal muscles, and pleura (Fig. 12-6). Once the pleura is penetrated by the forceps, a finger is placed through the site and the nearby thoracic structures are palpated. Palpation is done to ensure that there are no pleural adhesions that would misdirect the tube toward the lung and possibly cause the tube to penetrate the visceral pleura and enter the lung parenchyma. If adhesions are found, they may be gently broken down by the probing finger. The tube is clamped with a large Kelly forceps, placed through the site and then released from the clamp (Fig. 12-7). The tube is directed as desired and advanced until the most superficial perforation in the tube is at least 2 cm within the pleural space. The site is then sutured and dressed as below.

Advantages of this particular technique include the ability to manually palpate the pleura and break down adhesions. In addition, the direction of tube placement can more easily be controlled with this technique. For this reason, drainage of large loculated fluid collections would be ideally managed with this procedure, especially when many adhesions are present or the underlying lung tissue is felt to be more easily damaged. Should bleeding occur, it may be more easily controlled through an open site than with either of the closed site techniques. Disadvantages include the greater skin and intercostal muscle trauma, with greater risk of bleeding, however local control of bleeding can be more easily accomplished.

TROCAR GUIDED TUBE PLACEMENT

This technique involves the usual preparation and anesthesia. A skin incision is then made and a tube overlying a sharp trocar is placed through the inter-

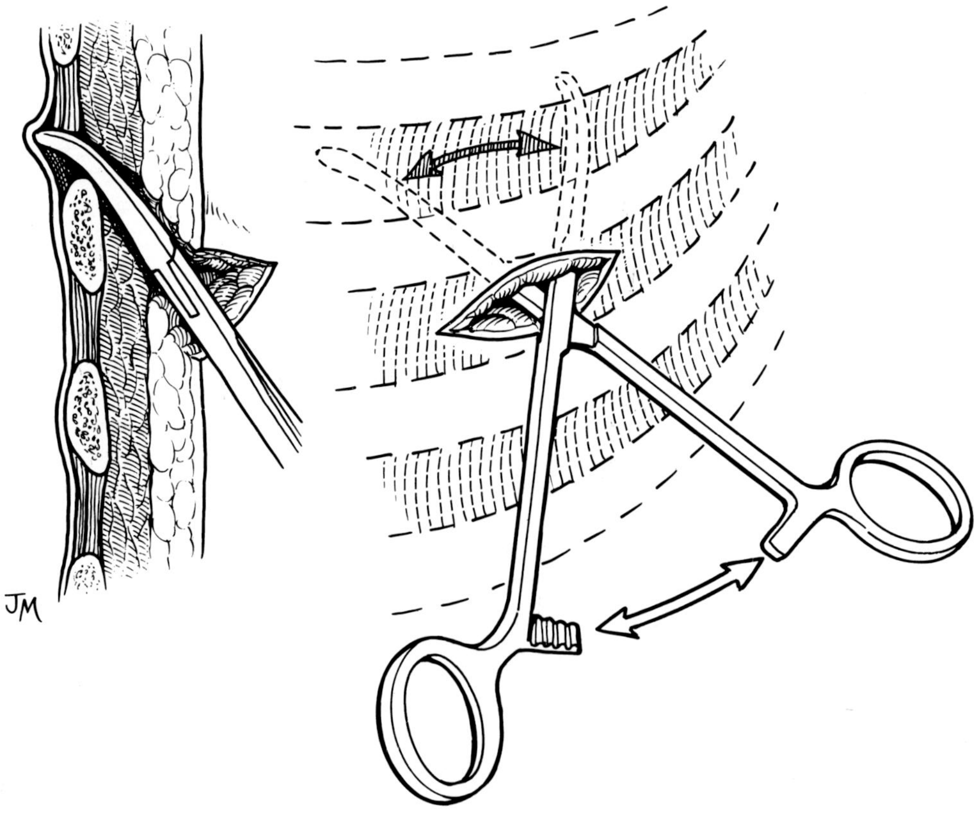

Figure 12-6

A Kelly forcep is used for blunt dissection through the subcutaneous tissues, intercostal muscles, and pleura.

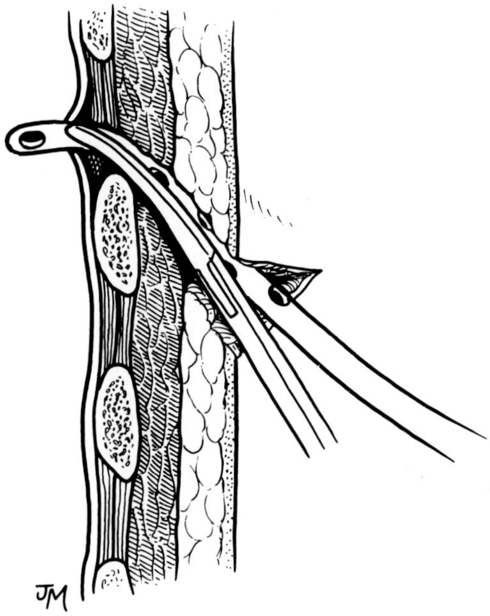

Figure 12-7

The tube is clamped with a large Kelly forceps, placed through the site, and then released from the clamp.

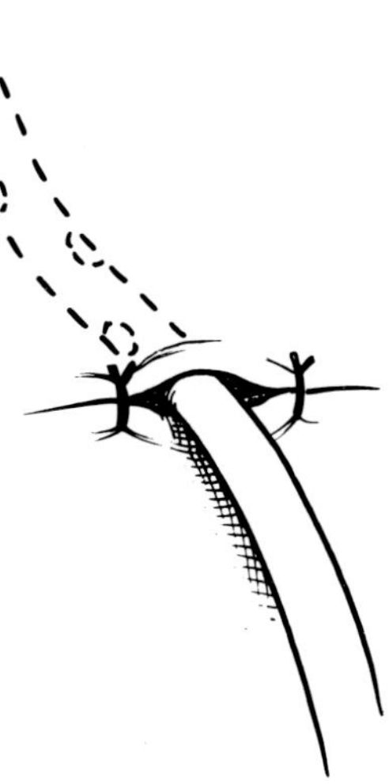

Figure 12-8

Two sutures placed, one on each side of the incision.

costal muscles and pleura under steady pressure. This particular technique has been complicated by multiple difficulties related to blind placement and the great forces used to penetrate the chest wall. Multiple inadvertent placements of tubes into the pulmonary parenchyma, great vessels, heart and abdominal organs have occurred and constitute reasons that this particular technique is rarely used today.[23]

SUTURING AND DRESSINGS

There are different methods of suturing used to affix chest tubes. While the actual positioning of sutures is variable, a few factors must be considered. The sutures must be nonabsorbable and of great enough tensile strength to firmly hold the tube in place. A reasonable choice is silk with sizes of 0 or 1-0, and for the smaller tubes, 2-0 silk may be used. Another consideration is that the loops through the skin must not compromise local perfusion or cause tissue necrosis. A few specific techniques warrant discussion. One method involves placement of two sutures, one at each end of the incision (Fig. 12-8). The first suture traverses across the incision, closing the incision around the tube. The knot in the suture is tied in the middle such that the free ends of the suture are each several inches long. The free ends are then wrapped tightly around the tube in opposite directions through two to three circumferences and then tied tightly around the tube. This is repeated with the other suture at the opposite end of the incision. When the tube is removed, both sutures are then cut at their passages through the skin and both are removed with the tube. The site is left open and dressed with gauze. The other commonly used suturing technique is designed so that there will be a "purse string" to close the site after removal of the tube. The "purse string" technique is somewhat more complicated to place and tie. A single suture is placed as above, but the tube is displaced in advance to fit tightly in one end of the incision. The suture is then wrapped and tied as above. A second suture is placed around the tube in horizontal mattress fashion and looped into a single throw of a surgeon's knot. The free ends are then wrapped around the tube and a bow knot is tied. When the tube is to be removed, the bow knot is untied and unwound from the tube. The initial suture is then cut and removed with the tube and the "purse string" suture is pulled taut and tied to close the thoracostomy site.

Dressing the chest tube is a very important aspect of placement. Initially a petroleum laden gauze with or without antiseptic is wrapped around the tube to seal the skin site. Drain sponges are then placed around the tube and gauze pads over the tube. Silk tape or other very adherent tape is then used to dress the entire site. Should the adherence of the tape to the skin be in question, a dressing preparation may be used (Benzoin). Care must be taken to adequately affix the chest tube to the skin without kinking the tube or drainage system.

COMPLICATIONS

Multiple complications of thoracostomy placement have been reported. The most common of the complications are minor and easily managed. Bleeding from skin, subcutaneous, or muscular vessels commonly occurs, and is managed by application of gentle pressure. Minor infection is not unusual and may necessitate antibiotic therapy until the tube can be removed. Rarely, more severe complications can occur. These may include: misplacement of the tube, major bleeding, lung laceration or puncture, and delayed complications of erosion into vital structures or severe infection. Multiple reports have documented placement of the tube in the subcutaneous tissues especially in the obese. Other sites of untoward placements include the lung, liver, spleen, diaphragm, heart, and great vessels. Intercostal artery, vein, or nerve injury can also occur. Obviously any of the above may endanger the patient significantly and may require emergent operative management.

Complications based on the position of the tube include compression of the intercostal nerve causing intercostal neuralgia or inadequate advancement of the tube leaving one of the holes in the subcutaneous tissue. Forceful injection of air into these tissues may cause subcutaneous emphysema. Based on the extent of the air insufflation of the subcutaneous tissues, the emphysema may be localized or may be severe, temporarily disfiguring and distressing to the patient's family and can even in extreme cases cause respiratory compromise. Complications may also occur due to inappropriate connections to the drainage system. For example, when a Heimlich valve is placed onto the tube in reverse, a tension pneumothorax may be created.[66]

Reexpansion pulmonary edema may also complicate chest tube drainage of a chronic large pleural fluid collection or pneumothorax. The usual situation is after rapid removal of fluid or air and reexpansion of the underlying lung. After a delay of 15 min to 2 h, the patient develops acute pulmonary edema of a noncardiogenic variety. It is thought that slower drainage of pleural fluid or air will prevent this complication.[67,68]

DRAINAGE SYSTEMS

Multiple drainage systems have been used to maintain the integrity of the pleural space. The goals have been to collect the fluids drained from the chest tube and at the same time either prevent the negative inspiratory intrathoracic pressures from causing airflow through the tube and into the pleural space or apply an external negative pressure to the pleural space. The early collection systems were glass and consisted of one to three bottles in series. A fluid collection chamber, present in all of the systems, allowed the fluid drained from the tube to be collected. In the single bottle system the collection bottle also acted as a water seal to prevent air influx into the pleural space. The water seal principle includes a chamber vented to the atmosphere with a long tube extending below the surface of a small amount of water in the chamber. This long tube is then attached to the chest tube. When drainage of air or fluid occurs, the substance freely passes into the chamber with little resistance. However, when negative pressure is generated in the thorax, the water is then siphoned up into the tube in the chamber until the height of the water column is equal to the negative intrathoracic pressure, thus preventing air influx into the pleural space. Of note, the small magnitude of negative pressure generated in the thorax is not sufficient to aspirate the water column into the chest unless the chamber is at or near the level of the chest. The water seal should thus be kept at a level below that of the patient's chest. The single bottle system is adequate for drainage of a simple pneumothorax, but if fluid drainage is excessive, the fluid collects in the single bottle and thus the water seal pressure increases as the fluid level in the bottle rises. A higher positive pressure is then necessary to generate flow of air or fluid from the chest and into the bottle.

The two bottle system includes separate bottles for collection of the drained fluid and for regulation of the water seal. This system corrected the problem of altered water seal pressure by accumulation of the drained fluids. The collection chamber is simply a bottle not vented to the atmosphere, but with two small tubes just entering through the lid of the chamber and not protruding below the fluid level. The collection chamber is connected to the system between the water seal and the thoracostomy tube itself. The two bottle system works sufficiently well for the drainage of simple air and fluid collections, however, occasionally a negative pressure placed on the throacostomy tube is needed to either forcefully remove collections of air or fluid, or expand a partially collapsed lung.

A suction pump can be placed on either the one or two bottle systems provided that the pump allows for a regulated negative pressure as is the case for the Emerson pump. This pump however is then dedicated to use on only a single patient at one time and is relatively clumsy and expensive. Most hospitals have installed a large-scale suction system throughout the hospital that is accessed through a specialized outlet. The difficulty in this situation is that this form of suction is at a much higher negative pressure than is appropriate for the pleural space and may also be highly variable. To correct for the high level and variability of wall suction, a third bottle is added to the system and acts as a suction regulator. This bottle is basically a manometer which uses a water or mercury column with an immersed tube exposed to the outside air. The regulator chamber lies between the wall suction and the water seal chamber. There are two short tubes protruding through the top of the chamber and not below the water level in the chamber. These are connected to the wall suction and the water seal. A third tube then is left open to the atmosphere and protrudes down into the fluid in the regulator chamber. When the suction is turned on, the air above the fluid in the regulator chamber is placed at a negative pressure. The suction is then increased to generate a flow of bubbles from outside the bottle, down the third tube and up into this air chamber. The depth of the longer tube within the fluid then corresponds to the negative pressure generated above the fluid level and transmitted to the water seal chamber and the collection chamber. The level of the fluid in the regulator chamber is adjustable and controls the negative pressure applied to the pleural space. The wall suction in this system must be set to high enough levels to generate a steady flow of bubbles through the regulator chamber. Higher levels of wall suction above this point will not generate a higher system vacuum, but will promote faster evaporation of the water in the regulator chamber. A seldom used variation on this system is to use mercury in the regulation chamber to more easily generate high negative pressures to be applied to the pleural space. Obviously, with the environmental hazards of mercury exposure and the limited usefulness of these excessive negative pressures, this practice has fallen into disfavor.

Many commercially prepared chest drainage systems are available. Most of these are variations on the three chamber system made as single use devices. The use of plastics has made these systems more durable. The majority of the systems are as described above and are graduated to allow for easy measurement of fluid drained. Use is relatively easy with the only necessary preparation being the filling of the water seal and pressure regulation chambers. One important variation on these systems is the replacement of the regulator chamber with a vacuum regulation valve. The valve allows fewer gradations of negative pressure, but does allow for higher negative pressures without the use of mercury, typically to -40 cmH_2O.

ASSESSMENT OF TUBE FUNCTION

Once the thoracostomy is placed, adequate placement within the thoracic cavity is verified either by fluid flow or by the development of condensation within the tube as air freely flows into and out of the tube from the thorax. Assessing placement with plain chest radiography is also essential. Ideally posteroanterior and lateral films should be checked to verify tube course within the thorax and verify that all of the holes in the tube lie within the chest cavity. The most superficial hole in the tube is marked by an interruption in the radiopaque line which makes the tube visible on radiographs. Progression of treatment for the pathologic process and tube placement are then assessed on a daily basis with serial films. In certain clinical circumstances computed tomography may be beneficial for assessment of the pathologic process, especially in the case of complicated parapneumonic effusions.

An essential part of the therapy for processes requiring thoracostomy placement is the diligent serial assessment of tube function. This is done by a serial assessment of clinical parameters (i.e., fever curve, level of leukocytosis, assessment of dyspnea, assessment of oxygenation and ventilation), but also by assessment of the function of the tube and drainage system. The clinician must evaluate for air bubbling in the water seal chamber, tidal movements in the water seal chamber, absence of large fluid collections in the tubing itself, and the description and amount of drainage. Chest radiography can also be very helpful.

Bubbling within the water seal chamber is a very important initial observation. This bubbling indicates one of several things: the intrathoracic air collection has not yet fully been removed by the tube, there exists a persistent communication between the tracheobronchial tree and the pleural space (a bronchopleural fistula), or there is an air leak outside of the patient and within the drainage system or associated tubing. Of note, if suction is not applied, an air leak in the system, external to the patient, will cause incomplete evacuation of air from the chest, but will not manifest necessarily as bubbling in the water seal chamber. Provided the patient's clinical situation has stabilized, air leaks within the drainage system may be ruled out by clamping the tube at the level of the skin with a forceps. If the bubbling in the water seal chamber stops then the air is coming from within the patient, if not, the drainage system should be evaluated for leaks. Chest radiography is of benefit at this time: If there is no visible pneumothorax, then a bronchopleural fistula exists. If pneumothorax is present with the patient on water seal, the system should be placed to suction in an attempt to reexpand the lung. If the chest tube has been on suction and the pneumothorax has not been reexpanded then a bronchopleural fistula exists or the chest tube is not properly working. In general the management of a bronchopleural fistula should include the titration of suction to both maximize expansion of the underlying lung and minimize the air flow across the bronchopleural communication. In some patients the flow is minimized while on water seal while other patients have decreased flow after the application of intermediate or high levels of suction, as much as -25 cmH_2O.[68]

The clinician must also observe the movements of the water column in the water seal chamber. This may be difficult if the tube has been placed to suction. The suction may be temporarily removed to assess tidaling. Tidal movements in the water seal chamber are indicative of transmission of the intrapleural pressures through the tube, similar to a manometer. During inspiration in typical negative pressure breathing, the fluid level is elevated and the opposite occurs during expiration. On the contrary, if the patient is on positive pressure breathing, in other words mechanical ventilation, the inspiratory phase will result in depression of the fluid level and expiration will cause elevation. Cough in either situation will depress the fluid level. The presence of tidal motion guarantees proper tube function, while absence of tidal motion indicates tube occlusion or kinking. Clearance of debris occluding a thoracostomy tube can be accomplished by "stripping." The connecting tubing is grasped and occluded near the thoracostomy tube with one hand, while the other hand is used to grasp the tube proximal to the first hand. The second hand then occludes the tube and is withdrawn in the direction of the drainage system. When the two hands are separated by one to two feet, the initial occlusion is released, and the first hand again occludes the tube beside the second hand. This motion is then repeated several times with the goal of creating suction within the tube and hopefully dislodging an occluding fibrin clot or other debris. Also some would advocate the instillation of streptokinase into the tube to dissolve any fibrin clot present. In the usual protocol 250,000 units of streptokinase in 100 cc of normal saline are instilled and left in the tube for several hours with the system clamped, then after unclamping, the chest tube is reassessed. Any nonfunctioning chest tube is of no benefit to the patient and does present significant cumulative risk of infection. Nonfunctioning tubes should be promptly removed. The decision must then be made as to whether another chest tube placement is indicated at another site. Chest tube placement at a relatively used site is not easily made sterile and presents significant risk for infection.

Recording the amount and description of fluid drainage is another matter of daily concern. The disposable drainage systems have a convenient method of measurement as the collection chambers are graduated, however the fluid level must be marked at least on a daily basis to more easily measure the daily output. For most indications the thoracostomy tube may be removed after the 24 h drainage is less than 50 to 100 cc. This however must be assessed in conjunction with plain chest radiography or computed tomography to ensure that the fluid collection is actually drained rather than loculated.

CHEST TUBE REMOVAL

The indications for removal of chest tubes placed for various pathological processes are as varied as the indications for tube placement. In general, absence of air leak and cessation of fluid flow are reasonable guidelines. A sterile occlusive dressing is placed on a small stack of gauze. The sutures are removed (or retained in the case of purse string suture). The tube is then removed while the patient performs a Valsalva maneuver to create positive pleural pressure and minimize the risk of air entry into the site during removal. The tube is removed with a steady tug, quickly. The occlusive dressing is held over the site as the tube is removed so that pressure may be applied over the site as the end of the tube is removed. If the purse string suture technique was used, the sutures are then retied. The occlusive dressing with gauze pad is taped into place and a plain chest radiograph taken to verify absence of pneumothorax.

SUMMARY

Thoracostomy tube placement is an essential component of management of several pathophysiologic entities within the routine clinical practice of pulmonary and critical care physicians. The American Board of Internal Medicine has mandated that physicians attempting board certification in critical care medicine be well versed in the placement and management of thoracostomy tubes. Hopefully this brief summary of the indications for chest tube placement, techniques of chest tube placement, and management of chest tubes will facilitate the attainment of clinical competence by pulmonary and critical care physicians and others who seek proficiency in this aspect of patient care.

REFERENCES

1. Hippocrates: *Genuine Works,* vol 2 (translated by Francis Adams). New York: William Wood and Company; 1886:266.
2. Playfair WS: On the treatment of empyema in children. *Obstet Trans* 1872; 14:4.
3. Brewer LA: Wound of the chest in war and peace, 1943–1968. *Ann Thorac Surg* 1969; 7:387.
4. Tape TG, Blank LL, Wigton RS: Procedural skills of practicing pulmonologist: A national survey of 1000 members of the American College of Physicians. *Am J Respir Crit Care Med* 1995; 282–287.
5. Light RW: *Pleural Diseases,* 2d ed. Philadelphia: Lea & Febiger; 1990; 237.
6. Garramone RR, Jacobs LM, Sahdev P: An objective method to measure and manage occult pneumothorax. *Surg Gynecol Obstet* 1991; 173:257.
7. Mathur R, Cullen J, Kinnear WJM, Johnston IDA: Time course of resolution of persistent air leak in spontaneous pneumothorax. *Respir Med* 1995; 89:129.
8. Blanco G: Spontaneous pneumothorax. *Hosp Med* 1975; March:40.
9. Flint K, Al-Hillawi AH, Johnson N McI: Conservative management of spontaneous pneumothorax. (letter) *Lancet* 1984; 1:687.
10. Clague HW, El-Ansary EH: Conservative management of spontaneous pneumothorax (letter). *Lancet* 1984; 1:688.
11. Delius RE, Obeid FN, Horst M, Sorensen VJ, Fath JJ, Bivins BA: Catheter aspiration for simple pneumothorax: Experience with 114 patients. *Arch Surg* 1989; 124:833.
12. Miller KS, Sahn SA: Chest tubes: Indication techniques, management and complications. *Chest* 1987; 91:758–764.
13. Sudduth CD, Sahn SA: Pleurodesis for nonmalignant pleural effusions: Recommendations. *Chest* 1992; 102:1855.
14. Vargas FS, Milanez JRC, Filomeno LT, Fernandez A, Jatene A, Light RW: Intrapleural talc for the prevention of recurrence in benign or undiagnosed pleural effusion. *Chest* 1994; 106:1771.
15. Zwillich SW, Pierson DJ, Creagh E, Sutton FD, Schatz E, Petty TL: Complications of assisted ventilation: A prospective study of 354 consecutive episodes. *Am J Med* 1974; 57:161.

16. Peterson GW, Baier H: Incidence of pulmonary barotrauma in a medical ICU. *Crit Care Med* 1983; 11:67.
17. DeLatorre FJ, Tomasa A, Klamburg J, Leon C, Soler M, Rius J: Incidence of pneumothorax and pneumomediastinum in patients with aspiration pneumonia requiring ventilatory support. *Chest* 1977; 72:141.
18. Kollef MH: Risk factors for the misdiagnosis of pneumothorax in the intensive care unit. *Crit Care Med* 1991; 19:906.
19. Light RW: Management of spontaneous pneumothorax. *Am Rev Respir Dis* 1993; 148:245.
20. Sahn SA: The pleura. *Am Rev Respir Dis* 1988; 138:184.
21. Symbas PN: Chest drainage tubes. *Surg Clin North Am* 1989; 69:41.
22. Iberti TJ, Stern PM: Chest tube. *Crit Care Clin* 1992; 8:879.
23. Millikan JS, Moore EE, Stiner E, Aragon GE, VanWay CW: Complications of chest tube for acute trauma. *Am J Surg* 1980; 140:738.
24. Etoch SW, Bar-Natan MR, Miller FB, Richardson JD: Chest tube: Factors related to complications. *Arch Surg* 1995; 130:521.
25. Ross IB, Fleiszer DM, Brown RA: Localized tension pneumothorax in patients with adult respiratory distress syndrome. *Can J Surg* 1994; 37:415.
26. Heffner JE, McDonald J, Barbieri C: Recurrent pneumothoraces in ventilated patients despite ipsilateral chest tubes. *Chest* 1995; 108:1053.
27. Peterson WP, Whiteneck GG, Gerhart KA: Chest tubes, lung entrapment, and failure to wean from the ventilator: Report of three patients with quadriplegia. *Chest* 1994; 105:1292.
28. Kollef MH, Dothager DW: Reversible cardiogenic shock due to chest tube compression of the right ventricle. *Chest* 1991; 99:976.
29. Gerard PS, Kaldawi E, Litani V, Lenora RA, Tessler S: Right-sided pneumothorax as a result of a left-sided chest tube. *Chest* 1993; 103:1602.
30. Singh KJ, Newman AJ: Pulmonary artery catheterization: An unusual complication of chest tube insertion. *Aust N Z J Surg* 1994; 64:513.
31. Salon JE: Reversible diaphragmatic eventration following chest tube. *Ann Emerg Med* 1995; 25:556.
32. Bald M, Balkier AA, German PS, Pascal GP, Skrbensky GT, Herold CJ: Complications after emergency chest tube: Assessment with CT. *Radiology* 1995; 195:539.
33. Quigley RL: Thoracentesis and chest tube drainage. *Crit Care Clin* 1995; 11:111.
34. Carney M, Ravin CE: Intercostal artery laceration during thoracentesis: Increased risk in elderly patients. *Chest* 1979; 75:520.
35. Picone AL: Nonsurgical management of bleeding secondary to chest tube: A case report (letter). *Chest* 1992; 102:1304.
36. Urschel JD: Balloon tamponade for hemorrhage secondary to chest tube insertion. *Respir Med* 1994; 88:549.
37. Sargent EN, Turner AF: Emergency treatment of pneumothorax: A simple catheter technique for use in the radiology department. *AJR* 1970; 109:531.
38. Peters J, Kubitschek KR: Clinical evaluation of a percutaneous pneumothorax catheter. *Chest* 1984; 86:714.
39. Crouch JD, Keagy BA, Delany DJ: "Pigtail" catheter drainage in thoracic surgery. *Am Rev Respir Dis* 1987; 136:174.
40. Conces DJ, Tarver RD, Gray WC, Pearcy EA: Treatment of pneumothoraces utilizing small caliber chest tubes. *Chest* 1988; 94:55.
41. Thal AP, Quick KL: A guided chest tube for safe thoracostomy. *Surg Gynecol Obstet* 1988; 167:517.
42. Semrad N: A new technique for closed thoracostomy insertion of chest tube. *Surg Gynecol Obstet* 1988; 166:171.
43. Guyton SW, Paull DL, Anderson RP: Introducer insertion of mini-thoracostomy tubes. *Amer J Surg* 1988; 155:693.
44. Parker LA, Charnock GC, Delany DJ: Small bore catheter drainage and sclerotherapy for malignant pleural effusions. *Cancer* 1989; 64:1218.
45. Delius RE, Obeid FN, Horst HM, Sorensen VJ, Fath JJ, Bivins BA: Catheter aspiration for simple pneumothorax: Experience with 114 patients. *Arch Surg* 1989; 124:833.
46. Molina PL, Solomon SL, Glazer HS, Sagel SS, Anderson DJ: A one-piece unit for treatment of pneumothorax complicating needle biopsy: Evaluation in 10 patients. *AJR* 1990; 155:31.
47. Samelson SL, Goldberg EM, Ferguson MK: The thoracic vent: Clinical experience with a new device for treating simple pneumothorax. *Chest* 1991; 100:880.
48. Kerr A, Vasudevan VP, Powell S, Ligenza C: Percutaneous catheter drainage for acute empyema: Improved cure rate using CAT scan, fluoroscopy, and pigtail drainage catheters. *NY State J Med* 1991; 91:4.
49. Pollak JS, Passik CS: Intrapleural urokinase in the treatment of loculated pleural effusions. *Chest* 1994; 105:868.
50. Seaton KG, Patz EF, Goodman PC: Palliative treatment of malignant pleural effusions: Value of small-bore catheter thoracostomy and doxycycline sclerotherapy. *AJR* 1995; 164:589.
51. Moulton JS, Benkert RE, Weisiger KH, Chambers JA: Treatment of complicated pleural fluid collections with image-guided drainage and intracavitary urokinase. *Chest* 1995; 108:1252.
52. Quinn SF, Demlow TA: Large-caliber (24-28-F) catheters for radiologically guided percutaneous procedures. *Radiology* 1993; 189:922.
53. van Sonnenberg E, Nakamoto SK, Mueller PR, Casola G, Neff CC, Friedman PJ, et al: CT-ultrasound-guided catheter drainage of empyemas after chest tube failure. *Radiology* 1984; 151:349.
54. Westcott J: Percutaneous catheter drainage of pleural effusion and empyema. *AJR* 1985; 144:1189.
55. Merriam MA, Cronan JJ, Dorfman GS, Lambiase RE, Haas RA: Radiographically guided percutaneous catheter drainage of pleural fluid collections. *AJR* 1988; 151:1113.
56. Sahn SA: Management of complicated parapneumonic effusions. *Am Rev Respir Dis* 1993; 148:813.
57. LeMense GP, Strange C, Sahn SA: Empyema thoracis: Therapeutic management and outcome. *Chest* 1995; 107:1532.
58. Moore KL: *Clinically Oriented Anatomy*. Baltimore: Williams and Wilkins; 1985:49–75.
59. Rice DC, Agasthian T, Clay RP, Deschamps C: Silicone thorax: A complication of chest tube in the presence of mammary implants. *Ann Thorac Surg* 1995; 60:1417–1419.
60. Miller KS, Sahn SA: Chest tubes: Indications, technique, management, and complications. *Chest* 1987; 91:258–264.
61. McVay PA, Toy PT: Lack of increased bleeding after paracentesis and thoracentesis in patient with mild coagulation abnormalities. *Transfusion* 1991; 31:164–171.
62. Galvin IF, Gibbons JRP, Magous M, Bowe P: Placement of an apical chest tube by a posterior intercostal approach. *Br J Hosp Med* 1990; 44:330–331.
63. Rowlingson JC: Intercostal nerve block. In Suratt PM, Gibson RS (eds): *Manual of Medical Procedures*. St. Louis: C. V. Mosby; 1982:250–255.
64. Heimlich HJ: Valve drainage of the pleural cavity. *Dis Chest* 1968; 53:282.
65. Thal AP, Quick KL: A guided chest tube for safe thoracostomy. *Surg Gyn Obstet* 1988; 167:517.
66. Bernstein A: Re-expansion pulmonary edema. *Chest* 1980; 77:708.
67. Janocik SE, Roy TM, Killeen TR: Re-expansion pulmonary edema: A preventable complication. *J Kentucky Med Assoc* 1993; 91:143–146.
68. Powner DJ, Cline CD, Rodman GH: Effect of chest tube suction on gas flow through a bronchopleural fistula. *Crit Care Med* 1985; 13:99–101.

C H A P T E R 1 3

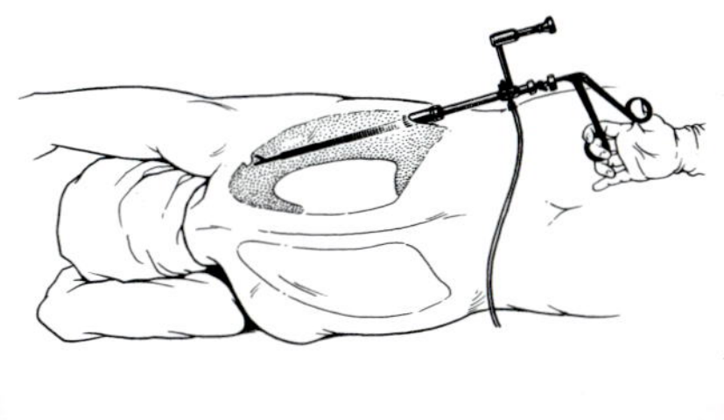

MEDICAL THORACOSCOPY: ROLE IN PLEURAL AND LUNG DISEASES

Praveen N. Mathur and Robert Loddenkemper

"Medical" thoracoscopy offers pulmonologists an invaluable tool for understanding and treating pleural diseases. Indeed, fluid collection, pneumothorax, and pleural thickening are frequently encountered in a pulmonary practice. Although the radiographic detection of pleural abnormalities may be obvious, determination of a specific diagnosis can represent a major challenge. Unfortunately, approximately 25 percent of pleural abnormalities remain undiagnosed[1–6] after thoracentesis and/or closed pleural biopsy. Clinicians in pursuit of a specific diagnosis must, therefore, choose an additional or alternative plan. Medical thoracoscopy has been successfully used for diagnosis and evaluation of several pleural and lung parenchymal disorders.

Historical Background

The initial effort to "endoscopically" view the pleural space was reported in 1910 by Jacobaeus, an internist.[7] He reported two cases of exudative pleurisy in which he performed a thoracoscopy for diagnostic purposes under local anesthesia. Later he reported 40 cases in which he used a modified cystoscope to lyse pleural adhesions, and 120 cases involving the diagnosis of pleural-based tumors.[8] During the next 40 years, thoracoscopy became widely used to lyse pleural adhesions to facilitate artificial pneumothorax, which was the mainstay of therapy for pulmonary tuberculosis. With the advent of antituberculous therapy, the number of thoracoscopies declined. In addition, the Abrams and Cope needle biopsies proved reasonably successful for the diagnosis of malignant and tuberculous pleural effusion,[9,10] thus precluding a major role for diagnostic thoracoscopy. With its decline in popularity, thoracoscopy, especially in the United States, became relegated to an occasional perioperative procedure performed by thoracic surgeons.[11]

Several different instruments, both rigid and flexible, have been employed to view the pleural space. In 1974, a small-caliber arthroscope was used by Ash and Manfredi for thoracoscopy.[12] Biopsies of the pleura were taken with Cope or Vim-Silverman needles through a separate puncture site. Similarly, Boushy[13] reported the use of a Tru-Cut biopsy needle under arthroscopic guidance for pleural biopsy. The arthroscope, with a relatively narrow angle optical system, does not accurately lend itself to visualize the large pleural cavity, which accounts for the lack of subsequent enthusiasm for this technique. Mediastinopleuroscopy[14] was described by Deslauriers and coworkers in 1976, using standard Carlens' technique. Attempts to utilize the mediastinoscope[15,16] for thoracoscopy through a lateral intercostal incision have found this instrument unwieldy to manipulate within the pleural space. The instrument provides relatively poor visualization, owing to the lack of an optical system.

With the introduction of fiberoptic technology, instruments such as the fiberoptic bronchoscope have been used for thoracoscopy. Initially, a thorough digital assessment through the interspace is necessary before introducing these relatively fragile instruments into the pleural cavity. Any adhesions may result in acute angulation with subsequent fracture of optical fibers. Additionally, flexible bronchoscopes are difficult to manipulate within a relatively wide pleural cavity. Various methods have been devised to control the flexible bronchoscope, including introducing the instrument through a chest tube,[17,18] with less than satisfactory results. Independent studies by Oldenburg and Newhouse[19] and Davidson and coworkers[20] have found the rigid thoracoscope to be superior to the flexible fiberoptic bronchoscope for examination of the pleural cavity. In addition, biopsy specimens are much smaller with the flexible bronchoscope compared with the rigid instrument, resulting in lower diagnostic yield.

The rigid thoracoscope is currently the most suitable instrument[3,4,20–25] for thoracoscopy, providing both excellent optical quality and ease in maneuverability within the pleural space. The skills for rigid instrument use are easily acquired.[19,20] Video camera attachments to these endoscopes allow recording capabilities and excellent magnification during the examination and greatly facilitate transthoracoscopic or video-assisted procedures. Probes for palpation, coagulation, needle or forceps biopsy, and insufflation of sclerosing agents can be placed through either a working channel within a scope or a separate interspace puncture site. When available, a rigid scope with a working channel and a bidirectional flexible tip purposefully made for examining the pleural cavity may combine advantages of both rigid and flexible thoracoscopy.

This recent thoracoscopy revival, performed both inside and outside the operation room,[24,25] has occurred because of the marked improvements in endoscopic video systems, permitting greater visualization of the pleural surfaces, and because of the development of local anesthetics and neuroleptic agents which preclude the need for general anesthesia in selected cases.

Differences between Video-Assisted Thoracic Surgery and Medical Thoracoscopy

Thoracoscopy offers the pulmonologist the ability to visualize and biopsy both pleural surfaces and provide better understanding of pleural diseases. The entire chest cavity and lung can be examined and on occasion, minute emphysematous blebs, responsible for pneumothoraces, can be seen. This information is not always detectable by CT scan. During thoracoscopy the intent of a pulmonologist is very different from that of a thoracic surgeon. The intent of a thoracic surgeon is to perform thoracic surgery in a minimally invasive manner. Video-assisted thoracic surgery (VATS) is performed in an operating room almost exclusively under general anesthesia and single-lung ventilation, which allow the collapse of the lung on the examined side. Usually multiple ports of entry and disposable instruments are used. An additional large incision may become necessary for the removal of larger tumors or pieces of tissue. VATS has been used to perform stapled lung biopsies, lobectomies, and pneumonectomies. It has also been used for pleurectomies, pericardial windows, sympathectomy, and vagotomy and for resection of peripheral benign and metastatic nodules.[26–29] In patients with malignant pulmonary nodules and poor pulmonary reserve, wedge resection with generous margins can be achieved without open thoracotomy. Long-term effects of this approach, including local recurrence rates, are being studied. Other successfully performed procedures include: repair of bronchopleural fistula and evaluation of mediastinal tumors or adenopathy.

In contrast, medical thoracoscopy is performed by a pulmonologist in a endoscopy suite or operating room, depending on the local availability of the appropriate facility, local anesthesia, and conscious sedation. One or two ports of entry are used along with simple, nondisposable instrumentation. The usual objective is to *diagnose* pleural diseases, but thoracoscopy also provides an effective method of performing pleurodesis. Lastly, thoracoscopy may lead to evaluation of innovative biologic therapies in the treatment of pleural diseases.

Diagnostic Thoracoscopy

Diagnostic thoracoscopy has been shown to be helpful in several pleural and lung pathologies. In tuberculosis and cancer, the reported diagnostic sensitivity of thoracoscopic biopsy and brush samples from the pleura vary from 93 to 97 percent.[19,20,23–25,30–38] In cases of breast or ovarian cancer, hormone receptor assays on thoracoscopically obtained material provide further important information for therapeutic decision making.[39] In bronchial carcinoma, thoracoscopy answers the important question of whether the tumor has spread to the pleura or whether the effusion is secondary to venous or lymphatic obstruction or is parapneumonic. As a result, it is possible to avoid exploratory thoracotomy and/or to determine operative eligibility. Weissberg and co-workers[16] performed thoracoscopies in 45 patients with lung cancer and pleural effusion. In 37 they found pleural invasion. Three patients had mediastinal disease. The remaining five had no metastatic disease and therefore no contraindication to resection.

PLEURAL EFFUSION

Algorithms for investigating pleural effusion of unknown etiology typically begin with thoracentesis. Pleural fluid is analyzed for chemistries, microbiology, and cytology. Cytologic examination, often with repeated examination of large amounts of pleural fluid, is diagnostic in only 60 to 80 percent of patients with metastatic disease,[40–43] and fewer than 20 percent of patients with mesotheliomas.[44,45] Moreover, there exists a low but real false-positive rate ranging from 0.5 to 1.5 percent. Repeat thoracentesis, if nondiagnostic, is followed by percutaneous pleural biopsies which have a diagnostic yield of 59 percent for malignant pleural effusion.[3,43]

Approximately 20 percent of pleural effusions remain idiopathic after several weeks of observation with sophisticated noninvasive techniques.[3,4,46] Morbidity not withstanding, investigation in these unexplained cases must continue and thoracoscopy is often decisive. Tubercle bacilli can be recovered from pleural fluid in 14 to 59 percent of cases. Cytologic diagnoses are usually obtained in 42 to 73 percent of malignant effusions. Since other tests seldom provide a specific diagnosis, the pathologic examination of pleural tissue plays an important role in the diagnosis and differential diagnosis of pleural exudates. In a prospective study comparing thoracoscopy, cytology, and needle biopsy in 208 cases of malignant effusion, diagnostic sensitivity was 95, 62 and 44 percent, respectively.[32] In another study, 250 patients with pleural effusions were examined in a prospective manner during a 4-year period. All underwent aspiration of pleural fluid, a closed pleural biopsy, and thoracoscopy. With the needle biopsy in patients with tuberculosis, 52 percent were diagnosed; in contrast only 35 percent in the tumor group were positive. This difference is probably due to the more widespread pleural involvement in tuberculosis. In contrast, the yield of thoracoscopic biopsy under visual control was twice as high, with positive results obtained in 92 percent of patients.

Boutin and coworkers[3] reported a large series of 1000 consecutive patients with pleural effusion, 215 of whom had pleural effusions lasting for more than 4 weeks without any proven etiology despite repeated thoracentesis and one or more percutaneous needle biopsies of the pleura. Following thoracoscopy, 150 patients were diagnosed with malignant pleural effusion, including 35 with mesothelioma. Other investigators have also found levels of diagnostic accuracy in excess of 88 percent.[15,19,29,30,33,46,47] The diagnostic accuracy of pleural disease by thoracoscopy[15,19,21,29,48] depends on the methods of diagnosis and the duration of follow-up. The diagnostic accuracy has been reported to be in the range of 90 to 100 percent. However, the follow-up was either not stated or was less than 6 months. Boutin and coworkers[3] have reported a false-negative rate of 15 percent with a 1-year follow-up. Enk and Viskum[22] reported a diagnostic accuracy of 69 percent among patients followed up to 5 years. However, in this study even after thoracotomy had established the diagnosis of benign pleural disease, within 6 months 25 percent of the patients were diagnosed with a malignancy. Menzies and Charbonneau,[30] in an elegant study, have reported a 96 percent accuracy with a sensitivity of 91 percent and a specificity of 100 percent. Thus the negative predicted value of 93 percent was obtained for the diagnosis of pleural malignancy with a follow-up of 1 year.

There are several reasons thoracoscopy may be diagnostic when cytologic examination of pleural fluid or a percutaneous needle biopsy fails to establish the diagnosis. For example, a positive cytology for malignant cells requires two factors to be present: (1) significant exfoliation of cells from the pleural surface into the pleural effusion and (2) cytologic characteristics sufficient to establish the diagnosis of malignancy. These may be absent in many malignant diseases of the pleura, especially in malignant mesothelioma. Another reason conventional methods may fail to establish a diagnosis is that malignant pleural disease is not always accessible to needle biopsy of the parietal pleura. Canto and coworkers[49] reported on 78 patients with proven metastatic disease to the pleura; only 53 percent had involvement of costoparietal pleural areas. In other series totaling 203 patients undergoing thoracoscopy,[49–51] 84 percent of the metastases were in the lower hemithorax, on the lung surface or the diaphragm, and were poorly accessible or totally inaccessible to closed-needle biopsy. Meyer,[52] in a series of 53 autopsies, demonstrated that 32 percent of these cases had involvement of the visceral pleura only. Similarly, Rodriguez-Panadero and coworkers,[53] in 191 autopsies, showed that the parietal pleura is less frequently involved with metastatic pleural disease than the visceral pleura. It appears that in patients with metastatic pleural disease, 32 to 47 percent have disease inaccessible to closed-needle biopsy.

Most cytology-negative pleural effusions associated with lung cancer are still the result of the malignancy. Few of these patients are ultimately found to have surgically resectable disease. Decker and coworkers[54] described 73 patients with lung cancer and ipsilateral cytologically negative pleural effusion and found only 6.1 percent had a completely resectable tumor. Fifty percent required an open thoracotomy to determine resectability. Thoracoscopy now appears to be a more desirable technique to identify the small group of patients who could potentially benefit from a surgical resection. Ideally, diagnostic thoracoscopy and surgical resection, if indicated, could be performed under the same general anesthesia. Obtaining the diagnosis in unresectable or metastatic cases using minimally invasive techniques will allow earlier institution of palliative therapy, which potentially may improve the length of survival. Certainly, the quality of life following thoracoscopy for obtaining and determining resectability is far superior to the prolonged recovery following exploratory thoracotomy in these patients with a predictably short life expectancy.

METASTATIC PLEURAL MALIGNANCIES

Needle biopsies are successful in only 50 percent of metastatic pleural malignancies.[24,25,32,55] Moreover, unlike thoracoscopy, closed pleural biopsies are of little value for diagnosing localized tumors or metastatic tumors confined to the diaphragmatic, visceral, or mediastinal pleura.[49] Similarly pleural fluid cytology exhibits variable success.[56,57] A yield of 50 to 60 percent from pleural fluid cytology is a representative figure.[40] The main advantage of diagnostic thoracoscopy is its ability to achieve an early diagnosis when pleural biopsy and pleural fluid cytology have failed[30–33] and to recover tissue for hormone receptor assay. This topic is discussed in detail in Chap.14.

MALIGNANT MESOTHELIOMA

Although malignant mesothelioma may be clinically suspected, it can be difficult to establish a diagnosis. Specimens from closed-needle biopsies are rarely of sufficient size to allow definite diagnosis of mesothelioma. In patients with suspected, but unproven mesothelioma, diagnostic thoracoscopy is indicated and may be performed under local anesthesia if surgical resection is not a consideration. Diagnosis of malignant mesothelioma depends foremost on histologic and immunohistologic findings. Obtaining biopsy samples for diagnosis of mesothelioma is one of the best indications for thoracoscopy. The sensitivity is above 90 percent.[3,58–62] By allowing direct visualization of lesions thoracoscopy facilitates the choice of biopsy sites and allows correlation of staging with survival (Figs. 13-1 to 13-4). In addition, the finding of pleural plaques (Fig. 13-5) supports the final diagnosis. This topic is discussed in detail in Chap. 14.

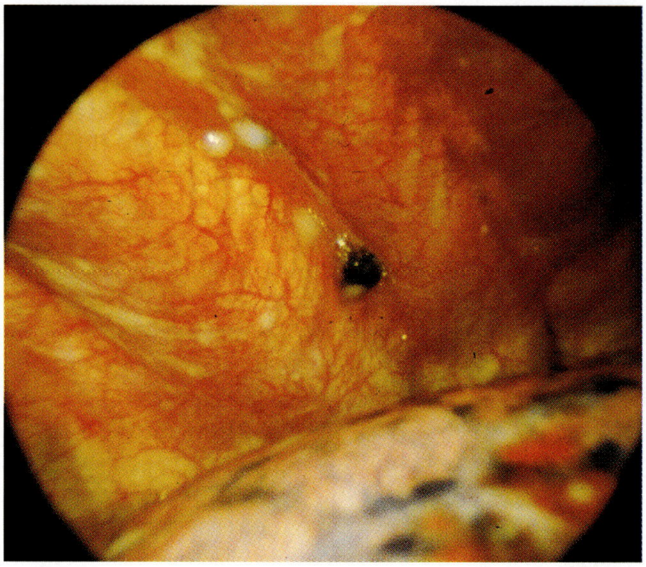

Figure 13-1

Small, whitish nodules on the parietal pleura (plus a black lymph node): metastatic adenocarcinoma (lung looks normal apart from anthracotic pigmentation).

TUBERCULOUS PLEURAL EFFUSIONS

Much less common than in past years, tuberculosis now accounts for less than 10 percent of all effusions. Although the yield of blind needle biopsy averages 69 percent with a range of 28 to 88 percent,[32,70] the diagnostic accuracy is much greater when the thoracoscope is used, because the pathologist is provided with multiple selected biopsies (Figs. 13-6 and 13-7). In a prospective study,[46] the immediate diagnosis in 100 tuberculosis cases could be established in 94 percent using thoracoscopy, compared with 38 percent by needle biopsy. In addition, the percentage of positive TB cultures was twice as high from thoracoscopic biopsies, including cultures from fibrinous adhesions (78 percent), as the percentage in pleural effusions and needle biopsies combined (39 percent), allowing bacteriologic confirmation of the diagnosis and sensitivity testing. In five of the 78 positive cases with tuberculosis (6.4 percent), a primary resistance against one or more antituberculous drugs was found, indicating that thoracoscopy had influence on both therapy and prognosis.

It is of interest that the chance of positive TB cultures is much higher in cases with fibrin production (87 percent). This manifests as a diffusely thickened pleura, multiple adhesions, and sometimes formation of encapsulating membranes with fluid loculation and was present in 75 percent of cases. By comparison, the picture of sago-like pleuritis with miliary tuberculous granulomas was seen in only 25 percent. Here, a positive TB culture was obtained from all materials in only 50 percent, a highly significant difference ($p < .0005$). In this study, the chance of positive TB cultures from pleural effusion was also, statistically, much better in cases with a pleural glucose < 50 mg/dL (59 percent positive versus 25 percent with glucose > 50 mg/dL $p < .005$); however, the first group comprised only 17 percent of the patients.

The endoscopic appearance of tuberculosis has been well described. It is characterized by grayish white granulomata blanketing the whole parietal and diaphragmatic pleura, especially in the area of the costovertebral gutter. Lesions have often lost their specific appearance by the time of thoracoscopy and may mimic a simple inflammatory process, with increased vascularity, a reddish color, a hemorrhagic fibrinous reaction, and numerous adhesions.

Hyaline and calcified asbestos pleural plaques have endoscopically distinctive characteristics (Fig. 13-5),

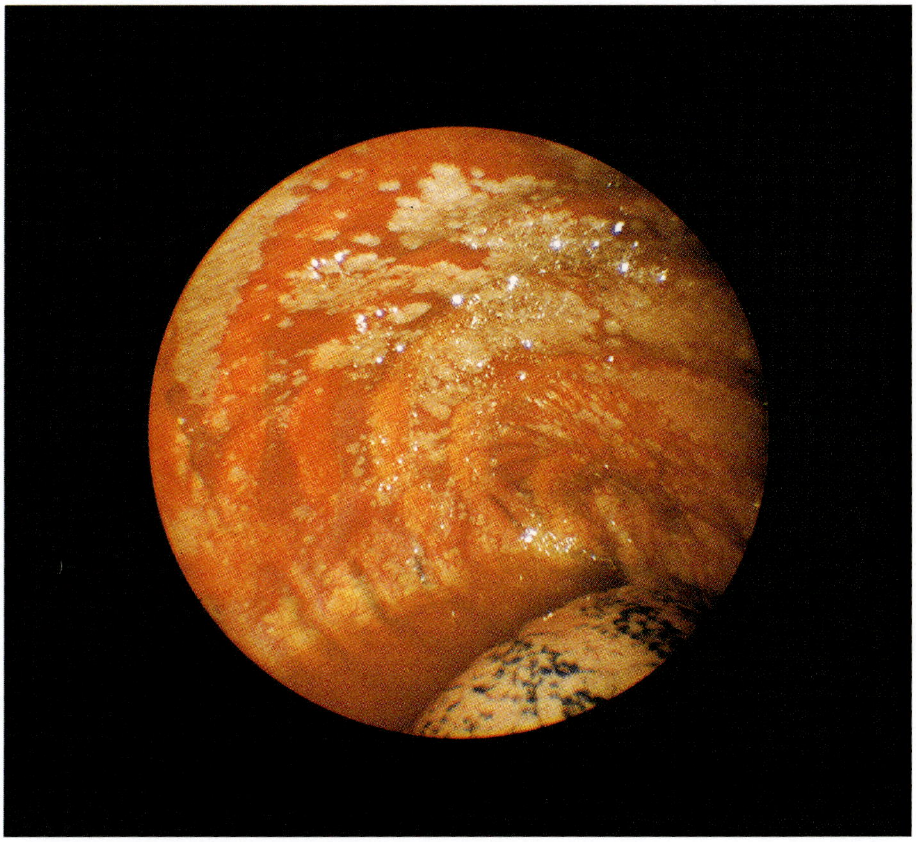

Figure 13-2

Diffuse malignant pleural mesothelioma of the chest wall pleura (lung normal, hemorrhagic effusion).

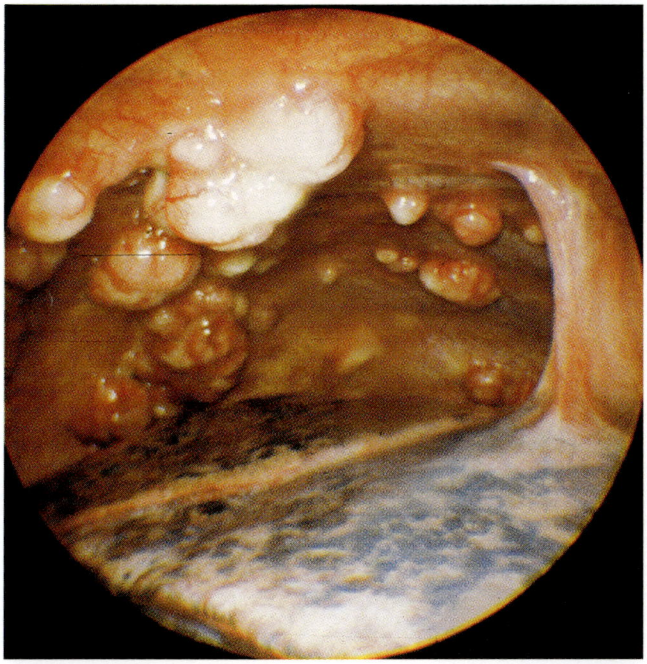

Figure 13-3

Nodular diffuse mesothelioma of the chest wall (adhesions between lung and chest).

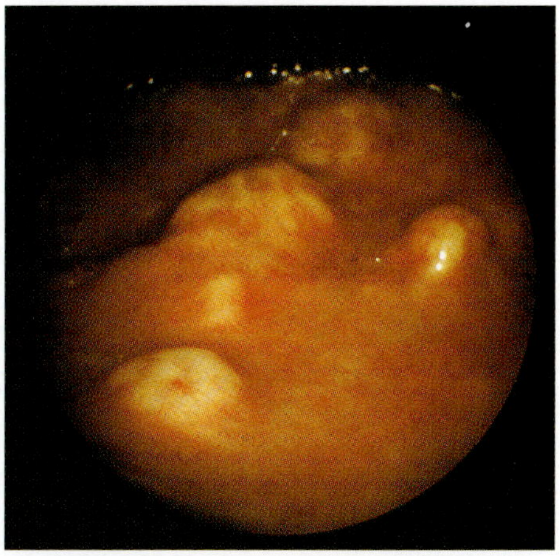

Figure 13-4

Fibronodular diffuse mesothelioma.

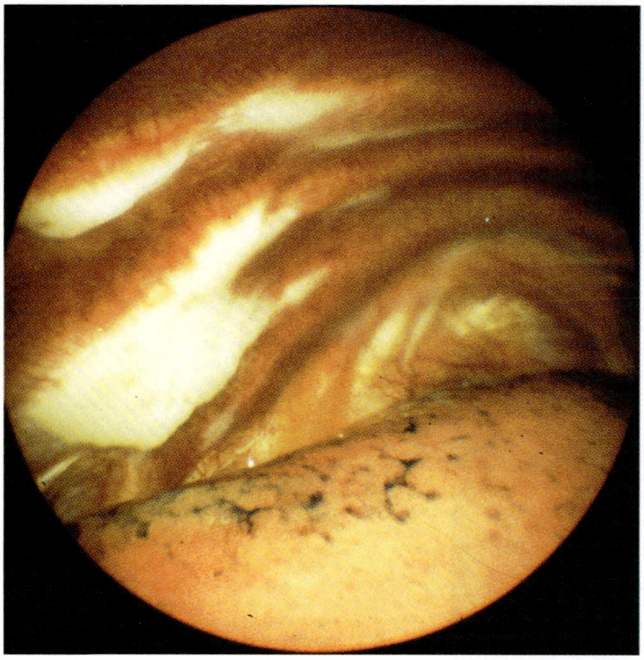

Figure 13-5

Pleural plaques.

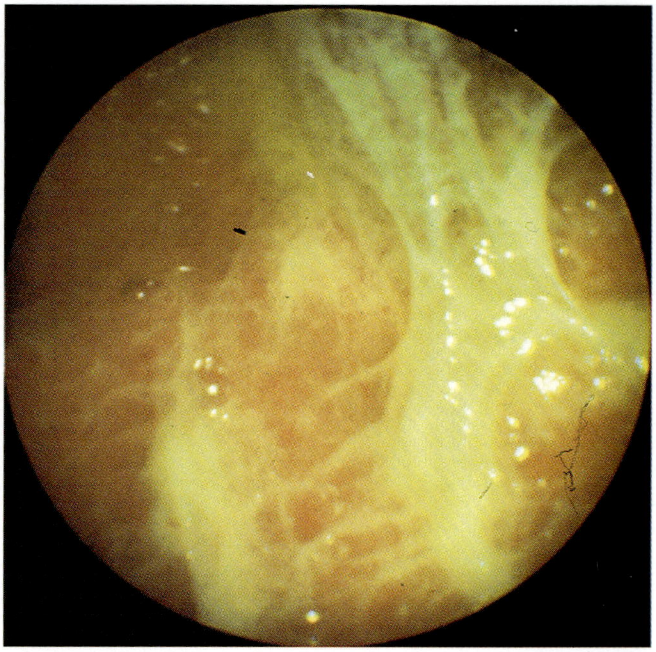

Figure 13-7

Fibrinous exudative tuberculous pleurisy.

appearing smooth and white. Direct biopsies are very difficult because of an extremely hard consistency. In rheumatoid effusion[69] the visceral surface shows nonspecific inflammation and the parietal surface has a "gritty" appearance (Fig. 13-8). Numerous small vesicles or granules have been identified on the parietal pleura. After appropriate pleural fluid assays are nondiagnostic, thoracoscopy may help to establish these benign diagnoses (Figs. 13-9 and 13-10) and, more importantly, eliminate the possibility of malignancy. Thoracoscopy should not replace pleural fluid chemistry, microbiology, cytology, and percutaneous needle biopsies as a preliminary diagnostic procedure.

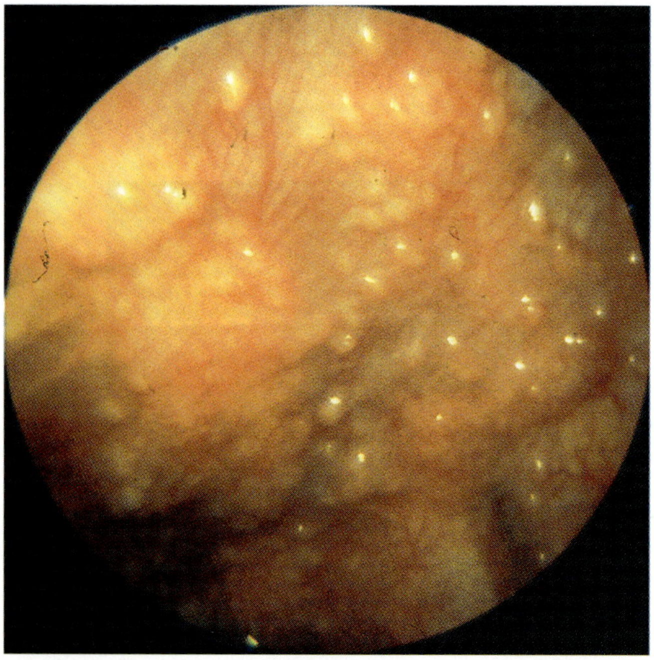

Figure 13-6

Sago-like early tuberculous pleurisy (chest wall).

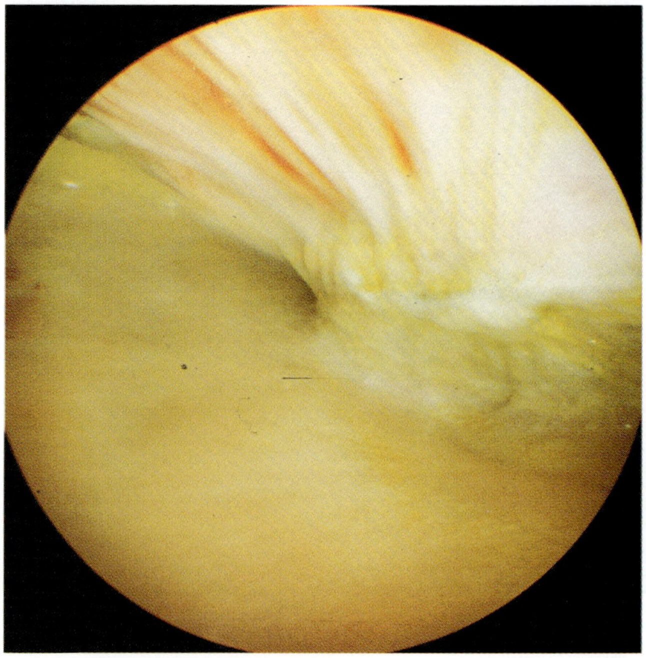

Figure 13-8

Chronic rheumatoid pleurisy.

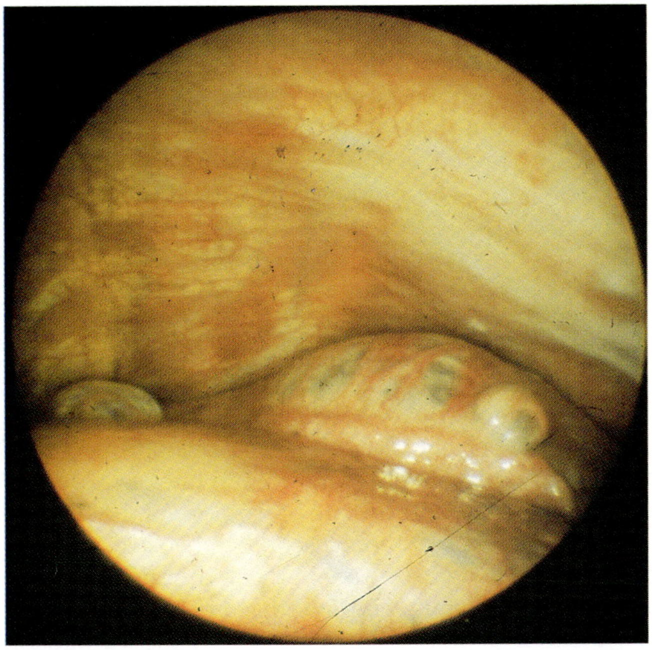

Figure 13-9

Bulla in the apex (spontaneous pneumothorax).

DIFFUSE PULMONARY DISEASE

Thoracoscope-Guided Lung Biopsy

Diffuse lung diseases, currently of great interest because of recent advances in therapy, provide an excellent indication for diagnostic thoracoscopy. Thoracoscopic lung biopsy has been advocated when less invasive techniques such as fiberoptic bronchoscopy with transbronchial biopsy, bronchoalveolar lavage, or fine needle aspiration biopsies have failed to establish a diagnosis.[65–71] It is possible to obtain sizable biopsies of the lung parenchyma during thoracoscopy. Thoracoscopic lung biopsy can be helpful in the diagnosis of diffuse pulmonary disease, pulmonary infection, and infiltrates or peripheral lesions of unknown etiology (Fig. 13-11). Boutin and coworkers[65] obtained pulmonary parenchymal specimens in 75 patients with both diffuse parenchymal diseases and localized parenchymal lesions using a biopsy forceps with cautery for hemostasis, which preserved the histologic structure of the biopsy specimen. Complications included pneumothorax in eight patients and low-grade fever in 11. The overall sensitivity was 92 percent, ranging from 70 percent for peripheral lesions to 100 percent for diffuse diseases. Similarly, Kapsenberg[68] performed 115 thoracoscopic lung biopsies in patients with diffuse pulmonary disease. Sensitivities ranged from 92 to 100 percent for diffuse lung disease, as compared with only 70 percent for peripheral localized opacities.

Rodgers and coworkers[69,70] performed 86 thoracoscopic lung biopsies in children, 42 of whom were immunocompromised, establishing a diagnosis of *Pneumocystis carinii* in 23, various bacterial infections in eight, viral infection in four, and interstitial fibrosis in seven. Bonniot and coworkers[71] have successfully obtained lung biopsies with excellent hemostasis and no air leakage in 18 patients using a cryoprobe to seal the biopsy site.

Most patients undergoing thoracoscopy can be discharged in a few days with negligible morbidity, pro-

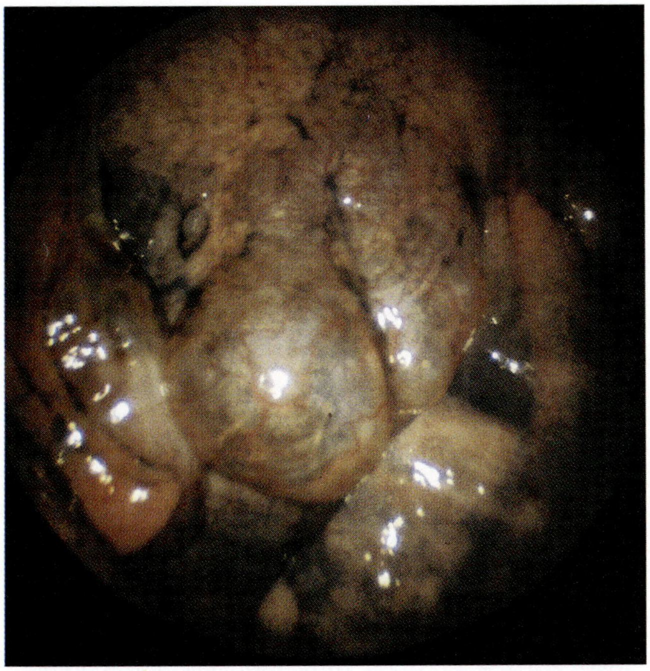

Figure 13-10

Multiple bullae (bullous emphysema)—spontaneous pneumothorax.

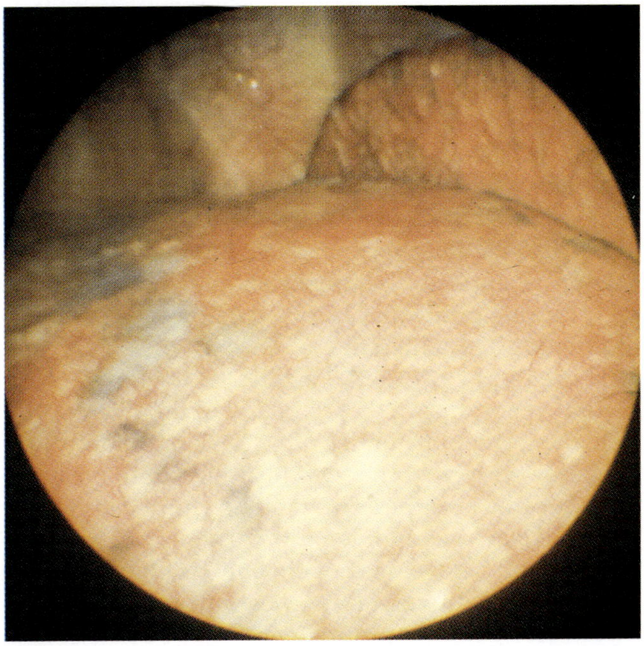

Figure 13-11

Sarcoidosis of the lung (granulomatous) with one nodule on the chest wall.

vided that cut pulmonary tissue has been adequately secured with staples or cautery and an air leak is not present.[65] This contrasts with a formal open lung biopsy, which carries an operative mortality of at least 1.7 percent.[72]

Thoracoscopic specimens are from peripheral lung tissue, and it is not known if the biopsies provide equivalent information to those obtained at open lung biopsy. At our institution, lung tissue obtained from thoracoscopic-guided forceps biopsies directly correlated with the histologic and microbiologic findings obtained by open lung biopsy in the same patients.[73] A clear advantage of obtaining lung biopsies by thoracoscopy, as opposed to bronchoscopy, is that larger pieces of representative lung tissue can be obtained. As thoracoscopy becomes more widely available, patients who require lung biopsy for either localized or diffuse disease may be offered a diagnostic approach, intermediate to that currently available from bronchoscopy and open lung biopsy.

Other reported indications for using diagnostic thoracoscopy-guided biopsy include suspected "nonsurgical" mediastinal tumors such as lymphoma, and for sampling subcarinal, as well as aorticopulmonary window lymph nodes.

Empyema

During the exudative phase of empyema, effusions are characteristically thin and adhesions have not yet formed. In this stage the fluid can drain with a chest tube. Beyond this stage, however, fluid is thick and multiple adhesions are formed, resulting in loculation. Thoracoscopic visualization may allow debridement of fibrinoid adhesions and permit evacuation of loculated fluid. Thoracoscopy can allow drainage of pus from the pleural space in patients with purulent empyema. After removal of pus from the cavity, adhesions are dissected to create a large, single cavity. Placement of a large-caliber drain in a clean, adhesion-free cavity ensures that the lung reexpands against the wall when suction is applied. Treatment should be carried out early during empyema before the adhesions become too fibrous and adherent.

Hutter and coworkers[74] suggested irrigation of the pleural space during thoracoscopy to debride and divide the loculations under direct vision. In this study, irrigation with two tubes was instituted until fluid cultures became negative. This method shortened the duration of stay and avoided a thoracotomy. If an organized "peel" develops, open empyectomy may be necessary. The timing of thoracoscopic intervention is, therefore, critical. Appropriateness may be determined by CT scanning and clinical history or even by early medical thoracoscopy at the time of the initial insertion of the chest tube.

Complications

Mortality has been reported to be an extremely rare event during thoracoscopy. Viskum and Enk[75] noted only one death in 8000 cases reviewed. In Boutin and coworkers' review of 4300 cases, the mortality rate was 0.09 percent.[76] The mortality rate for thoracoscopy is comparable with that of transbronchial lung biopsy (0.22 to 0.66 percent).[77,78] In his review, Viskum found that there was no mention of wound infection in any study, that empyema occurred in 12 of 652 cases from three studies, and that hemorrhage occurred in six of 256 patients in three other studies. Oxygen desaturation during thoracoscopy under local anesthesia occurs in less than 2 percent of cases.[20] Menzies and Charbonneau[30] reported a major complication rate of 1.9 percent and minor complication rate of 5.6 percent. Boutin and coworkers,[31] in 817 thoracoscopies, reported a persistent air leak of greater than 7 day's duration in 2 percent, subcutaneous emphysema in 2 percent, and postoperative fever in 16 percent. Of the 14 patients who died within 30 days following thoracoscopy, no deaths were attributed to the procedure. Although risks are low, precautions should include monitoring of cardiac rhythm and oxygenation. Adequate control of hemorrhage is essential after obtaining biopsies, but coagulation is rarely necessary. A concern often expressed regarding thoracoscopy is the risk of bleeding and the need for surgical backup. In this regard, the reported incidence of significant bleeding, that is, requiring transfusion or surgical intervention, is exceedingly low.[4,13,19,20,31] Specific procedures such as talc pleurodesis have been carefully evaluated for long-term sequelae from the procedure. For example, up to 35 years following talc pleurodesis, there was no evidence of malignancy, fibrosis, or adverse functional sequelae.[81,82]

Contraindications

The major contraindication is the lack of a pleural space owing to pleural adhesions. Other relative contraindications are uncontrolled cough, hypoxemia (not due to significant pleural effusion), coagulation disorder, and severe cardiac disease. When lung biopsy is being considered, contraindications would include pulmonary hypertension, honeycomb lung, and vascular tumors. As for any procedure, the risk and benefits of an intervention must be routinely evaluated. Oxygen desaturation can obviously occur in patients with severe underlying parenchymal lung disease, and severe lung disease is a relative contraindication to thoracoscopy under local anesthesia.[24,25] In these cases, video-assisted or open lung biopsies under general anesthesia in the operating room may be a safer alternative.

Summary

This overview of the indications for medical thoracoscopy is far from exhaustive, and new applications will surely be proposed. In conclusion, thoracoscopy provides the diagnosis of pleural-based malignancy or tuberculosis with a high degree of accuracy when routine cytology and closed-needle pleural biopsies have failed. In patients, in whom adequate visualization can be accomplished, an unequivocal pathologic diagnosis of benign disease can be made with a specificity approaching 100 percent. If transbronchial biopsy and bronchoalveolar lavage are inconclusive, VATS lung biopsy appears to be a safe alternative to open lung biopsy by thoracotomy for diagnosis of diffuse interstitial or infectious lung disease. Thoracoscopy is often effective in the management of malignant pleural effusion and spontaneous pneumothorax.

A close working relationship between pulmonary physicians and thoracic surgeons ensures that patients undergoing diagnostic thoracoscopy, under local anesthesia with intravenous sedation in the pulmonary endoscopy suite, are appropriate candidates for this procedure.[79,80] It is absolutely mandatory that physicians intent on performing this procedure be adequately trained. We believe that collaboration between thoracic surgeons and pulmonologists not only facilitates training in thoracoscopy, but also ensures that patients undergoing thoracoscopy will be carefully assessed from both perspectives.

HOW I DO IT

Indications

The major clinical utility for thoracoscopy is in the diagnosis of pleural disorders and pleurodesis. Indications for diagnostic thoracoscopy include exudative pleural effusion of an unknown etiology, mesothelioma, tuberculosis, and benign pleural disorders including empyemas. Pleurodesis is performed in malignant pleural effusion, spontaneous pneumothorax, and recurrent nonmalignant pleural effusion. Before thoracoscopy, a comprehensive workup should be performed, including biochemical, bacteriologic, and cytologic analysis of pleural fluid and one or two closed pleural biopsy specimens. Diagnostic thoracoscopy is usually considered in approximately 20 to 25 percent of patients with exudative pleural effusions.[3]

Contraindication

The only absolute contraindication to thoracoscopy is the lack of a pleural space owing to obliterative adhesions. The minimum pleural space required for insertion of a thoracoscope is approximately 6 to 10 cm in diameter; the lesion must also be within an accessible area. Relative contraindications are related to concerns about the general health of the patient: fever, uncontrolled cough, unstable cardiovascular status, hypoxemia (not due to a large pleural effusion), and incorrectable bleeding disorders. Refractory cough carries a high risk of subcutaneous emphysema.

Preprocedure

Routine chest films are frequently supplemented with bilateral decubitus films and a chest CT scan. The chest roentgenogram and/or CT scan provides the basis of determining the point of inserting the thoracoscope. The respiratory status is evaluated with blood gas analysis and pulmonary function tests. Routine blood tests, including coagulation parameters, and an electrocardiogram should be performed.

Equipment

We use a rigid thoracoscope (Karl Storz Endoscopy America Inc., Culver City, Calif.) (Fig. 13-12) with a working channel of 3 or 5 mm. A xenon light source satisfies the requirements for high-quality visual exploration and video documentation. Besides the biopsy forceps, needle biopsy, and suction catheter (Fig. 13-13), the working channel also accommodates electrocautery. The trocar consists of an obturator and cannula which should have a blunt conical tip. The

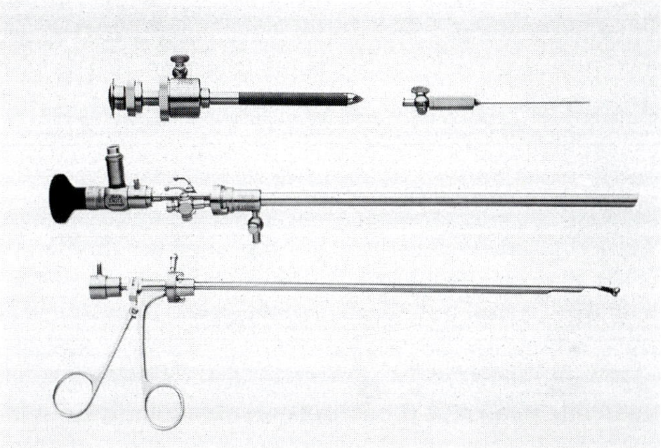

Figure 13-12

The Karl Storz rigid thoracoscope with the trocar (*upper left*) and a pneumothorax cannula (Veress) (*upper right*).

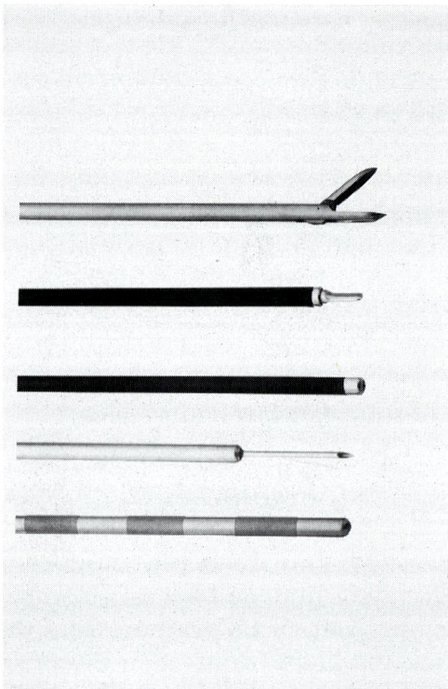

Figure 13-13

Accessories used through the working channel of the thoracoscope, including (*from above*) forceps, cautery probe, combined suction and cautery cannula, needle, and probe.

trocar is 10 mm in diameter. Unlike the instruments for laparoscopy this trocar does not have to be airtight. Air should be allowed to enter and leave the thoracic cavity freely. The examination may be limited by pain if the trocar is larger than 10 mm. Thoracoscopes are available with various angles of vision including 0, 30, 45, or 90 degrees. The direct viewing 0-degree telescope is more natural when moving the thoracoscope in a circular manner, and most of the thoracic cavity can be viewed. With an oblique thoracoscope, a panoramic view of the whole chest cavity can be obtained. We use a 3 or 5 mm (insulated) coagulating forceps through the working channel for biopsies.

Accessories

These include sterile sheets and gowns for the physicians (Laparotomy Pack IV Johnson & Johnson Medical Inc., Arlington, Tex.). Instruments include: needles, syringes, scalpel, sutures, compresses, forceps, needle holders, and hemostats. These are usually all available in a chest tube insertion tray. In addition, local anesthesia, a talc atomizer or aerosolized talc canister (Fig. 13-14), a chest tube between the sizes 24 and 32 Fr with an inner stylet (Dekentel Inc., Fall River, MA), anti fog solution, and an underwater drainage for pleural fluid are needed.

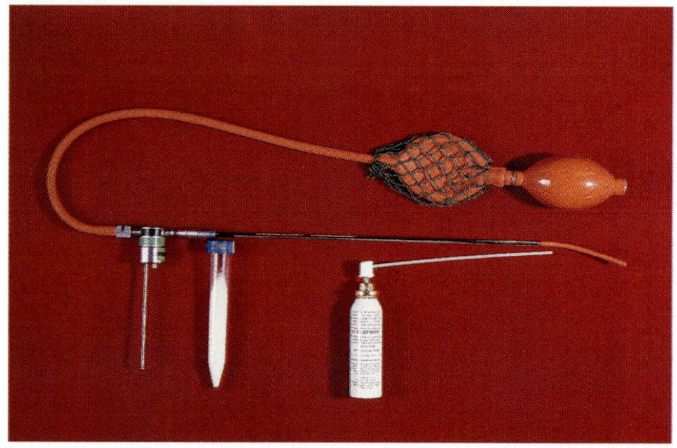

Figure 13-14

Talc atomizer and canister of aerosolized talc.

Endoscopy Room

We perform thoracoscopy in a fully equipped endoscopy suite. A light source, video camera, and recording equipment are placed on a mobile cart. The thoracoscopy is performed on a procedure table used for bronchoscopy, which is radiolucent in the thoracic area. A Mayo stand is placed sideways to hold the disinfecting scrub and chest tube insertion tray. On a separate sterile table, the thoracoscope, trocar, forceps, talc atomizer, and all other accessories are placed. Thoracoscopy must be carried out under strict sterile conditions. All the instruments including the trocar, thoracoscope, and forceps should be sterilized. All accessories, light conducting fiberoptic cable (and, if necessary, video camera), should be sterilized as well.

Point of Entry

An axillary point of entry is selected in most cases. The site of entry depends on either the anticipated location of the pathologic lesion to be biopsied or the indication for the procedure, such as talc pleurodesis. The entry in the midaxillary line at the level between the fourth or seventh intercostal space allows complete thoracic cavity inspection. In spontaneous pneumothorax, a third or fourth intercostal space entry is preferred to thoroughly evaluate the apex of the lung. Metastatic disease or mesothelioma is commonly found in the costovertebral angles and on the diaphragmatic surfaces.[49–51] Therefore, entry in the fifth to seventh intercostal space allows direct visualization of these lesions. In some cases, the point of entry can be determined with help of the CT scan.

Several important anatomic landmarks are essential and should always be kept in mind. The anteriomedial end of the second intercostal space is located by palpating the angle formed by the manubrium and the body of the sternum; the ribs can then be counted from top to bottom. In the axillary hollow the second intercostal space can be felt in a nonobese patient. In the lateral position, the ribs can be counted along the midaxillary line. The lowest that can be felt is the 10th; the 11th and 12th are floating ribs and are posterior. The ribs can be counted from the bottom upward. The internal mammary artery and vein are located just posterior to the ribs and about 16 to 18 mm lateral to the sternal margins. In the lateral decubitus position, the liver may reach the fifth or sixth intercostal space. The major fissure crosses the midaxillary line at the fourth intercostal space on the right, and the minor fissure begins on the fifth intercostal space on the left. The male nipple is generally situated near the level of the fourth rib.

The single puncture technique is the easiest method to learn and is commonly used by pulmonologists.[19,20,24,33,38] A double puncture method[3,4,25,31] increases the diagnostic and therapeutic benefit of the procedure in selected cases. With the double puncture method, the second site of entry is selected closer to the area of interest. This permits viewing of areas difficult to reach, such as the mediastinal pleural surfaces and the apex of the lung.

Performance of Thoracoscopy

The physician and assistant clean their hands with the standard surgical scrub technique and then put on a sterile gown and gloves. Every patient is monitored with automated blood pressure monitoring and cardiac and cutaneous oxygen saturation monitors. The patient's skin is prepared by shaving and disinfecting a large area from the sternum to the clavicle and across the axilla past the scapula to the spinous processes and down to the base of the thorax. The patient lies on the healthy side in a lateral decubitus position with the head resting on a pillow. Patient movement is minimized with cushioned support; the arm is raised over the head with the help of a sling. A rolled up sheet is placed on the table under the patient's thorax, which facilitates arching the vertebral column upward, thus enlarging the intercostal spaces.

We perform thoracoscopy under local anesthesia and conscious sedation. Our current practice is to premedicate the fasting patient with atropine 0.4 to 0.8 mg IV to minimize the chance of vasovagal reaction. The vital signs are monitored by a nurse, who also provides the intravenous sedation. This is accomplished by incremental increases in intravenous administration of a narcotic (morphine, hydrocodone) and a benzodiazepine (midazolam). Dosing is kept flexible according to the physician's wishes and patient's needs. Agents to reverse narcotics and benzodiazipines should be available at the time of the procedure. This approach effectively reduces discomfort and frequently creates amnesia for the procedure. It is essential to allay the patient's anxiety as much as possible by carefully explaining the procedure beforehand and announcing each step as thoracoscopy proceeds.

The physician stands on one side of the patient, while the assistant is across the table. The previously marked site of entry in the intercostal space is palpated with the index and middle finger of one hand. A small wheal is produced between the two fingers by a syringe with 20 ml of 2% lidocaine attached to a small bore needle for intradermal injection. The local anesthesia is infiltrated subcutaneously through intercostal muscle down to the parietal pleura. The path of the needle should be kept perpendicular to the chest wall to ensure that the entire path of the instruments is painfree. As the needle penetrates the parietal pleura, the patient may experience transient pain. Entry into the pleural cavity is confirmed by drawing back on the syringe, which will fill with air or fluid. The chest wall depth is established by withdrawing the needle until the gas bubbles are no longer obtained. This will be the depth for placement of the trocar. Approximately 8 to 10 ml of lidocaine is infiltrated at this location of the parietal pleura. With the scalpel a 10-mm incision is made through the skin and subcutaneous tissue parallel with and in the middle of the selected intercostal space. The incision is relatively small so that the trocar fits tightly. Bleeding through the incision is minimal owing to this compression. Blunt dissection is performed with a hemostat through the intercostal muscles and parietal pleura. The process is identical to inserting a chest tube with the exception that a tunnel is not created, since this would limit the mobility of the thoracoscope. Once the parietal pleura is opened, the index finger is inserted to examine the pleural cavity and confirm an adequate pleural space.

We have recently changed our technique and now use a modified Seldinger technique. After the local anesthesia, a skin and subcutaneous incision is made. A needle is introduced (Fig. 13-15), and once in the pleural space a soft tip guide wire is passed (Fig. 13-16). The needle is then removed. Several dilators of increasing diameter are then introduced over the wire (Figs. 13-17 and 13-18). For the 10-mm trocar-cannula, the 30 Fr (1 mm = 3 Fr) dilator provides a perfect opening. We find this technique to be bloodless and less traumatic to the patient.

The handle of the trocar should be held firmly in the palm of the hand, while the extended index finger limits the depth of insertion (Fig. 13-19). While fixating the intercostal space with two fingers the trocar is advanced in a corkscrew motion until a sudden release of resistance is felt. Once the trocar is in the pleural cavity, the operator can hear air movement into and out of the pleural cavity synchronous with the patient's breathing. Pressure equilibrium with the atmosphere occurs quickly. If the trocar is not handled carefully, it might injure the lung. The cannula should lie 1 to 3 cm

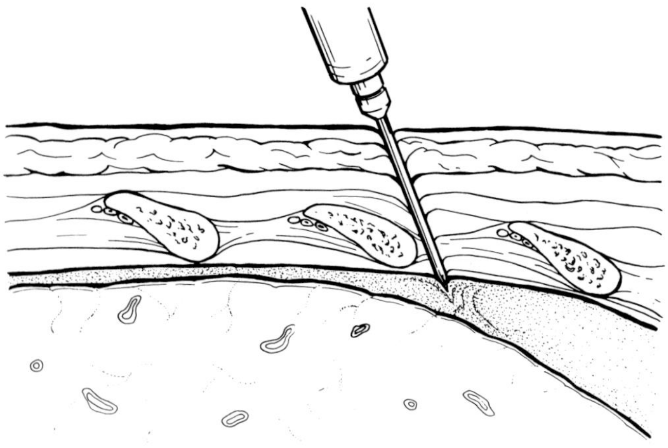

Figure 13-15

Needle entry into the pleural space.

within the pleural cavity and be held in position by the assistant. If the patient coughs, the assistant will withdraw the cannula within the chest wall. After removing the inner trocar, the thoracoscope with a 0 deg angle is placed in the cannula. The video camera is attached to the thoracoscope, which is advanced into the pleural cavity under direct vision (Figs. 13-20 and 13-21). The pleural fluid is removed with a suction catheter placed through the working channel. The thoracoscope is advanced toward the back and directed to the dependent area, toward the costophrenic angle. After completely removing the fluid, a systematic exploration of the chest cavity is performed by maneuvering the thoracoscope. In difficult cases, oblique telescopes are valuable to ensure adequate pleural inspection. The orientation is simple, although fine adhesions resembling spider webs may interfere with complete examination of the pleural cavity. These can be mechanically separated. Fibrous band or vascular adhesions should be avoided or cauterized by electrocautery. Air can be cautiously introduced to further collapse the lung and improve visualization. Extreme care must be taken to

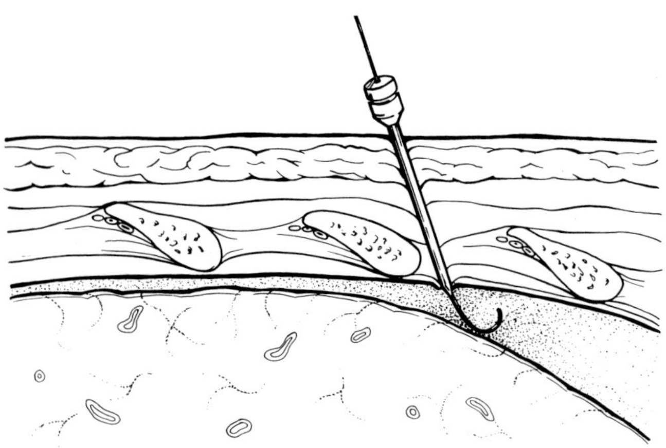

Figure 13-16

Guidewire passes through the needle.

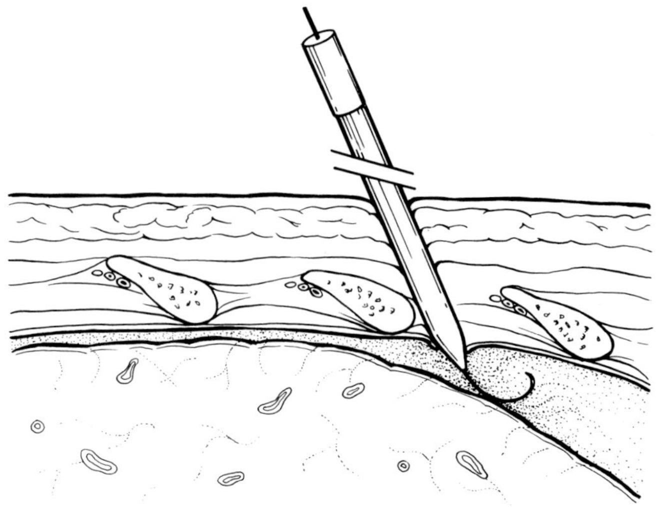

Figure 13-17

Dilator being placed over the guidewire.

avoid iatrogenic tension pneumothorax and subcutaneous emphysema when insufflating air into the pleural cavity.

It is mandatory that the endoscopist be knowledgeable with the anatomy of the thoracic cavity. Anatomic relationships and intrathoracic structures must be appreciated during thoracoscopy. The 0-degree optics are best for the initial overview. To prevent the lenses from fogging, the tip could be immersed in warm sterile saline or coated with a defogger agent. In the right chest orientation can be achieved by locating the point where the three lobes meet, the junction of the oblique fissure and horizontal fissure. On the left, the oblique fissure can be used for orientation. The diaphragm can be recognized by the respiration-related movement. Rib, intercostal muscle, fat, blood vessels, and nerves are usually well distinguished. The heart and the great vessels

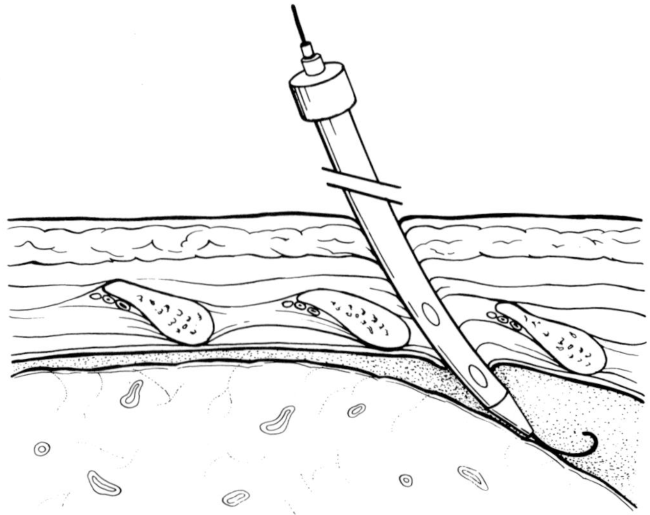

Figure 13-18

Chest tube and dilator being inserted over the guidewire.

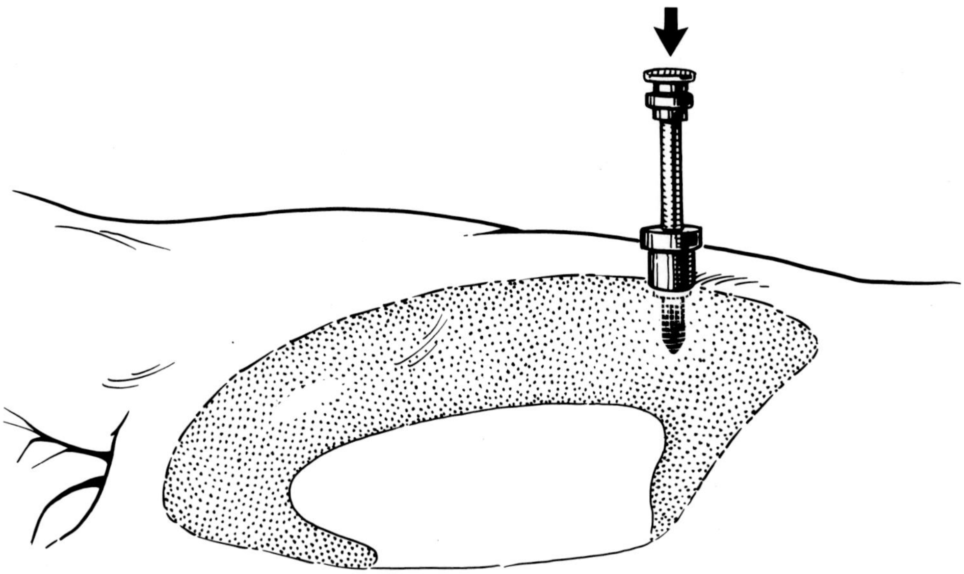

Figure 13-19

The trocar being placed in the chest cavity.

are identified by pulsations which are occasionally transmitted to adjacent parts of the lung. Visual exploration is carried out in a few minutes. A probe enables the physician to push aside any fibrinous strands interfering with clear view. The observation should be performed from a distance to obtain a panoramic view and then from a closer distance of 1 to 2 cm to inspect the cavity very carefully and to select the best biopsy sites.

In its normal state the pleura is transparent, allowing visualization of many structures through it. Variable amounts of anthracotic pigment can occasionally be seen within the parietal pleura. Fatty collections are often abundant in the pleura. These are long, yellowish plaques located along the ribs and around the pericardium and diaphragm. One of the hardest tasks for the endoscopist is to distinguish between innocuous inflammation and malignancy. It is almost impossible to tell the difference by inspection. Certain patterns of pleural lesions can be seen such as: lymphangitis, which appears as a fine reticular pattern, covering part of the pleura; granulomata, which are 1 to 3 mm in diameter and are seen with tuberculosis or sarcoidosis; and malignant nodules, which vary in size and shape.[24,25] Suspicious areas are biopsied through the working channel of the thoracoscope using either a 3- or 5-mm biopsy forceps.

Pleural Biopsy Techniques

Before pleural biopsy, the rib and intercostal space should be identified with a blunt probe. If the pleura is thick, the rib will feel hard compared with the spongy intercostal space. When the pleura is thick, the

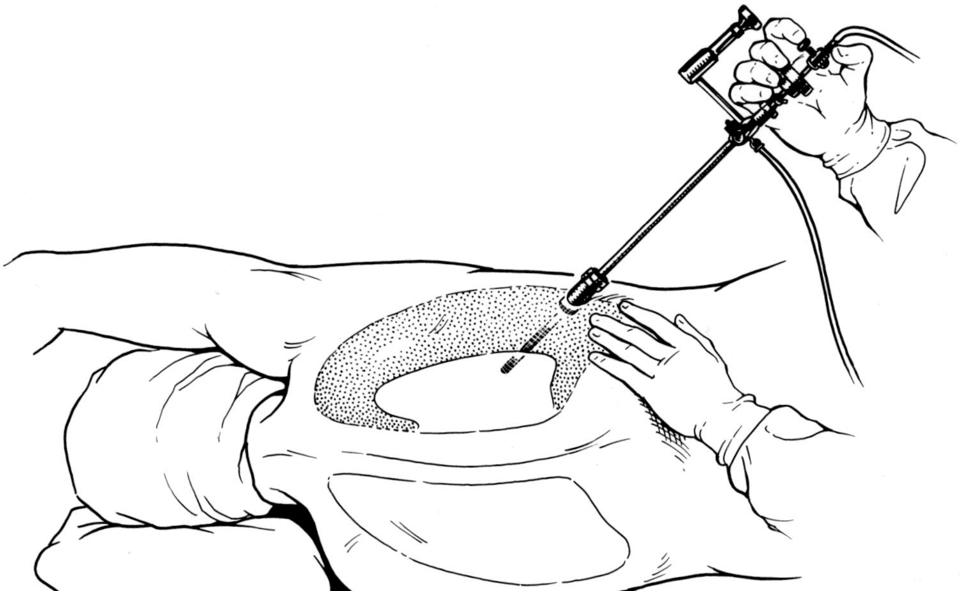

Figure 13-20

The thoracoscope is placed in the chest cavity through the cannula and the suction catheter is placed in the working channel.

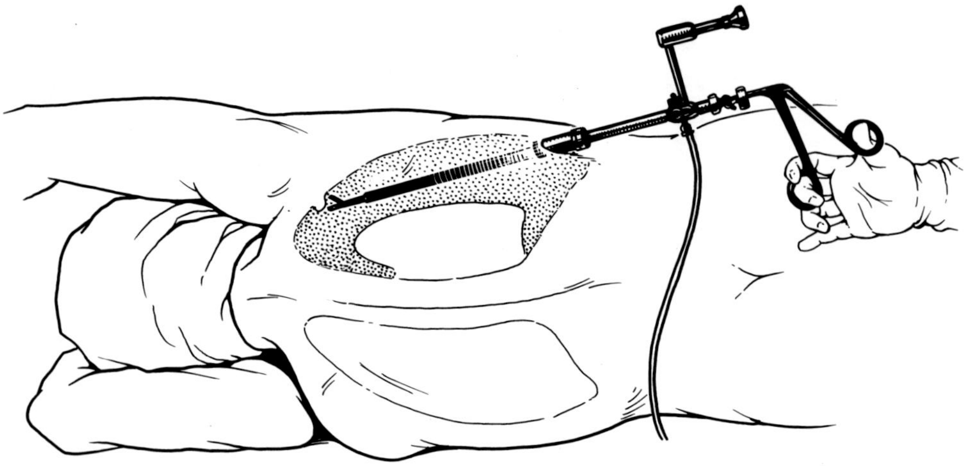

Figure 13-21

The biopsy forceps is placed through the working channel of the thoracoscope.

biopsy is simple, with minimal risk of injuring the intercostal arteries. In contrast, when the pleura is thin, the biopsy should be performed against one of the ribs. Typically four to six biopsies of a suspicious pleural lesion will establish a diagnosis. Sufficient quantities of tissue must be obtained, especially if hormonal receptor studies are required for tumors such as adenocarcinoma of the breast. When malignancy is suspected but the endoscopic findings are nonspecific, the number of biopsies should be increased to between 10 and 12 from a variety of areas on the pleural surface.[4,5] Attention should be paid to fibrinous nodules as they can mask malignant lesions. The fibrinous material should be removed with forceps and the biopsy taken from the base of the lesion. Intercostal hemorrhage is unusual and controlled with either local pressure with epinephrine-soaked gauze or coagulation with cautery. Following the procedure, insertion of a chest tube will bring the lung surface in apposition to the chest wall.

Lung

The lung is shaped like a cone, narrowing at the apex. Variable adhesions between the visceral and parietal pleura may be seen. When the lung is normal, the surface is pink and soft, with a reticular pattern demarcating the pulmonary lobules; black anthracotic pigment is scattered over the surface. The visceral pleural surface is transparent. Areas of atelectasis are purplish red with a clear edge. Malignant nodules are quite easily seen, as are emphysematous bullae protruding from the surface.

Talc Pleurodesis

Our preferred method for pleurodesis is insufflation of talc into the pleural cavity.[73,81,82] Following complete evacuation of the pleural fluid and lysis of any adhesions, 4 to 8 g of USP grade asbestos-free sterile talc is insufflated into the pleural space through a working channel of the thoracoscope. Uniform distribution of the talc on all pleural surfaces is confirmed by direct vision. Care must be taken to avoid talc abrasion of the glass lens of the thoracoscope.

Chest Tube Care

A chest tube is required after every procedure; the placement and duration varies with the indication. During a diagnostic procedure, when only parietal pleural biopsies are performed, a chest tube may be required for only a few hours. At the conclusion of the procedure, a chest tube (24 to 28 Fr) is placed through the same incision as the thoracoscope. It is directed cranially to evacuate the pneumothorax created during the procedure. A chest roentgenogram is performed immediately following the procedure. If the lung has completely reexpanded and there is no air leak, the chest tube is removed within 3 to 4 h after the procedure. If air continues to leak, the chest tube remains until the leak stops. Patients undergoing simple diagnostic thoracoscopy are typically discharged from the hospital within 24 h of the procedure.

When talc pleurodesis is performed, a second incision is required to place the chest tube in the lowest possible intercostal space. Before insufflating talc, the thoracoscope is directed toward the diaphragm. The assistant indents the intercostal spaces or puts a small needle into the chest cavity, while the physician documents the lowest intercostal space for entry of the chest tube. Before inserting a chest tube (28 to 36 Fr), extra holes are created along the radioopaque line to permit drainage of the entire hemithorax. The chest tube is pushed through the point of entry, perpendicular to the skin at first, then tunneled in the desired direction through the chest wall. The chest tube is directed posteriorly and then upward as close to the apex as possible. When the chest tube is left in place for drainage, sutures are applied to secure the tube to the skin. A purse string suture usually helps in closing the chest tube wound tightly. If the thoracoscopy is performed for pleurodesis, the chest tube should be left in place until the fluid drainage is less than 150 ml/day and no air leak is present, usually 3 to 6 days. A daily chest film is obtained while the chest tube is in place to assess chest tube position, fluid accumulation, and lung reexpansion. Patients requiring talc pleurodesis remain hospitalized for an average of 3 to 6 days.

Summary

In summary, thoracoscopy offers several advantages for diagnosis and therapy of pleural diseases. Thoracoscopy helps in the diagnosis of pleural-based malignancy or tuberculosis with a high degree of accuracy when routine studies and closed-needle pleural biopsies have failed. In patients in whom adequate visualization is possible, an unequivocal pathologic diagnosis of benign diseases can be made with a specificity approaching 100 percent.[30] Thoracoscopy is effective in the management of malignant pleural effusion[73] and spontaneous pneumothorax.[82]

REFERENCES

1. Poe RH, et al: Sensitivity, specificity, and predictive values of closed pleural biopsy. *Arch Intern Med* 1984; 144:325–328.
2. Gunnels JJ: Perplexing pleural effusion. *Chest* 1978; 74:390–393.
3. Boutin C, et al: Thoracoscopy in malignant pleural effusion. *Am Rev Resp Dis* 1981; 124:588–592.
4. Boutin C, et al: Thoracoscopy in the diagnosis of malignant effusion. *Endoscopy* 1980; 12:155–160.
5. Pugatch RD, et al: Differentiation of pleural lesions using computed tomography. *J Comput Assist Tomog* 1978; 2:601–606.
6. Feinsilver SH, et al: Fiberoptic bronchoscopy and pleural effusion of unknown origin. *Chest* 1986; 90:516–519.
7. Jacobaeus MC: Über die Möglichkeit, die Zystoskopie bei Untersuchung seröser Höhlungen anzuwenden. *Munch Med Wschr* 1910; 40:2090–2092.
8. Jacobaeus HC: The practical importance of thoracoscopy in surgery of the chest. *Surg Gynecol Obstet* 1922; 34:289–296.
9. Abrams LD: A pleural punch biopsy. *Lancet* 1958; 1:30–31.
10. Cope C: A new pleural biopsy needle-preliminary study. *JAMA* 1958; 167:1107–1108.
11. Alexander J: *The Collapse Therapy of Pulmonary Tuberculosis.* Springfield, Ill. Charles C Thomas, 1937:313–316.
12. Ash SR, Manfredi F: Directed biopsy using a small endoscope. Thoracoscopy and peritoneoscopy simplified. *N Engl J Med* 1974; 291:1398–1399.
13. Boushy SF, et al: Thoracoscopy: Technique and results in eighteen patients with pleural effusion. *Chest* 1974; 4:386–389.
14. Deslauriers J, et al: Mediastinopleuroscopy: A new approach to the diagnosis of intrathoracic diseases. *Ann Thorac Surg* 1976; 22:265–269.
15. Weissberg D, Kaufman M: Diagnostic and therapeutic pleuroscopy: Experience with 127 patients. *Chest* 1980; 78:732–735.
16. Weissberg D, et al: Pleuroscopy in clinical evaluation and staging of lung cancer. *Poumon Coeur* 1981; 37:241–243.
17. Senno A, et al: Thoracoscopy with the fiberoptic bronchoscope. A simple method of diagnosing pleuropulmonary diseases. *J Thorac Cardiovas Surg* 1974; 67:390–393.
18. Senno A, et al: Fiberoptic thoracoscopy. *NY St J Med* 1975; 75:51–56.
19. Oldenburg FA, Newhouse MT: Thoracoscopy. A safe, accurate diagnostic procedure using the rigid thoracoscope and local anesthesia. *Chest* 1979; 75:45–50.
20. Davidson AC, et al: Thoracoscopy: Assessment of a physician service and comparison of a flexible bronchoscope used as a thoracoscope with a rigid thoracoscope. *Thorax* 1988; 43:327–332.
21. Canto A, et al: Thoracoscopy in the diagnosis of pleural effusion. *Thorax* 1977;33:550–554.
22. Enk B, Viskum K: Diagnostic thoracoscopy. *Eur J Resp Dis* 1981; 62:344–351.
23. Newhouse MT: Thoracoscopy: Diagnostic and therapeutic indications. *Pneumologie* 1989; 43:48–52.
24. Brandt HJ, et al: *Atlas of Diagnostic Thoracoscopy.* New York, Thieme Inc, 1985.
25. Boutin C, et al: *Practical Thoracoscopy.* Springer Verlag, 1991.
26. Wakabayashi A: Expanded applications of diagnostic and therapeutic thoracoscopy. *J Thorac Cardiovasc Surg* 1991; 102:721–723.
27. Nathanson LK, et al: Videothoracoscopic ligation of bulla and pleurectomy for spontaneous pneumothorax. *Ann Thorac Surg* 1991; 52:316–319.
28. Lewis RJ, et al: Imaged thoracoscopic surgery: A new thoracic technique for resection of mediastinal cyst. *Ann Thorac Surg* 1992; 102:318–320.
29. Page RD, et al: Thoracoscopy: A review of 121 consecutive surgical procedures. *Ann Thorac Surg* 1989; 48:66–68.
30. Menzies R, Charbonneau M: Thoracoscopy for the diagnosis of pleural disease. *Ann Intern Med* 1991; 114:271–276.
31. Boutin C, et al: Thoracoscopy. In Chrétien J, et al (eds): *The Pleura in Health and Disease,* vol 30. New York, Dekker, 1985:587–622.
32. Loddenkemper R, et al: Prospective evaluation of biopsy methods in the diagnosis of malignant pleural effusions. Intrapatient comparison between pleural fluid cytology, blind needle biopsy and thoracoscopy. *Am Rev Resp Dis* 1983; 127(suppl 4):114.
33. Loddenkemper R: Thoracoscopy: Results in non cancerous and idiopathic pleural effusions. *Poumon Coeur* 1981; 37:261–264.
34. Bloomberg AE: Thoracoscopy in diagnosis of pleural effusions. *NY St J Med* 1970; 19:1974–1977.
35. Canto A: Diagnostic results in secondary malignant pleural effusions. *Pneumologie* 1989; 43:58–60.
36. Pepper JR: Thoracoscopy in the diagnosis of pleural effusions and tumors. *Br J Dis Chest* 1978; 72:74–75.
37. Rusch VW, Mountain C: Thoracoscopy under regional anesthesia for the diagnosis and management of pleural disease. *Am J Surg* 1987; 154:274–278.
38. Canto A, et al: Thoracoscopy in the diagnosis of pleural effusion. *Thorax* 1977; 32:550–554.
39. Levine MN, et al: Pleural effusion in breast cancer. Thoracoscopy for hormone receptor determination. *Cancer* 1986; 57:324–327.
40. Salyer WR, et al: Efficacy of pleural needle biopsy and pleural fluid cytopathology in the diagnosis of malignant neoplasm involving the pleura. *Chest* 1975; 67:536–539.
41. Dines DE, et al: The value of cells in the pleural fluid in the differential diagnosis. *Mayo Clin Proc* 1975; 50:571.
42. Light RW: *Pleural Diseases.* Philadelphia, Lea & Febiger, 1990.
43. Scerbo J, et al: A prospective study of closed pleural biopsies. *JAMA* 1971; 218:377.
44. Legha SS, Muggia FM: Pleural mesothelioma: Clinical features and therapeutic implications *Ann Intern Med* 1977; 87:613–621.
45. Martensson G, et al: Differentiation between malignant and non-malignant pleural effusion. *Eur J Resp Dis* 1985; 67:326–334.
46. Loddenkemper R, et al: Prospective individual comparison of blind needle biopsy and of thoracoscopy in the diagnosis and differential diagnosis of tuberculous pleurisy. *Scand J Respir Dis* 1978; 102(suppl):196–198.

47. Pepper JR: Thoracoscopy in the diagnosis of pleural effusion and tumors. *Br J Dis Chest* 1978; 72:74–75.
48. Wu MH, et al: Thoracoscopy in the diagnosis of pleural effusion. *Jpn J Clin Oncol* 1989; 19:116–119.
49. Canto A, et al: Points to consider when choosing a biopsy method in cases of pleurisy of unknown origin. *Chest* 1983; 84:176–179.
50. Canto-Armengod A: Macroscopic characteristics of pleural metastases arising from the breast and observed by diagnostic thoracoscopy. *Am Rev Resp Dis* 1990; 142:616–618.
51. Canto A, et al: Lung cancer and pleural effusion: Clinical significance and study of pleural metastatic location. *Chest* 1985; 87:649–651.
52. Meyer PC: Metastatic carcinoma of the pleura. *Thorax* 1966; 21:437–442.
53. Rodriguez-Panadero F, et al: Pleural metastatic tumors and effusion. Frequency and pathogenic mechanism in a postmortem series. *Eur Resp J* 1989; 2:366–369.
54. Decker DA, et al: The significance of cytologically negative pleural effusion in bronchogenic carcinoma. *Chest* 1978; 74:640–642.
55. Migueres J, et al: Intérêt de la ponction biopsie pleurale à l'aiguille dans le diagnostic des pleurésies non purulentes (à propos de 250 épanchements). *Rev Med Toulouse* 1974; 10:387.
56. Collins TR, Sahn SA: Thoracocentesis. Clinical value, complications, technical problems, and patient experience. *Chest* 1987; 91:817–822.
57. Ryan CJ, et al: The outcome of patients with pleural effusion of indeterminate cause at thoracotomy. *Mayo Clin Proc* 1981; 56:145–149.
58. Boutin C, et al: La thoracoscopie: Intérêt actuel. Sa place dans le diagnostic des pleurésies chroniques. *Poumon Coeur* 1979; 35:23–29.
59. Martensson G: Thoracoscopy in the diagnosis of malignant mesothelioma. *Poumon Coeur* 1981; 37:249–251.
60. Martensson G, et al: Diagnosis and prognosis in malignant pleural mesothelioma: A prospective study. *Eur J Resp Dis* 1984; 65:169–178.
61. Boutin C: Thoracoscopy in malignant mesothelioma. *Pneumologie* 1989; 43:61–65.
62. Boutin C, et al: Le mésotheliome malin: Facteurs pronostiques dans une série de 125 patients étudiés de 1973 à 1987. *Bull Acad Natl Med* 1992; 176:105–117.
63. Faurschou P, et al: Thoracoscopic, histological, and clinical finding in nine cases of rheumatoid pleural effusion. *Thorax* 1985; 40:371–375.
64. Loddenkemper R, et al: Diagnostik des tuberkulosen Pleuraergusses: Prospektiver Vergleich laborchemischer, bakteriologischer, zytologischer und histologischer Untersuchungsergebnisse. *Prax Klin Pneumol* 1983; 37:1153–1156.
65. Boutin C, et al: Thoracoscopic lung biopsy. Experimental and clinical preliminary study. *Chest* 1982; 82:44–48.
66. Brandt HJ: Biopsie pulmonaire sous controle visuel. *Poumon Coeur* 1981; 37:307–311.
67. Dijkman JH, et al: Transpleural lung biopsy by the thoracoscope route in patient with diffuse interstitial pulmonary disease. *Chest* 1982; 82:76–83.
68. Kapsenberg PD: Thoracoscopic biopsy under visual control. *Poumon Coeur* 1981; 37:313–316.
69. Rodgers BM: Thoracoscopy in children. *Poumon Coeur* 1981; 37:301–306.
70. Rodgers BM, et al: Thoracoscopy. Early diagnosis of interstitial pneumonitis in the immunologically suppressed child. *Chest* 1979; 75:126–180.
71. Bonniot JPA, et al: Pleural and lung cryobiopsies during thoracoscopy. *Chest* 1989; 95:492–493.
72. Wall CP, et al: Comparison of transbronchial and open biopsies in chronic infiltrative lung diseases. *Am Rev Resp Dis* 1981; 132:280–285.
73. Hartman DL, et al: Comparison of thoracoscopic lung biopsy with open lung biopsy in diffuse interstitial lung disorder. *Am Rev Resp Dis* 1992; 145:A750.
74. Hutter JA, et al: The management of empyema thoracis by thoracoscopy and irrigation. *Ann Thorac Surg* 1985; 39:517–572.
75. Viskum K, Enk B: Complications of thoracoscopy. *Poumon Coeur* 1981; 37:25–28.
76. Boutin C, et al: La thoracoscopie en 1980. Revue générale. *Poumon Coeur* 1981; 37:11–19.
77. Andersen HA, Fontana R: Transbronchoscopic lung biopsy for diffuse pulmonary diseases: Technique and results in 450 cases. *Chest* 1972; 62:125–128.
78. Zavala DC: Pulmonary hemorrhage in fiberoptic transbronchial biopsy. *Chest* 1976; 70:584–588.
79. Mathur P, Martin WJ: Clinical utility of thoracoscopy. *Chest* 1992; 102:3–4.
80. Loddenkemper R, Boutin C: Thoracoscopy: Present diagnostic and therapeutic indications. *Eur Resp J* 1993; 6:1544–1555.
81. Lange P, et al: Lung function 22–35 years after treatment of idiopathic spontaneous pneumothorax with talc or simple drainage. *Thorax* 1988; 43:559–561.
82. Almind M, et al: Spontaneous pneumothorax: Comparison of simple drainage, talc pleurodesis, and tetracycline pleurodesis. *Thorax* 1989; 44:627–630.

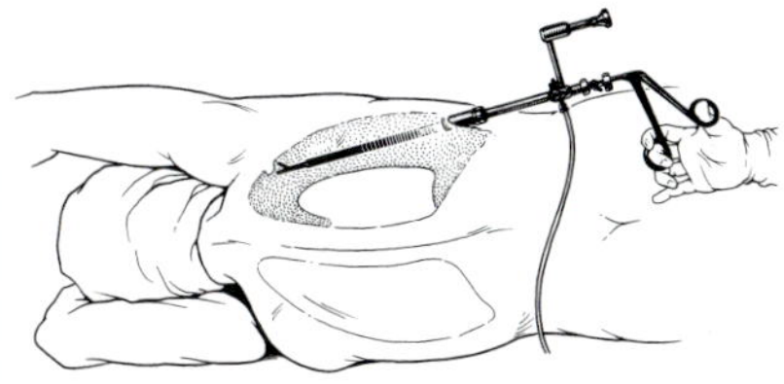

CHAPTER 14

THE ROLE OF THORACOSCOPY FOR THE DIAGNOSIS AND TREATMENT OF PLEURAL CANCERS

P. Astoul and C. Boutin

Medical thoracoscopy can be described as diagnostic and therapeutic exploration of the pleural cavity performed through one or several points of entry after artificial or spontaneous pneumothorax. The revival of thoracoscopy was made possible by the tremendous advances in endoscopy technology. Among all the indications, diagnosis of pleural exudates is the oldest indication for thoracoscopy and remains the most common one.

Indeed, despite complete nonsurgical evaluation, including thoracentesis and needle biopsy, approximately 20 percent of chronic exudates remain undiagnosed after several weeks of observation. A complete evaluation includes the following[1,2]: one or more thorough analyses of pleural fluid—biochemical, bacteriologic, cytologic, and immunologic[3]; one or two pleural biopsy attempts using a biopsy needle (Abrams, Vim-Silverman, or Cope); microbiologic and cytologic sputum analysis; Mantoux test, as well as fungal antigen tests in endemic areas; bronchoscopy; and a thorough clinical and radiologic assessment.

However, such a workup can be detrimental to the patient in that it can delay early treatment. Indeed, in mesotheliomas and adenocarcinomas of unknown origin, local treatment with biologic response modifiers (recombinant interleukin 2, interferon-γ, tumor necrosis factor) has been evaluated by several teams and has demonstrated a good response in patients with early stage diseases. Medical thoracoscopy allows insertion of an implantable access system for intrapleural instillation of chemotherapy or cytokines and also allows a second look for evaluation of response to treatment.

Diagnostic Thoracoscopy

In malignant pleural effusion, the reported diagnostic sensitivity of thoracoscopic biopsy and brush samples from the pleural surface varies from 93 to 97 percent.[4,5] In cases of breast or ovarian cancer, hormone receptor assays on thoracoscopically obtained biopsy material provide further important information for therapeutic decision making.[6] In bronchial carcinoma, thoracoscopy answers the important question of whether the tumor has spread to the pleura or whether the effusion is secondary to venous or lymphatic obstruction or is parapneumonic. Then it may be possible to avoid exploratory thoracotomy and/or to determine operative eligibility. Weissberg and coworkers[7] performed thoracoscopies in 45 patients with lung cancer and pleural effusion. In 37 they found pleural invasion, three patients had mediastinal disease, and the remaining five had no evident metastatic disease and therefore no contraindication to resection. Although the possibility of tuberculosis should not be ruled out, malignancy has been found more frequently in recent decades. Pleural cancer usually becomes evident at an advanced stage, and delay in diagnosis reduces the likelihood that intrapleural pleurodesis will be effective. Invasion of the visceral pleura creates a condition known as *trapped lung,* which is associated with an irreversible functional deficit.

METASTATIC PLEURAL MALIGNANCIES

Closed pleural needle biopsies are at best successful in 50 percent of metastatic pleural malignancies.[8,9] They are of little value with localized tumors (where thoracoscopy is highly sensitive). They are of no use in metastatic tumors confined to the diaphragmatic, visceral, or mediastinal pleura.[10] On the other hand, the more the tumor is widespread within the parietal pleura, the more closed biopsy is likely to be positive. Thus, centers which see more advanced disease have a higher yield with closed pleural biopsy alone.

Similarly, variable results are obtained from the cytology of pleural fluid.[11,12] In 95 cases of pleurisy, Salyer and coworkers[13] obtained 53 positive needle biopsy results and 69 positive cytologies, the combination of the two methods giving a positive yield in 86 patients (90 percent). This high yield is achieved only in the advanced stages of disease. A yield of 50 to 60 percent from pleural fluid cytology is a more representative figure.[14]

The value of thoracoscopy is in making an early diagnosis when the two conventional methods of pleural biopsy and pleural fluid cytology have failed.[4,15,16] The endoscopic appearance of the pleura is suggestive of malignancy in more than 86 percent of cases (Table 14-1) and discloses the following aspects:

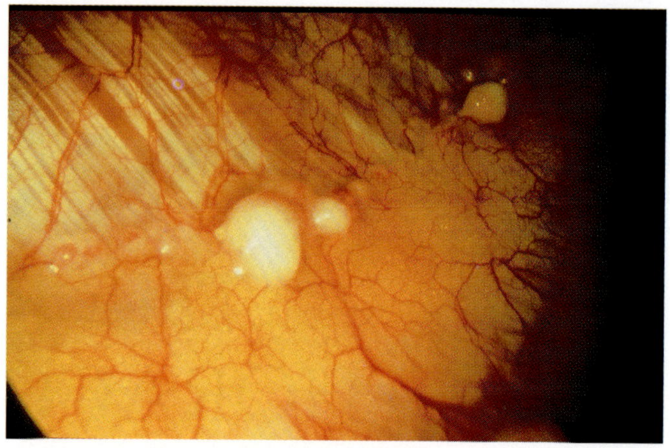

Figure 14-1

Metastases in the intercostal space. The rib is covered with a fatty yellow plaque. The internal intercostal muscle fibers are clearly visible. There are metastatic nodules all along the lymphatic vessels running through the intercostal space. An Abrams biopsy is unlikely to be successful in sampling such localized processes.

1. Nodules which are 1 to 5 mm in diameter (Fig. 14-1)
2. Polypoid lesions of somewhat larger dimensions (Fig. 14-2)
3. Still larger localized tumoral masses (Figs. 14-3 and 14-4)
4. Malignant thickening of the pleura, whitish in color, with an irregular, pebbly surface; hard pachypleuritis with little vascularity (Fig. 14-5)
5. Localized white "candle wax drops"

Table 14-1
ENDOSCOPIC APPEARANCE OF PLEURAL CANCERS

Patients (n)	*Metastasis* 100	*Mesothelioma* 100	*p*
Nodules-masses	40	35	NS
Pleural thickening	30	20	NS
Combinations of the above	10	12	NS
Grapelike appearance	3	23	<.01
Lymphangitis	6	2	NS
Nonspecific abnormalities	11	8	NS

NOTE: NS, not significant.

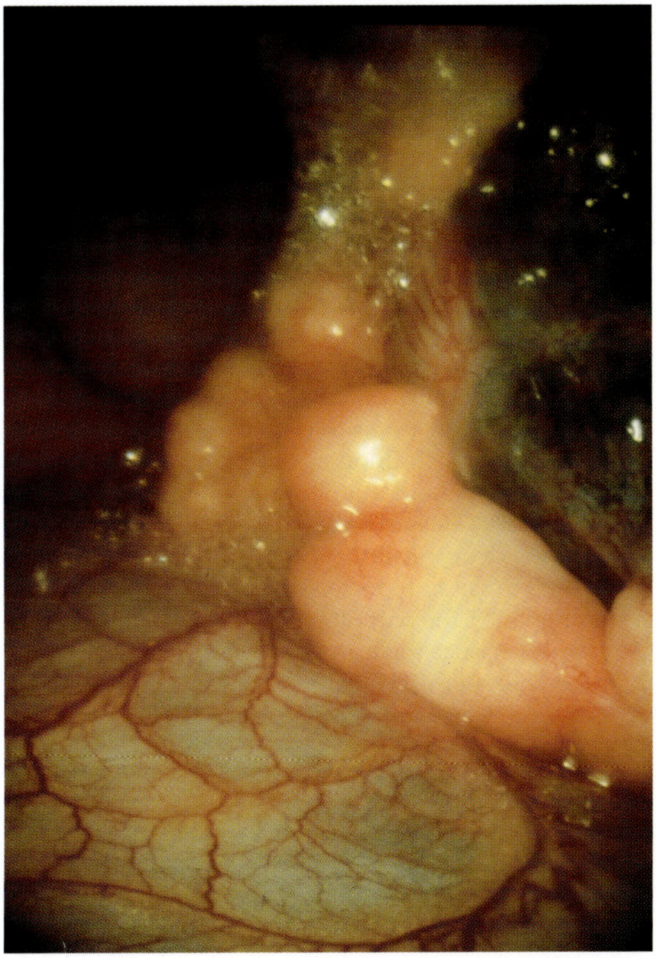

Figure 14-2

Pulmonary and diaphragmatic metastases. Malignant nodules: the diaphragm, which is normal, can be seen at the bottom. The lung is on the right, and has brownish patches of anthracotic pigment. It is attached to the diaphragm and covered with white metastases. These lesions are inaccessible to closed pleural needle biopsy techniques.

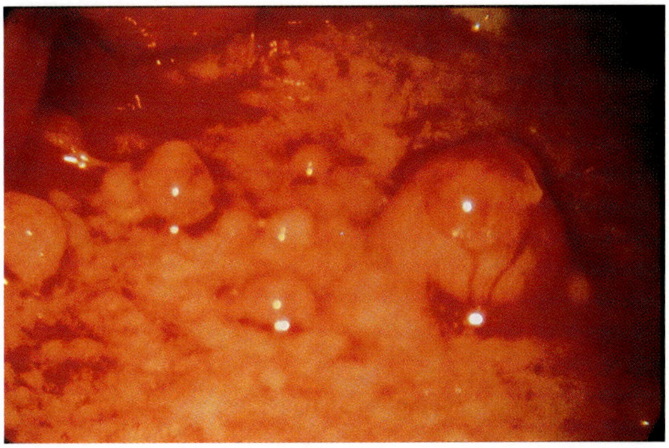

Figure 14-3

Nodules of various size arising from a background of malignant thickening of the parietal pleura. No normal structures of the intercostal space are visible.

The clinician should not be satisfied, however, with the macroscopic appearance alone, since this can be misleading. Some malignancies look like nonspecific inflammation and, conversely, certain inflammatory lesions can look like tumors (Fig. 14-6). Even mesotheliomas, which often have a fairly characteristic grapelike nodular form, can look like ordinary inflammation. Endoscopic appearance, therefore, gives only a general impression and must always be confirmed by microscopic examination of biopsy material.

Topography

The topography of pleural malignancies was studied by Canto and coworkers.[17] In 94 percent of their patients the lower half of the pleural cavity was affected, which justifies a low point of entry, either the sixth or seventh intercostal space. In 28 percent of patients,

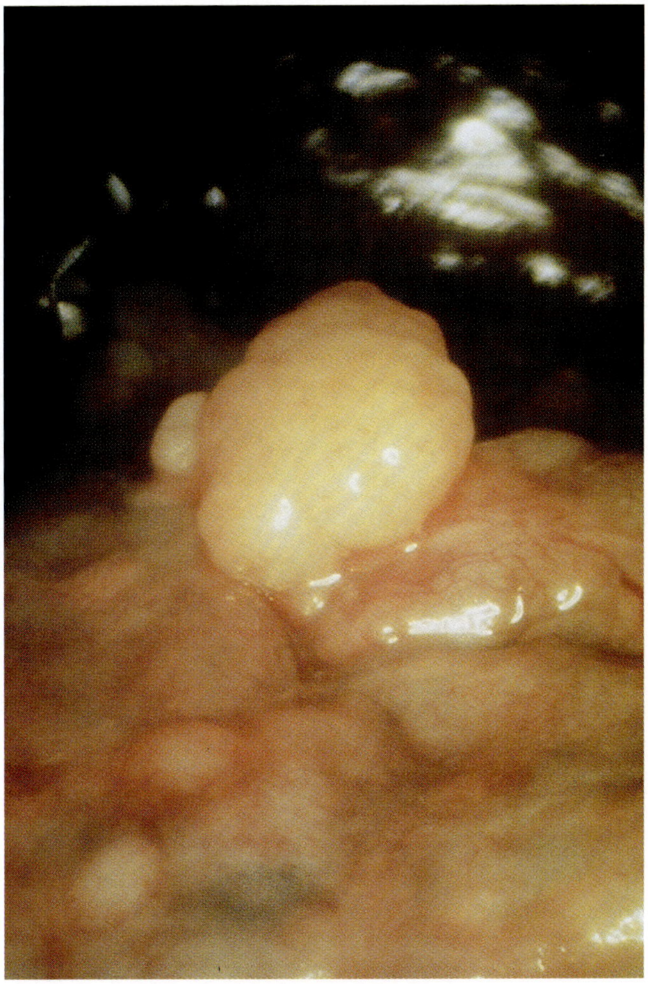

Figure 14-4

Cancerous nodules and thickening of the diaphragmatic pleura.

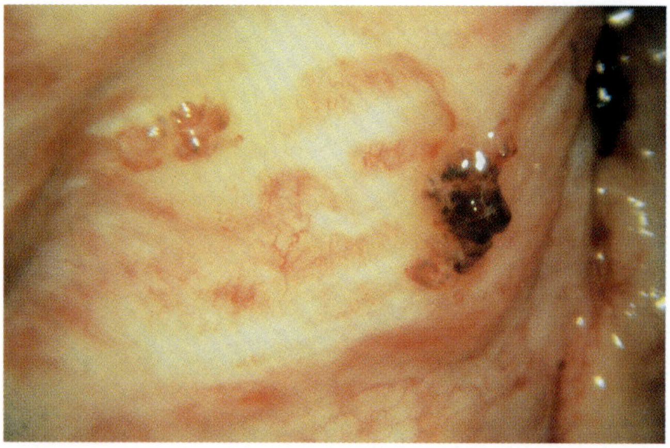

Figure 14-5

Tumoral thickening of the parietal pleura.

only the visceral pleura was involved; hence, closed-needle biopsy could not succeed. In breast cancer, lesions frequently occur on the anterior ipsilateral parietal pleura.

Histopathology

Histopathologic results are the only criteria for definitive diagnoses. In our series the sensitivity of biopsy has increased with the years, rising from 78 percent early in our experience to 97 percent after we had perfected the thoracoscopic equipment and gained greater experience.[18]

We have reviewed[19] 4301 reported cases of diagnostic thoracoscopy using rigid instruments in cases of chronic pleural effusion from 21 different studies. Of 1472 cancer cases, 1333 correct pathologic diagnoses (92.5 percent) were achieved from thoracoscopic specimens. But why are 7.5 percent of thoracoscopic biopsies negative? Several answers have been advanced:

1. In some patients with cancer, pleural effusion is due not to malignant pleural invasion but to malignant obstruction of mediastinal or pulmonary lymphatics which were not biopsied.
2. Rarely, an effusion is a late consequence of lymphatic obstruction due to mediastinal radiotherapy which occurred in 1 percent of patients in our series.
3. The thoracoscopist learns with experience and has a suboptimal yield initially.
4. Multiple biopsies must be taken systematically. There is no such thing as too many. The costovertebral gutter and diaphragm must be routinely sampled. Metastases can sometimes not be recognized endoscopically.
5. If the biopsy is reported as negative in suspected malignancy, the pathologist should be asked to section all tissue, including "deepers," and to completely review all slides. This has enabled us to obtain additional diagnoses in several cases.
6. Sometimes the pleura is covered with a fibrinous, necrotic layer which requires removal to biopsy the parietal pleura behind it.
7. The major stumbling block of thoracoscopy lies in cases of adherent pleura (Fig. 14-7). Once again the experience of the physician is paramount in being able to biopsy after dividing and cutting adhesions. There are, however, cases where this is impossible. In our routine experience, where we have

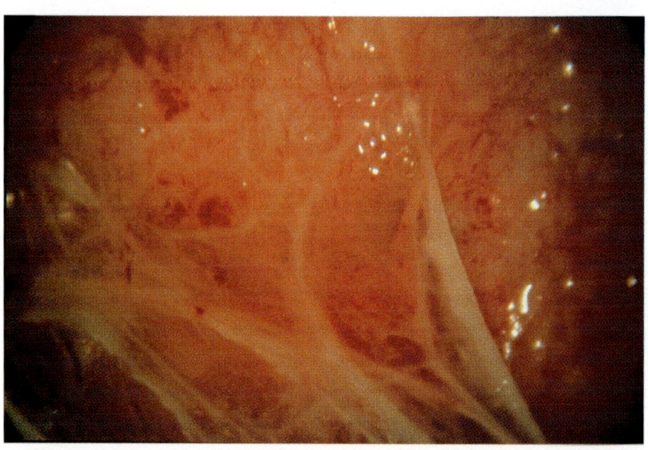

Figure 14-6

Inflammation and congestion of the parietal pleura with fibrinous network of loose and avascular adhesions between parietal and visceral pleura.

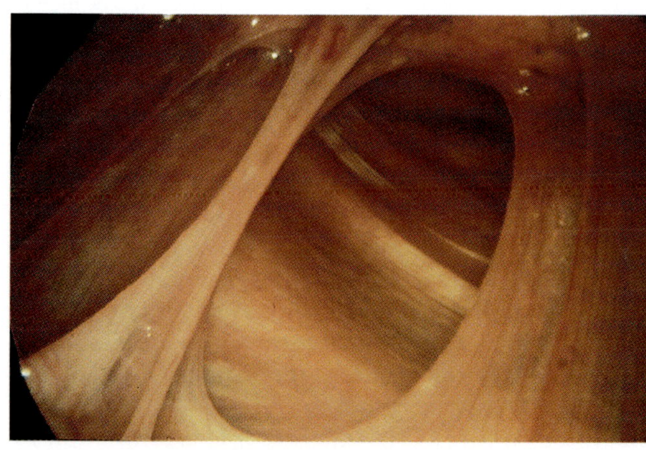

Figure 14-7

Inflammatory adhesions. Some adhesions are thin, almost transparent. Vessels may be seen running along their length. The adhesions should be cut close to the ribs to avoid damaging the lung. They are divided using a laser or an electrocautery loop to ensure hemostasis of the vessels. Adhesions like these are often found in recurrent spontaneous pneumothorax along the pathway of an anterior chest tube; they do not bind the lung tightly enough to the chest wall to prevent relapses.

managed to achieve 97 percent sensitivity in cancerous effusions, false-negative findings were universally due to adhesions which denied access to the neoplastic tissue.

MESOTHELIOMA

Malignant mesothelioma is a disease for which no treatment has been proved to be effective. Pleural mesothelioma is particularly refractory, because chemotherapy has no effect, radiation therapy simply provides palliation against pain, and surgery is controversial.

However this pessimism belies the fact that certain forms have a better prognosis when diagnosed early. To better ascertain prognostic factors, multifactorial studies using the Cox model have been performed (Table 14-2[20–26]). A new staging system[27] takes into account the importance of visceral pleural invasion as a prognostic factor (Table 14-3). Thus mesothelioma is one of the best indications for thoracoscopy. It allows the evaluation of the visceral and parietal pleura for determining early stage disease.[28]

The diagnosis of malignant mesothelioma depends foremost on histologic findings. The reported sensitivity of pleural fluid cytology ranges from 0 to 64 percent. Likewise the sensitivity of needle biopsy varies from 6 to 38 percent. Herbert and Gallagher[29] claimed that the value of both these methods is limited and advocated surgical biopsy. With thoracoscopy, we have achieved results similar to those of surgery and better than fluid cytology or Abrams' needle biopsy (Table 14-4).

Pleural endoscopy is much less invasive than thoracotomy and allows equally good tissue sampling for pathologic examination, which is crucial to diagnosis. In the past, pathologists were reluctant to establish a diagnosis of mesothelioma without an autopsy to bolster their findings. Now, with the increased incidence of this disease and the availability of immunohistochemistry techniques, pathologists are more forthcoming. By permitting direct visualization of lesions, thoracoscopy facilitates the choice of biopsy sites. In addition, thoracoscopy is the only examination that now allows accurate assessment of the degree of involvement of the diaphragmatic, parietal, visceral, and mediastinal pleura. Pulmonary biopsies are also necessary to document significant prior exposure to asbestos.

Thoracoscopic Findings

In 137 of our 188 patients,[28] the pleural cavity was completely free or displayed only loose or fibrinous adherences that did not impede thoracoscopic examination. In the other 51 patients, the procedure was hindered by adhesions, and electrocoagulation or a yttrium-aluminum-garnet (YAG) laser was required to sever adhesions and obtain a cavity of at least 10 cm. Although complete examination was not possible in these cases, biopsy samples were almost always obtained from malignant lesions on the parietal or visceral pleura.

The following lesions were observed in the parietal pleura or diaphragm:

- Nodules or masses ranging from 5 to 10 mm in 92 patients (49 percent) (Fig. 14-8). In 25 patients (13 percent), a grapelike aspect characteristic of mesothelioma was noted (Fig. 14-9).
- Thickening of the pleura in 21 patients (11 percent). This thickening was more or less regular, with elevated, pale, hard, poorly vascularized tissue that suggested malignancy.
- Malignant-looking pachypleuritis in association with nodules or masses in 63 patients (33.5 percent).
- Nonspecific inflammatory appearance with fine granulations (1 to 2 mm in diameter), lymphangitis (Fig. 14-10), congestion, hypervascularization, or local thickening of the pleura in 12 patients (6.5 percent) (Figs. 14-11 and 14-12).

The sensitivity of thoracoscopic biopsy was 98 percent (185 positive biopsies out of 188 patients). In the three failed cases, thick adhesions prevented adequate specimen collection, and the tissue obtained demonstrated only mesothelial hyperplasia. Conclusive sampling was obtained by Abrams needle biopsy (one patient), repeat thoracoscopy (one patient), and surgical biopsy (one patient). In 135 cases (72 percent), the histologic type of mesothelioma was epithelial; in 38 cases (20 percent) it was mixed; and in 15 cases (8 percent) it was fibrosarcomatous.

Mineralogic Study

Thoracoscopic lung biopsy has proved to be highly useful in detecting asbestos fibers in the lung. We studied thoracoscopic lung biopsy first in animals and then in humans, demonstrating a high diagnostic yield with low morbidity.[30] Our technique is the same as that published by Dijkman.[31] Biopsies were obtained using coagulating forceps introduced through a second point of entry under direct vision (Fig. 14-13). One to eight specimens were taken in each session. The high-frequency coagulation allowed perfect hemostasis and aerostasis (Fig. 14-14). The pleural drainage usually lasted for 48 h.

A 1989 review of 10 different series, covering a total of 1031 patients, revealed very few complications following thoracoscopic lung biopsy (Table 14-5[32–40]). Only one death was attributed to the procedure. Although larger specimens may be taken using the new Endo-GIA stapler (Ethicon-Endo Surgery, Inc., Cincinnati, OH), this device is not absolutely necessary to obtain tissue for asbestos fiber counts.

Table 14-2

MULTIFACTORIAL ANALYSIS OF PROGNOSTIC FACTORS FOR MALIGNANT PLEURAL MESOTHELIOMA

Author	*Chahinian et al.*[20]	*Alberts et al.*[21]	*Antman et al.*[22]	*Calavrezos et al.*[23]	*Spirtas et al.*[24]	*Ruffie et al.*[25]	*Rush et al.*[26]	*Boutin et al.*[28]
Year	1982	1988	1988	1988	1988	1989	1991	1993
No. of patients	57	262	136	93	1197	170	83	188
Classified favorable prognostic factors[a]	Epithelial type	PS	PS	PS	Age < 50	Stage I	None	Epithelial type
	Age < 65	Medical treatment	Epithelial type	Epithelial type	Stage I	Platelets < 400,000		No weight loss
	PS	White race	Absence of chest pain	Age 50	Treatment	No weight loss		Localized tumor
	Surgery	SDg > 6 mo	SDg > 6 mo	No chest pain	Geographic origin			No visceral pleura invasion
	Response to chemotherapy	Stage I	Surgery	Stage I + II Multimodal treatment				Stage I

[a]Favorable prognostic factors are listed in each column according to their statistical significance in each study.
NOTE: PS, Performance status; SDg, interval between first system and diagnosis.

Table 14-3
NEW INTERNATIONAL STAGING SYSTEM FOR DIFFUSE MALIGNANT PLEURAL MESOTHELIOMA[27]

T1	T1a	Tumor limited to the ipsilateral parietal pleura, including mediastinal and diaphragmatic pleura No involvement of the visceral pleura
T1	T1b	Tumor involving the ipsilateral parietal pleura, including mediastinal and diaphragmatic pleura Scattered foci of tumor also involving the visceral pleura
T2		Tumor involving each of the ipsilateral surfaces (parietal, mediastinal, diaphragmatic, and visceral pleura) with at least one of the following features: • Involvement of diaphragmatic muscle • Confluent visceral pleural tumor (including the fissures) or extension of tumor from visceral pleura into the underlying pulmonary parenchyma
T3		Locally advanced but potentially resectable tumor Tumor involving all of the ipsilateral surfaces (parietal, mediastinal, diaphragmatic, and visceral pleura) with at least one of the following features: • Involvement of the endothoracic fascia • Extension into the mediastinal fat • Solitary, completely resectable focus of tumor extending into the soft tissues of the chest wall • Nontransmural involvement of the pericardium
T4		Locally advanced, technically unresectable tumor Tumor involving all the ipsilateral pleural surfaces (parietal, mediastinal, diaphragmatic, and visceral) with at least one of the following features: • Diffuse extension or multifocal masses of tumor in the chest wall, with or without associated rib destruction • Direct transdiaphragmatic extension of tumor to the peritoneum • Direct extension of tumor to the contralateral pleura • Direct extension of tumor to one or more mediastinal organs • Direct extension of tumor into the spine • Tumor extending through to the internal surface of the pericardium with or without a pericardial effusion or tumor involving the myocardium

In a group of 25 control patients who had not been in known contact with asbestos, thoracoscopy carried out for reasons unrelated to asbestos exposure revealed the following fiber counts (Table 14-6):

Table 14-4
SENSITIVITY OF DIAGNOSTIC METHODS IN MALIGNANT MESOTHELIOMA[a]

	No. of patients	*Sensitivity, %*
Surgery	9/9	100
Thoracoscopy	185/188	98
Fluid cytology	49/175	28
Needle biopsy	33/135	24

[a]Thoracoscopic biopsies were positive in every case in which they were feasible (135 patients).[28]

$1.4 \pm 0.3 \times 10^6$ chrysotile fibers per gram of dry tissue
$1.0 \pm 0.4 \times 10^6$ amphibole fibers per gram of dry tissue

These figures contrast sharply with the following values obtained in subjects with known asbestos exposure:

$19.5 \pm 11.5 \times 10^6$ chrysotile fibers per gram of dry tissue
$10.8 \pm 2.6 \times 10^6$ amphibole fibers per gram of dry tissue

These findings confirm that the pulmonary asbestos burden is correlated with asbestos exposure and suggest that thoracoscopy permits differentiation between occupational and environmental mesothelioma.[30] Contrary to the opinion of Churg and Wood,[41] thoracoscopic pulmonary biopsy seems to be an excellent method for mineralogic studies of the peripheral lung.

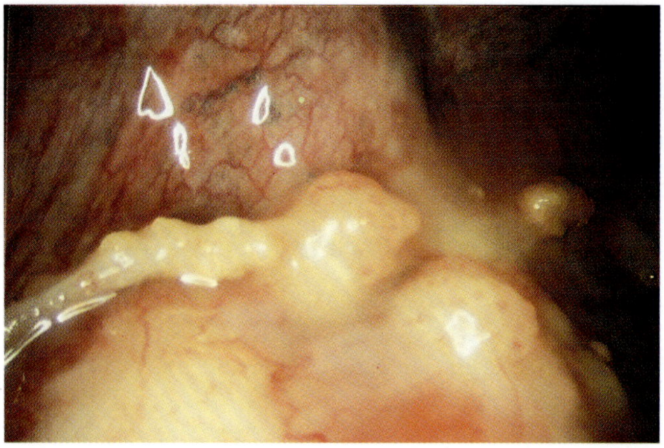

Figure 14-8

Mesothelioma. Nodules of various diameter (ranging from 5 to 15 mm) invading the diaphragm (*bottom*) and the lung (*top*).

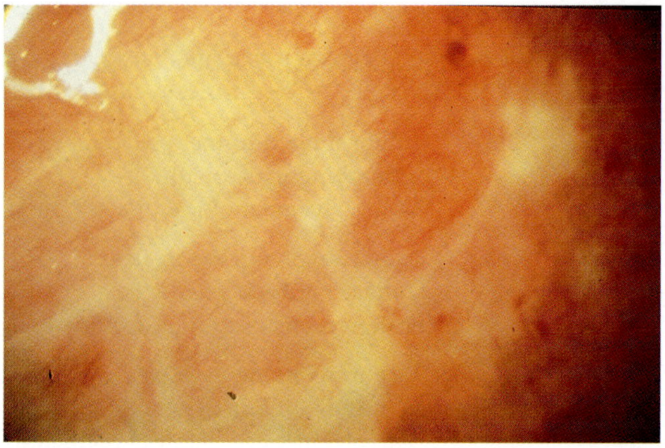

Figure 14-10

Mesothelioma—appearance of lymphangitis. An irregular, white "network" can be seen; in some places it gets thicker, resembling candle wax droppings. When biopsied, the lesions cut cleanly and do not hemorrhage. This was a case of invasion of the pleura by chronic lymphoid leukemia. At an early stage of mesothelioma, such an aspect of lymphangitis may be observed. The photo was taken using high magnification; each lymphatic vessel has a diameter of 0.5 to 1 mm.

Therapeutic Thoracoscopy

About half of all pleural effusions are malignant, and most of these prove to be chronic, recurrent, and disabling for the patient. A minority of patients will benefit from systemic therapy. Although thoracenteses may be repeated to relieve dyspnea, the resulting depletion in ions, liquids, and proteins contributes to the degradation of the general status of the patient.

In most cases, the treatment of malignant pleural effusions is purely palliative, with the goal of patient comfort, that is, preventing recurrent effusion and obtaining the longest possible survival with the best quality of life.

Among the sclerosing agents used, talc powder (Fig. 14-15) seems to be the best for obtaining pleurodesis. Permanent pleurodesis may be achieved after the thoracoscopic examination, by spraying 6 to 10 ml (3 to 5 g) talcum powder (Figs. 14-16 to 14-18) into the pleural space. A chest tube is inserted, and all air is aspirated from the chest cavity. A final chest x-ray is taken to assess the position of the tube and to confirm full reexpansion of the lung. Drainage or aspiration under negative pressure (50 to 100 mmHg) is maintained for 4 to 6 days.

More specific antineoplastic intracavitary chemotherapy or immunotherapy can be offered to patients with minimal pleural disease. To avoid pleural infection, we insert a subcutaneous implantable access system for delivering the drugs.

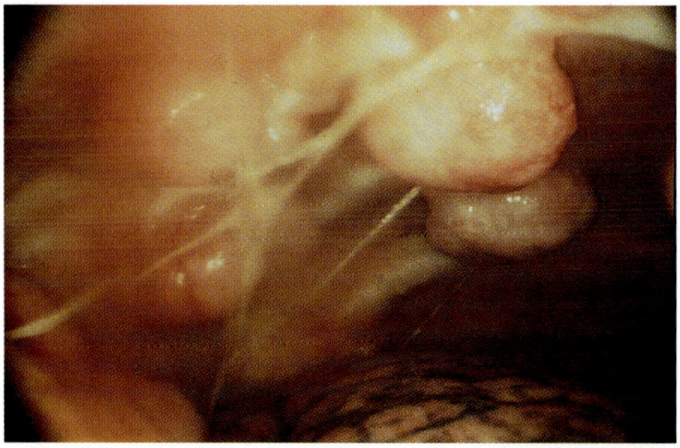

Figure 14-9

Mesothelioma—mixed tumoral involvement of the parietal pleura: small nodules and diffuse thickening. The surface of the lung is clearly visible (*bottom*).

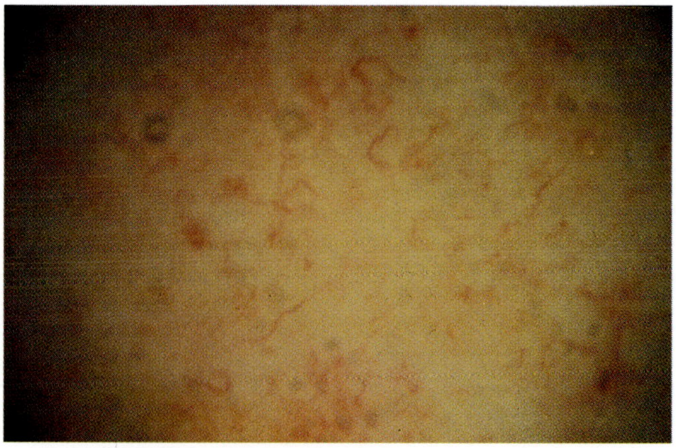

Figure 14-11

Nonspecific appearance. The pleura is uniformly thickened, white with very small vessels. This is frequently seen in chronic idiopathic effusions. Numerous biopsies in different areas of the pleura are necessary to obtain the correct diagnosis; in this case the histopathologic diagnosis was mesothelioma.

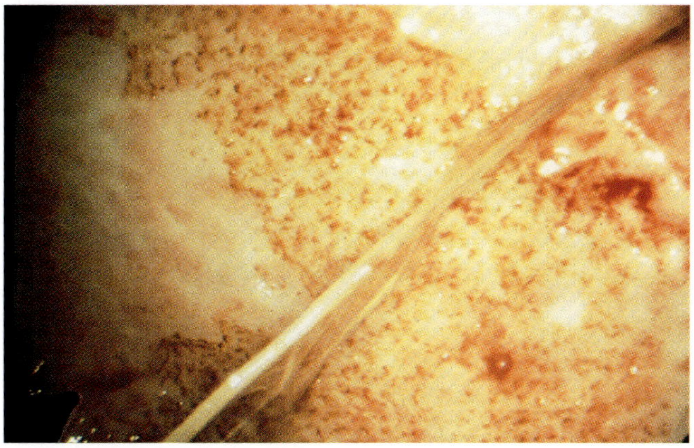

Figure 14-12

Mesothelioma—parietal lymphangitis associated with fibrohyalin pleural plaques. A fibrinous adhesion runs diagonally across the foreground of the photo. There are white, asbestotic, fibrohyalin pleural plaques on the top right and the left. Diffuse parietal malignant lymphangitis can be seen between these plaques.

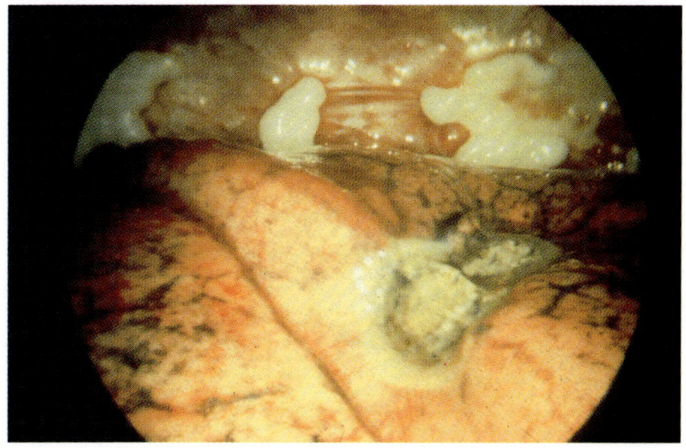

Figure 14-14

Pulmonary biopsy. This patient, formerly exposed to asbestos, presented with asbestotic, fibrohyaline pleural plaques. Note that these plaques are situated exclusively on the parietal pleura and that the lung appears normal. Since all sputum tests for ferruginous bodies were negative, two pulmonary biopsies were taken: one for pathologic diagnosis of asbestosis and one for an asbestos fiber count under an electron microscope, using Sebastien's technique.[19] This sample contained 19×10^6 amphibole fibers and 6.7×10^6 chrysotile fibers per gram of dry pulmonary tissues. Coagulating forceps were used to ensure hemostasis and aerostasis of the lung; the biopsy scar can be seen in the center of the photograph. Several biopsies can be taken from different areas. Chest tube drainage brings the lung back to its position against the chest wall. The drain is usually removed on the third day.

TALC POUDRAGE PLEURODESIS

In North America, the standard pleurodesis procedure has been chest tube administration of tetracycline.[42] However, during the past decade, reported experience with tetracycline, which actually is no longer available, shows that the technique of pleurodesis has its own complications and results in a significant percentage of early and late failures.[43,44]

Conversely, in Europe and neighboring countries, thoracoscopic talc poudrage is widely used. However, the recommendation of various pleurodesis agents is frequently based on English language literature only, thus omitting much of the wide and well established European experience dating back to Bethune.

In a series of 360 patients (88 with malignant mesothelioma and 272 with pleural metastases), thoracoscopic talc poudrage achieved immediate pleurodesis in 90.2 percent.[45] Of the 327 evaluable patients at 1 month, 295 had an immediate response. Of these, 265 could be followed until death with a mean survival of 12 months (2 to 120 months). Twenty-one relapses (7.9 percent) occurred at a mean time from talc pleurodesis of 10.2 ± 2.2 months (2 to 45 months) (Table 14-7). Finally, taking into account the immediate failures and the observed relapses, 82.1 percent of patients had a lifetime pleural symphysis, including, respectively, 74.1 percent of patients having mesothelioma and 85.4 percent having pleural metastases. The median survival of the whole cohort was 6.4 months, 9 months for patients having mesothelioma and 5.2 months for patients having metastases. Median survival differed significantly depending on response and was 7.6 months in responders and 2.6 months in nonresponders ($p < .001$). In this series, 32 deaths (9.2 percent) occurred within 4 weeks after talc poudrage. All were caused by critical illnesses that were present before the procedure.

The mean drainage time was 5.3 ± 0.2 days. The drainage time was longer than 7 days in 6.1 percent of patients, and in one patient the chest tube had to be

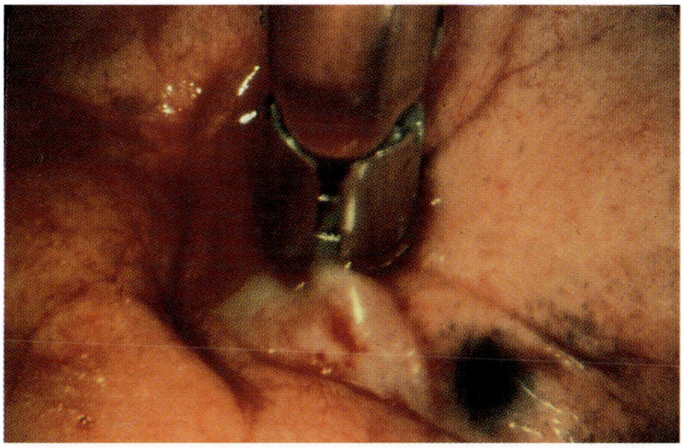

Figure 14-13

Pulmonary biopsy. The biopsy area is grasped with a coagulating forceps perpendicular to the pulmonary surface. We use a unipolar double spoon forceps; the lung tissue outside the biopsy is coagulated, ensuring airtightness and hemostasis. The structure of the piece of lung inside the forceps is not damaged during the biopsy.

Table 14-5
DIAGNOSTIC YIELD AND COMPLICATIONS OF PULMONARY BIOPSIES BY THORACOSCOPIC ROUTE

Authors	*Diagnostic yield, %*	*No. of patients*	*Pneumothorax*	*Hemorrhage*	*Infection*	*Death*
Boutin[32]	96	170	7	—	1	—
Brandt[33]	87	467	—	1	—	—
Dijkman[31]	98	65	10	1	2	1
Faurschou[34]	100	7	—	—	—	—
Guy[35]	100	14	3	6	—	—
Janik[36]	100	17	—	—	—	—
Kapsenberg[37]	95	115	6	—	—	—
Rodgers[38]	94	81	4	3	—	—
Voellmy[39]	75	32	—	—	—	—
Wetzer[40]	89	63	—	—	—	—
Total	93	1031	30	5	3	1

replaced. Two patients had significant subcutaneous emphysema that resolved spontaneously. Some pleural effusion was left at the removal of the chest tube (100 to 500 ml). These patients (4.3 percent) were considered to have had a partial response.

Pain was almost always experienced during the first 24 h after the procedure, though much less intense than after talc poudrage for pneumothorax. Pain was managed systematically with drugs ranging from acetaminophen to morphine sulfate, depending on the needs of the patients. Fever above 101.3°F occurred in 9.8 percent of patients and lasted for an average of 1 day. It was easily managed with acetaminophen. An empyema occurred in 2.5 percent of patients, and 0.8 percent had a pulmonary infection.

These results are similar to those of the largest series reported by Boniface and Guerin[46] (270 patients, 93 percent responses), Ladjimi and coworkers[47] (218 patients, 78 percent responses), Weissberg and Ben-Zeev[48] (169 patients, 92.2 percent responses), Canto

Table 14-6
FIBER COUNTS IN PULMONARY BIOPSIES PERFORMED BY THORACOSCOPY

	Chrysotile	*Amphiboles*
Control patients ($n = 25$)	1.4 ± 0.3	1 ± 0.41
Occupational exposure ($n = 30$)	19.5 ± 11.5 (NS)[a]	10.8 ± 2.6 ($p < .001$)[b]
Northern Corsican environmental exposure ($n = 8$)	2.7 ± 1.5 (NS)[b]	20.1 ± 8.1 ($p < .001$)[b]

[a]Biopsy samples were analyzed by electron microscopy according to the Sebastien technique: pulmonary asbestos burden correlates with known asbestos exposure, whether occupational or environmental (patients from northern Corsica).

[b]Student's test versus mean fiber counts in control (unexposed) patients.

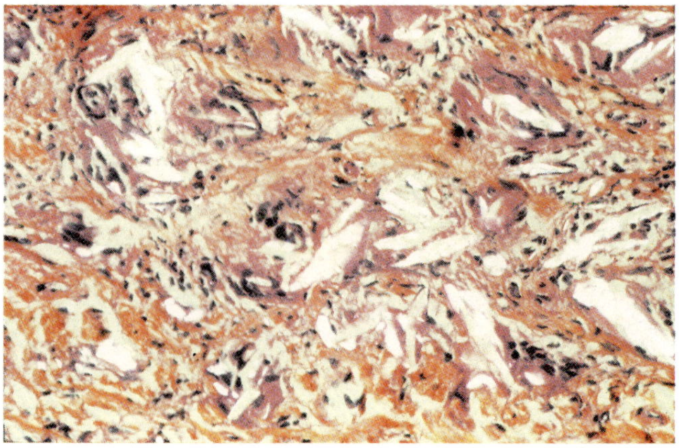

Figure 14-15

Talc powder. Under electron microscope magnification, talc particles range from between 8 and 10 to between 20 and 30 μm. Talc is asbestos-free.

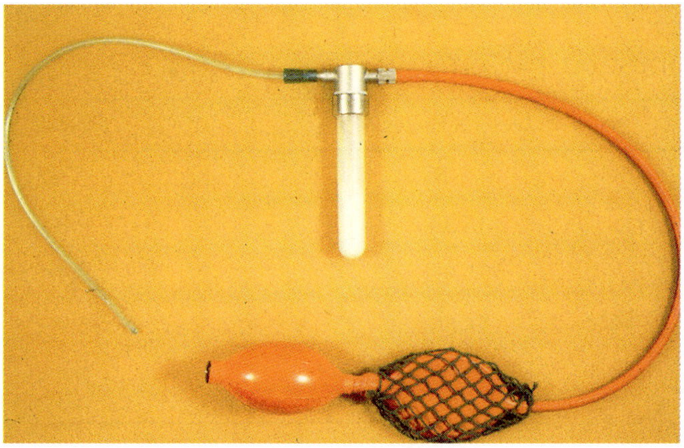

Figure 14-16

Talc atomizer. To spray out the talc particles, the simplest device consists of a double-balloon pump, a plastic tube containing 2 to 6 ml of talc and a small catheter. During insufflation the catheter is rotated in all directions ensuring a uniform distribution of talc throughout the pleural cavity.

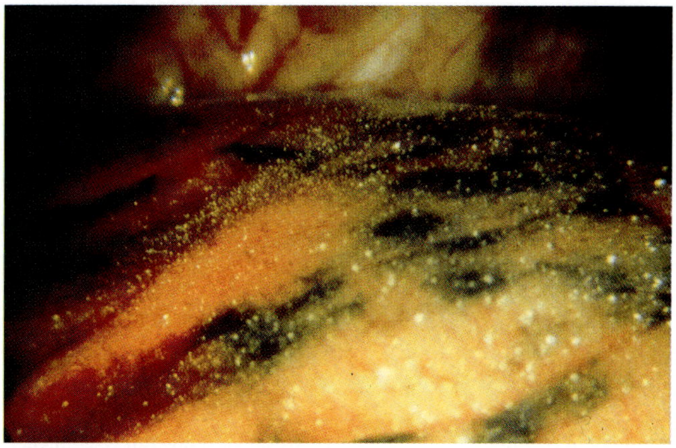

Figure 14-18

Talc poudrage. Talc particles spread over the pleural surface induce a permanent fibrosis. At autopsy these particles may easily be found on microscopic sections. Induced pleurodesis is permanent. Tetracycline-induced pleurodesis may be transient, since tetracycline is soluble and may disappear.

and coworkers[49] (128 patients, 86 percent responses), and Sanchez-Armengol and Rodriguez-Panadero[50] (119 patients, 87 percent responses). Recent reviews of the literature in English also confirmed the superiority of talc when compared with other pleurodesis agents, including tetracycline and bleomycin (Table 14-8).[51–55] The same conclusion can be drawn from randomized controlled trials, despite the frequent limited number of patients included. Experimental studies by Bresticker and coworkers[56] also demonstrated the superiority of talc versus tetracycline, the former being as effective as mechanical abrasion.

The quality of pleurodesis depends on a perfect drainage technique. The chest tube should be large (28 to 32 Fr) and must be inserted as low as possible in the thorax. Additional holes made in the lower part of the tube help drain most of the pleural cavity. We consider that trapped lung is a contraindication to thoracoscopic talc poudrage since pleurodesis is satisfactory in only 50 percent of cases. Boniface and Guerin[46] obtained similar results but consider an attempt at thoracoscopic talc poudrage to be worthwhile because of the lack of alternative therapy. Sanchez-Armengol and Rodriguez-Panadero[50] also achieved only 50 percent positive results in 22 patients with massive lesions invading the visceral pleura.

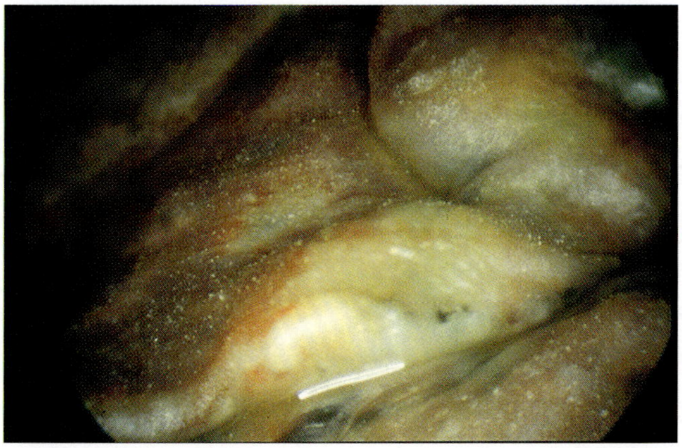

Figure 14-17

Talc poudrage. Between 5 and 6 ml of talc is generally sufficient to induce a good pleurodesis. Excellent distribution of talc over the pleural surface is seen in the picture. Talc slurry never produces this result.

Talc pleurodesis has been associated with acute respiratory failure; all reported observations were following talc slurry that delivered high doses (10 g) of talc.[57–59] Talc slurry does not allow a good distribution of talc all over the pleural surface. Talc poudrage performed after a thorough aspiration of all pleural effusion gives much better results with limited quantities of talc.[60]

INTRAPLEURAL TREATMENT

Talc pleurodesis is a purely palliative procedure that enhances the functional and general status of the patient by eliminating the need for repeated thoracentesis. A more specific approach can be attempted in some patients utilizing intrapleural chemotherapy as a sclerosing or antimitotic agent. Effectiveness is proportional to the sclerosing effect, which itself depends on the cytotoxic effect.

The need to insert a catheter or chest tube for the administration of intrapleural chemotherapy poses a high risk of infection. Markman and associates[61] treated eight patients with malignant mesothelioma

Table 14-7
RESULTS OF TALC PLEURODESIS AT 1 MONTH[a]

	Pleural metastases	*Mesotheliomas*	*Overall*
No. evaluable patients	242	85	327
Failure	5.8%	15.3%	9.8%
Partial response	3.7%	5.9%	4.3%
Complete response	88.5%	78.8%	85.9%
Total	100%	100%	100%

[a]Complete response, normal or subnormal radiograph; partial response, some liquid left (< 500 ml), not requiring further tapping; failure; all other cases.

with intrapleural cisplatin (100 mg/m^2 in 250 ml of saline). Only one patient showed a response; however, these patients had extensive disease, which severely limited the diffusion of drug throughout the pleural cavity. Two out of seven patients treated with cisplatin combined with cytarabine intrapleurally demonstrated a response. A Lung Cancer Study Group Trial published by Rush and colleagues[62] included 46 patients. The overall response rate was 49 percent. Intrapleural immunotherapy is also available and can be administered after thoracoscopic placement of an implantable access system connected to a catheter in the pleural cavity.[63] It minimizes the risk of pleural infection and ensures proper placement of the catheter to apply the drug directly to the lesions. Indeed, in an earlier study concerning intrapleural immunotherapy for pleural cancer carried out in our department, pleural infection occurred in 64 percent of our 18 patients.

IMPLANTABLE ACCESS SYSTEM FOR INTRAPLEURAL TREATMENT

The implantable access system (IAS) was designed for repeat access to the vascular system. It consists of a stainless steel portal chamber, a silicone catheter, and

Table 14-8
PLEURODESIS IN MALIGNANT EFFUSION: LITERATURE REVIEW

Technique	*Series*	*No. of patients*	*Positive response, %, at* 0–1 month	3 months	6 months	12 months
Talc poudrage (691 patients)	Boniface and Guerin[46]	270	93			80
	Fentiman et al.[51]	12	—	—	—	92
	Hartman et al.[52]	33	97	95		
	Marchandise et al.[53]	33	87		76	
	Viallat et al.[64]	327	90.2	88.9	87.5	84.8
Bleomycin (69 patients)	Hartman et al.[52]	37	64	70		
	Ostrowski[54]	32	69	54		
	Boutin et al.[45]	20	80	75	50	
Cyclines (212 patients)	Fentiman et al.[51]	21	—	—	—	48
	Hartman et al.[52]	36	33	47		
	Heffner et al.[43]	27	78	65		
	Sherman et al.[55]	108	94	49		

a cath-shield connector to firmly connect the catheter to the chamber.

Based on our experience, we now recommend this IAS for prolonged administration of intrapleural medication. Our experience includes more than 100 patients and shows an overall response rate of 22 percent using interferon-γ and interleukin 2 (Table 14-9). The main indications for intrapleural immunotherapy are stage I mesothelioma, pleural adenocarcinoma of unknown origin, and metastatic cancer that has become resistant to conventional chemotherapy.[64–66] In the latter indication interleukin 2 or interferon-γ may restore the response to chemotherapy. In stage I mesothelioma, nearly 40 percent of patients respond to interferon-γ or interleukin 2.

Another indication for thoracoscopy is assessment of tumor response. Follow-up can be accomplished using repeated pleural fluid cytology, but when there is no more liquid, cytology is not feasible. Although others judge response on the decrease in the amount of fluid, it appears that a second thoracoscopy is the most effective means of visualizing tumor response. We perform a thoracoscopy and CT scan before treatment to establish diagnosis and staging. Then 15 to 30 days after treatment, we repeat the CT scan after fluid removal. If the scan shows that the lesions have stabilized or regressed, we repeat the thoracoscopy to confirm response. In five cases, we have observed complete regression with negative biopsies. Thus, thoracoscopy appears to be an excellent method for evaluating tumor response.

Complications

Thoracoscopy is one of the safest pneumonologic examinations; Viskum and Enk[67] noted only one death in 8000 cases reviewed. In our own review of 4300 cases, the mortality rate was 0.09 percent. In his review, Viskum found that there was no mention of wound infection in any study, that empyema occurred in 12 out of 652 cases from three studies, and that hemorrhage occurred in six patients of 256 reported in three other studies. O_2 desaturation during thoracoscopy under local anesthesia is reportedly less than 2 percent.

In our initial series we observed the following complications:

- A persistent (more than 7 days) postoperative air leak in 2 percent of patients with chronic spontaneous pneumothorax. This complication probably resulted from the disease rather than from the procedure.
- Subcutaneous emphysema in 0.5 percent of cases.
- Seeding of the chest wall along the pathway of the thoracoscope in eight patients with mesothelioma. Since we began performing local radiotherapy to the puncture site, this has no longer been observed.
- Two cases of hemorrhage. Both occurred during our early experience. Since the introduction of diathermocoagulation we have observed no more bleeding.
- Benign cardiac arrhythmias.
- Low-grade hypotension.
- Brief hyperthermia [100.4 to 101.3°F (38.0 to 38.5°C)] for 12 to 24 h postoperatively in 15 percent of the cases.

Complications can best be prevented by observing the following rules:

1. Measure arterial blood gases or oxygen saturation during the procedure.
2. Monitor cardiac rhythm by simultaneous ECG.
3. Postpone thoracoscopy for several days if the patient has a severe cough.
4. Ensure that the patient is adequately oxygenated during thoracoscopy.
5. Coagulate and ensure hemostatis if hemorrhage exceeds 20 ml.
6. Insert a chest tube (at least until the lung fully expands) to prevent subcutaneous emphysema.
7. Start chest physiotherapy on the day of thoracoscopy to mobilize the diaphragm and avoid accumulation of secretions and airway obstruction.
8. To prevent invasion of the trocar tract in cases of mesothelioma, administer radiation therapy of 21 Gy (7 Gy/day for 3 days) to the scar area beginning on postoperative day 10.

Table 14-9
INTRAPLEURAL IMMUNOTHERAPY: OBJECTIVE RESPONSES (CR + PR) ACCORDING TO STAGE AND CYTOKINES (BOUTIN[65] AND ASTOUL[63])

Stage	*IFN*	*IL-2*	*IFN + IL-2*	*Total*
IA	7	1	1	9/17
IB	6	0	1	7/17
II	9	10	1	20/125
III + IV	0	0	0	0/6

Contraindications

Contraindications are uncommon and rarely absolute. The main limitation is the size of free pleura space; this must be at least 10 cm in diameter. If extensive adhesions are present, an extended thoracoscopy exploration (that is without first creating a pneumothorax) can be carried out, but this requires special skills and should not be undertaken without special training.

Several factors may make it necessary to delay thoracoscopy but are rarely prohibitive. These are cough, hypoxemia, hypocoagulability (prothrombin time less than 60 percent and/or platelet count less than 60,000 per cubic millimeter), and cardiac abnormalities. The thoracoscopist must evaluate the benefit-risk ratio in each case.

Contraindications for pulmonary biopsy are:

1. Mean pulmonary arterial pressure greater than 35 mmHg
2. A chest x-ray film with a honeycomb pattern of the lung or end-stage interstitial fibrosis
3. Suspicion of arteriovenous pulmonary aneurysm
4. Hydadid cyst
5. Vascular tumor

Summary

Medical thoracoscopy is safe and efficient.[68–70] It can be described as a diagnostic and a therapeutic procedure. This means that in addition to inspection of the thoracic cavity this technique allows (1) collection of biopsy specimens from the pleura and also from the lung, (2) section of adhesions, (3) coagulation of bleeding lesions, and (4) pleurodesis and finally insertion of a thin catheter under visual control for intrapleural treatment.

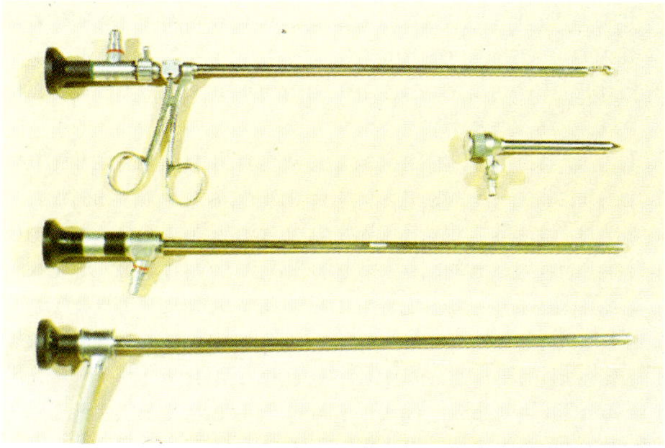

Figure 14-19

Telescopes and trocars for medical thoracoscopy. From top to bottom: (1) optical biopsy forceps for parietal or diaphragmatic pleural biopsy under direct vision using a single entry site; (2) trocar 7 mm in diameter with a lateral port for aspiration of fluid or insufflation of air; (3) direct viewing (0-degree) telescope; (4) oblique viewing (50-degree) telescope.

Equipment Needs

The revival of thoracoscopy was made possible by the advances in endoscopic technology. Endoscopic telescopes of very small diameter now provide extremely high optical resolution. New endoscopic instrumentation (forceps, scalpels, staples, laser fibers, and video cameras) has an ever-increasing number of applications. New anesthetic methods also permit a wide range of operative alternatives from outpatient procedures to selective double-lumen intubation under general anesthesia.

A rigid thoracoscope with a cold light source is used in most cases. Some authors have tried to use a flexible fiberoptic bronchoscope,[71] but comparative studies have documented the superiority of the rigid system.

The major equipment requirements for rigid thoracoscopy are trocars, telescopes, and forceps (Fig. 14-19). Trocars consist of an obturator and a cannula. To facilitate examination, trocars should not be too large; with a 7-mm trocar, insertion is an easy and painless procedure—pressure against the ribs is minimal. Unlike the airtight instruments used for laparoscopy, our thoracoscopic trocar allows air to enter and leave the pleural cavity freely. Telescopes are available with various angles of vision including 0 degrees (straightforward) and 50 or 90 degrees (oblique). Using the oblique telescope like a periscope, a superb panoramic view of the whole inner chest wall can be obtained, including the area around the point of entry. Although direct viewing may be more natural, the practitioner very quickly becomes a customed to "retrovision." Illuminated forceps are ideal for biopsy of the parietal pleura under direct vision using a single point of entry. For biopsy of the diaphragmatic pleura or fibrous pleural lesions, including asbestotic pleural plaques, and for sampling the visceral pleura and the lung, a 5-mm coagulating forceps introduced via a 5-mm insulated trocar through a second point of entry is a more suitable device (Fig. 14-20).

Thoracoscopy can be performed either in a properly equipped operating room or in an endoscopy suite. The room must contain the following:

1. A procedure table. A simple operating table is adequate, but ideally it should allow height adjustment and have a back so that the patient can be placed in a semisitting position. Tables that can be adjusted laterally along a longitudinal axis allow the patient to be repositioned easily. More sophisticated tables are available but are by no means essential.

2. Suction equipment for the pleural fluid. The volume of the collecting bottles should be at least 2 liters, and pressure must be adjustable.
3. Simple anesthetic equipment with air feed and oxygen.
4. An overhead light with adjustable brightness.
5. A Mayo stand for placing a large instrument tray directly over the patient.
6. A 150-W high frequency (HF) scalpel for electrocauterry or an Nd:YAG laser.

Thoracoscopy must be carried out under sterile conditions. The thoracoscopy room should be sterilized in the same way as an operating room. The trocar, telescopes, forceps, connecting wires, fiberoptic fibers, and all other accessories are sterilized after careful cleaning. Talc is sterilized by autoclaving at 160°C.

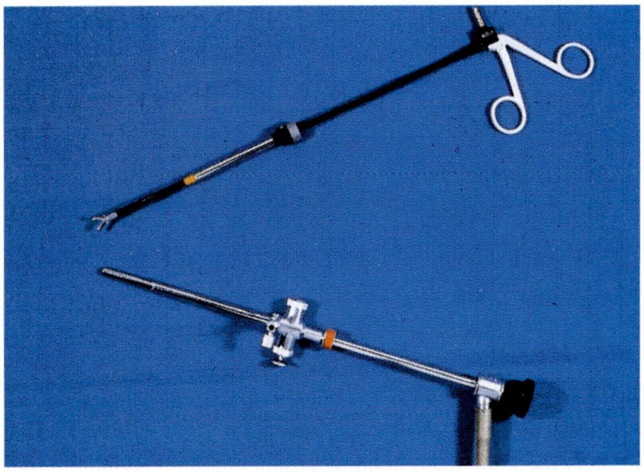

Figure 14-20

Double-puncture technique. The practitioner holds the direct or oblique viewing telescope in one hand and the coagulating forceps in the other. The assistant holds the trocar cannulas firmly in place. The distance between the two trocars is generally 10 to 15 cm.

HOW I DO IT

Implantable Access System

After local anaesthesia to the placement site with 10 ml of 2% lidocaine, an incision approximately 2 cm long is made and a pocket is created by blunt dissection 1 cm below the skin surface. The IAS is placed over a rib to provide support during injection. In most cases, the most suitable location is the third or fourth rib on the midclavicular line.

The next steps involve guide wire insertion and pleural catheter placement. A trocar is used to make a tunnel, approximately 5 cm long, from the pocket to the site of entry and to puncture the parietal pleura. When the IAS is placed during thoracoscopy, pleural puncture and guide wire insertion can be performed under visual control. Direct insertion of the guide wire into the pleura is also possible without thoracoscopy if pleural fluid is present. However, if thoracoscopy is not used and there is no pleural fluid, the pleural space must first be punctured with a 2-mm-diameter trocar. In this case, penetration of the trocar into the pleural space is detected by negative pressure readings on a manometer during breathing. The guide wire is introduced into the pleural space through the trocar, which is then removed. After insertion of the guide wire, the pleural catheter is threaded under the skin into the pleural cavity.

Finally the IAS is placed in the subcutaneous pocket, and its corners are sutured to the underlying muscle fascia. The catheter is attached by the cath-shield connector. A small suction drain with several openings is placed in the pocket to prevent any fluid collection. The pocket is then closed. The IAS should not be situated directly under the incision.

Injection and Maintenance

The treatment can be started as soon as the incision has healed. After cleansing the skin with an antiseptic, injection is performed with a Huber needle. To avoid injection of the subcutaneous tissue, the needle should be inserted through the top of the dome to the bottom of the chamber. To maintain the patency of the IAS, the IAS and catheter should be flushed with heparinized saline once every month. Immediate and complete pleural dispersion usually follows the instillation of the medication. Intracavitary injection of technetium-99m-labeled macroaggregates through the IAS has shown that instillation is followed by complete and instant diffusion. Indeed, intrapleural treatment does not obliterate the pleural space, and thus pleural distribution remains satisfactory in most patients until the end of treatment.

Using the IAS, local treatment can be an ambulatory procedure. IAS placement takes only a few minutes longer than placement of a chest tube. Patient tolerance is excellent (Fig. 14-21). In our series, most patients did not feel the device between treatment sessions. Unlike open chest tubes, which require daily cleansing of the stoma and rinsing of the tube, IAS requires minimal maintenance.

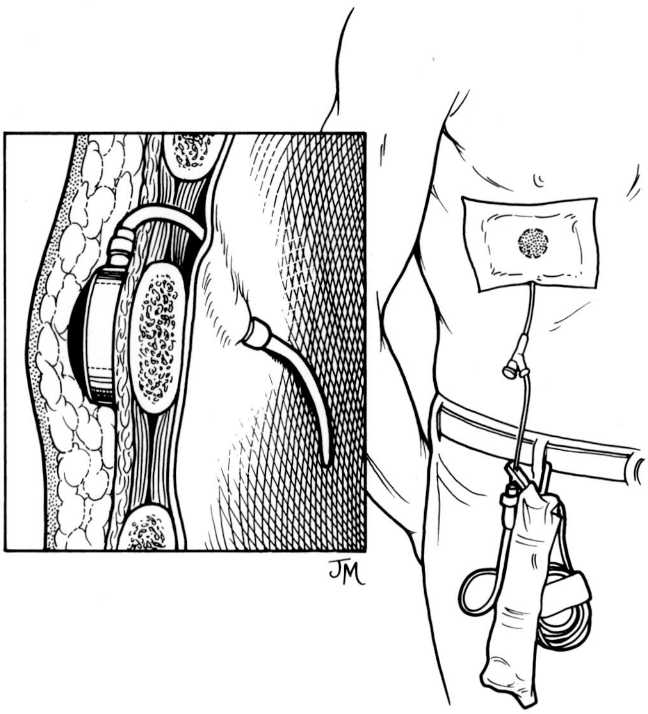

Figure 14-21

An intrapleural catheter is inserted during a thoracoscopy and connected to an implantable access system placed in a subcutaneous pocket. Using a Huber needle an infusor allows an ambulatory treatment.

Medical Thoracoscopy

POSITION OF THE PATIENT

The patient should lie comfortably in the lateral decubitus position with the healthy side down. A bolster or rolled-up sheet is placed under the patient's thorax to spread the intercostal spaces on the exposed side of the chest wall. The head is lowered and the arm positioned to a bar at a right angle to the head with gauze or a sling (Fig. 14-22). The patient is electrically grounded by placing a metal plate between the table and one buttock. The physician usually faces the patient, while the assistant stands across the table behind the patient's back (Fig. 14-23).

ANESTHESIA

Local anesthesia is always preferred if the thoracoscopy procedure is to be brief in a low-risk patient whose pleural cavity is free of adhesions. Local anesthesia is also preferable to general anesthesia in high risk patients exhibiting poor general health, compromised respiratory function, or cardiac insufficiency. Local anesthesia permits the patient to remain conscious as long as reasonably possible and ensures prompt recovery as soon as the lung has reexpanded.

General anesthesia may be necessary in some cases. It is the technique of choice for procedures requiring selective double-lumen intubation and lung immobilization such as laser resection and cauterization of pleural blebs in spontaneous pneumothorax. General anesthesia may be delivered by mask with spontaneous ventilation or after double-lumen intubation.

In the past we and many others performed thoracoscopy using general anesthesia after endotracheal intubation. This method was more comfortable for patient and physician alike, since it allowed time for multiple biopsies, section of extensive adhesions, and use of electrocautery as well as time for high-quality photographs and video films.

We now prefer to use a "light" anesthesia technique combining local anesthesia and a neuroleptanalgesia. This technique is simple and has practically no contraindications. Modern drugs that combine the properties of sedation, analgesia, and amnesia are excellent adjunctive medications. Suitable neuroleptanalgesics include droperidol (5 to 10 mg), propofol (400 mg), pethidine (5 to 10 mg), diazepam (5 to 10 mg) and fentanyl (5 μg).

POINT OF ENTRY

The procedure site is usually in the midaxillary zone between the third and sixth intercostal space because pleural adhesions are uncommon in this area (Fig. 14-22). However, choice of the point of entry can vary depending on the indication for thoracoscopy. In patients with spontaneous pneumothorax, the offending leak is usually in the upper lobe so the best location is between the third and fourth intercostal spaces. In patients with pleural effusion the fifth, sixth, or seventh intercostal spaces are the best sites for entry. The last two spaces allow access to most metastatic tumors and mesotheliomas and provide excellent visualization of the diaphragm and the costovertebral gutter. Pulmonary biopsies are facilitated by entry through the fourth or fifth intercostal space.

INDUCTION OF PNEUMOTHORAX

To insert the thoracoscope into the pleural cavity, pneumothorax must first be induced. A specially designed pleural trocar (Fig. 14-24) 2 to 3 mm in diameter and 100 mm in length should be used. The pointed obturator is used to pass through the skin and intercostal muscles without prior incision, and the blunt obturator is then inserted to pass safely through the parietal pleura without risk of puncture of the lung or diaphragm. A characteristic sound is heard when the pleura is transgressed. The blunt obturator is then removed, and air can be heard whistling into the cavity. Intrathoracic pressure must remain negative; insuf-

Figure 14-22

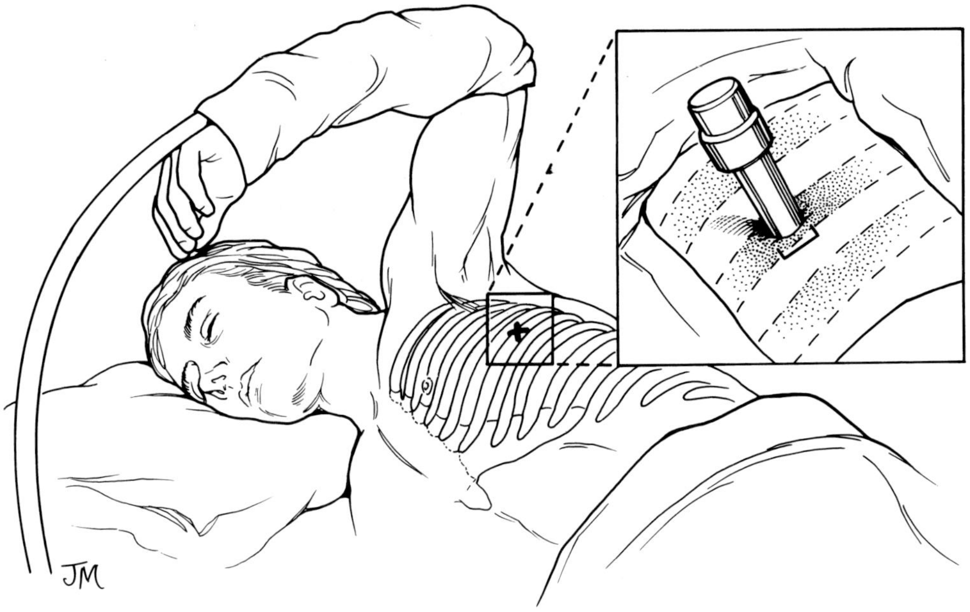

Position of the patient. The patient is lying on the healthy side. The skin is prepared by disinfecting a large area. The upper arm is raised at a right angle. The forearm is attached to a supple metal cradle or held up in a sling.

flating air under positive pressure may induce mediastinal shifts, compromise cardiovascular performance, and cause pain. A pneumothorax apparatus or a similar set up is used to measure the quantity of air allowed to enter the thoracic cavity. Although other pleural needles can be used instead of a trocar for entering the pleural cavity, ordinary thoracentesis needles are hazardous since their pointed tips risk perforating the lung, especially as it reexpands during fluid removal.

Once the trocar is in place, 200 to 300 ml of fluid is aspirated; then the valve is opened to allow an equivalent amount of ambient air to enter the cavity. As soon as the lung is in a state of equilibrium, the pleural

Figure 14-23

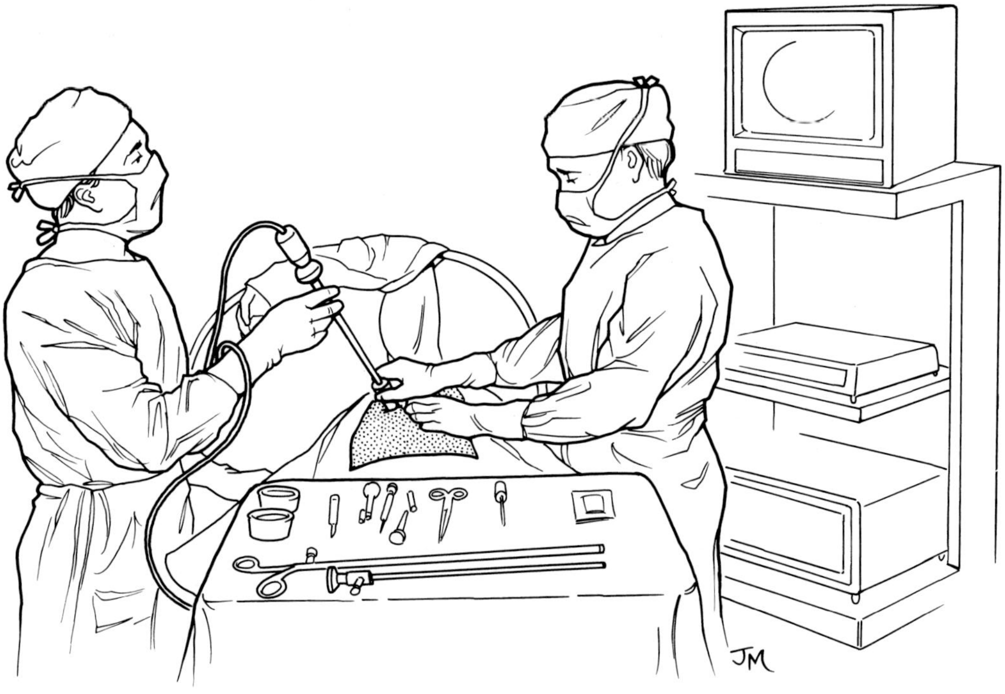

The endoscopy room. The operator is usually facing the patient. The assistant is across the table, behind the patient's back. A video camera and video screen allow the procedure to be observed not only by the operators but also by the anesthesiologist and the nurse. Video recording is also suitable for educational purposes.

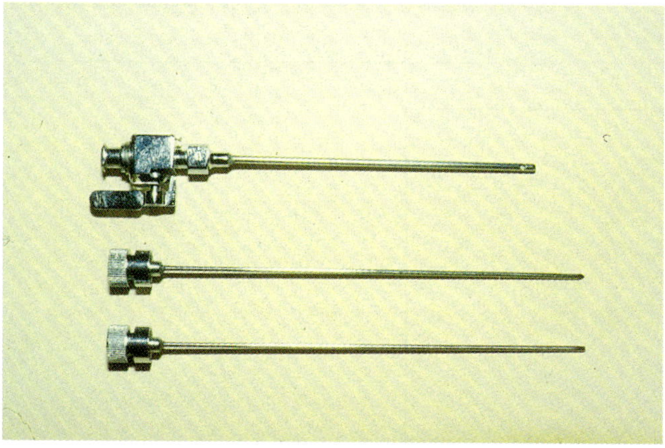

Figure 14-24

Pleural trocar. From *top* to *bottom,* pleural trocar 3 mm in diameter with a valve for control of air exchange; pointed obturator to pass through the skin and intercostal muscles; and blunt obturator used to pass safely through the parietal pleura without risk to the lung.

trocar is removed. Equilibrium is achieved when an equal amount of air, or CO_2 if it has been insufflated, is heard entering and exiting the pleura during inhalation and exhalation.

It is sometimes useful to consider performing pneumothorax the day before thoracoscopy. This allows time for the thoracoscopist to study posteroanterior, lateral and oblique radiographs or biplane fluoroscopy views taken after induction of pneumothorax (Fig. 14-25). Areas showing pleural adhesion can be identified. Performing pneumothorax the day before thoracoscopy can also be helpful because it often reveals pleural tumors not previously visualized. The practitioner can then select the optimal site to biopsy.

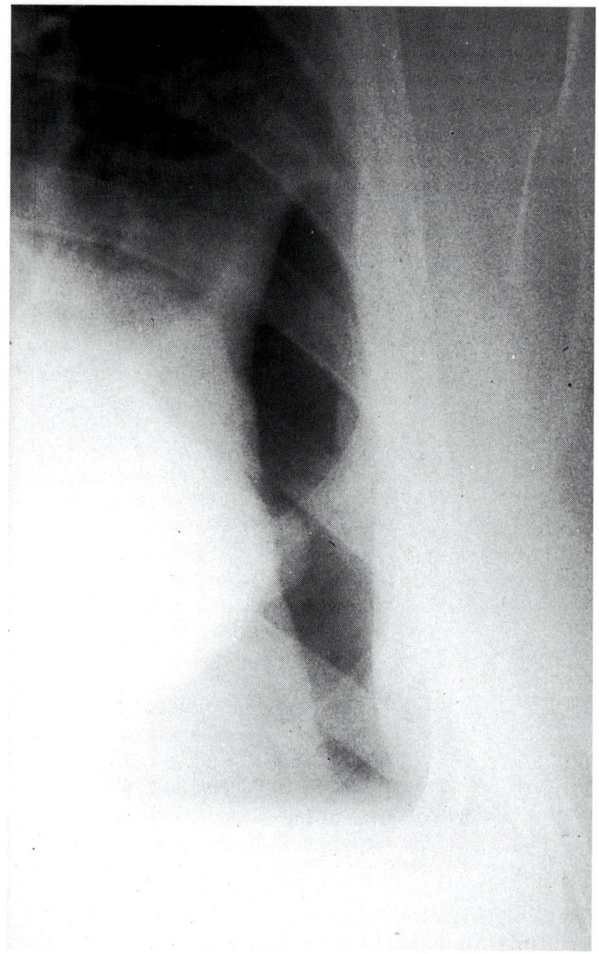

Figure 14-25

An artificially induced pneumothorax a few hours before thoracoscopy allows visualization of the volume of the cavity and sometimes of adhesions. Selection of the best site of entry may be determined.

EXAMINATION

Almost complete visualization of the parietal and visceral pleura is possible; only the posterior and the mediastinal sides of the lung cannot be seen. Using a 50-degree telescope as an inverted periscope, the endoscopist can obtain a circular panoramic view of the entire cavity (Fig. 14-26). Practice brings knowledge of how to move the endoscope in all directions without pushing against the ribs; this is particularly important since contact with the ribs can be painful to patients under local anesthesia. Fine adhesions resembling spider webs can hinder examination; they can be severed easily using a blunt probe, forceps, or electrocautery (Figs. 14-27 and 14-28).

Inspecting the pleura and performing biopsies are the two essential steps of the examination. Perfect knowledge of normal and pathologic endoscopic anatomy is mandatory. Biopsy can be performed using illuminated forceps through a single point of entry. Biopsy of the parietal pleura poses no problem.

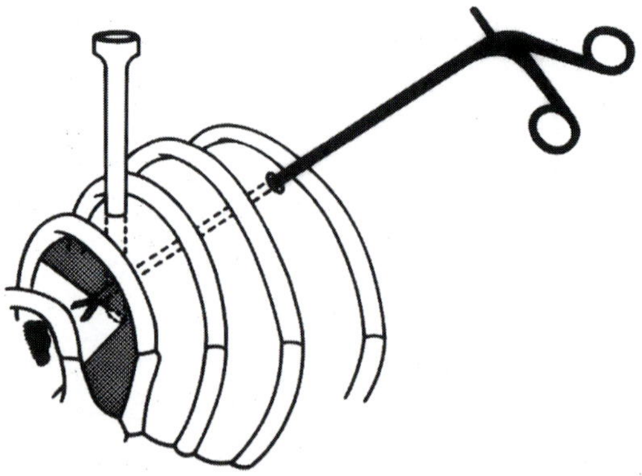

Figure 14-26

Exploration of the pleural cavity. An oblique vision telescope allows panoramic viewing of the cavity. Using 50- and 0-degree telescopes virtually eliminates all blind spots during examination. The lung biopsy is performed with a 5-mm-diameter coagulating forceps under vision through a second port of entry. Exploration and biopsy using a 50-degree telescope.

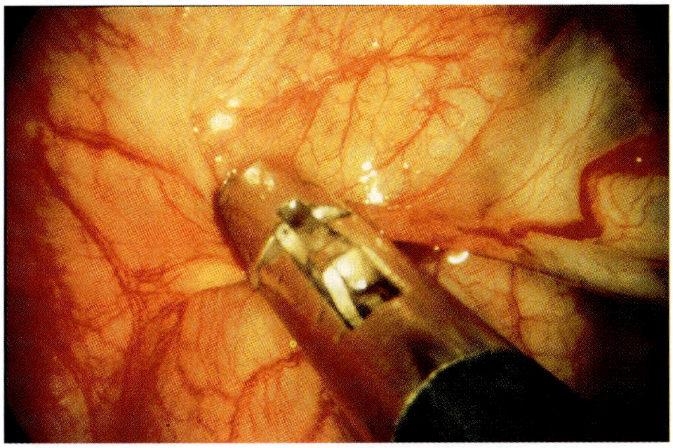

Figure 14-27

Section of small adhesions. Under direct vision adhesions can be cut with a coagulating forceps to avoid bleeding of small vessels frequently running from the lung to the parietal pleura. Double puncture technique is the best, easiest, and safest method to sever adhesions.

When the pleura is thin, specimens should be taken against the rib to avoid injuring the intercostal neurovascular bundle. In this regard it is noteworthy that the main danger for the beginner is hemorrhage from an intercostal vessel. A well trained thoracoscopist can quickly create a second point of entry if there is need for additional instrumentation to sever adhesions, take lung biopsies using a YAG laser, coagulate bleeding vessels, or introduce a stapler or snare.

At the end of the thoracoscopy a chest tube is inserted and air-aspirated. After a diagnostic procedure for pleural effusion, the tube can be removed as soon as the lung has reexpanded against the chest wall, and the patient can be discharged the same day. However, after lung biopsy, chest tube suction must be prolonged for 24 to 48 h. After a therapeutic procedure, especially after talc pleurodesis, pleural drainage should be maintained until the lung has reexpanded, bubbling has stopped, and the volume of fluid collected is less than 100 ml/day. This may take 2 to 5 days.

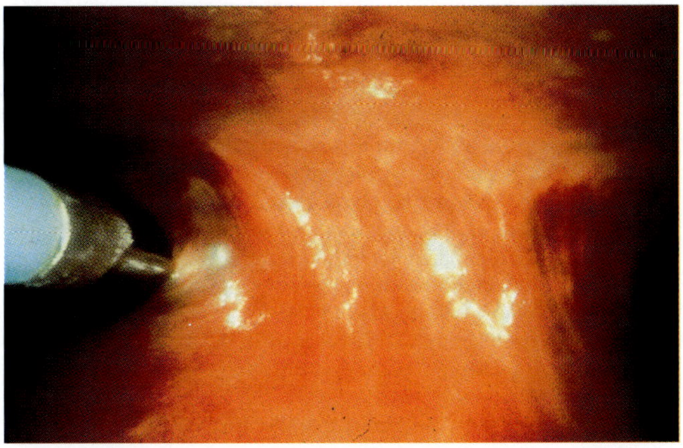

Figure 14-28

Section of large adhesions. Large adhesions may be severed by means of a hook. High-frequency coagulation ensures perfect hemostasis. The section must be performed as close as possible to the parietal pleura to avoid injuring the lung.

THE SECOND POINT OF ENTRY

Although a single point of entry is generally sufficient, a second point of entry is necessary in the following circumstances:

- When the first port of entry does not allow complete and/or satisfactory inspection of the pleural cavity. In this case the second port of entry should be made in proximity to the structure requiring closer scrutiny.
- When the first port of entry does not allow safe collection of a biopsy specimen from the pleura. Such is often the case when the pleura has become immobile and as a result there is a risk of tearing rather than cutting with the optical forceps. Safe biopsy may also be limited due to the hemorrhagic risk in cases where it is impossible to locate the intercostal artery by palpating the wall. This can occur when the pleura has thickened so that outline of the rib is no longer visible or the space has lost its flexibility (Fig. 14-11).
- When it is necessary to control hemorrhage after biopsy. Biopsy of the parietal pleura or budding tumor can lead to bleeding from small vessels. Hemostasis should be done before further biopsy.

For the puncture a trocar consisting of an obturator and cannula with a blunt conical tip is used. The initial trocar accommodating the telescope is 7 mm in diameter and 100 mm in length. For the second puncture a trocar that is 5 mm in diameter and 100 mm in length is used. It is made of electrically insulated plastic, which avoids accidental burns. This trocar accommodates biopsy forceps, brushes, needles, and laser fibers. The 5-mm double-spoon insulated coagulating forceps is used through this second site for pleural or lung biopsies. Power should be sufficient to coagulate the cut surface of the lung without destroying the histologic features of the specimen. A setting of approximately 100 W is usually used.

REFERENCES

1. Light RW: Management of pleural effusions. In Chretien J, et al: (eds): *The Pleura in Health and Disease.* New York, Dekker, 1985:789–809.
2. Sahn SA: The pleura. *Am Rev Respir Dis* 1988;138:184–234.
3. Rossi GA, et al: Symptomatic treatment of recurrent malignant pleural effusions with intrapleurally administered *Corynebacterium parvum. Am Rev Respir Dis* 1987;135:885–890.

4. Boutin C, et al: Thoracoscopy in the early diagnosis of malignant pleural effusions. *Endoscopy* 1980;12:155–160.
5. Martensson G, et al: Differentiation between malignant and non malignant pleural effusion. *Eur J Resp Dis* 1983;67:311–334.
6. Levine MN, et al: Pleural effusion in breast cancer—Thoracoscopy for hormone receptor determination. *Cancer* 1986; 57:324–327.
7. Weissberg D, et al: Pleuroscopy in clinical evaluation and staging of lung cancer. *Poumon Coeur* 1981;37:241–243.
8. Huguenin-Dumittan S, Dottrens A: Resultats de la biopsie à l'aiguille. *Poumon Coeur* 1981;37:35–50.
9. Fentiman IS, et al: Pleural effusion in breast cancer. A review of 105 cases. *Cancer* 1981;47:2087–2095.
10. Canto A, et al: Lung cancer and pleural effusion. Clinical significance and study of pleural metastatic locations. *Chest* 1985;87:649–652.
11. Collins TR, Sahn SA: Thoracentesis. Clinical value, complications, technical problems, and patient experience. *Chest* 1987;91:817–822.
12. Johnston WW: The malignant pleural effusion. A review of cytopathologic diagnosis of 584 specimens from 472 consecutive patients. *Cancer* 1985;56:905–909.
13. Salyer WR, et al: Efficacy of pleural needle biopsy and pleural fluid cytopathology in the diagnosis of malignant neoplasm involving the pleura. *Chest* 1975;67:536–539.
14. Dines DE, et al: The value of cells in the pleural fluid in the differential diagnosis. *Mayo Clin Proc* 1975;50:571–572.
15. Weissberg D, et al: Pleuroscopy in patients with pleural effusion and pleural masses. *Ann Thorac Surg* 1980;29:205–208.
16. Wihlm JM, et al: Résultats comparés de la ponction, de la biopsie à l'aiguille, de la pleuroscopie et de la thoracotomie dans le diagnostic des pleurésies chroniques. *Poumon Coeur* 1981;37:57–60.
17. Canto A, et al: Points to consider when choosing a biopsy method in cases of pleurisy of unknown origin. *Chest* 1983;84:176–179.
18. Boutin C, et al: Thoracoscopy in Chretien J, et al: (eds): *The Pleura in Health and Disease*. New York, Marcel Dekker, 1985;587–622.
19. Boutin C, et al: Indications actuelles de la thoracoscopie. *Rev Fr Mal Resp* 1981;9:309–318.
20. Chahinian APh, et al: Diffuse malignant pleural mesothelioma (prospective evaluation of 69 patients). *Ann Intern Med* 1982;96:746–755.
21. Alberts AS, et al: Malignant pleural mesothelioma: A disease unaffected by current therapeutic maneuvers. *J Clin Oncol* 1988;6:527–535.
22. Antman K, et al: Malignant mesothelioma: Prognostic variables in a registry of 180 patients. The Dana Farber Cancer Institute and Brigham and Women's Hospital experience over two decades, 1965-1985. *J Clin Oncol* 1988;6:147–153.
23. Calavrezos A, et al: Malignant mesothelioma of the pleura. *Klin Wochen Schr* 1988;66:607–613.
24. Spirtas R, et al: Survival patterns for malignant mesothelioma: The seer experience. *Int J Cancer* 1988;41:525–530.
25. Ruffie P, et al: Diffuse malignant mesothelioma of the pleura in Ontario and Quebec: A retrospective study of 332 patients. *J Clin Oncol* 1989;7:1157–1168.
26. Rush VW, et al: The role of extra pleural pneumonectomy in malignant pleural mesothelioma. A Lung Cancer Study Group trial. *J Thorac Cardiovasc Surg* 1991; 102:1–9.
27. International Mesothelioma Interest Group: A proposed new international TNM staging System For Malignant Pleural Mesothelioma. *Chest* 1995;108:1122–1128.
28. Boutin C, et al: Thoracoscopy in pleural malignant mesothelioma: A prospective study of 188 consecutive patients. *Cancer* 1993;72:394–404.
29. Herbert A, Gallagher PJ: Pleural biopsy in the diagnosis of malignant mesothelioma. *Thorax* 1982;37:816.
30. Boutin C, et al: Black spots concentrate oncogenic asbestos fibers in the parietal pleura. *Am J Respir Crit Care Med* 1996;153: 444–449.
31. Dijkman JH: Thorakoskopie bei immunsupprimierten patienten. *Pneumologie (Stuttg)* 1989;43:116–118.
32. Boutin C, et al: Practical thoracoscopy. Berlin, Springer-Verlag, 1991.
33. Brandt HJ: Biopsie pulmonaire pour contrôle visuel. *Poumon Coeur* 1981; 37:307–311.
34. Faurschou P: Diagnostic thoracoscopy in pleural pulmonary infiltrates without pleural effusion. *Endoscopy* 1983;17:21–25.
35. Guy P, et al: Biopsies pulmonaires par thoracoscopie. *Poumon Coeur* 1983;39:179–181.
36. Janik NS, et al: Thoracoscopic evaluation of intrathoracic lesions in children. *J Thorac Cardiovasc Surg* 1982;83:408–413.
37. Kapsenberg PD: Thoracoscopic biopsy under visual control. *Poumon Coeur* 1981;37:313–316.
38. Rodgers BM: Thoracoscopy in children. *Poumon Coeur* 1981;37:301–306.
39. Voellmy W: Résultats diagnostiques de la thoracoscopie dans les affections du poumon et de la plèvre. *Poumon Coeur* 1981;37: 67–73.
40. Wetzer K, et al: Die thorakoskopishe Lungenbiopsie. *Z Erkrank Atmungsorgane* 1980;152:82–88.
41. Churg A, Wood P: Observations on the distribution of asbestos fibers in human lungs. *Environ Resp* 1983;31:374–380.
42. Walker-Renard PB, et al: Chemical pleurodesis for malignant pleural effusions. *Ann Intern Med* 1994;120:56–64.
43. Heffner JE, et al: Clinical efficacy of doxycycline for pleurodesis. *Chest* 1994;105:1743–1747.
44. Heffner JE, Unruh LC: Tetracycline pleurodesis. Adios, farewell, adieu. *Chest* 1992;101:5–7.
45. Boutin C, et al: Etude randomisée de l'efficacité du talcage thoracoscopique et de l'instillation de tetracycline dans le traitement des pleurésies cancéreuses récidivantes. *Rev Fr Mal Respir* 1985;2:374.
46. Boniface E, Guerin JC: Intérêt du talcage par thoracoscopie dans le traitement symptomatique des pleurésies récidivantes. A propos de 302 cas. *Rev Mal Respir* 1989;6:133–139.
47. Ladjimi S, et al: Résultats du talcage pleural sous thoracoscopie au cours des pleurésies néoplasiques. *Rev Mal Respir* 1989;6: 147–150.
48. Weissberg D, Ben Zeev I: Talc pleurodesis. Experience with 360 patients. *J Thorac Cardiovasc Surg* 1993;106:689–693.
49. Canto A, et al: Pleural effusion of malignant etiology. Thoracoscopic use of talc as an effective method of pleurodesis. *Med Clin* 1985;84:806–808.
50. Sanchez-Armengol A, Rodriguez-Panadero F: Survival and talc pleurodesis in metastatic pleural carcinoma; Revisited report of 125 cases. *Chest* 1993;104:1482–1485.
51. Fentiman IS, et al: A comparison of intracavitary talc and tetracycline for the control of pleural effusions secondary to breast cancer. *Eur J Cancer Clin Oncol* 1986;22:1079–1081.
52. Hartman DL, et al: Comparison of insufflated talc under thoracoscopic guidance with standard tetracycline and bleomycin pleurodesis for control of malignant pleural effusions. *J Thorac Cardiovasc Surg* 1993;106(2):743–748
53. Marchandise FX, et al: Thoracoscopy in the diagnosis and management of chronic pleural effusions. *Acta Clin Belg* 1993; 48:5–10.
54. Ostrowski MJ: An assessment of the long-term results of controlling the reaccumultation of malignant effusions using intracavitary bleomycin. *Cancer* 1986;57:721–727.
55. Sherman S, et al: Clinical experience with tetracycline pleurodesis of malignant pleural effusions. *Southern Med J* 1987; 80:716–719.
56. Bresticker MA, et al: Optimal pleurodesis: A comparison study. *Ann Thorac Surg* 1993;55:364–366.

57. Factor SM: Granulomatous pneumonitis. A result of intrapleural instillation of quinarcine and talcum powder. *Arch Pathol* 1975;99:499–502.
58. Rinaldo JE, et al: Adult respiratory distress syndrome following intrapleural instillation of talc. *J Thoraco Cardiovasc Surg* 1983;85:523–526.
59. Bouchama A, et al: Acute pneumonitis with bilateral pleural effusion after talc pleurodesis. *Chest* 1984;86:795–797.
60. Aelony Y, et al: Thoracoscopic talc poudrage pleurodesis for chronic recurrent pleural effusions. *Ann Intern Med* 1991;115:778–82.
61. Markman M, et al: High dose intracavitary cisplatin with intravenous thiosulfate: Low incidence of serious neurotoxicity. *Cancer* 1985;56:2364–2368.
62. Rush, VW, et al: Intrapleural cisplatin and cytarabine in the management of malignant pleural effusions a Lung Cancer Study Group trial. *J Clin Oncol* 1991;9:313–319.
63. Driesen P, et al: Implantable access system for prolonged intapleural immunotherapy. *Eur Respir J* 1994;7:1889–1892.
64. Astoul P, et al: Intrapleural recombinant IL-2 in passive immunotherapy for malignant pleural effusion. *Chest* 1993; 103:209-213.
65. Viallat JR, et al: Intrapleural immunotherapy with escalating doses of IL-2 in metastatic pleural effusions. *Cancer* 1993; 71:4067–4071.
66. Boutin C, et al: Intrapleural treatment with gamma-interferon in early stage malignant pleural mesothelioma. *Cancer* 1994; 74:2460–2467.
67. Viskum K, Enk B: Complications of thoracoscopy. *Poumon Coeur* 1981;37:25–28.
68. Boutin C, et al: The role of thoracoscopy in the evaluation and management of pleural effusions. *Lung* 1990;75:45–50.
69. Mathur P, Martin WJ: Clinical utility of thoracoscopy. *Chest* 1992;102:2–4.
70. Colt HG: Thoracoscopy. A prospective study of safety and outcome. *Chest* 1995;108:324–329.
71. Davidson AC, et al: Thoracoscopy: Assessment of a physician service and comparison of a flexible bronchoscope used as a thoracoscope with a rigid thoracoscope. *Thorax* 1988; 43:327–332.

CHAPTER 15

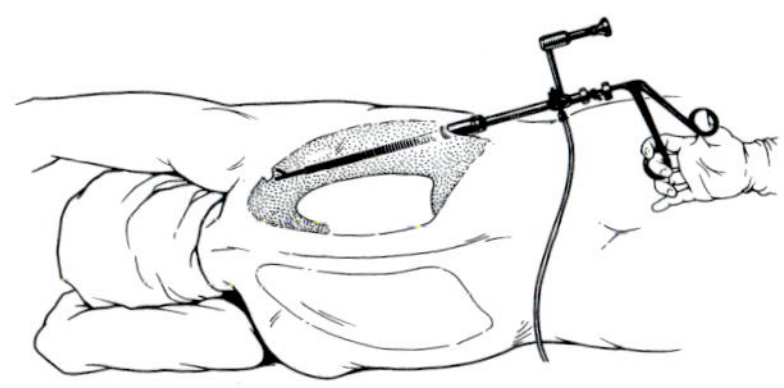

THORACOSCOPIC MANAGEMENT OF PNEUMOTHORAX

Henri G. Colt

Pneumothorax is a condition for which the benefits and risks of thoracoscopic management must be carefully weighed against other therapeutic alternatives. Decisions are based not only on the etiology of the pneumothorax but also on the patient's underlying illness and general functional status and the chance for failure or success of therapeutic intervention. During thoracoscopy, several techniques of pleurodesis and air-leak closure can be considered. Unfortunately, there are few clear guidelines on which to base management decisions. Before proceeding to diagnostic or therapeutic thoracoscopy, therefore, careful consideration is given to the potential consequences of each treatment modality. Often, interventional pulmonologists find it helpful to closely collaborate with primary care physicians, thoracic surgeons, and interventional radiologists to best ascertain proper patient management. In this chapter the indications and techniques of thoracoscopic management of pneumothorax, as well as the changing role of thoracoscopic diagnosis and management for patients with spontaneous pneumothorax, are described.

Historical Perspectives

Collection of air within the pleural cavity has been known to exist for centuries. In 1803, Itard was the first to suggest the term *pneumothorax,* which is still in general use today. Additional contributions during the 19th century were made by Laennec, Bell, and Trousseau, who also described many of the physical signs associated with air in the pleural space.[1] In 1901, the first radiographic picture of pneumothorax was described by Martin. The rest of the 20th century has brought many new developments to the study of pneumothorax. Initially, for example, spontaneous pneumothorax was thought to be associated with tuberculosis. Indeed, most patients with pneumothorax were treated as if they had this infectious disease. It was not until 1926 that Miller described emphysematous blebs and bullae and suggested that pneumothorax occurred in nontuberculous patients. In a historic doctoral thesis published in 1932, Kjaerjard further established that pneumothorax was a condition entirely separate from tuberculosis.[2] Subsequently, pneumothorax has been readily characterized by a battery of symptoms, signs, and radiographic appearances. Computed tomography scans can often reveal blebs, bullae, and emphysematous changes within the lung parenchyma. Open thoracic surgery techniques have been extremely successful for air-leak closure. Open resection of blebs and pleural abrasion techniques are almost 100 percent successful for preventing recurrence.[3] Less invasive methods for pleurodesis have also been widely used, including watchful waiting if the pneumothorax is small and the patient is asymptomatic, chest tube insertion and negative drainage, and chemical pleurodesis to prevent recurrence.[4] Thoracoscopy, a minimally invasive surgical technique by which the pleural and pulmonary anatomy can be examined and pathologic abnormalities detected, was widely used in patients with pneumothorax in Europe through the 1980s. Before then, it was frequently advocated by individuals such as Swierenga, Keller, Sattler, and Bloomberg.[5–8] Thoracoscopy became popular in the United States, however, only in the 1990s.[9]

Today, many chest physicians and surgeons have incorporated thoracoscopy into their management algorithms, resulting in a great benefit to their patients. Because of improved instrumentation, thoracoscopy today allows the performance of procedures identical with those previously performed only during an open thoracotomy. Thus, many thoracic surgeons and interventional pulmonologists believe that thoracoscopy should and can be performed earlier in the course of hospitalization of patients with persistent pneumothoraces, and some even advocate thoracoscopic exploration and management as routine and primary therapy (Table 15-1).[10–14] There is no doubt this stance is controversial. It is noteworthy that despite multiple studies and review papers, however, there is little worldwide consensus regarding the use of specific therapeutic interventions in patients with pneumothorax.

Indications for Thoracoscopy

CLINICAL PRESENTATION

Today it is known that pneumothorax occurs either spontaneously or secondary to an underlying illness, trauma, or diagnostic or therapeutic intervention. Patients may present with acute onset of pleuritic chest pain, shortness of breath, or hemoptysis. From a physiologic standpoint, the primary findings are hypoxemia and decreased vital capacity. A chest radiograph reveals partial or total collapse of the lung. "Tension" physiology is suspected if patients have tachypnea, tachycardia, malaise, or hypotension. Tension can also be suspected when chest radiographs demonstrate substantial mediastinal shift to the contralateral side. Chest tube insertion usually results in resolution of clinical symptoms and partial lung reexpansion. Both small-bore and large-bore chest tubes inserted under local anesthesia can be used effectively for initial treatment.[15] Smaller tubes may be most beneficial when pneumothoraces are iatrogenic in origin or when a prolonged air leak is unlikely. Larger tubes are warranted in patients at risk for prolonged air leak. These include patients with AIDS or *pneumocystis carinii* pneumonia, trauma victims, patients with asthma, and patients with known or suspected bullous lung disease such as those with chronic obstructive pulmonary disease (COPD).

PRIMARY SPONTANEOUS PNEUMOTHORAX

Spontaneous pneumothorax usually is defined as a pneumothorax that occurs abruptly and without any history of previous intervention or trauma. Spontaneous pneumothoraces are further defined as primary and secondary. Primary spontaneous pneumothorax occurs in healthy, often young individuals without any known etiology. These usually occur in tall, thin males, who often have uncomplicated, asymptomatic, small (less than 20 percent of the hemithorax) pneumothoraces. Chest drainage is usually unnecessary, and patients need only be carefully observed. The current trend is increasingly toward outpatient management, with patients returning to their physicians for follow-up chest radiographs until resolution of the pneumothorax is noted. Most patients are instructed to avoid strenuous physical activity, air travel, and scuba diving. Most experts agree that an increase in size of the pneumothorax or development of symptoms should prompt tube thoracostomy. Open surgical or even thoracoscopic procedures may be indicated, however, in patients who are at extremely high risk for

Table 15-1
POTENTIAL ADVANTAGES OF THORACOSCOPY OVER OTHER TREATMENT MODALITIES IN PATIENTS WITH PNEUMOTHORAX

Pleuropulmonary anatomy is assessed and abnormalities noted. Presence of blebs or bullae allow grading severity of lung disease and may help predict response to pleurodesis and risk of recurrence.
Chest tubes inserted under direct guidance enhance lung reexpansion and successful pleurodesis.
Ruptured as well as intact blebs and bullae can be electrocauterized, photocoagulated, or resected to seal air leaks and prevent recurrence.
Adhesions maintaining traction around visceral pleural tears can be severed.
Certain iatrogenic pneumothoraces (accidental chest tube insertion into lung, for example) are rapidly diagnosed and managed.
Possibly less morbidity than open thoracic surgery. Potential greater visibility and access to entire pleural space and lung than limited axillary thoracotomy.

recurrence, or in those who have occupations that require them to experience substantial changes in atmospheric pressure, or in those who live in areas without access to medical care.[16]

Primary spontaneous pneumothorax has been noted to occur in 7 to 9 per 100,000 people each year.[17] In one study,[18] at least 18 percent of the patients reported did not seek medical attention for more than a week. There is no doubt, therefore, that the incidence of spontaneous pneumothorax is probably underestimated. Risk factors for spontaneous pneumothorax are still unclear, but may include smoking, existence of localized abnormalities of the visceral pleura such as small congenital cysts, and HLA-A2B40 phenotype.[19]

The usual treatments for primary spontaneous pneumothorax are bed rest, repeated needle aspiration, tube thoracostomy with or without suction, and intervention with pleurodesis, pleurectomy, thoracotomy, or thoracoscopy.[20–25] Recurrence rates after tube thoracostomy alone are reportedly 20 to 50 percent. Usually, recurrence happens within the first 2 years after the initial event, and occurs on the same side as the initial pneumothorax.[15]

It is noteworthy that none of the conservative management modalities attempt to irradicate the cause of the pneumothorax, or help elucidate its potential etiology and presence of visceral pleura abnormalities. Thoracoscopy, on the other hand, allows careful inspection of the pleural space and lung to determine the cause of the pneumothorax as well as immediate treatment. Most experts agree that an operative procedure is indicated if a patient has had two or more occurrences. Although thoracoscopy has been advocated as part of routine management of a first episode of primary pneumothorax[10] the benefits of this approach have not yet been demonstrated. In addition, it is unclear whether thoracoscopic appearance predicts likelihood of recurrence.[26,27]

SECONDARY SPONTANEOUS PNEUMOTHORAX

Secondary pneumothorax is almost always associated with underlying lung disease such as COPD.[4] Pneumothorax can also occur in patients with fibrotic lungs, as in those with interstitial lung disease, or infectious cavitary lung disease (tuberculosis). Either primary or secondary spontaneous pneumothoraces may be unilateral, bilateral, or associated with hemothorax, hydropneumothorax, or tension physiology. Other etiologies for secondary spontaneous pneumothorax include cancer, asthma, all forms of interstitial lung disease, collagen vascular disease, Marfan's syndrome, cystic fibrosis, hydatid disease, histiocytosis X, lymphangiomyomatosis, and pulmonary alveolar proteinosis.[28–30] Catamenial pneumothorax occurs in young women, usually at the time of menses, and may be related to endometriosis. Pneumothorax also occurs in patients with AIDS who often have underlying *P. carinii* pneumonia.[31–33]

Immediate therapeutic intervention is usually indicated in patients with secondary spontaneous pneumothorax. Indeed, it appears that the risk of recurrence is higher in this population, and mortality rates of 5 to 20 percent have been reported. Most patients require initial large-bore chest tube drainage. Many have persistent air leaks lasting more than 3 to 5 days. It is in this particular patient population that early referral for thoracoscopy may be particularly indicated.[34] It is noteworthy, however, that thoracoscopic treatment of pneumothorax in this population may be less effective than in patients with primary spontaneous pneumothorax.[35–38] The site of air leaks may be difficult to find, and therapeutic treatment in and of itself, such as endoscopic stapling, may further tear an already fragile lung parenchyma. In selected patients, thoracoscopic pleurodesis may be, therefore, the procedure of choice. It appears that recurrence rates after secondary spontaneous pneumothorax are similar to those seen after primary spontaneous pneumothorax. Because of the increased morbidity and mortality of prolonged air leaks and recurrence in this patient population, however, an aggressive therapeutic strategy is often desirable. Bedside chest tube pleurodesis, thoracoscopic exploration and management, or open surgery by limited axillary or lateral thoracotomy should be considered early in the course of hospitalization. Table 15-2 outlines the current indications for thoracoscopic treatment of spontaneous pneumothorax.

CHRONIC PNEUMOTHORAX

Although most pneumothoraces resolve after proper chest-tube management, some air leaks may persist. Persistence of a pneumothorax for several weeks or even months can be associated with significant morbidity. Usually, these patients have a permanent bronchopleural fistula. Primary repair of the parenchymal laceration is often necessary and can be achieved by open thoracotomy. Other patients respond well to chronic small-bore chest tube drainage and discharge from the hospital with a one-way Heimlich valve. This technique has been increasingly used in patients with AIDS and in those with prolonged air leaks following lung-volume-reduction surgery. In others, an early thoracoscopic approach is warranted. Sometimes, adhesions maintaining the patency of the bronchopleural fistula can be lysed and the fistula closed. In others, laceration of a bulla or bleb may be noted, and the diseased area of lung can be satisfactorily resected using electrocautery, Nd:YAG laser photocoagulation, or endoscopic stapling. In many cases, pleurodesis is also

Table 15-2
INDICATIONS FOR THORACOSCOPIC TREATMENT OF SPONTANEOUS PNEUMOTHORAX

Persistent air leak >72 h after chest tube insertion
First recurrence of spontaneous pneumothorax
Initial pneumothorax in patients with occupations at high risk of recurrence or difficult access to medical care
Initial pneumothorax in patients with history of contralateral pneumothorax
Initial pneumothorax in patients who wish to know status of underlying lung and potentially minimize risk of recurrence compared with chest tube drainage alone
Patients at high risk for thoracotomy

achieved by thoracoscopic talc insufflation, pleurectomy, or thoracoscopic mechanical abrasion.[39–48] From large numbers of patients undergoing thoracoscopic treatment of pneumothorax as part of the VATS Study Group, it appears that thoracoscopic treatment has little mortality and minimal morbidity when compared with open thoracic surgery.[49] Still, it is unclear how thoracoscopic management compares with limited axillary thoracotomy, for example.[35,50] Before proceeding to thoracoscopy, the interventional pulmonologist must recognize this procedure's potential difficulties and limitations, and be ready and equipped to deal with any suspected or unsuspected operative findings.

Thoracoscopic Diagnosis

Thoracoscopy allows complete evaluation of the pleural space and lung. A complete inspection may result in detection of a lung parenchymal laceration, an entirely free pleural cavity despite chest-tube drainage, a malpositioned chest tube within lung parenchyma responsible for a continued air leak, or visceral and parietal pleural abnormalities such as endometriosis, congenital cysts, and cavitating or nodular lesions in patients with granulomatous disorders. The most likely abnormalities, of course, are blebs and bullae. A relatively large percentage (up to 30 percent) of patients may have normal findings on thoracoscopy.[26] Whether this is because of inadequate exploration or unsatisfactory technique or because currently available telescopes are not yet capable of detecting minute visceral pleural abnormalities is unclear.

The general treatment plan should probably be based on a thorough understanding of the underlying cause of the spontaneous pneumothorax. It appears that the most common cause of spontaneous pneumothorax is subpleural blebs. These are usually smaller than 1 cm in diameter and confined to the apex of the lung, as well as along the edges of the lower lobe or anterior segment of the upper lobe. Several classifications have been proposed, including those of Wakabayashi[37] and Vanderscueren[36] (Table 15-3). Whether risk of recurrence can be predicted based on thoracoscopic appearance is still unclear.

Many patients with spontaneous pneumothorax undergoing thoracoscopy have normal visceral pleura. This had been noted by Sattler in 1937[7] and still holds true today. Electron microscopy of the visceral pleura has demonstrated that mesothelial cells are often replaced by small 10 to 20-μm diameter pores that cannot be seen with the naked eye.[10] Certainly, these unseen lesions may account for recurrence despite resection of bullae in certain patients. This underscores the potential usefulness of blind apical stapling or extensive pleurodesis in patients with thoracoscopically normal lungs.

During thoracoscopy, it is essential to optimize visualization of pleuropulmonary abnormalities responsible for pneumothorax. When procedures are performed under general anesthesia with selective bronchial intubation, positive pressure ventilation can be used after the lung has been collapsed to detect the area of air leak by submerging the lung in normal saline. If performed under local anesthesia without intubation, blebs or bullae may become visible if the patient performs a valsalva maneuver or if positive airway pressure is applied by laryngeal mask or Ambu bag hand ventilation. During any form of lung insufflation, small, previously flat blebs will inflate, appearing as tiny bubbles on the visceral pleural surface. In spontaneously breathing patients, bullae and large blebs can also be seen when air enters the pleural cavity from the atmosphere through the pleural trocars. As the lung deflates spontaneously, these areas of trapped gas remain inflated and are easily differentiated from the rest of the lung parenchyma. Areas of air leak, however, may be difficult to locate. For this reason, some thoracoscopists have advocated inhalation of fluoresein dye by aerosol[10] or inhalation of methylene blue, which can also be administered bronchoscopically prior to thoracoscopy. Methylene blue can also be administered through the endotracheal tube in mechanically ventilated patients. It is this au-

Table 15-3
THORACOSCOPIC FINDINGS IN SPONTANEOUS PNEUMOTHORAX

Vanderschueren Classification[36]	
Type I	Endoscopically normal lung
Type II	Pleuropulmonary adhesions
Type III	Small blebs or bullae <2 cm in diameter
Type IV	Large bullae >2 cm in diameter
Wakabayashi Classification of Bullae[37]	
Blebs	Subpleural, translucent, <1 cm in diameter, most often confined to apex but also along edges of anterior segment of upper lobe, edges of middle lobe or lingula, and edges of superior segment of lower lobe. Probably the most frequent cause of pneumothorax.
Type I bullae	Thin-walled cyst with little communication with bronchial system. No trabeculae. Any size possible. May compress normal adjacent lung.
Type II bullae	Conglomerates of small to medium size intraparenchymal bullae with smooth internal lining and no trabeculae. Thick fibrous wall. Adjacent lung tissue is normal.
Type III bullae	Large bullae with numerous trabeculae, often diffuse. Adjacent lung is abnormal. Usually found in patients with COPD. Rupture causes large air leaks.

thor's experience, however, that dyes tend to dissiminate within the pleural space and are not always useful for air-leak detection. It is noteworthy that the utility of either of these procedures has yet to be demonstrated by prospective studies.

Thoracoscopic Management

EQUIPMENT

Successful thoracoscopy requires special equipment that enhances diagnosis and treatment of patients with spontaneous pneumothorax. Although direct visualization through the eyepiece of the thoracoscope can be performed, video technology today allows excellent visualization, as long as satisfactory light and resolution are provided. Thoracoscopists need to be familiar with the various manifestations of adhesions, fibrin deposition on visceral pleura, and early stage of spontaneous visceral pleural healing. Sometimes the site of visceral pleural laceration or bleb rupture may be covered by blood or fibrin. Instruments that facilitate thoracoscopic diagnosis include 0 degree and angled (usually 30 to 50 degrees) telescopes, pleural trocars of various diameters (usually 5, 7, 10, and 12 mm) to allow insertion of working instruments, an atraumatic suction catheter or Yankauer suction device, a suction-irrigation instrument, equipment for thoracoscopic talc insufflation, a set of atraumatic grasping forceps, biopsy forceps, electrocautery instrumentation, and endoscopic scissors for lysis of adhesions (Fig. 15-1). Most instruments are available in 5- or 7-mm diameters, although thoracoscopy can be also performed without pleural trocars in selected instances using specially designed or routine thoracic surgery instruments (Fig. 15-2).

Although large blebs, bullae, or areas of torn lung parenchyma can be resected using a ready-to-use suture such as the Endoloop (U.S. Surgical), most operators prefer endoscopic stapling for lung resection. Disposable endoscopic stapling devices come in various sizes, usually 12 to 15 mm in diameter, with staple lines ranging from 3 to 6 cm in length. These staplers resect and staple simultaneously, although the cutting blade can be removed. Adjustable angled distal extremities can be rotated to facilitate placement. Endoscopic staplers may be used through reusable or disposable trocars, or are inserted directly through small skin incisions into the pleural space. In patients with particularly fragile lung parenchyma, bovine pericardium strips can be used over the endoscopic stapling device. These strips are used routinely when thoracoscopic lung resections are performed for volume-reduction lung surgery.[51,52]

ANESTHESIA

General anesthesia with double-lumen endobronchial intubation is the most desirable technique for complete exploration and management of patients with pneumothorax, especially if endoscopic stapling is to be performed. During anesthesia, continuous positive air-

Figure 15-1

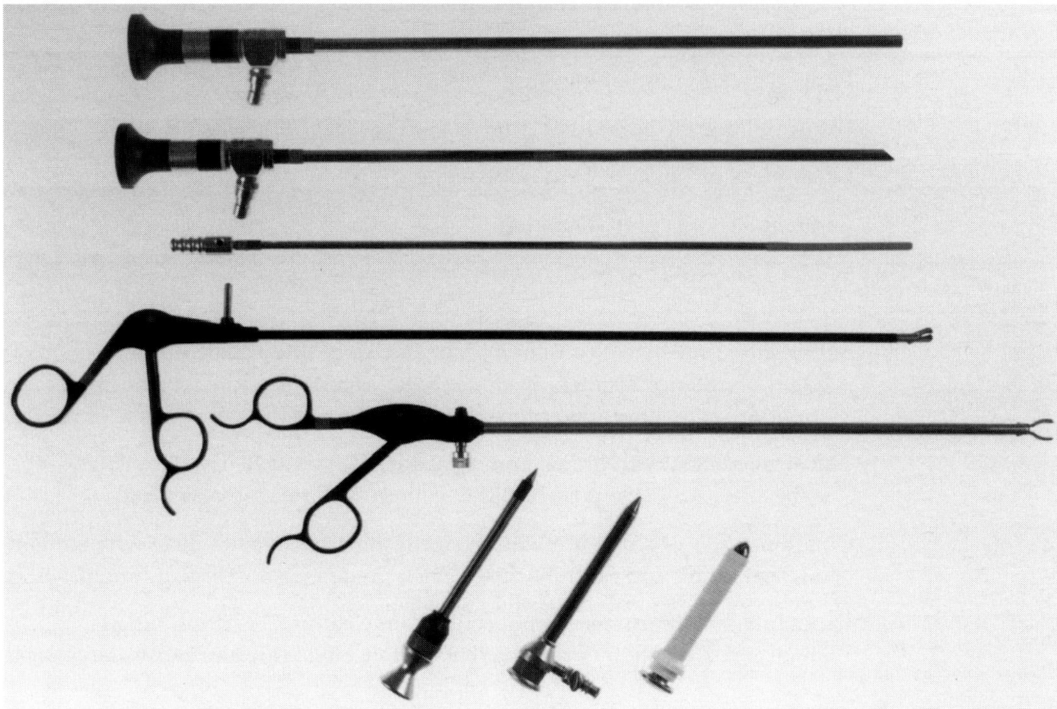

Instrumentation. Basic reusable instruments necessary for thoracoscopic management of spontaneous pneumothorax (Richard Wolf Company, Vernon Hills, IL): pleural trocars (5, 7, 10 mm), scissors, straight and angled telescopes, 7-mm grasping forceps, suction-irrigation device.

way pressure is often applied to the ipsilateral lung (the lung being operated on). This helps prevent hypoxemia, and slight inflation of the lung is helpful to identify blebs, bullae, or air leaks. Thoracoscopic evaluation may be difficult in patients who do not tolerate single-lung ventilation or in cases where endotracheal tubes are poorly placed. It is imperative that any interventional pulmonologist performing thoracoscopy with double-lumen endobronchial intubation be fully acquainted with the techniques of intubation and methods of precise tube placement.[53] A close working relationship is always required with the anesthesiology team.

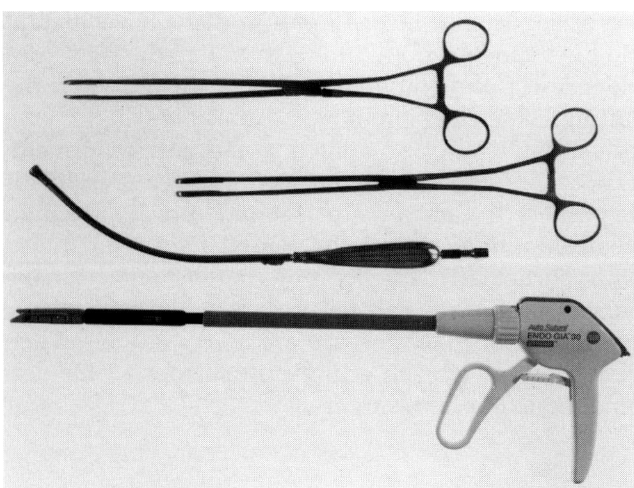

Figure 15-2

Instrumentation. Additional reusable and disposable instruments useful for bleb or bullae resection: grasping forceps (Pilling, Fort Washington, PA), Yankaur suction, Endo GIA 30 (U.S. Surgical).

Thoracoscopy can also be performed using single-lumen intubation and spontaneous assisted ventilation maintained by intravenous propofol or neuroleptic analgesia. In these cases, the lung cannot be deflated voluntarily, and lung collapse occurs on entry into the pleural space. Because the extent of lung inflation cannot be controlled, endoscopic stapling is more dangerous and is probably not warranted in this setting. Electrocauterization of blebs and small bullae, Nd:YAG laser photocoagulation, and pleurodesis, however, are easily achievable.

Conclusion

Thoracoscopy is an excellent therapeutic alternative for patients with pneumothorax and evidence of bleb or bullous lung disease (Table 15-4). Thoracoscopic exploration should probably be performed early in the

Table 15-4
SELECTED PUBLISHED STUDIES OF THORACOSCOPIC TREATMENT OF SPONTANEOUS PNEUMOTHORAX

Author	*Year*	*# Patients*	*Methods*[a]	*% Recurrence*	*Comments*
Swierenga et al.[8]	1974	136	1,3	8	17% with lesions >2 cm
Guerin and Boniface[69]	1985	109	4	5	41% with lesions >2 cm
Almind et al.[20]	1989	85	4	8	17% with lesions >2 cm
Olsen and Orbaeck[70]	1992	483	1,5	16	40% with lesions >2 cm
Bagnato[47]	1992	17	1	0	Bullectomy without pleurodesis
Van Brekel et al.[25]	1993	622	1,3	12	103 had COPD, normal exam in 41% of total, talc successful in 88%, thoracotomy done in 40, successful in 97%
Hazelrigg et al.[23]	1993	26	2,3,6	0	Better than historical axillary thoracotomy, follow-up 8 months
Janssen et al.[67]	1994	43	1,4,6	5	Normal exam in 34%, bullae >2 cm in 54%
Inderbitzi et al.[58]	1994	79	1,2,6	7	Follow-up 3 months
Waller et al.[35]	1994	22	1,2	18	Cases of secondary pneumothorax, minimal follow-up 2 months
Liu et al.[12]	1995	82	1,3,4	0	Follow-up 22 months, blebs or bullae in 83%, Endoloop ligation also used
Naunheim et al.[63]	1995	113	1,2,3,5,6	4	65 recurrent, stapling in 105, 23% recurrence if no blebs seen
Yim and Ho[64]	1995	100	1,3,6	3	Apical bullae 87%, follow-up 17 months

[a]Methods used: (1) bullectomy, (2) pleurectomy, (3) pleural abrasion, (4) talc, (5) chemical pleurodesis, (6) others.

hospital course of a functional patient with persistent air leak, before the morbidity of prolonged bed rest, persistent pneumothorax, and ineffective chest tube drainage take their toll. Thoracoscopy should always be considered in patients with persistent air leaks and radiographic evidence of incomplete lung reexpansion. The value of other imaging studies versus thoracoscopic exploration and their overall effect on management decisions and outcome has not been fully addressed.

Thoracoscopy allows detection of bronchopleural fistulae, air-leak repair or resection, and recurrence prevention. Occasionally, however, localization of air leaks may be extremely difficult. In these cases, blind apical stapling or thoracoscopic pleurodesis have been advocated. Thoracoscopic talc insufflation may be particularly indicated in patients who are not open surgical candidates, present high risk for general anesthesia, or have poor functional status. Obviously, the risks and benefits of thoracoscopic pleurodesis must be weighed against those of simple chest tube pleurodesis.

Regardless of the thoracoscopic technique employed, careful inspection of the pleural space and lung is necessary. This requires an experienced thoracoscopist. Successful thoracoscopic management of patients with spontaneous pneumothoraces often requires the collaborative efforts of the chest physician, anesthesiologist, and thoracic surgeon. How thoracoscopic management and particularly video-assisted thoracic surgery techniques compare with limited axillary thoracotomy requires further study. Comparative studies of the effects of thoracoscopic techniques such as talc insufflation, mechanical abrasion, and endoscopic stapling on success of air-leak repair, frequency of recurrence, and outcome are also warranted.

In patients with a recurrent or persistent pneumothorax, thoracoscopy usually permits diagnosis, detection, and closure of the responsible air leak. Pleurodesis helps avoid recurrence. It is likely that future outcome-based research will demonstrate that simple chest tube drainage is no longer warranted in patients with recurrent pneumothorax. In patients with persistent pneumothorax despite chest tube drainage, early

Table 15-5

MANAGEMENT DECISION TREE FOR SPONTANEOUS PNEUMOTHORAX

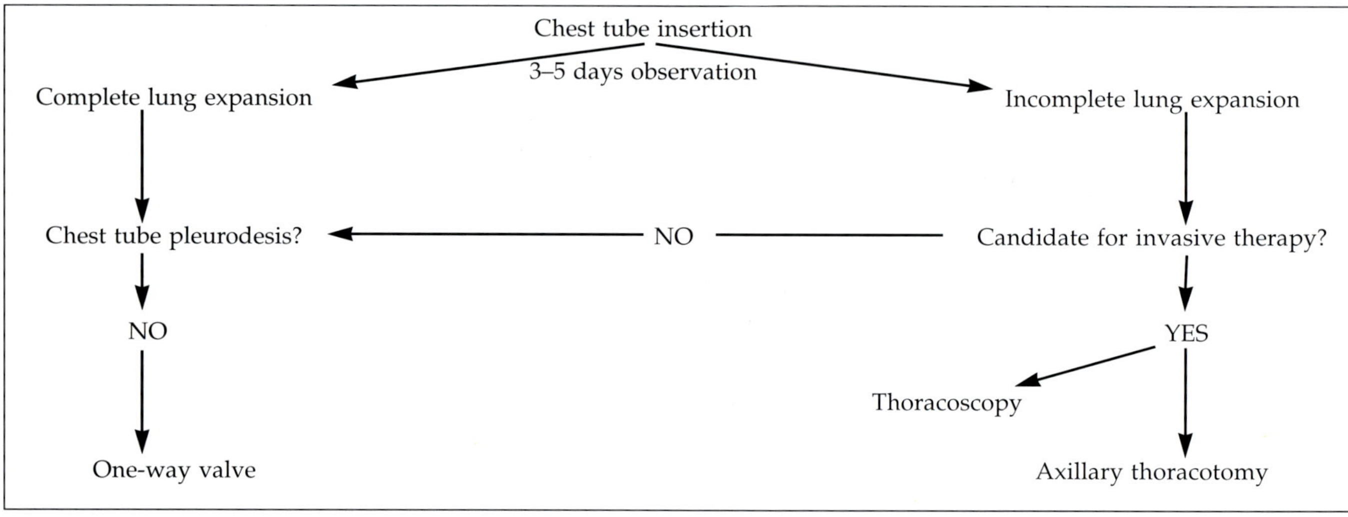

thoracoscopy (performed within 3 to 5 days of initial hospitalization), may significantly contribute to management decision making. Thoracoscopy also permits examination of underlying lung and pleura, so that patients and their families may be informed of the normal or pathologic findings. In selected patients with persistent air leaks or at high risk for recurrence, immediate decisions regarding performance of a formal open thoracotomy, simple pleurodesis, or one-way valve insertion and hospital discharge can be made based on a complete evaluation of thoracoscopic findings. How thoracoscopic appearance impacts on therapeutic management and affects outcome in all patients with primary or secondary spontaneous pneumothorax, however, requires further study. Although thoracoscopy avoids the morbidity of open thoracotomy, its role versus that of a limited axillary thoracotomy must also be defined. With so many advances having been made these past 200 years, future work should be devoted to providing answers to these questions. For now the approach outlined in Table 15-5 must suffice.

HOW I DO IT

PATIENT PREPARATION

After careful preoperative evaluation (Table 15-6) procedures are performed in the operating room or in a specially equipped endoscopy suite. Patients are fully monitored by electrocardiography, blood pressure checks, and oxygen saturation measurements. When double-lumen intubation techniques are employed, an arterial line is often warranted. Patients are usually placed in the full lateral decubitus position. Skin preparation and draping are carried out as for routine thoracoscopy and thoracotomy. A wide field is desirable with drapes below the scapula posteriorly and below the nipple anteriorly. If apical blebs are suspected, the initial trocar should be placed in the third or fourth intercostal space in the midaxillary line. An anterior trocar may be inserted in the fourth intercostal space in the anterior axillary line for introduction of a grasping instrument. If an endoscopic stapling device is to be used, a third trocar is usually necessary posteriorly, optimally within the ausculatory triangle just below the scapula. Trocar sizes and sites may be determined after the initial trocar entry and inspection. Depending on the need for complete evaluation and treatment, the thoracoscope can be inserted through any of the incision sites.[54]

It is essential that careful attention be paid to positioning of the ipsilateral arm. The arm should be abducted at right angles and kept relatively low to allow easy trocar insertion into the intraspaces of the upper chest. If patients have chest tubes in place, these tubes should probably be left inserted during anesthesia induction, intubation, and positioning to avoid risk of tension pneumothorax. The chest tube can be removed during sterile prepping, or, if necessary, immediately prior to trocar insertion. In selected instances, and especially, if intraparenchymal chest tube insertion is suspected, it is helpful to keep the tube in place until the pleural space has been entered and inspected.

Table 15-6

POTENTIAL CONTRAINDICATIONS FOR THORACOSCOPIC MANAGEMENT OF SPONTANEOUS PNEUMOTHORAX

Inexperienced thoracoscopist
Patients with large or prolonged air leak, suspected type II bullae, or severe COPD. (Limited axillary thoracotomy or simple thoracoscopic talc insufflation may be preferable.)
Patients with large trabeculated type III bullae. Resection may require bovine pericardium and/or associated lung reduction. Adhesions, often abundant, may be vascularized.
Patients unable to tolerate single-lung ventilation (large air leaks in mechanically ventilated patients, for example)
Patients at high-risk for general anesthesia (patients with severe cardiac disease, recent myocardial infarction, or sepsis, for example)
Patients with coagulopathy or very poor functional status (patients with malnutrition or advanced AIDS, for example)

TROCAR PLACEMENT AND INSPECTION

Once the lung is deflated, saline solution is introduced through suction tubing or through a suction irrigation device while the ipsilateral lung is gently reinflated. Bubbling demonstrates the site of the air leak and underlying bleb or bullous disease. If necessary, the operating table can be tilted inferiorly or the patient can be placed into the Trendelenberg position to pool saline solution in the superior aspect of the pleural space. This may improve visualization of the air leak without requiring complete reinflation of the lung. It should be remembered that whenever the lung is reinflated, thoracoscopic visualization is impaired. Once the air leak has been discovered, the saline solution can be removed by gentle suction. Excess negative pleural pressure prompts rapid lung reexpansion and obscures the visual field, and risks increasing the size of the visceral pleural tear.

If apical bleb disease is not found or has been otherwise not suspected, it is prudent to place one of the larger points of entry at the sixth or seventh intercostal space on the midaxillary line. By placing the telescope through this point of entry, complete examination can be made of the lung base and parenchyma near the fissures (Figs. 15-3 to 15-6). Substantial adhesions should be sectioned because visceral tears are often found adjacent to these adhesions. Removing adhesions may also facilitate lung manipulation, exploration, discovery of additional air leaks, bleb electrocauterization, and air-leak repair using the endoscopic stapler.

AIR-LEAK REPAIR USING THE ENDOSCOPIC STAPLER

After discovery of the air leak, the endoscopic stapler is placed through the anterior or posterior trocar and fired across the base of the bleb (Fig. 15-7). Often, it is

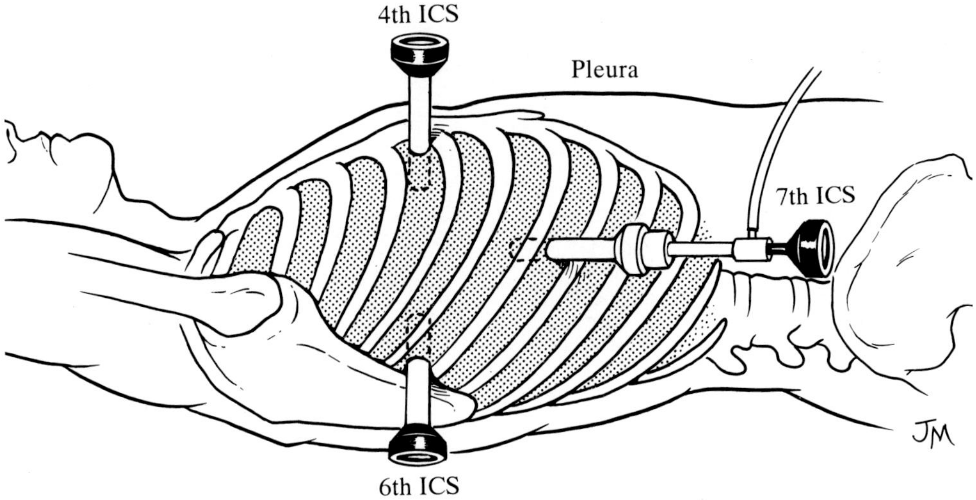

Figure 15-3

Trocar Placement. Trocar insertion for exploration and management of apical blebs. Trocars are placed in the fourth intercostal space on the anterior and midaxillary lines, and in the sixth intercostal space on the posterior axillary line. Telescope is inserted through a midaxillary incision, endoscopic stapler through the posterior incision, and the grasping forceps through the anterior incision. Trocar insertion for complete exploration and air-leak repair in lower lobe. At least one trocar is placed more inferiorly (seventh intercostal space) for the telescope.

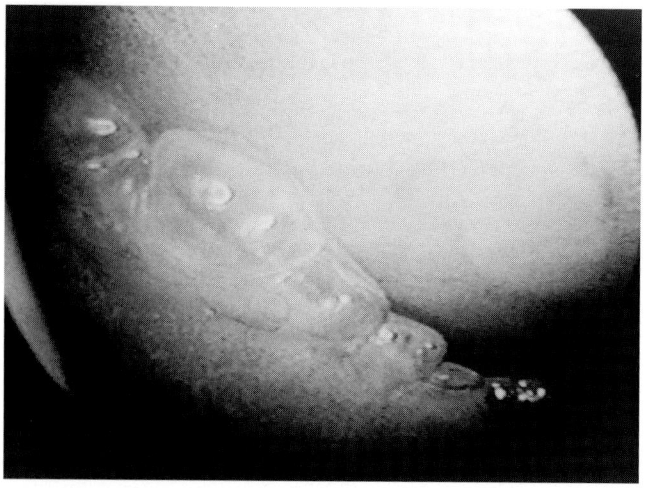

Figure 15-4

Blebs. Small translucent blebs on superior edge of middle lobe.

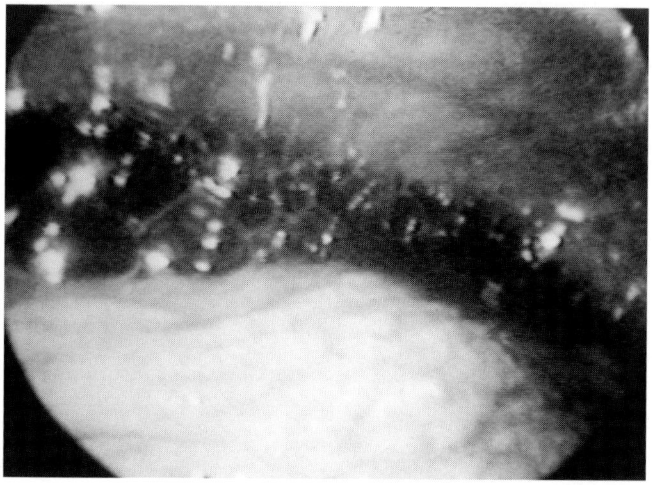

Figure 15-6

Air Leaks. Air leak demonstrated by bubbling when lung is submerged in normal saline solution

necessary to fire the stapler more than once. If the goal of the procedure is to seal the air leak and not resect blebs or bullae, the knife blade can be removed from the stapler. This excludes the bleb from the remaining lung parenchyma and decreases likelihood of air leak at the level of the staple line.

Caution is advised when using any endoscopic stapling device. A thorough working knowledge of the risks and complications of this intervention is essential. Staplers should never be fired blindly, nor used in proximity to large vascular structures. Staplers may misfire, fail to open once closed, or cut unsatisfactorily. Thoracoscopists should be experienced, particularly if nonsurgeons. An excellent working relationship should be developed with thoracic surgery colleagues so that disagreements regarding "turf" issues, privileges, competence, and patient safety are avoided. Close collaboration between thoracic surgeons and medical thoracoscopists is possible, and has already been demonstrated in many institutions in the United States and Europe. Indiscriminate use of endoscopic stapling and lung resection by inexperienced or insufficiently trained, nonsurgeon thoracoscopists should be discouraged. The thoracoscopist must be prepared to deal with complications should the need arise. If certain rules of safety are followed, however, and caution is applied, thoracoscopic staple resection of blebs or small bullae is extremely safe. Once stapling has been achieved, saline is again introduced into the pleural space to partially cover the lung and staple line. The lung is gently reinflated, and the absence of air leak or bleeding confirmed.

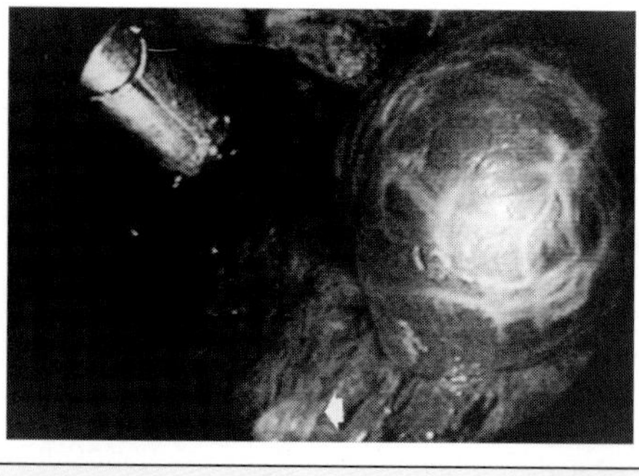

Figure 15-5

Bullae. Large bullae with adjacent small bleb.

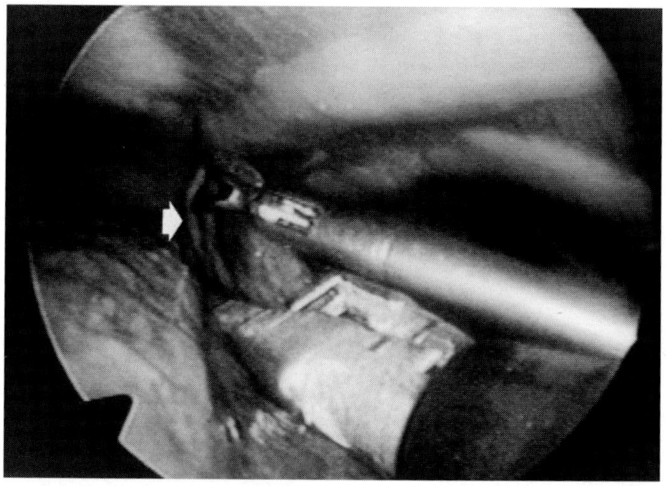

Figure 15-7

Endoscopic stapler. Ruptured bullae covered with fibrin (white plaque beneath tip of grasping forceps) being resected with Endo GIA stapler.

AIR-LEAK REPAIR USING ELECTROCAUTERY, LASER PHOTOCOAGULATION, AND PLEUROLYSIS

When fibrous adhesions are encountered, they can be severed using a combination of sharp and blunt dissection techniques (pleurolysis). Endoscopic scissors may be useful and should always be attached to electrocautery. Adhesions can also be freed by gentle traction or cut using electrocautery or laser photocoagulation. When using electrocautery or laser, it may be necessary to remove smoke or laser plume with a suction device. Blebs are effectively removed by electrocautery. Often, a ruptured or even intact bleb may be covered with a small amount of fibrin. Air leaks may or may not be observed, and occasionally, some bleeding around the area of the ruptured bleb is noted. The area of visceral tear is cauterized using electrocautery forceps or an electrocautery probe. This prompts retraction of the visceral pleura. Care is taken to avoid excessive power or duration of electrocautery, since this would promote tissue necrosis and increased air leak. Inflated blebs are easily cauterized by placing the electrocautery device on the bleb. The Nd:YAG laser is used either in the free beam or contact mode. No studies have demonstrated superiority of the laser compared with electrocautery alone. Excessive power and duration should be avoided because substantial visceral and lung parenchymal necrosis may occur.[55–57] Nd:YAG laser energy is preferentially absorbed by pigmented tissues. Laser-tissue interactions, therefore, depend on pigmentation of lung parenchyma (often emphysematous lungs are relatively dark), water content, and power density.

THORACOSCOPIC PLEURODESIS

It is generally believed that pleurodesis significantly decreases the likelihood of recurrent pneumothorax.[15] A limited pleurodesis can be performed at the apex of the pleural cavity, or diffuse pleurodesis may be performed at all visceral and parietal pleural surfaces. Pleurodesis may be performed thoracoscopically using a variety of methods and can be achieved alone or in conjunction with air-leak repair. Mechanical abrasion is accomplished by using a folded gauze or small gauze peanut and grasping forceps placed through the pleural trocar. A Kittner sponge can be placed on a curved Kelly clamp and introduced into the pleural cavity as well. Mechanical abrasion is performed carefully to avoid complete disruption of the parietal pleura. Some oozing of blood will occur as mechanical abrasion is accomplished. Usually, the entire apex is abraded under thoracoscopic visualization. The subclavian vessels should be avoided. A thorough knowledge of pleuropulmonary anatomy is essential. Of course, mechanical abrasion should be performed gently around intercostal neurovascular bundles since intercostal neuralgia or bleeding may occur.

An alternative to thoracoscopic mechanical abrasion is pleurectomy.[58] This, too, can either be localized or extensive. Usually an apical pleurectomy is sufficient but this technique should probably be avoided by pulmonologists because of the risk of laceration of underlying vasculature. The pleura is grasped with forceps and gently cut away from underlying intercostal muscle using a combination of sharp and blunt instruments. Dissection of the parietal pleura away from the chest wall can be facilitated by the subpleural injection of saline solution. Usually, apical pleurectomy is begun by making a small incision of the parietal pleura at the level of the third and fourth intercostal space and peeling the parietal pleura away from the underlying intercostal muscles. Complications include intercostal neuralgia, laceration of intercostal neurovascular bundles, and extensive bleeding.

Mechanical abrasion can also be performed using specially designed commercially available pleural abraders. One such instrument designed by the Richard Wolf Company (Illinois) is a curved, stainless steel instrument with a 5- or 7-mm grooved burr head. When using this abrader, laceration of the parietal pleura and intercostal neurovascular bundles is avoided by rubbing it along the rib surface rather than within the intercostal space.

Thoracoscopic pleurodesis is also accomplished by thoracoscopic talc insufflation or by injection into the pleural space of chemical irritants such as doxycycline or minocycline. The use of antimitotic agents should be avoided in patients with pneumothorax. Talc pleurodesis is often warranted in patients with secondary spontaneous pneumothorax in whom air leaks are difficult to detect or when air leaks are not entirely controlled by endoscopic stapling. Talc pleurodesis allows secondary closure of the bronchopleural fistula and obliteration of the pleural cavity. The results of thoracoscopic talc insufflation have been excellent, but it is unclear whether this procedure should be used in younger patients with primary, recurrent spontaneous pneumothorax. Arguments against talc pleurodesis have included the possibility of these patients developing a pulmonary neoplasm and the need for thoracic surgery years later, and the potential risk of restrictive lung disease due to talc. Neither of these arguments is defensible in previously published literature. Another question that has been of concern in the past pertains to the fibrogenicity of talc and potential development of malignant mesothelioma. This fear is unfounded when asbestos-free talc is used. Several studies have demonstrated that talc is safe, does not induce permanent radiographic alterations, and results in only minor functional sequellae.[59–61]

ENDING THE PROCEDURE

At the end of the thoracoscopic procedure, it is necessary to place one or two chest tubes to accelerate lung reexpansion, remove residual air from pleural cavity, and enhance effective pleurodesis. In the absence of talc pleurodesis, a 20 to 32 Fr straight silicone chest tube is sufficient. The chest tube may be placed through the anterior or midaxillary entry site and directed anteriorly and superiorly. Occasionally, a new incision made especially for chest tube insertion is desirable. Incisions should be kept small to avoid subcutaneous emphysema and facilitate healing. If talc pleurodesis is performed, a large-bore (usually 32 Fr) chest tube is warranted because talc can cause substantial fibrin formation which can obstruct a smaller caliber tube. The chest tube is fixed with 0 silk sutures, and resting sutures are placed for use upon chest tube removal. The other trocar entry sites can be closed in layers. The skin may be closed using separate nylon sutures or a subcuticular stitch. Chest tubes are attached to a negative suction device. A chest radiograph will confirm chest tube position and lung reexpansion. If no postoperative air leak is detected, chest tubes can be removed in 24 to 48 h. This is often the case after thoracoscopic bleb or bullae resection.[62] Postoperatively, chest tube drainage must be monitored carefully. Some tubes need to be milked or stripped to avoid clogging with blood or fibrin. Usually a trial of water-seal drainage is advocated prior to chest tube removal. The average length of time from thoracoscopy to discharge has been 2 to 3 days in most series.[63–68]

REFERENCES

1. Joseph M, et al: Spontaneous pneumothorax: Historical review. *Med J Aust* 1964; 1:1–5.
2. Greene R, et al: Pneumothorax. *Sem Roentgenol* 1977; 4:313–325.
3. Getz SB, Beasley WE: Spontaneous pneumothorax. *Am J Surg* 1983; 145:823–827.
4. Jenkinson SG: Pneumothorax. *Clin Chest Med* 1985; 6:153–161.
5. Bloomberg AE: Thoracoscopy in perspective. *Surg Gynec Obstet* 1978; 147:433–443.
6. Keller R, et al: Die behandlung des persistierenden pneumothorax durch thorakoskopische Mahnahmen. *Thoraxchirugie* 1974; 22:457–460.
7. Sattler A: Zur behandlung des spontanpneumothoraxmit besonder berucksichtigung der thorakoskopie. *Bietr Klin Tuberk* 1937; 89:395–408.
8. Swierenga J, et al: The value of thoracoscopy in the diagnosis and treatment of disease affecting the pleura and lung. *Pneumologie* 1974; 151:11–18.
9. Colt HG: Thoracoscopy: New frontiers. *Pulmonary Perspec* 1992; 9:1–5.
10. Boutin C, et al: Thoracoscopy in the diagnosis and treatment of spontaneous pneumothorax. *Clin Chest Med* 1995; 16: 497–503.
11. Cole FH, et al: Video-assisted thoracic surgery: Primary therapy for spontaneous pneumothorax. *Ann Thorac Surg* 1995; 60:931–935.
12. Liu HP, et al: Thoracoscopic surgery as a routine procedure for spontaneous pneumothorax: Results from 82 patients. *Chest* 1995; 107:559–562.
13. Rivas de Andres JJ, Lanzas LT: Thoracoscopy and spontaneous pneumothorax. *Ann Thorac Surg* 1993; 55:807–814 (letter).
14. Schoenenberger RA, et al: Timing of invasive procedures in therapy for primary and secondary spontaneous pneumothorax. *Arch Surg* 1991; 126:764–766.
15. Light RW: Management of spontaneous pneumothorax. *Am Rev Respir Dis* 1993; 143:245–248.
16. Killen DA, Gobbel WG: *Spontaneous Pneumothorax,* 1st ed. Boston, Little, Brown, 1968.
17. Melton LJ, et al: Incidence of spontaneous pneumothorax in Olmstead County, Minnesota 1950–1974. *Am Rev Respir Dis* 1979; 120:1379–1382.
18. Seremetis MG: The management of spontaneous pneumothorax. *Chest* 1970; 57:65–68.
19. Sharpe IK, et al: Familial spontaneous pneumothorax and HLA antigens. *Chest* 1980; 78:264–268.
20. Almind M, et al: Spontaneous pneumothorax: Comparison of simple drainage, talc pleurodesis, and tetracycline pleurodesis. *Thorax* 1989; 44:627–630.
21. Daniel TM, et al: Thoracoscopy and talc poudrage for pneumothoraces and effusions. *Ann Thorac Surg* 1990; 50:186–189.
22. Donahue DM, et al: Resection of pulmonary blebs and pleurodesis for spontaneous pneumothorax. *Chest* 1993; 104: 1767–1769.
23. Hazelrigg SR, et al: Thoracoscopic stapled resection for spontaneous pneumothorax. *J Thorac Cardiovasc Surg* 1993; 105: 389–393.
24. Light RW, et al: Intrapleural tetracycline for the prevention of recurrent spontaneous pneumothorax. *JAMA* 1990; 164: 2224–2230.
25. Van de Brekel JA, et al: Pneumothorax: Results of thoracoscopy and pleurodesis with talc poudrage and thoracotomy. *Chest* 1993; 103:345–347.
26. Janssen JP, et al: Videothoracoscopic appearance of first and recurrent pneumothorax. *Chest* 1995; 108:330–334.
27. Schramel FM, et al: Prognostic cators in patients with spontaneous pneumothorax treated with video-assisted thoracoscopy. *Diag Therapeut Endosc* 1995; 2:1–5.
28. Noyes BE, Orenstein DM: Treatment of pneumothorax in cystic fibrosis in the era of lung transplantation. *Chest* 1992; 101:1187–1188.
29. Tanaka F, et al: Secondary spontaneous pneumothorax. *Ann Thorac Surg* 1993; 55:372–376.
30. Spector ML, Stern RC: Pneumothorax in cystic fibrosis: A 26 year experience. *Ann Thorac Surg* 1994; 47:204–207.
31. Wait MA, Dal Nogare AR: Treatment of AIDS-related spontaneous pneumothorax. *Chest* 1994; 106:693–696.
32. Slabbynck H, et al: Thoracoscopic findings in spontaneous pneumothorax in AIDS. *Chest* 1994; 106:1582–1586.
33. Metersky ML, et al: AIDS-related spontaneous pneumothorax. *Chest* 1995; 108:946–951.
34. Weissberg D: The surgical management of recurrent or persistent pneumothorax: Pleuroscopy and talc poudrage. In Kittle CF (ed): *Current Controversies in Thoracic Surgery.* Philadelphia, Saunders, 1986:46–50.
35. Waller DA, et al: Videoassisted thoracoscopic surgery versus thoracotomy for spontaneous pneumothorax. *Ann Thorac Surg* 1994; 58:372–377.
36. Vanderschueren RG: The role of thoracoscopy in the evaluation and management of pneumothorax. *Lung* 1990; 168: 627–630.
37. Wakabayashi A: Thoracoscopic ablation of blebs in the treatment of recurrent or persistent spontaneous pneumothorax. *Ann Thorac Surg* 1989; 48:651–653.

38. Jancovici R, et al: Complications of video-assisted thoracic surgery: A five year experience. *Ann Thorac Surg* 1996; 61: 533–537.
39. Brestiker MA, et al: Optimal pleurodesis: A comparison study. *Ann Thorac Surg* 1993; 55:364–367.
40. Maggi G, et al: Pleural abrasion in the treatment of recurrent or persistent spontaneous pneumothorax. Results of 94 consecutive cases. *Int Surg* 1992; 77:99–101.
41. Nathanson LK, et al: Videothoracoscopic ligation of bulla and pleurectomy for spontaneous pneumothorax. *Ann Thorac Surg* 1991; 52:316–319.
42. Nkere UU, et al: Pleural abrasion: A new method of pleurodesis. *Thorax* 1991; 46:596–598.
43. Torre M, Belloni P: Nd:YAG laser pleurodesis through thoracoscopy: New curative therapy in spontaneous pneumothorax. *Ann Thorac Surg* 1989; 47:887–889.
44. Tschopp JM, et al: Successful closure of chronic BPF by thoracoscopy after failure of endoscopic fibrin glue application and thoracoplasty. *Chest* 1990; 97:745–746.
45. Wakabayashi A, et al: Thoracoscopic treatment of spontaneous pneumothorax using carbon dioxide laser. *Ann Thorac Surg* 1990; 50:786–790.
46. Hansen MK, et al: Spontaneous pneumothorax and fibrin glue sealant during thoracoscopy. *Eur J Cardiovasc Surg* 3:512–514.
47. Bagnato VJ: Treatment of recurrent spontaneous pneumothorax. *Surg Laparos Endosc* 1992; 2:100–103.
48. Hazelrigg SR, et al: Video-assisted thoracic surgery study group data. *Ann Thorac Surg* 1993; 56:1039–1044.
49. Murray KD, et al: A limited axillary thoracotomy as primary treatment for recurrent spontaneous pneumothorax. *Chest* 1993; 103:137–142.
50. Cooper JD, Patterson GA: Lung volume reduction surgery for severe emphysema. *Semin Thorac Cardiovasc Surg* 1996; 8:52–60.
51. McKenna RJ, et al: A randomized prospective trial of stapled lung reduction versus laser bullectomy for diffuse emphysema. *J Thorac Cardiovasc Surg* 1996; 111:317–322.
52. Benumof JL: Double lumen tube intubations. *J Bronchol* 1995; 2:59–68.
53. Landreneau RJ, et al: Videoassisted thoracic surgery: Basic technical concepts and intercostal approach strategies. *Ann Thorac Surg* 1992; 54:800–807.
54. Brenner M, et al: Animal model for thoracoscopic laser ablation of emphysematous pulmonary bullae. *Las Surg Med* 1996; 18:191–196.
55. Vanderschueren RG: Le talcage pleural dans le pneumothorax spontanc. *Poumon-Coeur* 1981; 37:273–276.
56. Brenner M, et al: CO_2 and Nd:YAG laser induced pulmonary parenchymal lung injury in a rabbit model. *Am J Respir Crit Care Med* 1996; 153:1136–1140.
57. Sawabata N, et al: In vitro study of ablated lung tissue in Nd:YAG laser irradiation. *Ann Thorac Surg* 1996; 61:164–169.
58. Inderbitzi RGC, et al: Three years' experience in video-assisted thoracic surgery (VATS) for spontaneous pneumothorax. *J Thorac Cardiovasc Surg* 1994; 107:1410–1415.
59. Viskum K, et al: Long term sequelae after talc pleurodesis for spontaneous pneumothorax. *Pneumologie* 1989; 43(2):105–106.
60. Research committee of the British Thoracic Association and the Medical Research Council pneumoconiosis unit. The survey of long term effects of talc and kaolin pleurodesis. *Br J Dis Chest* 1979; 73:285–288.
61. Lange P, et al: Lung function 22–35 years after treatment of idiopathic spontaneous pneumothorax with talc poudrage or simple drainage. *Thorax* 1988; 43:559–561.
62. Hazelrigg SR: Thoracoscopic management of pulmonary blebs and bullae. *Sem Thorac Cardiovasc Surg* 1993; 6:327–331.
63. Naunheim KS, et al: Safety and efficacy of video-assisted thoracic surgical techniques for the treatment of spontaneous pneumothorax. *J Thorac Cardiovasc Surg* 1995; 109:1198–1204.
64. Yim APC, Ho JKS: 100 consecutive cases of video-assisted thoracoscopic surgery for spontaneous pneumothorax. *Surg Endosc* 1995; 9:332–336.
65. Yim APC, Liu HP: Complications and failures of video-assisted thoracic surgery: Experience from two centers in Asia. *Ann Thorac Surg* 1996; 61:538–541.
66. Liu HP, et al: Video-assisted thoracic surgery: Manipulation without trocar in 112 consecutive procedures. *Chest* 1993; 104:452–454.
67. Janssen JP, et al: Treatment of patients with spontaneous pneumothorax during videothoracoscopy. *Eur Respir J* 1994; 7:1281–1284.
68. Melvin WS, et al: Thoracoscopic management of spontaneous pneumothorax. *Chest* 1992; 102:1875–1876.
69. Guerin JC, Boniface E: Les methodes de pleurodese. *Rev Prat* 1990; 40:1854–1856.
70. Olsen PS, Orbaeck AH: Long term results after tetracycline pleurodesis in spontaneous pneumothorax. *Ann Thorac Surg* 1992; 53:1015–1017.

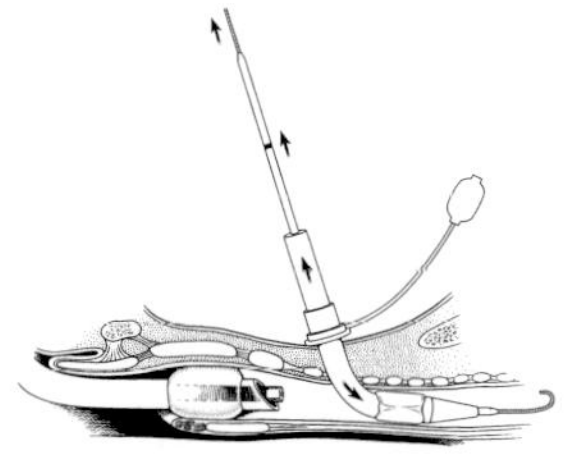

OTHER PROCEDURES

CHAPTER 16

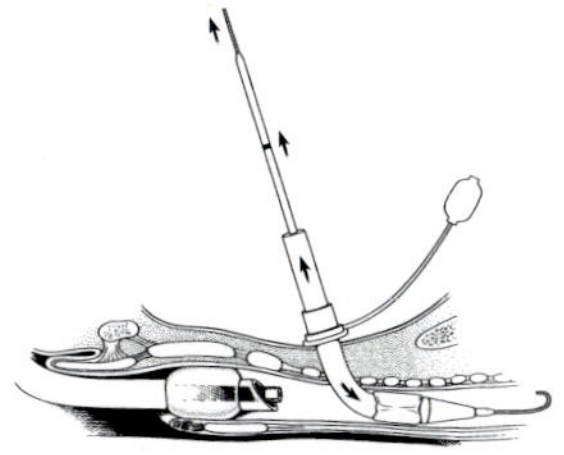

THORACENTESIS AND CLOSED PLEURAL BIOPSY

Raja G. Ogirala and Fiona Meller Azrieli

Thoracentesis

DIAGNOSTIC THORACENTESIS

Indications

Thoracentesis is indicated in every pleural effusion of unclear etiology. Whereas the presence of a pleural effusion is often first noted on a chest radiograph, decubitus views should almost always be performed prior to thoracentesis to confirm that there is indeed a layering effusion. Generally, when the thickness of the layering fluid is at least 10 mm, thoracentesis can be safely performed.[1]

Ultrasound-guided thoracentesis has been shown to significantly improve the yield of fluid in both small loculated and free-flowing pleural effusions but did not reduce the complication rate in large or small effusions.[2] When the clinical impression is fairly certain and the patient is afebrile and without pleurisy, such as a patient with congestive heart failure and bilateral effusions, a thoracentesis can be deferred and the patient treated and observed. It has been suggested, however, that if cardiomegaly is not present in the above circumstance, other possibilities should be explored.[3]

Contraindications

Besides not performing the procedure in an uncooperative patient, there are no absolute contraindications to performing thoracentesis.[4] Relative contraindications include a hemostatic defect, especially in patients receiving anticoagulants and thrombolytics, a cutaneous infection overlying the area to be penetrated, insufficient quantity of fluid, and an unstable medical condition. Attempts to correct a significant coagulopathy should be made before thoracentesis is attempted. Thoracentesis can be performed on mechanically ventilated patients as long as the benefits outweigh the possible risks. In a study of 32 such patients, of whom 11 were receiving positive end-expiratory pressure ranging from 5 to 25 cm H_2O, pneumothoraces occurred in two patients (6 percent). Both patients were on assist-control ventilation but were not receiving positive end-expiratory pressure.[5]

Pleural Fluid Analysis

The first major decision to make in analyzing the etiology of a pleural effusion is to determine if it is a transudate or an exudate. The distinction is made according to Light's criteria. Exudates have at least one of the following (and transudates none): (1) pleural fluid protein to serum protein ratio of >0.5, (2) pleural fluid lactate dehydrogenase (LDH) to serum ratio >0.6, (3) pleural fluid LDH level greater than 200 IU. Light points out that to separate exudates from transudates, the use of the protein and LDH levels simultaneously is superior to either alone[6] (Table 16-1).

Transudates are caused by increased hydrostatic pressure or decreased oncotic pressure. There is no abnormality of the pleural surfaces. Such conditions include congestive heart failure, liver cirrhosis with ascites, and nephrotic syndrome. Such systemic disor-

Table 16-1
CHARACTERISTICS OF PLEURAL EFFUSIONS

Diagnosis	*Color*	*Predominant cell type*
Transudates CHF, cirrhosis, nephrotic syndrome, peritoneal dialysis, urinothorax	Straw colored	Lymphocytes, mesothelial cells, mononuclear cells
Exudates		
Infection		
Parapneumonic (uncomplicated)	Turbid/purulent	PMNs
Empyema	White	PMNs
Tuberculosis	Straw colored/ serosanguinous	Acute—PMNs, chronic—lymphocytes
Amoebic liver abscess	Anchovy colored	PMNs
Aspergillosis	Black	Lymphocytes, mesothelial cells
Malignancy		
Lung cancer Breast cancer	Serous/bloody	Lymphocytes, macrophage, mesothelial cells
Lymphoma	Serous	Few lymphocytes
Mesothelioma	Serous/bloody/ viscous	Mononuclear cells
Connective tissue disease		
SLE	Serous/bloody	PMNs
Rheumatoid arthritis	Yellow-green	Lymphocytes
Miscellaneous		
Pulmonary embolism	Straw colored/ bloody	PMNs
Pancreatitis	Serosanguinous/bloody	PMNs
Chylothorax	Milky/bloody/ turbid/serous	Lymphocytes
Esophageal rupture	Early—serous, late—turbid/purulent	PMNs
Asbestos exposure	Serosanguinous	PMNs, mononuclears, eosinophils

NOTE: PMN, polymorphonuclear leukocytes; PD, peritoneal dialysis; LDH, lactate dehydrogenase; ADA, adenosine deaminase; CEA, carcinoembryonic antigen; EMA, epithelial membrane antigen; ANA, antinuclear antibody; RF, rheumatoid factor.

pH	Diagnostic features	Comments
>7.40	PD—glucose > 300 mg/dl, urinothorax—pleural/serum creat. >1, ammonia odor	Cirrhosis—right sided > 70% Urinothorax—effusion ipsilateral to obstructed kidney
≥7.30	LDH < 500 U/liter Glucose > 60 mg/dl	Resolves with appropriate antibiotics
<7.10 or 0.3 units less than arterial pH	Glucose < 40 mg/dl, LDH > 1000 Pus, positive Gram's stain or culture	Requires antibiotics and immediate drainage
Always <7.40 20% <7.30	Positive AFB smear, culture, ADA > 70 U/liter in absence of empyema/rheum. arthritis	Pleural fluid + tissue → 90 to 95% diagnostic, < 5% Mesothelial cells
	Positive amoebic gel diffusion test	Requires tube drainage
	Positive pleural fluid culture	Brown clumps hyphae suggestive
> or <7.30	Positive cytology/pleural tissue	CEA, B72.3, EMA are all positive in adenocarcinoma
≥7.30 20% <7.30	Positive cytology/flow cytometry	
<7.30	Tissue diagnosis	Increased hyaluronic acid supportive; CEA, B72.3, EMA are all negative
Usually ≥7.30 20% <7.30	Positive LE cells	Low complement Pleural ANA ≥ 1:160, increased immune complexes
<7.20	Glucose < 30 mg/dl	RF ≥ 1:320, low complement
≥7.30	None	Bloody effusion not contra-indication to anticoagulation
7.30–7.35	Pleural fluid/serum amylase > 1	60% left-sided effusions
>7.40	Triglyceride > 110 mg/dl positive chylomicrons	Trauma/surgery or lymphoma
Early ≥7.30, late <7.30	pH 6.00, elevated amylase	May see gross food particles
≥7.30	Presumptive	Often recurrent

ders require medical treatment of the underlying disorder and no further evaluation of the pleural fluid, per se, is warranted.

In contrast, exudative effusions result from increased permeability of the pleural surfaces to protein, impaired lymphatic drainage, or decreased pressure in the pleural space (trapped lung).[7] Exudative effusions require further evaluation to secure a diagnosis and initiate appropriate treatment. Pneumonia, pulmonary malignancy, and pulmonary embolism together account for more than 80 percent of all exudative effusions. Parapneumonic effusions (those associated with bacterial pneumonia or lung abscess) are probably the most common cause of exudative effusions.[4,8]

Parapneumonic effusions evolve through three stages known as the exudative, fibropurulent, and organizing stages; the greater the delay in medical treatment or institution of appropriate antibiotics, the more advanced the stage of the effusion at the time of diagnosis. At first, a subpleural focus of pneumonia with a polymorphonuclear infiltrate causes an increase in pulmonary and pleural capillary permeability with subsequent leakage of a protein-rich sterile fluid into the pleural space. At this early stage, the fluid contains a moderate amount of polymorphonuclear cells, has a normal pH and glucose and LDH <1000 U/liter.[9,10]

Within a few days, without appropriate antibiotics, bacteria invade the pleural space, followed by more polymorphonuclear cells and activated clotting factors which serve as a nidus for collagen deposition. Fibrin sheets cover the visceral and parietal pleura, and loculations form to contain the infection. At this stage, the fluid contains more polymorphonuclear cells, pH and glucose are decreased, LDH is increased, bacterial Gram's stain and culture are positive, and chest tube drainage becomes difficult.[1,11] Unchecked, fibroblasts grow from both pleural surfaces and create an inelastic membrane called a pleural peel, making the underlying lung nonfunctional. At this organizational stage, the pleural fluid is thick pus and an empyema exists.

Parapneumonic effusions are exudates with white blood cell counts >10,000 per microliter with predominantly polymorphonuclear cells.[9] Uncomplicated parapneumonic effusions resolve spontaneously with antibiotics and have the following characteristics: pH $\geq$ 7.30, glucose > 60 mg/dl, LDH < 500 U/liter.[4] Complicated parapneumonic effusions, on the other hand, require chest tube drainage in addition to antibiotics. They are defined by pH < 7.10 and/or glucose < 40 mg/dl, LDH > 1000 U/liter, and positive Gram's stain or culture and may be frankly purulent (empyema).[9] Because pleural fluid pH is influenced by arterial pH, arterial pH should be measured and the pleural fluid pH should be at least 0.30 U less than the arterial pH to qualify for chest tube placement.[12] If the fluid is loculated, thrombolytics may be required in addition to chest tube drainage and, ultimately, a decortication may be necessary.[13–16]

The nature of the effusion cannot be distinguished on clinical grounds alone. Because a parapneumonic effusion can advance quite rapidly, it is imperative that the thoracentesis be performed as early as possible and, if indicated, a chest tube placed immediately. Serial thoracenteses may be required for effusions with a pH between 7.10 and 7.29 to monitor progress and the possible need for chest tube placement if pH decreases.[4] Of note, a low pH as an indiction for chest tube drainage applies only to parapneumonic effusions.

Tuberculous pleurisy may be due to primary tuberculosis or reactivation. Patients are usually febrile and often present with a nonproductive cough and pleuritic chest pain. On presentation 30 percent are purified protein derivative (PPD) negative, but most will convert the skin test 6 to 8 weeks later.[17] The probable explanation for the initial negative PPD is that antigen-reactive T lymphocytes become sequestered in the pleural space during the acute phase of the illness.[18] The tuberculous effusion is usually serous with total protein > 4.0 g/dl, white blood cell count <5000/μl with 90 to 95 percent lymphocytes, and pH < 7.40, and it contains a scarcity (<5 percent) of mesothelial cells.[6,17] Mesothelial cells are lacking in pleural fluid when there is a heavy deposition of fibrin over the mesothelium or destruction of the mesothelium by diffuse inflammation. This prevents the shedding of mesothelial cells into the pleural space.[19] Mesothelial scarcity can also be seen in chronic empyema or malignant tumors.[20] Although the yield from an acid-fast bacillus (AFB) smear is low, pleural fluid culture is positive in 25 to 75 percent of cases.[4,17] A combination of pleural fluid and pleural tissue studies yields a diagnosis in 90 to 95 percent of cases of tuberculous pleuritis.[4]

Pleural effusion due to aspergillosis is uncommon but may be seen in patients who have undergone lobectomy or pneumonectomy for tuberculosis or lung cancer (usually with a bronchopleural fistula), those treated with pneumothorax therapy for tuberculosis in the past, immunosuppressed hosts with systemic aspergillosis and in association with allergic bronchopulmonary aspergillosis.[21–25] Pleural fluid is black if due to *Aspergillus niger* but can also be serous or serosanguinous.[26] The diagnosis is suggested by brown clumps of fungal hyphae on Gram's stain and confirmed by culture.[21] Treatment involves surgical resection and intravenous amphotericin B or chest tube placement with intrapleural amphotericin B.[21,22,25]

Amoebic hepatic abscesses may cause pleural effusions by either diaphragmatic irritation leading to a sympathetic right-sided effusion or direct rupture of the abscess through the diaphragm into the pleural space.[27,28] With the latter, the pleural fluid is thick brown or anchovy colored. The parasite usually cannot be isolated, and the diagnosis is confirmed by a positive amoebic gel-diffusion test.[28] Treatment consists of drainage with a large chest tube and metronidazole.[28] It is important to note that one-third of these patients have a coexisting bacterial infection that also requires treatment.[4]

Malignant pleural effusions are most commonly due to primary lung cancer, followed by breast cancer, with ovarian and gastric cancer representing 5 percent and unknown primary sites responsible for 7 percent.[29] Malignant effusions may be serous, serosanguinous, or grossly bloody. Primary lung cancer may extend directly to the pleura (grossly bloody effusion) or cause endobronchial obstruction with trapped lung and a resultant paramalignant effusion.[4] Effusions due to other primary cancers are usually due to tertiary spread to the pleura from existing liver metastases.[30] Commonly malignant effusions have red blood cell counts of 30,000 to 50,000 per microliter and, half the time, have 50 percent lymphocytes.[31,32] Five percent of patients with lung cancer have paramalignant effusions, which are due to the malignancy but are not due to direct pleural involvement, or effusions from another cause. These patients may be operative candidates.[33]

When the differential diagnosis is narrowed to malignancy and tuberculosis, pleural biopsy can often make the distinction. Adenosine deaminase may also provide a basis for discrimination as a level >30 IU/liter indicates a tuberculous effusion and <30 IU/L a parapneumonic or malignant pleural effusion.[34]

Lymphomas account for about 10 percent of malignant pleural effusions. Effusions are more commonly due to non-Hodgkin's lymphoma (direct pleural infiltration) than Hodgkin's (impaired lymphatic drainage).[4,29,35] Up to 25 percent of the pleural effusions secondary to lymphoma are chylous.[36]

Pleural effusions due to both malignant mesothelioma and benign asbestos pleurisy are usually unilateral (mesotheliomas being right-sided 60 percent of the time), may be serous, serosanguinous or bloody, and have low leukocyte counts.[31,37–40] Malignant mesotheliomas are associated with asbestos exposure (dose-dependent relationship unknown), have a long latency (>30 years), and usually present with symptoms.[37,41,42] The benign exudative pleural effusion associated with asbestos exposure has a strong dose-dependent relationship with asbestos exposure and a short latency and is often asymptomatic at presentation.[39,43] High hyaluronic acid levels cause a viscous pleural effusion and support a diagnosis of malignant mesothelioma, whereas elevated eosinophil counts (up to 50 percent) support a diagnosis of benign exudative pleural effusion associated with asbestos exposure.[40,44] Eosinophil counts > 10 percent are also seen with pneumothorax, blood in the pleural space, and resolving infection.[8]

It is difficult to distinguish benign from malignant mesothelioma cells cytologically, and often thoracotomy or thoracoscopy is required to provide enough tissue to diagnose malignant mesothelioma.[45–47] Benign exudative pleural effusion associated with asbestos exposure is diagnosed presumptively in an appropriate clinical setting. These benign effusions usually resolve after 3 to 4 months with residual costophrenic angle blunting and possible diffuse pleural thickening; follow-up for 2 to 3 years is usually required to exclude mesothelioma.[39,43,48]

Lupus pleuritis is the presenting manifestation in 5 percent of patients with systemic lupus erythematosis (SLE) but there is pleural involvement (pleural effusion or pain) in 50 to 75 percent of patients during the course of the disease.[49–51] Lupus pleuritis is usually associated with a lupus exacerbation and accompanied by pleuritic chest pain and fever.[52] Patients with rheumatoid pleurisy usually have moderate to severe arthritis and subcutaneous nodules and are not commonly febrile.[52,53] Effusions due to both lupus and rheumatoid pleuritis have white blood cell counts ranging from several hundred to 20,000 cells per microliter with an early polymorphonuclear predominance and later lymphocyte predominance.[52,54,55] Lupus effusions may be serous, bloody, or turbid.[4] Rheumatoid effusions may be turbid with a yellow-green tint or milky (chyliform or pseudochylous effusion) owing to cholesterol or appear to contain debris and frequently have LDH > 1000 U/liter.[55–58] Rheumatoid effusions generally have low glucose and pH with two-thirds having glucose < 30 mg/dl at first evaluation.[54,56,59,60] In contrast, lupus effusions usually have a normal glucose and pH. If LE cells are seen, they are diagnostic.[52,61]

Pleural fluid with antinuclear antibodies (ANA) ≥ 1:160 or pleural fluid/serum ANA ≥ 1 is likely secondary to lupus pleuritis, whereas a negative pleural fluid ANA or ANA titer less than serum titer in a patient with SLE signifies an effusion from another etiology.[52] Rheumatoid factor levels up to 1:160 may be seen in infectious and malignant effusions, but titers ≥ 1:320, or at least as high as the serum titer, are generally only seen in rheumatoid pleural effusions.[8,62]

Both rheumatoid and lupus effusions have low total hemolytic complement and low complement component levels.[55,62,63] Both also have higher pleural fluid immune complex levels than in effusions of other causes.[62–64] Although there are no controlled studies regarding the use of corticosteroids or NSAIDs in rheumatoid pleurisy, active lupus pleuritis responds dramatically to corticosteroids and spontaneous resolution does not usually occur.[51,63]

Pleural effusions occur in 30 to 50 percent of patients with pulmonary embolism. These are often exudates, but transudates have been described in 20 percent of patients with pulmonary embolism.[65–67] More than 35 percent of patients with pulmonary embolism but no radiographic evidence of infarction have hemorrhagic effusions, and if infarction is present, more than 80 percent of patients have bloody effusions.[65] The effusion is usually small, unilateral, and accompanied by ipsilateral chest pain, even though the emboli may be bilateral.[65] The effusion may or may not be accompanied by infiltrate.[65] Without consolidation, the effusions usually resolve in less than 1 week, but with consolidation, the effusion is usually larger and takes longer to resolve.[65] Pleural fluid analysis is highly variable and nondiagnostic in pulmonary embolism.[4] An initial bloody effusion is not a contraindication to full-dose anticoagulation.[67]

An elevated pleural fluid amylase occurs in three conditions: pancreatitis, malignancy, and esophageal perforation.[68] In acute pancreatitis the effusion is usually small; 60 percent are left-sided. The initial pleural amylase level may be normal but will subsequently rise to the level where pleural fluid/serum amylase > 1. These effusions are probably due to lymphatic transport of amylase from the peritoneal to the pleural cavity, impaired lymphatic drainage from the pleural space, and increased amylase clearance by the kidney.[4,68,69] Pleural white blood cell counts may be up to 50,000 cells per microliter with a polymorphonuclear predominance; glucose level is the same as serum, and pH is between 7.30 and 7.35.[68] In chronic pancreatitis, the effusion may be massive and the amylase is always elevated, occasionally reaching > 1000 U/liter.[70,71] Management involves treatment of the underlying condition, with thoracentesis and possible chest tube placement for the effusion.[4]

In esophageal perforation, the pleural fluid amylase is markedly elevated and is of salivary origin from swallowed saliva.[72–74] In 75 percent of patients with spontaneous esophageal rupture, pneumothorax occurs due to violation of the mediastinal pleura; 70 percent are on the left side.[75] Pleural effusion occurs in 75 percent of perforations with or without pneumothorax.[76] When mediastinal pleural rupture has occurred, anaerobic organisms from the mouth seed the pleural space, amylase is very high, and the pH decreases to 6.00 secondary to pleural fluid leukocyte metabolism.[77] When the mediastinal pleura is intact, the pleural fluid is sterile, polymorphonuclear cells predominate, and the amylase and pH are normal.[73]

Milky pleural fluid may be due to a chylothorax, pseudochylothorax, or an effusion with a large number of leukocytes. Increased lipid is confirmed by a cloudy supernatant after centrifugation. A chylothorax occurs when either the thoracic duct is ruptured and lymph leaks into the pleural space or chylous ascites moves into the pleural space.[78] Etiologies include mediastinal malignancies (50 percent), especially lymphoma, thoracic surgery (20 percent), and trauma (<5 percent).[79–83] The fluid is usually milky but may be bloody, turbid, or serous (malnourished patients), has a lymphocytic predominance, pH > 7.40, and glucose level equal to that of serum.[4,79]

Several features distinguish chylothorax from pseudochylothorax. Patients with chylothorax are usually acutely ill, have a large unilateral effusion with total lipid > 400 mg/dl, cholesterol 65 to 220 mg/dl, triglyceride > 110 mg/dl, and triglyceride greater than twice serum triglyceride. Chylomicrons, if seen, are diagnostic.[4,79,80,84,85] Patients with pseudochylothorax are more chronically ill, with effusions due to rheumatoid or tuberculous pleurisy of long duration (average 5 years), increased total lipids, high cholesterol due to degeneration of cells, triglyceride level < 50 mg/dl, and no chylomicrons but have lecithin globulin complexes.[79,86–88] Treatment for chylothorax is conservative, with an aim toward maintaining adequate nutrition. Pleural space drainage is indicated to relieve dyspnea.[80,82–84] If fluid persists or increases, thoracic duct ligation or pleurodesis may be necessary.[89,90] Treatment of pseudochylothorax involves treating the underlying condition, and, if necessary, therapeutic thoracentesis and possible decortication.[91,92]

It is important to distinguish bloody fluid caused by a traumatic thoracentesis from a frankly bloody effusion, since merely 1 to 2 ml of peripheral blood in 1000 ml of pleural fluid will cause red discoloration.[7] Peripheral blood in pleural fluid should clot within a few minutes, whereas blood secondary to pleural disease will not clot since it defibrinates with time.[7] A bloody effusion can be confirmed with a pleural fluid to peripheral blood hematocrit ratio greater than 0.5.

Proper technique for acquisition and handling of pleural fluid is most important. Pleural fluid for pH analysis needs to be anaerobically handled and maintained on ice. For cytologic analysis, as much fluid as possible should be submitted, minimum 25 to 50 ml. If a therapeutic thoracentesis is performed, several hundred milliliters can be submitted. Heparin needs to be added to the fluid to prevent clotting and optimize cytologic analysis. It is important to remember, however, that if a pleural biopsy may be required, only the minimal amount of pleural fluid necessary for diagnostic testing should be removed so as not to increase the risk of or possibly even preclude the pleural biopsy.

Complications

The most common major complication associated with thoracentesis is pneumothorax, with occurrence rates between 3 and 20 percent.[93] The air is introduced into the pleural space either from within, due to a puncture of the lung, or from without, as a consequence of air being allowed to leak through the needle or catheter. Most of these pneumothoraces do not require chest tube placement.[93,94] Factors that have been found to correlate with an increased risk of pneumothorax include malignancy, cough during the procedure, and therapeutic thoracentesis where large bore needles are used and there is more manipulation of equipment.[94] There may be an increased incidence of pneumothorax in patients with underlying chronic obstructive pulmonary disease (COPD).[95]

Other common complications include cough, pain at the site, dry tap, and vasovagal reactions.[93,94] Much less common complications include infection of the pleural space; intercostal artery laceration; lacerations of kidney, liver, and spleen; air embolism; catheter fragment left in the pleural space; tumor seeding of needle tract; and abdominal hemorrhage.[1,7,8,94,96–99]

THERAPEUTIC THORACENTESIS

Indications

A therapeutic thoracentesis is indicated to relieve the symptom of dyspnea due to a large pleural effusion often secondary to an underlying malignancy. While hypoxemia is frequently exacerbated for several hours after the procedure, the relief from the sensation of dyspnea may be due to the reduction in size of the thoracic cage.[100,101] In addition, a large-volume thoracentesis allows the underlying lung to be properly evaluated. It also can temporarily relieve dyspnea in conditions with large pleural effusions that are usually treated medically but are refractory to treatment, such as congestive heart failure, cirrhosis with ascites, and nephrotic syndrome. These effusions, however, tend to reaccumulate rapidly and the additional protein losses associated with fluid removal are usually ill-afforded.

When dyspneic patients with radiographic features suggestive of a large pleural effusion do not tolerate the removal of even small amounts of fluid, the possibility of an underlying trapped lung should be considered. Measuring pleural pressures to determine the time to terminate the procedure not only makes this simple procedure more cumbersome but also increases the cost of the procedure. Simple measures, such as questioning the patient regarding symptoms and monitoring closely for certain signs, are adequate to determine when to stop the procedure. Onset of cough and chest tightness are important warning signs to end the procedure. If the procedure is continued in the presence of these signs, patients will usually develop shortness of breath and further distress.

Complications

Besides those listed for diagnostic thoracentesis, therapeutic thoracentesis has the additional complications of reexpansion pulmonary edema, hypovolemia, and hypoxemia. The former two are seen when more than 1000 to 1500 ml of pleural fluid is removed in a single thoracentesis.[1,102,103] Supplemental oxygen during and for several hours after the procedure alleviates the hypoxemia.[100]

Closed Pleural Biopsy

HISTORICAL BACKGROUND

The introduction of needle biopsy of the parietal pleura by De Francis and coworkers in 1955[104] was followed 3 years later by the introduction of the Abrams and the Cope pleural biopsy needles.[105,106] This began the era of the closed pleural biopsy, providing a safe and easy bedside procedure to evaluate patients suspected of having pleural disease.

INDICATION

Pleural biopsy is indicated for the definitive evaluation of an exudative effusion of unknown origin.

CONTRAINDICATIONS

The procedure should not be attempted in a combative and uncooperative patient. It is also contraindicated in patients with pyoderma or herpes zoster involving the area of proposed procedure site. The procedure should not be performed in patients with empyema. A severe coagulation defect would be a relative contraindication; however, following correction of the coagulopathy, the procedure can be performed safely. In patients with limited respiratory reserve and a large exudative effusion of unclear etiology, the procedure may actually provide immediate benefit if the pleural biopsy is followed by therapeutic thoracentesis. However, a complication such as a pneumothorax can be especially problematic in these patients; therefore, prior to starting the procedure, one must ensure that prompt measures to deal with unwanted complications are available.

COMPARISON OF THE NEEDLES

The yield of positive pleural specimens using the Cope or the Abrams needles is variable, and the reported success rate of obtaining pleural tissue was about 70 percent in previous studies.[107–112] Skill of the operator performing the procedure,[113] biopsies close to the diaphragm,[114] performing multiple biopsies,[115] and altering the position of the Abrams needle to lie parallel to the parietal pleural can improve the yield of pleural tissue.

To decrease patient discomfort, multiple biopsies can be performed with the Abrams or the O&S pleural biopsy needles (between 3 o'clock and 9 o'clock positions) during a single entry into the pleural space. In contrast, it is necessary to repeat the maneuver several times while using the Cope pleural biopsy needle because only one specimen can be obtained during a single entry.

Because of the closed system, the risk of pneumothorax with the Abrams and the O&S biopsy needles is decreased during biopsy. In comparison, the Cope biopsy needle is an open system, and inadvertent leak of outside air into the pleural space is more likely during biopsy. After obtaining biopsies with the Abrams and the O&S biopsy needles (unlike the Cope biopsy needle), therapeutic thoracentesis can also be performed. The O&S biopsy needle's inner trochar point, which faces the lung, is relatively blunt compared with that of the Abrams biopsy needle, thus making fluid removal safer with the former needle.

The external diameter of the O&S biopsy needle is 3 mm compared with 4 mm of the Abrams pleural biopsy needle. An animal study showed the O&S biopsy needle to be safe, and despite its smaller external diameter, to yield a significantly larger pleural specimen compared with the Abrams biopsy needle.[116] In patients with pleural effusions, the O&S biopsy needle was again noted to yield a significantly larger pleural tissue sample, and also to significantly increase the diagnostic yield of pleural biopsies compared with the Abrams pleural biopsy needle.[117] When comparing the Abrams and Cope needles, the diagnostic yields are similar, but the former provides larger specimens and is superior in detecting mesothelial cells.[118]

In view of the above studies, and until results of other ongoing studies are available delineating the role of existing pleural biopsy needles, we advocate the use of the O&S pleural biopsy needle as the needle of choice in the evaluation of parietal pleura in patients with exudative pleural effusions. The Abrams pleural biopsy needle still has an important role. It should be used in elderly patients with poor tissue turgor and in patients with markedly crowded intercostal spaces (such as those with severe kyphosis or kyphoscoliosis). In patients with loss of tissue turgor, the biopsy flap of the O&S needle may become embedded too deeply in the subpleural tissue, and in patients with distorted and extremely narrowed intercostal spaces (since the biopsy flap opens beyond the cross-sectional area of the needle) there is a remote possibility of danger to the intercostal vessels or the nerve.

COMPLICATIONS

Pleural biopsy is a safe procedure, especially in experienced hands. In our experience complications have been quite rare, and we believe this can be achieved by careful screening of the patients, proper understanding of the technique and instruments, and meticulous implementation of the procedure. The reported frequency of pneumothorax is between 3 and 15 percent.[119] In asymptomatic patients with small pneumothoraces, these most probably represent leakage of atmospheric air into the pleural space via the biopsy instrument or through the incision site. In symptomatic patients with large pneumothoraces, these probably denote laceration of a lung during the procedure. Rare reported complications in the literature include injury to the intercostal vessels resulting in hemothorax,[119] development of an arteriovenous fistula,[120] and finally injury to the adjacent structures such as kidney, liver, and spleen.[121] In patients with malignant pleural effusion undergoing pleural biopsy, subsequent tumor seeding of the biopsy tract has also been noted.[122]

HOW I DO IT

Technique for Thoracentesis

The procedure needs to be explained carefully to the patient and informed consent obtained. The physician should talk to the patient during the procedure, explaining what is about to take place each step of the way. This will help to allay any fears and relax the patient. Always have 1.0 mg atropine readily available for emergent use should the patient develop a vasovagal reaction. Wait for the injection of local anesthetic to take effect, and try not to rush through the procedure, as this can occasionally result in unwanted complications. The patient should be comfortably seated on the edge of the bed, near the foot end with the procedure site closest to the foot of the bed. The bed should be raised with the patient's feet supported on a footstool, the head and arms resting on an adjustable table. This position enables the patient to sit upright and the operator to work unencumbered. During the entire procedure the patient's back should remain straight to prevent the pleural fluid from drifting anteriorly.

During the procedure, the following steps are recommended:

1. The procedure site is determined with the help of the radiograph and by locating the fluid on physical examination. After identifying the area of entry, the patient's chest wall is cleansed thoroughly with an antiseptic solution, and a sterile drape with a central hole is taped over the area. The needle should be inserted a few centimeters lateral to the spine, in the intercostal space, just above the superior margin of the rib below, to avoid the intercostal vessels and nerve that run in the inferior sulcus of each rib. The skin, subcutaneous tissue, and muscle are infiltrated with 2% lidocaine, first raising a superficial wheal with a short and small gauge needle (e.g., 25 gauge), then penetrating deeper with a larger needle (e.g., 21 gauge, 1.5 in. long). Before each injection aspiration is attempted to ensure the anesthetic agent is not injected into a blood vessel. The area of anesthesia is extended beyond the rib into the pleura.

2. Allow some time for the anesthetic agent to take effect. To the same needle attach a 50- to 60-ml syringe with 1-ml heparin (1000 U/ml). Heparin is added to prevent the occasional formation of a coagulum in the pleural fluid sample, since this can result in underestimation of the pleural fluid constituents especially the pleural fluid protein. The needle is gently pushed through the parietal pleura, aspirating while advancing. A sudden lessening of the force necessary to advance the needle ("give in") is often a clue to entry into the pleural space along with the aspiration of pleural fluid (Fig. 16-1).

3. If no pleural fluid is obtained after entering the pleural space, the following should be considered: the pleural fluid is too viscous, and a larger needle (e.g., 19 gauge or larger) is required; the needle is too short and does not reach the pleural space (in this case a longer needle or a 2 in. angiocath can be used); the needle is at a higher level than the fluid meniscus, and air bubbles may be aspirated indicating the needle's entry into the lung; the needle shaft is occluded by pleural fluid debris, intercostal muscle, or thickened pleura (this can be confirmed by noting that the syringe cannot be filled with air after removing the syringe needle assembly from the pleural space); and, finally, there is too low an entry. If air is obtained with a small needle, it is usually of no consequence and the procedure should be continued with the needle inserted at a different site.

4. Once the fluid is obtained, the needle is removed and the site covered with a bandage.

Technique for Therapeutic Thoracentesis

The technique of performing therapeutic thoracentesis is similar to that described for diagnostic thoracentesis; however, since a larger amount of fluid is to be aspirated and the inadvertent puncture of the reexpanding lung must be prevented, it is preferable to use plastic or Teflon catheters. If the larger, rigid, and reusable needles are used, care should be taken to at least secure a surgical clamp to the needle at its entry site to avoid unnecessarily deep penetration. We prefer to use the 2-in.-long, 18- or 16-gauge angiocath, attached to a syringe and introduced into the pleural space. Once pleural fluid is aspirated into the syringe, the catheter is advanced into the pleural space, the needle removed, and its protruding orifice immediately occluded with a finger. The catheter is now connected to a syringe via a three-way stopcock. The side port of the latter is connected to a vacuum bottle through high-pressure plastic tubing, and the fluid is allowed to drain.

When using the vacuum bottles, we advocate using the 1-liter bottle first, and if further fluid is to be removed, the 500-ml bottle, which exerts less pressure, should then be used. We have found that the rapid removal of fluid during the terminal portion of the procedure can exacerbate respiratory symptoms. In addition, if on connection to the vacuum bottle, there is no flow of fluid, it is worth trying another vacuum bottle, since occasionally the bottles are defective. On completion, the catheter is removed and an adhesive bandage immediately applied.

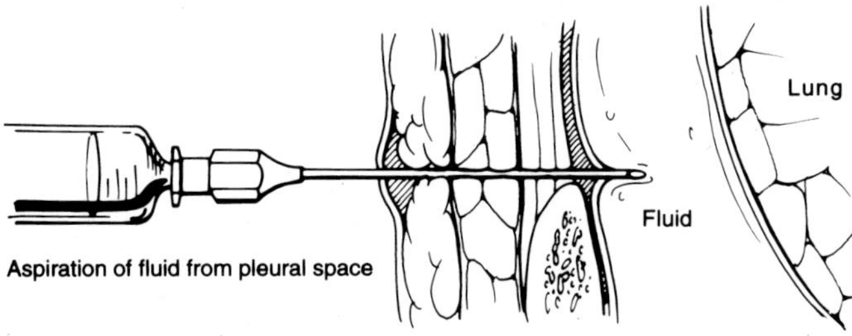

Figure 16-1

Thoracentesis.

Equipment

Commercially available thoracentesis kits are becoming popular because they are all reasonably and comparably priced (ranging from $30 to $35), especially when purchased in bulk; they are all disposable; and finally, they contain all the necessary items for thoracentesis. The only additional items one needs along with these kits are a pair of sterile gloves and a vacuum bottle. We have evaluated the kits described below and our impressions are included in their brief descriptions. One should also carefully read the well written instruction manuals accompanying these kits and become acquainted with the components contained within them.

The only major drawback to most of these kits is that a skin incision, and sometimes a rather deep incision, has to be made to allow passage of the catheter assembly. We have noticed an initially clear straw-colored effusion occasionally turns into a hemorrhagic effusion in a subsequent thoracentesis. This may be related to the deep scalpel incision made during the initial thoracentesis. If the incision site has not been properly sealed, pleural fluid also tends to continue to leak, even after the procedure has been completed. We have described the technique of applying the bandage to seal the incision site in the pleural biopsy section. The slightest bleeding into the pleural space can also materially affect such studies as the cell count, color, protein, and LDH. So, these kits should *not* be used for diagnostic thoracentesis. In procedures combining diagnostic with therapeutic thoracentesis, first remove 60 ml using a 21-gauge needle for diagnostic purposes before proceeding with the therapeutic thoracentesis using the kits. The introducer needle should never be advanced back into the catheter after it has been partially withdrawn from the pleural space since the catheter sheath may be sheared off into the pleural space. Our evaluations and impressions of commercially available thoracentesis kits follows:

1. *The Arrow-Clarke Thoracentesis Kit.* This includes an 8 Fr multiorificed soft catheter mounted on a long introducer needle. A deep incision is made to facilitate the introduction of the needle into the pleural space. Once fluid is aspirated, confirming entry into the pleural space, the catheter is advanced into the pleural space and the needle removed. Once the needle is removed, the pleuraseal valve prevents the needle from being reinserted. A black marking band on the catheter denotes that the most proximal side hole is 1 cm away in the pleural space. During the procedure, ensure that the catheter does not come out of the chest wall beyond the black marking band; otherwise air can leak into the pleural space. The procedure can be completed using the tubes provided which have flow-directing valves. The tubing can be connected to either the collection bag or the vacuum bottle.

The only minor problem we encountered with the kit was that if the skin incision was not deep and wide enough, the catheter's proximal end occasionally failed to traverse along with the introducer needle and became curled up on the needle in the intercostal muscles. In such instances the catheter fails to advance over the needle into the pleural space despite the aspiration of pleural fluid into the syringe. The proximal end of the catheter is softer compared with the remaining stiff catheter. A larger and deeper incision usually rectifies this problem.

2. *The Argyle Turkel Safety Thoracentesis System.* This includes a 12.5-cm catheter mounted on a 16-gauge needle. The needle has a spring-incorporated safety cannula which withdraws into the shaft of the needle during penetration through the chest wall, and once in the pleural space it extends beyond the sharp needle, thus protecting the underlying lung from inadvertent puncture. There are also safety color features in the needle hub: it turns red when the sharp needle tip is advanced through tissue and green when the safety cannula extends beyond the needle bevel. The shaft also has a one-way valve. As mentioned above, during aspiration do not withdraw the catheter from the chest wall beyond the 1-cm mark, since outside air may leak into the pleural space through the side holes situated at the proximal end of the catheter. Safety features of the tubing and technique are similar to the earlier described kit.

3. *Pharmaseal Thoracentesis Catheter Tray.* This includes a 7-in. flexible radiopaque catheter introduced through a short 2-in. needle and a one-way fluid direction valve. After the catheter has been introduced into the pleural space, the needle is withdrawn and the needle hub snapped into place. It is extremely important to place the butterfly clamp over the needle point to protect the catheter from accidental shearing.

4. *Baxter Thoracentesis Catheter.* This incorporates an 18-gauge introducer needle with an 8 Fr catheter and has similar safety features as the Arrow Clarke needle. The technique of using this kit is the same as described above.

Thoracentesis in Special Settings

Thoracentesis can be adapted to the following special settings:

1. Debilitated and sick patients. The procedure can be performed with the patient lying in bed, on the side containing the pleural effusion, in the lateral decubitus position near the edge of the bed. Alternatively, in a hospital bed where the head of the bed has been maximally elevated, the patient can lie with the side of the body not undergoing thoracentesis leaning against the raised head of the bed.

2. Intubated patients on a mechanical ventilator. Always use catheters in this situation. During introduction of the needle, if the patient is not positive end-expiratory pressure (PEEP) sensitive, transiently remove PEEP, if possible, or decrease the tidal volume by 50 to 100 ml and temporarily increase the inspired fraction of oxygen. Also, if toward the end of the procedure, the lung is felt to touch the catheter, the procedure should be terminated.

3. Ultrasound-guided thoracentesis. This should always be performed at the same time as the ultrasound guidance is provided. Marking the area and sending the patient to a different area for the procedure or a time delay is not recommended, since even slight movement of the marked area on the skin or shift of the fluid can result in a dry tap or even a pneumothorax.

4. Simple aspiration of the spontaneous pneumothorax. Since its introduction in 1981, this procedure has gained increasing acceptance.[123] Simple aspiration of the pneumothorax has been noted to be effective in 42 of 64 patients.[124] Spontaneous pneumothorax can be aspirated using the above-described thoracentesis kits or, alternatively, using the Argyle Turkel Safety Pneumothorax System, especially designed for this purpose. During this procedure, there is no need to use a vacuum bottle; aspirated air from the pleural space can be expelled into the atmosphere manually.

Technique for Pleural Biopsy

The positioning of the patient, aseptic preparation of the procedure site, and instillation of local anesthesia are the same as described in the thoracentesis section of this chapter. However, there are two additional caveats for performing a pleural biopsy. One should not do pleural biopsies close to the diaphragm on the left side, since there have been previous reports of splenic hematoma and laceration of the spleen requiring splenectomy.[121,125] Also, a liberal amount of lidocaine should be used to anesthetize the area beyond the rib into the pleura. Once inside the pleural space, with the 21-gauge needle, the presence of pleural fluid should be confirmed by aspirating before making the skin incision. The following technique is recommended:

1. An incision is made through the skin and subcutaneous tissue using a no. 11 scalpel blade. The skin incision should be wide and deep enough to allow easy passage of the biopsy needle.

2. The biopsy needle is advanced through the incision. Applying firm pressure with a twisting motion, the biopsy needle is gradually "popped" through the parietal pleura. During this maneuver, the needle should be firmly supported with the free hand close to the skin to prevent accidental penetration injury to the lung. Alternatively, the index finger of the operating hand placed along the shaft of the needle also provides better leverage.

3. The biopsies can then be performed using one of the biopsy needles described below. Occasionally in patients with narrowed interspaces, difficulty may be encountered pushing the biopsy needle into the pleural space. Maneuvers to widen the interspace such as raising the ipsilateral shoulder and positioning the patient's arm above the head should be tried to enable passage of the needle into the pleural space.[1]

4. Once biopsy specimens have been obtained, the biopsy needle is withdrawn and the incision site immediately occluded with the finger to prevent outside air from leaking into the pleural space. The adhesive half wing of a bandage is anchored on one side of the skin incision, then pulled across the incision while pinching the skin on either side of the incision together; the remaining adhesive half wing is then firmly attached to the skin on the other side of the incision. This causes the incision site to be well puckered between the skin folds. This method obviates the need for skin sutures even in patients with poor tissue turgor. The remainder of the skin is cleansed with alcohol to remove the antiseptic solution which may be irritating to some patients.

5. Following completion of the procedure, the patient should be informed about the availability of analgesics if any pain should develop. In addition, the patient's vital signs are also monitored, and a chest radiograph is obtained and reviewed.

ABRAMS NEEDLE

The Abrams needle (Fig. 16-2) has two concentric tubes and an inner solid stylet. The large outer trocar has a diameter of 4 mm and a short trocar point that is sharp enough to penetrate the chest wall after a scalpel incision has been made through the skin, but will not puncture the lung if the effusion is completely aspirated. The outer trocar has a small hollow lateral opening at its distal end, the biopsying orifice. The inner cutting cannula (inner tube) fits into the outer trocar, and both tubes have proximal hexagonal collars (hand grips). The indicator knob on the outer trocar's hexagonal collar indicates the position of the biopsy orifice. Twisting the inner cutting cannula clockwise or counterclockwise in the outer trocar will close or open the biopsy orifice of the outer trocar (Fig. 16-3*A*). The Abrams biopsy needle is assembled with the stylet inside the inner cutting cannula and the outer trocar mounted over the inner cannula.

CONVENTIONAL TECHNIQUE

When using the conventional technique, the following steps are recommended:

1. Following entry into the pleural space, the inner stylet is removed and a 20-ml syringe attached to the Luer fittings of the inner cutting cannula.

2. The biopsy orifice is now opened by turning the inner cutting cannula counterclockwise, and fluid is aspirated into the syringe to confirm its position in the

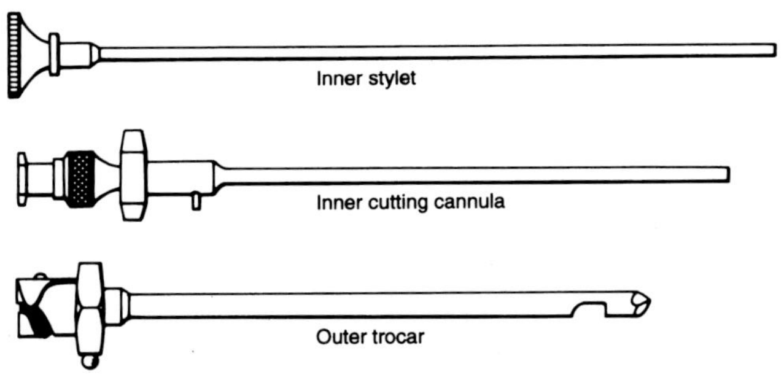

Figure 16-2

Abrams biopsy needle.

pleural space. Rotate the entire pleural biopsy needle and the syringe assembly so that the knob in the hexagonal collar is in the caudad position, that is, the biopsying orifice is facing the rib below (Fig. 16-3*B*). Now withdraw the entire needle assembly until a tug or resistance is felt, and at this point raise the needle to a 30-degree angle to the pleura (Fig. 16-3*C*). Holding the outer trocar firmly, the inner cannula is twisted clockwise, cutting off the pleura specimen while closing the biopsy orifice.

3. The biopsy specimen can then be aspirated with the pleural fluid into the syringe, and multiple biopsies can be performed before withdrawing the pleural biopsy needle. Alternatively, individual biopsies can be obtained with repeated needle entries.

MODIFIED TECHNIQUE

Although this method of pleural biopsy is slightly complicated, the increased yield of pleural specimen makes the technique well worth mastering.[126,127] The technique becomes less cumbersome if a glass syringe is used. This method is more commonly used in England. The technique uses the following steps:

1. Once inside the pleural space the Abrams needle's biopsying orifice is opened and fluid aspirated to confirm its position. The instrument is then slowly withdrawn while slight traction is applied to the plunger of the 50-ml glass syringe until the point is reached where fluid is no longer aspirated.

2. The apparatus is advanced again about 1 cm into the effusion and is then tilted laterally through 90 degrees until the syringe and needle lie parallel to the ribs. In this position the knob on the collar of the Abrams needle should be pointing toward the operator, indicating that the orifice is now facing the parietal pleura and pleural fluid can be aspirated.

3. The collar of the Abrams needle is held firmly between the thumb and index finger of the left hand with the barrel of the syringe lying loosely in the palm. With traction applied to the plunger, the apparatus is then tilted even further laterally until fluid can no longer be aspirated. The orifice is now lying against the parietal pleura.

4. The traction is maintained on the plunger to draw parietal pleura into the orifice, and the biopsy is completed by twisting the syringe clockwise, to advance the cutting edge.

5. The apparatus is returned medially through 90 degrees and advanced about 1 cm to tear off the biopsy specimen, if it has not been completely severed by the cutting edge. The biopsy needle is then withdrawn from the pleural space.

O&S BIOPSY NEEDLE

The O&S biopsy needle, which was formerly called the Raja needle, has a unique self-opening biopsy flap that has been designed to scrape parietal pleura into the biopsy orifice. The biopsy flap opens beyond the cross-

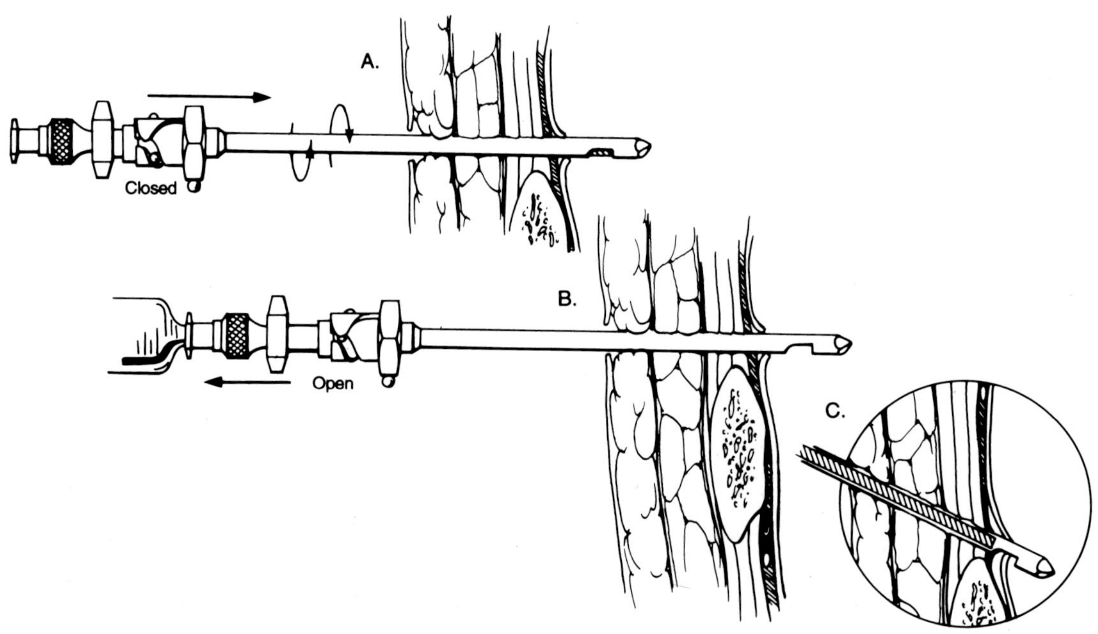

Figure 16-3

Abrams biopsy needle.

sectional area of the needle, and results in larger biopsy specimens.

COMPONENTS

Figure 16-4 shows the four-piece assembly of the O&S Biopsy Needle. The instrument consists of a biopsy harvester, an obturator, and two concentric stainless steel tubes, an inner tube and a hollow outer tube. The inner tube, with its trocar point, has a unique self-opening stainless steel biopsy flap, and a Luer lock. The hinge connecting the biopsy flap to the inner tube has safety features that prevent the biopsy flap from extending beyond 60 degrees, and the biopsy flap also opens beyond the cross-sectional area of the needle. The outer tube is mounted over the inner tube. Both tubes have knurled circular collars, each with one flat surface. The orientation of the biopsying orifice is indicated by the orientation of the flat surface of the proximal knurled circular collar (proximal to the patient).

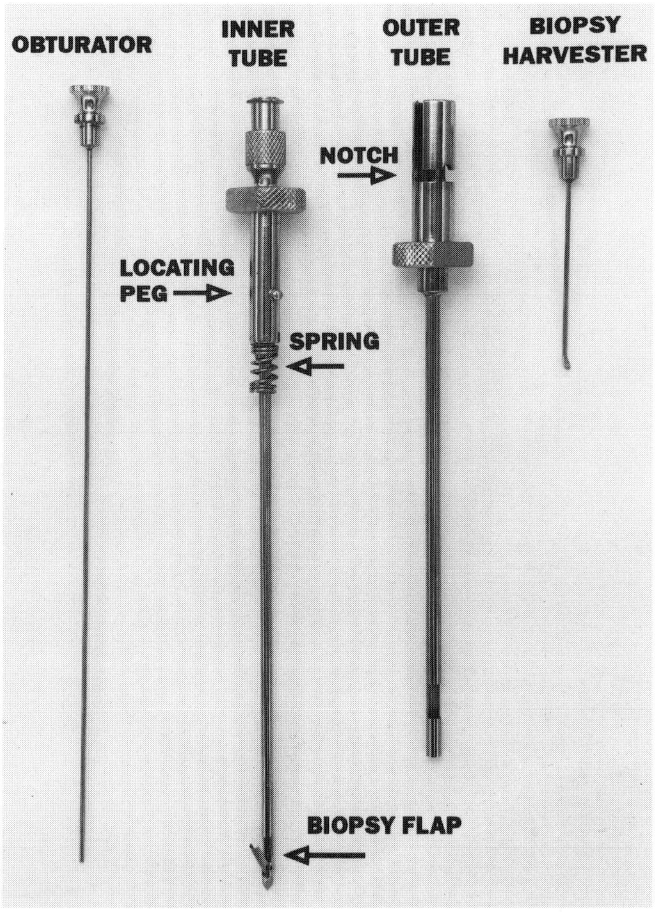

Figure 16-4

The components of the O&S pleural biopsy needle (*from left*): biopsy harvester, outer cannula, inner cannula with biopsy flap, and obturator.

It is important that only the proximal knurled circular collar (proximal to the patient) be manipulated to open or close the biopsying orifice.

The O&S Biopsy Needle has two positions—closed and open as detailed below.

Familiarization with setting the closed and open positions of the O&S biopsy needle is essential before using this instrument.

The closed and open positions are defined as follows:

1. In the closed position flat surfaces on the knurled circular collars are 60 degrees opposed, with the peg in the notch of the outer slot. A spring is incorporated to keep the peg in this position.

2. In the open position flat surfaces on the knurled circular collars are facing the same way and have been moved apart.

OPERATION

Operation of the O&S biopsy needle should proceed as follows:

1. After making the skin incision as described above, the O&S pleural biopsy needle, with the obturator removed and the syringe attached to its Luer fitting, is advanced in the closed position into the pleural space (Fig. 16-5*A*).

2. Once in the pleural space, the proximal knurled circular collar is twisted clockwise to bring the needle to the open position and advanced toward the patient until the peg reaches the distal end of the closed vertical slot. Pleural fluid is aspirated to confirm the needle is both in the open position and in the pleural space (Fig. 16-5*B*).

3. Orient the biopsy orifice by rotating the needle so that the flat portions of the knurled collars face the superior aspect of the rib below, that is, the biopsy flap is open and facing down.

4. The needle in the open position is slowly withdrawn until the biopsy flap is felt to engage the parietal pleura (Fig. 16-5*C*).

5. While firmly holding the knurled circular collar distal to the patient, the needle is brought to a closed position by withdrawing the proximal knurled circular collar. This maneuver scrapes the pleural specimen into the biopsy orifice (Fig. 16-5*D*). The proximal collar is then twisted counterclockwise to lock the locating peg of the inner tube into the notch of the horizontal slot of the outer tube. (Trying to bring the needle to closed position by moving the distal knurled circular collar will result in the biopsy flap moving away from the pleura, thus resulting in a negative biopsy).

NOTE: Increased resistance may occasionally be encountered when the needle is being brought to the

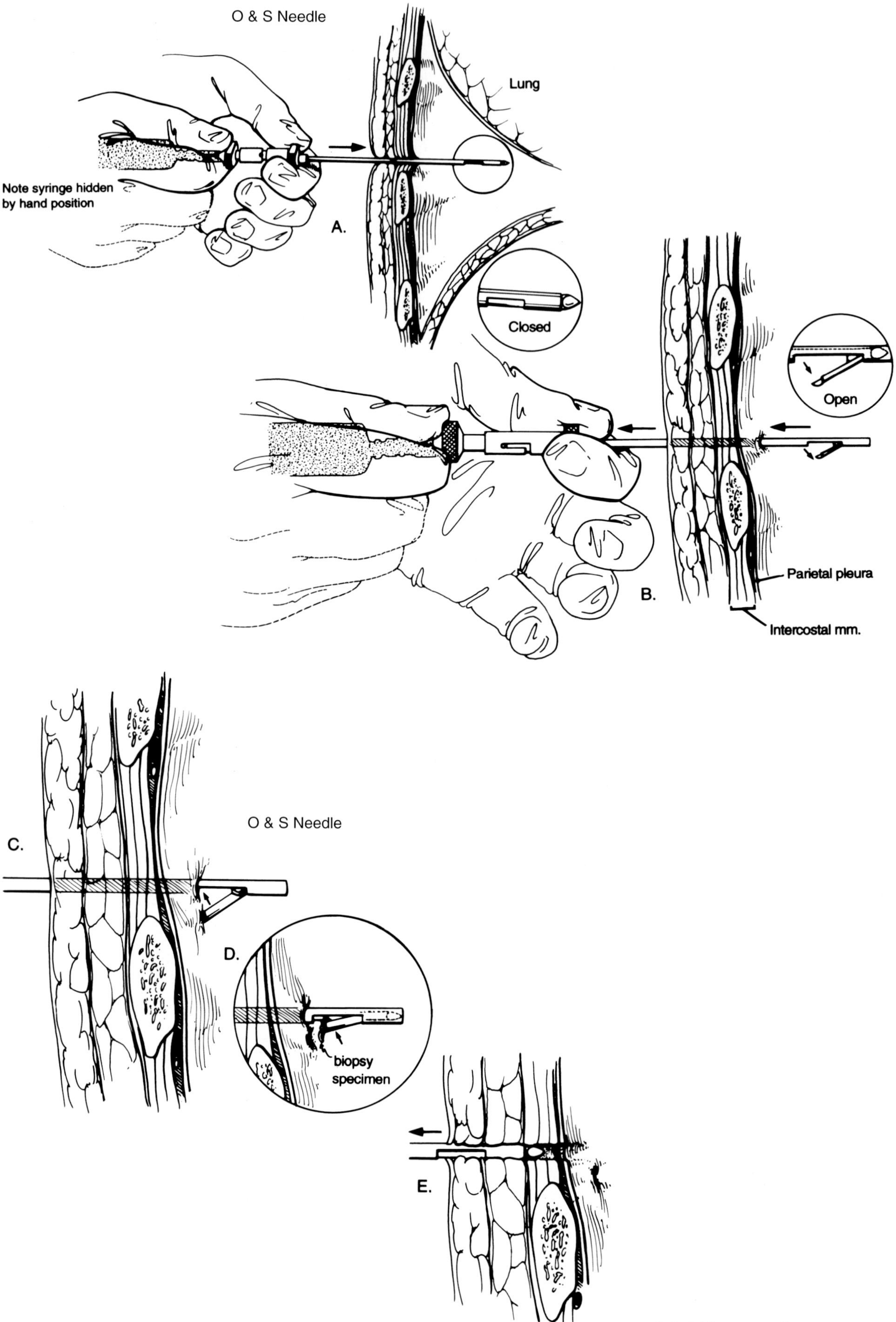

O & S biopsy needle.

closed position, owing to either of the following: (1) The biopsy flap is embedded too deeply in the subpleural tissue or (2) the biopsy flap is lying against the rib. If either happens, without withdrawing the needle reintroduce the entire syringe and needle assembly into the pleural cavity, or in the latter case lift the needle slightly away from the rib and perform the pleural biopsy, as outlined above.

6. Return the needle to the closed position and withdraw the entire biopsy needle from the patient (Fig. 16-5*E*). Care should be taken not to separate the knurled collars during withdrawal of the biopsy needle.

RULES TO OBSERVE

The following important rules must be observed for this procedure:

1. Check the biopsy flap before the procedure.

2. The flat surfaces on both knurled circular collars must be aligned while performing the biopsy.

3. *Always* move the outer tube (knurled circular collar proximal to the patient) for opening or closing the O&S biopsy needle.

4. The biopsy needle should be in the closed position when inserting or withdrawing the instrument from the pleural cavity.

COPE BIOPSY NEEDLE

The Cope pleural biopsy needle (Fig. 16-6) has four components: a large concentric tube (the outer cutting cannula) with a guard; a solid stylet; a hollow beveled trocar into which the solid stylet can be locked; and a hollow, blunt-tipped hooked biopsy trocar. The hooked biopsy trocar has a biopsy hook at its distal end, and a right-angled indicator projection near its hub to orient the direction of the distal biopsy hook.

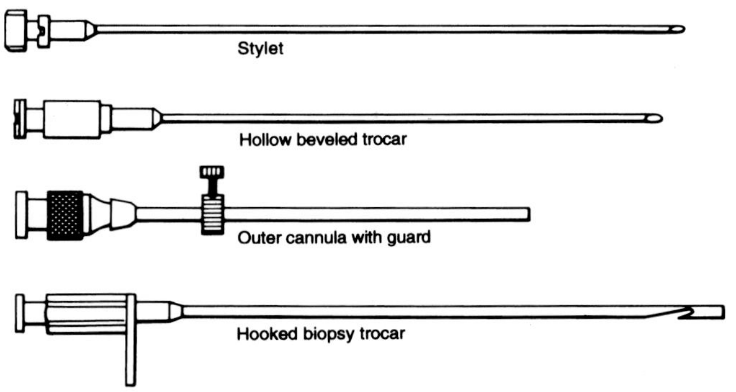

Figure 16-6

Cope biopsy needle.

The stylet is locked into the hollow beveled trocar, and the outer cannula is mounted onto the hollow beveled trocar. Following a small skin incision, the above assembled three components of the needle are introduced into the pleural space. With the patient holding his or her breath in expiration, the hollow beveled trocar along with its stylet is removed, the orifice of the outer cannula is occluded with a finger, and a 20-ml syringe is quickly attached to the outer cannula. Pleural fluid is then aspirated to confirm entry into the pleural space and also for diagnostic purposes. The guard on the outer cannula is loosened and the guard advanced to lie adjacent to the skin and tightened in that position. Again the patient is asked to hold his or her breath in end expiration, the syringe is removed from the outer cannula, and the hooked biopsy trocar attached to a syringe (or a stopcock closed to the pleural space) is introduced inside the outer cannula. During the brief periods between the changing of the components of the needle, always occlude the orifice of the outer cannula to prevent inadvertent air leak into the pleural space.

The biopsy needle is now rotated so that the right-angled indicator projection is facing the rib below. The needle assembly (along with the outer cannula) is now withdrawn until a tug is felt (Fig. 16-7*A*). Although the biopsy is usually performed at 90 degrees, to obtain better pleural yield the needle is raised to a 30-degree angle (Fig. 16-7*B*). The hooked biopsy trocar is held firmly in this position with one hand, while the outer cannula is advanced into the pleural space with a twisting motion of the other hand, to sever the entrapped

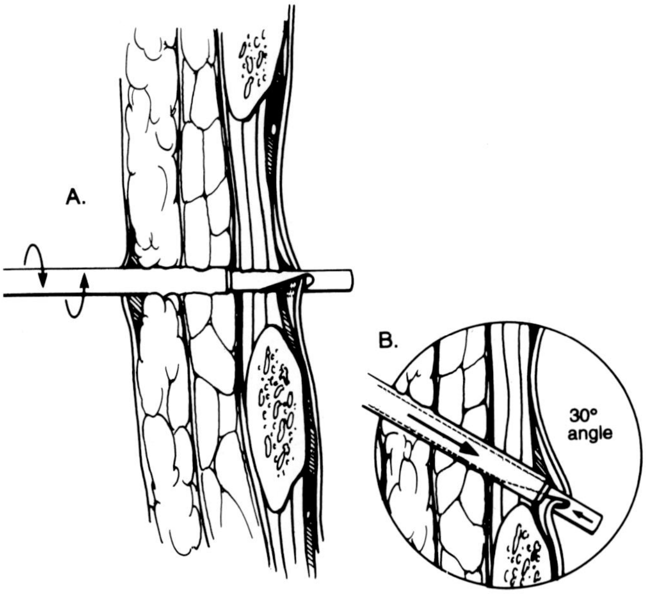

Figure 16-7

Biopsy utilizing the Cope hooked biopsy trocar.

pleura. Since only one specimen can be obtained during a single entry, the above maneuver needs to be repeated to obtain several specimens.

Biopsy Specimens

Four to five pleural biopsies should be taken. Use care while retrieving the specimens from the biopsy needle. The pleural fluid from the syringe can be used to flush out the biopsy specimen or, if the specimen is stuck in the biopsy needle, it can be retrieved with either the obturator/stylet or the biopsy harvester. Hypodermic needles used to scoop out the biopsy specimens can lead to fragmentation or crush artifacts. Pleural tissue is recognized by its whitish or whitish gray appearance. One biopsy specimen should be placed in a sterile tube with 3 ml of normal saline for culture of fungi and acid-fast bacilli. The remaining three to four biopsies should be immersed in formalin for histopathologic examination. If the pathologist reports only the presence of muscle and adipose tissue, additional deeper cuts of the remaining specimens should be requested. The deeper tissue embedded in the paraffin blocks may occasionally contain the actual pleural component of the specimen.

To purchase the kits and biopsy needles:

1. *Arrow-Clark Thoracentesis Kit.* 1-800-233-3187.

2. *Argyle Turkel Safety Thoracentesis System.* 1-800-428-4400.

3. *Pharmaseal Thoracentesis Catheter Tray.* 1-800-422-9837.

4. *Baxter Thoracentesis Catheter.* 1-800-422-9837.

5. *Biopsy Needles.* Popper & Sons, Inc., Biomedical Instrument Division, 300 Denton Avenue, New Hyde Park, NY 11040.

REFERENCES

1. Light RW: Thoracentesis (diagnostic and therapeutic) and pleural biopsy. In Light RW (ed.): *Pleural Diseases.* Philadelphia, Lea & Febiger, 1995.
2. Kohan JM, et al: Value of chest ultrasonography versus decubitus roentgenography for thoracentesis. *Am Rev Respir Dis* 1986; 133:1124–1126.
3. Rabin CB, Blackman NS: Bilateral pleural effusion: Its significance in association with a heart of normal size. *J Mt Sinai Hosp* 1957; 24:45–53.
4. Sahn SA: The pleura. *Am Rev Respir Dis* 1988; 138:184–234.
5. Godwin JE, Sahn SA: Thoracentesis: A safe procedure in mechanically ventilated patients. *Ann Intern Med* 1990; 113:800–802.
6. Light RW, et al: Pleural effusions: The diagnostic separation of transudates and exudates. *Ann Intern Med* 1972; 77:507–513.
7. Jay SJ: Diagnostic procedures for pleural disease. *Clin Chest Med* 1985; 6:33–48.
8. Kinasewitz GT, Fishman AP: Pleural dynamics and effusions. In Fishman AP (ed): *Pulmonary Diseases and Disorders,* 2d ed. New York, McGraw-Hill, 1988:2117–2138.
9. Light RW, et al: Parapneumonic effusions. *Am J Med* 1980; 69:507–512.
10. Light RW: Management of parapneumonic effusions. *Arch Intern Med* 1981; 141:1339–1341.
11. Potts DE, et al: Pleural fluid pH in parapneumonic effusions. *Chest* 1976; 70:328–331.
12. Light RW, et al: Diagnostic significance of pleural fluid pH and P_{CO_2}. *Chest* 1973; 64:591–596.
13. Tillet WS, et al: Use of streptokinase-streptodornase in treatment of postpneumonic empyema. *J Thorac Surg* 1951; 21:275–297.
14. Geha AS: Pleural empyema: Changing etiologic, bacteriologic, and therapeutic aspects. *J Thorac Cardiovasc Surg* 1971; 61:626–635.
15. Bergh NP, et al: Intrapleural streptokinase in the treatment of hemothorax and empyema. *Scand J Thorac Cardiovasc Surg* 1977; 11:265–268.
16. Ogirala RG, Williams MH Jr: Streptokinase in a loculated pleural effusion: Effectiveness determined by site of installation. *Chest* 1988; 94:884–886.
17. Berger HW, Mejia E: Tuberculous pleurisy. *Chest* 1973; 63:88–92.
18. Ellner JJ: Pleural fluid and peripheral blood lymphocyte function in tuberculosis. *Ann Intern Med* 1978; 89:932–933.
19. Spriggs AI, Boddington MM: Absence of mesothelial cells from tuberculous pleural effusions. *Thorax* 1968; 15 :169–171.
20. Hirsch A, et al: Pleural effusion: Laboratory tests in 300 cases. *Thorax* 1979; 34:106–112.
21. Krakowka P, et al: Infection of the pleura by *Aspergillus fumigatus. Thorax* 1970; 25:245–253.
22. Hillerdal G: Pulmonary aspergillus infection invading the pleura. *Thorax* 1981; 36:745–751.
23. Walsh TJ, Bulkley BH: Aspergillus pericarditis: Clinical and pathologic features in the immunocompromised patient. *Cancer* 1982; 49:48–54.
24. Murphy D, Land DJ: Pleural effusion in allergic bronchopulmonary aspergillosis: Two case reports. *Br J Dis Chest* 1981; 75:91–95.
25. Colp CR, Cook WA: Successful treatment of pleural aspergillosis and broncho-pleural fistula. *Chest* 1975; 68:96–98.
26. Mitzger JB, et al: Pulmonary oxalosis caused by *Aspergillus niger. Am Rev Respir Dis* 1984; 129:501–502.
27. Ibarra-Perez C: Thoracic complications of amebic abscess of the liver: Report of 501 cases. *Chest* 1981; 79:672–676.
28. Cameron EWJ: The treatment of pleuro-pulmonary amebiasis with metronidazole. *Chest* 1978; 73:647–650.
29. Sahn SA: Malignant pleural effusions. In Fishman A (ed): *Pulmonary Diseases and Disorders,* 2d ed. New York: McGraw-Hill, 1988:2159–2170.
30. Meyer PC: Metastic carcinoma of the pleura. *Thorax* 1966; 21:437–443.
31. Sahn SA: Malignant pleural effusions. *Clin Chest Med* 1985; 6:113–125.
32. Yam LT: Diagnostic significance of lymphocytes in pleural effusions. *Ann Intern Med* 1967; 66:972–982.
33. Decker DA, et al: The significance of a cytologically negative pleural effusion in bronchogenic carcinoma. *Chest* 1978; 74:640–642.
34. Piras MA, et al: Adenosine deaminase activity in pleural effusion: An aid to differential diagnosis. *Br Med J* 1978; 4:1751–1752.
35. Blank N, Castellino RA: The intrathoracic manifestations of the malignant lymphomas and leukemia. *Semin Roentgenol* 1980; 15:227–245.
36. Bruneau R, Rubin P: The management of pleural effusions and chylothorax in lymphoma. *Radiology* 1965; 85:1085–1092.

37. Hillerdal G: Malignant mesothelioma 1982; review of 4710 published cases. *Br J Dis Chest* 1983; 77:321–343.
38. Heller RM, et al: The radiological manifestations of malignant pleural mesothelioma. *Am J Roentgenol* 1970; 108:53–59.
39. Epler GR, et al: Prevalence and incidence of benign asbestos pleural effusion in a working population. *JAMA* 1982; 247:617–622.
40. Mattson SB: Monosymptomatic exudative pleurisy in persons exposed to asbestos dust. *Scand J Respir Dis* 1975; 56:263–272.
41. Selikoff IJ: Cancer risk of asbestos exposure. In Hiatt HH, et al (eds): *Origins of Human Cancer.* Cold Spring Harbor, NY, Cold Spring Harbor Laboratory, 1977:1765–1784.
42. Taryle DA, et al: Pleural mesotholiomas—An analysis of 18 cases and review of the literature. *Medicine* 1976; 55:153–162.
43. Hillerdal G: Non-malignant asbestos pleural disease. *Thorax* 1981; 36:669–675.
44. Rasmussen KN, Faber V: Hyaluronic acid in 247 pleural fluids. *Scand J Respir Dis* 1967; 48:366–371.
45. Elmes PC, Simpson JC: The clinical aspects of mesothelioma. *Quart J Med* 1976; 45:427–429.
46. Oels HC, et al: Diffuse malignant mesothelioma of the pleura: A review of 37 cases. *Chest* 1971; 60:564–570.
47. Legha S, Muggia FM: Pleural mesothelioma: Clinical features and therapeutic implications. *Ann Intern Med* 1977; 87:613–621.
48. Gaensler EA, Kaplan AI: Asbestos pleural effusions. *Ann Intern Med* 1971; 74:178–191.
49. Alarcon-Segovia D, Alarcon DG: Pleuro-pulmonary manifestations of systemic lupus erythematosus. *Dis Chest* 1961; 39:7–17.
50. Harvey AM, et al: Systemic lupus erythematosus: Review of the literature and clinical analysis of 138 cases. *Medicine* 1954; 33:291–437.
51. Winslow WA, Ploss LN, Lotman B: Pleuritis in systemic lupus erythematosus: Its importance as an early manifestation in diagnosis. *Ann Intern Med* 1958; 49:70–88.
52. Good JT Jr, et al: Lupus pleuritis: Clinical features and pleural fluid characteristics with special reference to pleural fluid antinuclear antibodies. *Chest* 1983; 84:714–718.
53. Walker WC, Wright V: Pulmonary lesions and rheumatoid arthritis. *Medicine* 1968; 47:501–520.
54. Sahn SA, et al: Rheumatoid pleurisy. Observations on the development of low pleural fluid pH and glucose level. *Arch Intern Med* 1980; 140:1237–1238.
55. Pettersson T, et al: Chemical and immunological features of pleural effusions: Comparison between rheumatoid arthritis and other diseases. *Thorax* 1982; 37:354–361.
56. Lillington GA, et al: Rheumatoid pleurisy with effusion. *Arch Intern Med* 1971; 128:764–768.
57. Ferguson GC: Cholesterol pleural effusion in rheumatoid lung disease. *Thorax* 1966; 21:577–582.
58. Nosanchuk JS, Naylor B: A unique cytological picture in pleural fluid from patients with rheumatoid arthritis. *Am J Clin Path* 1968; 50:330–335.
59. Carr DT, Mayne JG: Pleurisy with effusion in rheumatoid arthritis, with reference to the low concentration of glucose in pleural fluid. *Am Rev Respir Dis* 1962; 85:345–350.
60. Sahn SA: Pleural fluid pH in the normal state and in diseases affecting the pleural space. In Chretein J, et al (eds): *The Pleura in Health and Disease.* New York, Marcel Dekker, 1985:253–266.
61. Good JT Jr, et al: The diagnostic value of pleural fluid pH. *Chest* 1980; 78:55–59.
62. Halla JT, et al: Immune complexes and other laboratory features of pleural effusions: A comparison of rheumatoid arthritis and systemic lupus erythematosus. *Ann Intern Med* 1980; 92:748–752.
63. Hunder GG, et al: Pleural fluid complement in systemic lupus erythematosus and rheumatoid arthritis. *Ann Intern Med* 1972; 76:357–362.
64. Andrews BS, et al: The role of immune complexes in the pathogenesis of pleural effusions. *Am Rev Respir Dis* 1981; 124:115–120.
65. Bynum LJ, Wilson JE III: Radiographic features of pleural effusions in pulmonary embolism. *Am Rev Respir Dis* 1978; 117:829–834.
66. Worsley DF, et al: Chest radiographic findings in patients with acute pulmonary embolism: Observations from the PIOPED study. *Radiology* 1993; 189:133–136.
67. Bynum LJ, Wilson JE III: Characteristics of pleural effusions associated with pulmonary embolism. *Arch Intern Med* 1976; 136:159–162.
68. Light RW, Ball WC: Glucose and amylase in pleural effusions. *JAMA* 1973; 225:257–259.
69. Kaye MD: Pleuropulmonary complications of pancreatitis. *Thorax* 1968; 23:297–306.
70. Pottmeyer EW III, Frey CF, Matsuno S: Pancreaticopleural fistulas. *Arch Surg* 1987; 122:648–654.
71. Anderson WJ, et al: Chronic pancreatic pleural effusions. *Surg Gynecol Obstet* 1973; 137:827–830.
72. Sherr HP, et al: Origin of pleural fluid amylase in esophageal rupture. *Ann Intern Med* 1972; 76:985–986.
73. Maultiz RM, et al: The pleuropulmonary consequences of esophageal rupture: An experimental model. *Am Rev Respir Dis* 1979; 120:363–367.
74. Abbott OA, et al: Atraumatic so-called "spontaneous" rupture of the esophagus. *J Thorac Cardiovasc Surg* 1970; 59:67–83.
75. O'Connell ND: Spontaneous rupture of the esophagus. *Am J Roentgenol* 1967; 99:186–203.
76. Flavell G: *The Oesophagus.* London, Butterworth, 1963.
77. Good JT Jr, et al: The pathogenesis of the low pleural fluid pH in esophageal rupture. *Am Rev Respir Dis* 1983; 127: 702–704.
78. Nix JT, et al: Chylothorax and chylous ascites: A study of 302 selected cases. *Am J Gastroenterol* 1957; 28:40–53.
79. Staats BA, et al: The lipoprotein profile of chylous and nonchylous pleural effusions. *Mayo Clin Proc* 1980; 55:700–704.
80. Roy PH, Carr DT, Payne WS: The problem of chylothorax. *Mayo Clin Proc* 1967; 42:457–467.
81. Bower GC: Chylothorax: Observations in 20 cases. *Dis Chest* 1964; 46:464–468.
82. Williams KR, Burford TH: The management of chylothorax. *Ann Surg* 1964; 160:131–140.
83. Strausser JL, Flye MW: Management of non-traumatic chylothorax. *Ann Thorac Surg* 1981; 31:520–526.
84. Bessone LN, Ferguson TB, Burford TH: Chylothorax. *Ann Thorac Surg* 1971; 12:527–550.
85. Seriff NS, et al: Chylothorax: Diagnosis by lipoprotein electrophoresis of serum and pleural fluid. *Thorax* 1977; 32: 98–100.
86. Bower GC: Chyliform pleural effusion in rheumatoid arthritis. *Am Rev Respir Dis* 1968; 97:455–459.
87. Coe JE, Aikawa JK: Cholesterol pleural effusion. *Arch Intern Med* 1961; 108:763–774.
88. Ferguson GC: Cholesterol pleural effusion in rheumatoid lung disease. *Thorax* 1966; 21:577–582.
89. Lampson RS: Traumatic chylothorax—A review of the literature and report of a case treated by mediastinal ligation of the thoracic duct. *J Thorac Surg* 1948; 17:778–791.
90. Adler RH, Levinsky L: Persistent chylothorax and treatment by talc pleurodesis. *J Thorac Cardiovasc Surg* 1978; 76:859–863.
91. Hillerdal G: Chyliform (cholesterol) pleural effusion. *Chest* 1985; 88:426–428.
92. Goldman A, Burford TH: Cholesterol pleural effusion: A report of three cases with a cure by decortication. *Dis Chest* 1950; 18:586–594.
93. Seneff MG, et al: Complications associated with thoracocentesis. *Chest* 1986; 90:97–100.

94. Collins TR, Sahn SA: Thoracocentesis: Clinical value, complications, technical problems and patient experience. *Chest* 1987; 91:817–822.
95. Brandstetter RD, et al: Pneumothorax after thoracentesis in chronic obstructive pulmonary disease. *Heart Lung* 1994; 23:67–70.
96. Carney M, Ravin CE: Intercostal artery laceration during thoracocentesis. Increased risk in elderly patients. *Chest* 1979; 75:520–522.
97. Sue DY, Lam K: Retention of catheter fragment after thoracentesis. *Postgrad Med* 1982; 72:101–106.
98. Agurlar-Torres FG, et al: Subcutaneous implantation of an adenocarcinoma following thoracocentesis. *Wis Med J* 1977; 76:19–21.
99. Heffner JE, Sahn SA: Abdominal hemorrhage after perforation of a diaphragmatic artery during thoracentesis. *Arch Intern Med* 1981; 141:1238.
100. Brandstetter RD, Cohen RP: Hypoxemia after thoracentesis. A predictable and treatable condition. *JAMA* 1979; 242:1060–1061.
101. Estenne M, et al: Mechanism of relief of dyspnea after thoracocentesis in patients with large pleural effusions. *Am J Med* 1983; 74:813–819.
102. Rhodes ML: Thoracentesis. In Jay SJ, Stonehill RB (eds): *Manual of Pulmonary Procedure.* Philadelphia, WB Saunders, 1980:1–11.
103. Light RW, et al: Observations on pleural fluid pressures as fluid is withdrawn during thoracentesis. *Am Rev Respir Dis* 1980; 121:799–804.
104. De Francis N, Klosk E, Albano E: Needle biopsy of the parietal pleura. *N Engl J Med* 1955; 252:948.
105. Abrams LD: A pleural-biopsy punch. *Lancet* 1958; 1:30–31.
106. Cope C: New pleural biopsy needle. *JAMA* 1958; 167:1107–1108.
107. Heller P, et al: Needle biopsy of the pleura. *N Engl J Med* 1956; 255:684–690.
108. Donohoe RF, Katz S, Mathews MJ: Aspiration biopsy of the parietal pleura. *Am J Med* 1957; 22:883–893.
109. Hyde RW, Hall CB, Hall WJ: New pulmonary diagnostic procedures. *Am J Dis Child* 1973; 126:292–295.
110. Leggat P: Needle biopsy of parietal pleura in malignant disease. *Br Med J* 1959; 2:478–479.
111. Kettel LJ, Cuggell DW: Pleural biopsy. *JAMA* 1967; 200:317–320.
112. Von Hoff DD, Livolsi V: Diagnostic reliability of needle biopsy of the parietal pleura. *Am J Clin Pathol* 1975; 64:200–203.
113. Walsh LJ, et al: Audit of pleural biopsies: An argument for a pleural biopsy service. *Respir Med* 1994; 88:503–505.
114. Canto A, et al: Points to consider when choosing a biopsy method in cases of pleurisy of unknown origin. *Chest* 1983; 84:176–179.
115. Mungall IPF, et al: Multiple pleural biopsy with Abrams needle. *Thorax* 1980; 35:600–602.
116. Ogirala RG, et al: Raja pleural biopsy needle: A comparison with the Abrams needle in experimental pleural effusion. *Am Rev Respir Dis* 1989; 139:984–987.
117. Ogirala RG, et al: Comparison of the Raja and the Abrams pleural biopsy needles in patients with pleural effusion. *Am Rev Respir Dis* 1993; 147:1291–1294.
118. Morrone N, et al: Pleural biopsy with Cope and Abrams needles. *Chest* 1987; 92:1050–1052.
119. Poe RH, et al: Sensitivity, specificity, and predictive values of closed pleural biopsy. *Arch Intern Med* 1984; 14:325–328.
120. Lai JH, et al: Intercostal arteriovenous fistula due to pleural biopsy. *Thorax* 1990; 45:976–978.
121. Bhandari S, Sellars L: Splenic hematoma complicating pleural biopsy. *Postgrad Med J* 1995; 71:319.
122. Schachter EN, Basta W: Subcutaneous metastasis of an adenocarcinoma following a percutaneous pleural biopsy. *Am Rev Respir Dis* 1973; 107:283–285.
123. Raja OG, Lalor AJ: Simple aspiration of the pneumothorax. *Br J Dis Chest* 1981; 75:207–208.
124. Light RW: Pneumothorax. In Light RW (ed): *Pleural Diseases.* Philadelphia, Lea & Febiger, 1995.
125. Mearns AJ: Iatrogenic rupture of the spleen. *Br Med J* 1973; 1:395–396.
126. Raja OG, Lalor AJ: Modification to the technique of percutaneous pleural biopsy using Abrams' needle. *Br J Dis Chest* 1980; 74:285–286.
127. Dhillon DP, Spiro SG: Malignant pleural effusions. *Br J Hosp Med* 1983; 29:506–510.

CHAPTER 17

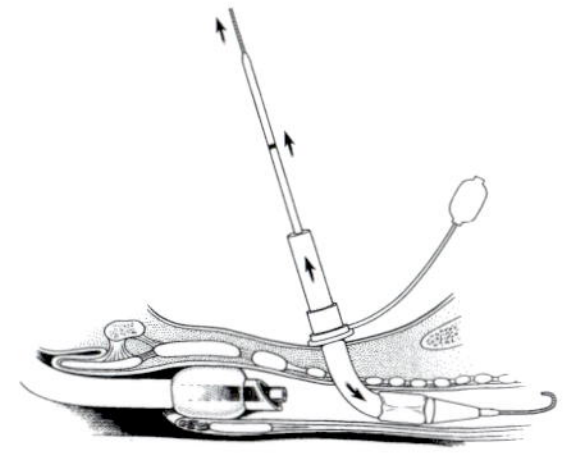

TRANSBRONCHIAL NEEDLE ASPIRATION

Atul C. Mehta, Asok Dasgupta, and Ko-Pen Wang

Historical Perspectives

The technique of transbronchial needle aspiration (TBNA) has opened new boundaries in the practice of flexible bronchoscopy (FB). Schieppati, acknowledged as "the father of TBNA," described the technique of subcarinal puncture as early as 1949.[1] He presented his data to the Argentine Congress of Bronchoesophagology and later published it in the *Review of the Argentine Medical Association.* This, however, did not receive much attention until his subsequent publication in English.[2] Using a 1-mm-diameter and 50-cm-long needle through a rigid bronchoscope (RB), 83 patients were subjected to mediastinal punctures through the carina. Positive aspirates were obtained in 26 of 69 patients (38 percent) suspected of bronchogenic carcinoma. At about the same time, Brouet and coworkers and Euler and coworkers in Europe were experimenting with TBNA of the mediastinal lymph nodes.[3,4] In 1962, Schiessle described his technique and experience with TBNA in the diagnosis of mediastinal tumors and adenopathy.[5] Knowing the status of the carinal lymph node in patients with lung cancer to decide inoperability was believed to be important by these early pioneers. Versteegh and Swierenga obtained 25 (16 percent) positive malignant transcarinal aspirates in 150 patients, and in 14 of them TBNA was exclusively diagnostic. In all these patients inoperability was confirmed by thoracotomy. They found that only half of patients with positive aspirates had an abnormal carina.[6] Fox and colleagues, using a modified Vim Biegeleisen biopsy needle, were able to get a core of tissue in a series of 50 patients. Carcinoma or lymphoma was diagnosed in 40 percent, with lymph node tissue being present in 65 percent of these specimens.[7] Bridgeman and coworkers used a Vim Silverman needle to perform transbronchial left atrial punctures for ventriculography. They used the same needle to perform subcarinal lymph node biopsies and were able to diagnose cancer in 12 of 50 patients (24 percent). In four of these patients the subcarinal biopsy was exclusively diagnostic. They concluded that "obtaining adequate subcarinal lymph node material can be of considerable aid in making a diagnosis, in determining the extent of disease, and helping us avoid an unnecessary thoracotomy, particularly in patients who are poor operative risks."[8] Wang and coworkers were the first in North America to sample mediastinal and hilar lymph nodes using a long, rigid esophageal varices needle through the RB.[9,10] Subsequently, in 1983, they adapted this procedure through the FB for the diagnosis and staging of bronchogenic carcinoma.[11] Shure and Fedullo further extended the use of TBNA, through the FB, to increase the diagnostic yield of peripheral masses.[12] Now TBNA can be used not only for diagnosing mediastinal and lung parenchymal lesions but also for staging lung cancer in a noninvasive fashion.

Despite the sensitivity and ease of use by some experts, TBNA has not been widely accepted. In an American College of Chest Physicians (ACCP) survey of 871 bronchoscopists, Prakash and colleagues showed that only 11.8 percent and 2.3 percent of all pulmonologists use TBNA routinely for the workup of patients with malignant and nonmalignant diseases, respectively. Although damage to the FB was a concern, the lack of effective training and the inability to retrieve adequate specimens were the major reasons cited against its use.[13]

We hope this chapter will alleviate some of the concerns related to this important diagnostic tool and thus increase it usage.

Anatomy

The role of TBNA is to sample tissues from outside the confines of the airways, such as lymph nodes or masses close to the airway. A proper understanding of the anatomy of the lymph nodes and the related major vascular structures is essential.

The esophagus lies posterior to the trachea. The aortic arch lies anterior and to the left of the distal one-third of the trachea and makes an easily recognizable pulsatile imprint on the anterolateral wall of the trachea.[14] The aortic arch and the innominate artery lie directly anterior to the trachea above the level of the main carina. The superior vena cava and the azygos vein lie anteriorly and to the right of the distal third of the trachea. The right pulmonary artery lies immediately in front of the right main bronchus and the origin of the upper lobe bronchus. Similarly the left pulmonary artery is in close approximation (3 to 5 mm) to the left main bronchus anteriorly and to the left upper lobe bronchus superiorly.

Use of contrast CT of the mediastinum is ideal to delineate the lymph node anatomy and particularly to subdivide them into several groups that are accessible to TBNA (Tables 17-1 and 17-2).[15] The selection of a particular site for TBNA is facilitated by viewing the interior of the tracheobronchial tree as if looking at a clock face and using the bifurcations of the tracheobronchial tree as reference points. With the bronchoscopist standing behind the patient lying in the supine position, the *right paratracheal* chain is easily accessed at 2 cm or two tracheal rings proximal to the carina at 1 to 2 o'clock position avoiding the azygos veins (3 o'clock) and the mediastinal reflection of the pleura.[16] The *subcarinal nodes* are sampled 3 to 5 mm below on either side of the main carnia in an infero-

Table 17-1

LOCATION OF MEDIASTINUM AND HILAR LYMPH NODES FOR TBNA (DEFINED BY CT SCAN)

	Lymph node	Location
1.	Anterior carina lymph node	In front and between the proximal portion of the right and left main bronchus
2.	Posterior carina lymph node	Behind and between the proximal portion of the right and left main bronchus, or directly behind the right main bronchus
3.	Right paratrachea lymph node	Behind the superior vena cava and in front of the anterolateral aspect of the lower trachea near the azygous arch
4.	Left paratrachea lymph node (Aortopulmonary window)	Lateral to the trachea near the tracheobronchial angulation, below the aortic arch and above the left main pulmonary artery
5.	Right main bronchus lymph node	In front of the right main bronchus
6.	Left main bronchus lymph node	In front of the left main bronchus
7.	Right upper hilar lymph node	In front and between the right upper lobe bronchus and the bronchus intermedius
8.	Subcarina lymph node	Between the right and left main bronchus, at or near the level of the right upper lobe bronchus
9.	Right lower hilar lymph node	Nodes lateral or in front of the bronchus intermedius, at or near the level of the right middle lobe bronchus
10.	Sub-subcarina lymph node	Between the bronchus intermedius and the left main bronchus, at or near the level of the right middle lobe bronchus
11.	Left hilar lymph node	Between the left upper lobe and left lower lobe bronchus

SOURCE: Wang KP: Staging of bronchogenic carcinoma by bronchoscopy. In Wang KP, Mehta AC (eds): *Flexible Bronchoscopy.* Cambridge, Blackwell Science, 1995:211, with permission.

medial direction. The *right hilar* lymph nodes may be approached through the bronchus intermedius at 3 o'clock position, avoiding the anterior wall and damage to the right pulmonary artery. The *left hilar* nodes are reached through the secondary carina where the left upper lobe bifurcates from the left main-stem bronchus. The *left paratracheal* or aortopulmonary window node is approached by drawing an imaginary line from the carina to the lateral wall of the left main-stem bronchus with aspirations performed from the lateral aspect of this wall at 9 o'clock position.[17] A CT scan can also identify other high-risk areas such as the right posterolateral tracheal wall and posterior wall of right main bronchus where the lung is in close approximation. Similarly the posterior trachea and the left main-stem bronchi are separated from the esophagus by only 2 to 3 mm.[18]

Indications and Results

Indications for TBNA have evolved over the years (Table 17-3). Its primary importance lies with the diagnosis and staging of bronchogenic carcinoma. The advent of the larger needle (19 gauge) to obtain a core of tissue for histologic analysis has not only improved the yield for lung cancers but also helped to establish the diagnosis of lymphoma and granulomatous conditions involving the mediastinum.

STAGING OF CARCINOMA

Lung cancer has become the most common cause of all cancer mortality in the United States. Surgical resection offers the only hope for cure. However, only 20 to 25 percent of lung cancers are resectable, mainly

Table 17-2

TBNA SITE FOR MEDIASTINUM AND HILAR LYMPH NODES (DEFINED BY BRONCHOSCOPY)

Lymph node	Site
1. Anterior carina lymph node	First and second intercartilage interspace from the lower trachea at about the 12–1 o'clock position
2. Posterior carina lymph node	Posterior portion of the carina at about the 5–6 o'clock position
3. Right paratrachea lymph node	Second to fourth intercartilage interspace of the lower trachea at about the 1–2 o'clock position
4. Left paratrachea lymph node (AP window)	First or second intercartilage interspace from the lower trachea at about the 9 o'clock position
5. Right main bronchus lymph node	First or second intercartilage interspace from the proximal right main bronchus at about the 12 o'clock position
6. Left main bronchus lymph node	First or second intercartilage interspace from the proximal left main bronchus at about the 12 o'clock position
7. Right upper hilar lymph node	Anterior portion of the right upper lobe spur
8. Subcarina lymph node	Medial wall of the right main bronchus at about the 9 o'clock position, proximal to the level of the right upper lobe orifice
9. Right lower hilar lymph node	Lateral of anterior wall of the bronchus intermedius at about the 3 o'clock position and the 12 o'clock position near or at the level of the right middle lobe orifice
10. Sub-subcarina lymph node	Medial wall of the bronchus intermedius at about the 9 o'clock position, proximal to the level of the right middle lobe orifice
11. Left hilar lymph node	Lateral wall of the left lower lobe bronchus at about 9 o'clock, at the level of the superior segment orifice of the left lower lobe

SOURCE: Wang KP: Staging of bronchogenic carcinoma by bronchoscopy. In Wang KP, Mehta AC (eds): *Flexible Bronchoscopy.* Cambridge, Blackwell Science, 1995:212, with permission.

Table 17-3
INDICATIONS FOR TBNA

Major	Mediastinal or hilar adenopathy To establish diagnosis For staging of known or suspected lung carcinoma
	Extrinsic compression of the airway by peribronchial process
	Submucosal disease
	Peripheral nodules
Minor	Endobronchial lesion Necrotic tumor Hemorhagic tumor Predicting line of surgical resection
	Follow-up of small cell tumor
	Mediastinal cysts Diagnosis Drainage
	Mediastinal abscess

because of metastasis either to the mediastinal lymph nodes or to extrathoracic structures.[19] The goal of preoperative staging is to identify those patients who do not have mediastinal involvement. Thus, in physiologically acceptable patients with no evidence of distant metastasis curative surgery can be offered. Mediastinal lymph node sampling can be done either through cervical mediastinoscopy (CME), anterior thoracotomy, or TBNA. A positive aspirate from N2 nodes by TBNA would not only preclude curative surgery but also save the patient from the morbidity of mediastinoscopy. Thus, TBNA would obviate the need for surgical staging at a considerable cost saving.[20–23]

Positive transcarinal aspirates have been used as early as the 1960s in deciding unresectability of lung cancer.[6] Wang obtained 18 malignant aspirates in 32 patients using an esophageal varices needle through the rigid bronchoscope, 20 of whom were ultimately documented to have bronchogenic carcinoma.[10] The same authors had a 76 percent yield using FB in patients with proven mediastinal disease.[24] Shure and Fedullo studied 110 consecutive patients with bronchogenic carcinoma and reported a 15 percent transcarinal yield without CT localization of carinal adenopathy. They noted that the presence of an endobronchial lesion or a widened carina with erythema or visible tumor was predictive of a positive aspirate.[20] In another study, Schenk and associates had 19 positive aspirates (43 percent) in 44 patients with CT-proven mediastinal adenopathy; TBNA was negative in the other 44 patients who had a normal mediastinum by CT.[25] Similar increase in diagnostic yield based on radiographic evidence of mediastinal adenopathy or, bronchoscopic evidence of carinal abnormality has been reported by Utz and coworkers.[26] Recently Harrow and colleagues analyzed their experience with TBNA in the staging of lung cancer and tried to correlate these results with bronchoscopic and roentogenographic findings. A positive TBNA involving N2 nodes was associated with the presence of mediastinal adenopathy on chest radiograph ($p < .0055$), a subcarinal node size greater than 20 mm on CT scans ($p < .01$), carinal widening ($p < .001$) and endobronchial disease ($p < .005$), particularly of the right upper lobe[27] (Tables 17-4 and 17-5).

All the above studies were done using the cytology (21-gauge) needles. Using the 19-gauge histology needle, Schenk and coworkers studied 25 patients with proven bronchogenic carcinoma and mediastinal adenopathy on CT and were able to obtain diagnostic aspirates in 20 of these patients. In 12 patients both the histology and flush specimens from the 19-gauge needle were positive. However, in six patients only the histology specimen and in two other patients only the flush solution was exclusively diagnostic. There were two false-positive results and overall sensitivity was judged to be 80 percent.[28] Schenk and coworkers also compared sensitivity of 22- and 19-gauge needles in the staging of lung cancer. In 55 patients with mediastinal adenopathy, TBNA identified 47 patients with the 19-gauge needles and 29 patients with the 22-gauge needles. In two patients the 22-gauge needle was exclusively diagnostic, and in 20 patients involvement was proved solely by the 19-gauge needle. Futhermore,

Table 17-4

DIAGNOSTIC YIELD FROM TBNA FOR STAGING OF LUNG CANCERS AS REPORTED IN THE LITERATURE

Reference	*No. of Pts. or Aspirate with Proven Carcinoma*	*No. of Pts. with Proven Mediastinal Disease*	*TBNA +ve No. of Pts.*	*TBNA +ve % of Pts.*	*Comments*	*PPV*
Wang and Terry[11]	10	6	5	83	1 sclc	100
Wang et al.[24]	40	25	19	76	3 sclc	100
Shure and Fedullo[20] [a,b]	110	?	16	15		100
Utz et al.[26] [a]	88	?	32	36	12 sclc	100
Harrow et al.[21,69]	547	?	127	23	2 false positive	98
Schenk et al.[25]	88	44	19	43	2 false positive	89
Schenk et al.[28] [c]	25	25	20	80		100

[a]Denotes transcarinal aspirates only.

[b]CT chest not available.

[c]18 gauge TBNA for histology.

NOTE: sclc, small cell lung cancer; PPV, the positive predictive value.

cytologic analysis of the flush solution from the 19-gauge needle had a sensitivity of 64 percent as compared with 53 percent with the 22-gauge cytology needle. Sensitivity from combined cytology and histology obtained by the 19-gauge needle was 86 percent and was statistically higher ($p < .001$) than that obtained by the 22-gauge needle.[29] They calculated the cost of mediastinoscopy or invasive staging to be approximately $3000 and demonstrated significant savings using TBNA as the staging procedure.

Review of the above studies collectively suggests that TBNA has great value in identifying mediastinal involvement from bronchogenic carcinoma, as follows:

- When mediastinal lymphadenopathy is seen on the CT scan or there is blunting of the carina, sensitivity could be as high as 100 percent. However, a normal imaging study or a normal carina does not preclude a positive aspirate.
- Histology needle has a higher yield than cytology needle by either histology or cytology (flush) specimen and minimizes the problem of false-positive results.
- TBNA can establish a diagnosis of bronchogenic carcinoma as well as perform staging during a single outpatient procedure that is associated with a significant cost saving. Moreover, it also saves the

Table 17-5

DIAGNOSTIC YIELD OF TBNA BASED ON BRONCHOSCOPIC FINDINGS OF CARINAL ABNORMALITY AS REPORTED IN THE LITERATURE

		CARINAL ABNORMALITY					
		PRESENT			ABSENT		
	Total No. of Pts	*No.*	*TBNA positive*	*% positive*	*No.*	*TBNA positive*	*% positive*
Utz et al.[26]	88	30	13	43	58	19	33
Shure and Fedullo[15]	110	21	8	38	89	8	9
Wang et al.[24]	40	14	10	71	26	9	35

patient from the morbidity of a more invasive procedure.[20,30]

- On occasion, TBNA, especially with the cytology needle, can identify micrometastasis. In selected patients with squamous cell carcinoma and ipsilateral small and limited mediastinal lymph node involvement, surgery could still be beneficial. Under such circumstances use of information provided by TBNA should be individualized.
- TBNA has a high positive predictive value but a low negative predictive value, that is, a negative TBNA does not rule out metastatic involvement, and these patients should have surgical staging.
- Sensitivity of diagnosing small cell carcinoma by TBNA is higher than non-small cell carcinoma.[21,25,27]

PERIBRONCHIAL AND SUBMUCOSAL DISEASE

Central tumors may present either as an exophytic growth visible endoscopically, as submucosal spread (evident as erythema, thickening, or loss of mucosal markings and bronchial narrowing), or as a predominant peribronchial disease presenting as extrinsic compression.[31] Although exophytic growth is readily diagnosed with forceps biopsy,[32] both submucosal disease and extrinsic compression pose difficulty in establishing a diagnosis. Tita and colleagues performed TBNA in 50 patients having extrinsic compression as the sole endobronchial finding. Thirty-five of these patients were eventually proved to have bronchogenic carcinoma, 20 (57 percent) by FB. In four patients the diagnosis was exclusively based on TBNA, increasing the diagnostic yield of FB by 25 percent.[33–35] Shure and Fedullo similarly studied 31 patients presenting with endoscopic abnormalities suggestive of submucosal and peribronchial disease. All patients underwent washings, brushings, forceps biopsy, and TBNA. Forceps biopsy was positive in 55 percent, TBNA in 71 percent, both together in 89 percent and the combination of all procedures was diagnostic in 97 percent. Thus TBNA can significantly increase the diagnostic yield of FB when dealing with submucosal disease or extrinsic compression.[31]

PERIPHERAL NODULES OR MASSES

Transbronchial needle aspiration using the cytology needle has also been useful in establishing the diagnosis of peripheral nodules and masses. Based on its relationship with the adjacent bronchus, Tsuboi and coworkers[36] have classified solitary pulmonary nodules (SPN) into four different types: (I) the bronchial lumen is patent up to the tumor; (II) the bronchus is contained in the tumor mass; (III) the bronchus is compressed and narrowed by the tumor, but the bronchial mucosa is intact; and (IV) the proximal tree is narrowed by peribronchial or submucosal spread of the tumor or by enlarged lymph nodes (Fig. 17-1). It is thus obvious that in a type III or IV lesion, washings, brushings, or forceps biopsy have a minimal diagnostic yield and the yield might be increased by TBNA.

Wang and associates reported their findings in 20 patients, 15 with SPN and 5 with peripheral masses. The diagnosis of malignancy was made in 55 percent of patients overall, and TBNA was exclusively diagnostic in 35 percent. The yield from TBNA was significantly higher than that with forceps biopsy or washings either alone or in combination. In this small study, bronchoscopy was nondiagnostic in patients with lesions smaller than 2 cm in diameter.[37] In a similar study by Shure and Fedullo on 42 patients, addition of TBNA to washings, brushings, and forceps biopsy increased the diagnostic yield from 48 to 69 percent. Diagnostic yield was higher for lesions larger than 2 cm in diameter (76 percent versus 33 percent). In the subset of patients where forceps could be passed just to the border of the mass but not into it (Tsuboi type IV), transbronchial needle aspiration was positive in 80 percent (Table 17-6).[12] Schenk and coworkers published data on 91 consecutive patients with bronchogenic carcinoma, 42 of whom had SPN or peripheral masses, and obtained a yield of 40 percent in this subset.[25] In another study comparing TBNA with transthoracic needle aspiration (TTNA), Wang and colleagues reported an overall diagnostic yield of 46 percent for peripheral masses with TBNA when limited to parenchyma and 89 percent when concomitant mediastinal involvement was present and sampled. They recommended FB as the procedure of choice, when both parenchymal and mediastinal lesions coexisted. However if a benign etiology is suspected or the lesion is less than 2 cm in size and peripheral, TTNA should be done first since the yield with TBNA is limited.[38] Similar diagnostic sen-

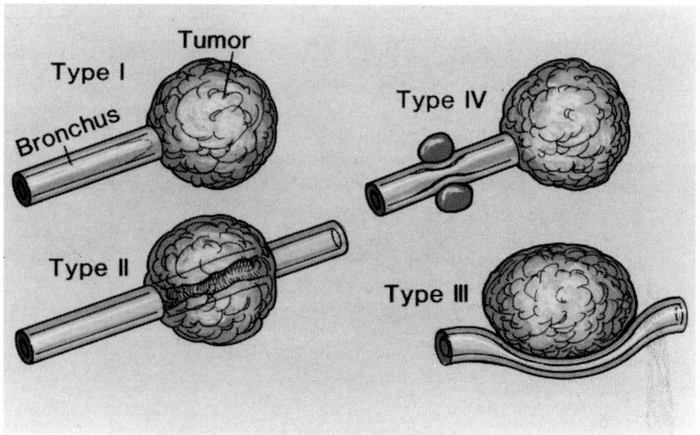

Figure 17-1

Schematic representation of tumor-bronchial relationship; see text. (*Modified from Tsuboi et al.*[36])

Table 17-6

DIAGNOSTIC YIELD OF TBNA FOR PERIPHERAL NODULES AND MASSES AS REPORTED IN THE LITERATURE

Reference	*Patients, n*	*TBNA Positive, n*	*TBNA Positive, %*	*TBNA Exclusively Diagnostic, n*
Wang et al.[37]	20	11	55	7[b]
Shure and Fedullo[12] [a]	42	22	52	8[b]
Castella et al.[82] [a]	45	31	69	12
Katis et al.[83] [a]	37	23	62	8
Wang and Britt[84]	22	8	36	2
Gasparini et al.[39]	349	242	69	67
Wang et al.[38]	160	73	46	—

[a]Addition of TBNA increased diagnostic yield by 21, 27, and 24 percent, respectively.
[b]At least.

sitivity (69 percent for TBNA) has been reported by Gasparini and associates who in their large study of 1027 patients concluded that 75 percent of those with malignant peripheral nodules or masses could have had their condition diagnosed using forceps biopsy and TBNA rather than the percutaneous route.[39] TBNA is also associated with a significantly lower rate of complications than TTNA. Wang and colleagues also suggested that TBNA had a higher yield over forceps biopsy in the case of solitary metastases of hematogenous origin, since these are likely to be type III lesions.[37]

ENDOBRONCHIAL LESIONS

In the presence of an obvious endobronchial lesion, the yield of forceps biopsy as the initial diagnostic procedure in a number of different studies has been between 67 and 100 percent.[40–44] Buirski and coworkers used intralesional needle aspiration in the case of endobronchial tumors and reported a diagnostic yield of 80 percent as compared with 67 percent by forceps biopsy alone.[44] However, Lundgreen and associates, reporting on a similar number of patients, had a diagnostic yield of 65 percent by TBNA and 85 percent by forceps.[43]

Despite these conflicting results, there exist a number of situations where TBNA could be helpful. If the surface of the airway lesion is necrotic, forceps biopsy may be negative and TBNA may help obtain viable tumor tissue from the center of the lesion and establish a diagnosis. Extensive crush artifacts in endobronchial biopsy specimens are often reported in small cell cancer. Needle aspiration has been critical in establishing a diagnosis in these cases.[45] When an endobronchial lesion is likely to bleed (e.g., carcinoids), TBNA can be safely performed to obtain a tissue diagnosis.[46,47]

MISCELLANEOUS

Management of Lung Cancer

Needle aspiration has also been used to follow response to therapy in patients with small cell cancer.

York and coworkers have performed submucosal needle aspiration proximal to an endobronchial tumor and found it useful to predict the line of surgical resection in patients with non-small cell carcinoma.[48]

In patients with a bleeding diathesis where mediastinoscopy is contraindicated, TBNA may provide the only means for diagnosis.[49]

Lymphoma

A number of studies have been reported where lymphoma was diagnosed using either the cytology or the histology needles.[16,17,50,51] The use of flow cytometry to analyze TBNA aspirates has helped diagnose lymphoma in cases where standard cytologic analysis has been negative.[52]

Mediastinal Cysts and Abscess

Mediastinal masses have been both diagnosed and therapeutically aspirated using the transbronchial route.[53–55] McDougall and Fromme describe a patient with a cystic subcarinal mass who encountered severe airway obstruction and gas-exchange problems during anesthesia. Decompression of the cyst using TBNA allowed for a safe anesthesia and subsequent resection.[56] Wang and colleagues reported a patient with a right paratracheal mass on CT scan consistent with a diagnosis of carcinoma. TBNA demonstrated serosanguinous fluid suggestive of a sterile abscess with no recurrence on later scans.[57] Sclerosing hemangioma, a relatively benign tumor, was diagnosed by Hiryano and associates following a 21-gauge needle aspiration.[58]

Sarcoidosis

Histology needles have further extended the ability to diagnose granulomatous conditions involving the mediastinum. Pauli and coworkers report their findings in 193 patients with suspected sarcoidosis. Using a rigid bronchoscope and a larger needle than that used in flexible scopes, they were able to show noncaseating granulomas in 66 percent of their patients, irrespective of the stage of the disease. When TBNA was combined with forceps biopsy, the yield increased to 78 percent.[59] Wang and associates, using an 18-gauge needle and FB, were able to reveal noncaseating granulomas in 18 of 20 sarcoid patients with a sensitivity of 90 percent. They attributed their increased sensitivity to the high density of granulomas seen in lymph nodes when compared with lung tissues.[60] In another study of 51 patients with the 19-gauge needle, Morales and coworkers showed that the addition of TBNA to transbronchial lung biopsy (TBLB) increased the diagnostic yield from 60 to 83 percent for stage I, and from 76 to 86 percent for stage II disease; 23 percent of stage I and 10 percent of stage II patients were exclusively diagnosed by TBNA.[61] Considering that patients with negative TBLB were hitherto referred for mediastinoscopy, the availability of TBNA provides a less invasive, safe, and economical means for obtaining a definitive diagnosis.

Infections

A number of other benign disorders have been diagnosed using TBNA. Diagnosis of mediastinal tuberculous adenitis by TBNA, both in immunocompromised and immunocompetent hosts, has been described.[62–65] Transbronchial needle aspiration has helped diagnose *Pneumocystis carinii* pneumonia and cryptococcal infection in patients with AIDS.[66]

Complications

Extensive use of TBNA by many bronchoscopists has confirmed the safety of needle aspiration. After more than two decades of use, reported complications have included two pneumothoraces, one pneumomediastinum, and one hemomediastinum.[10,24,32,67] Inadvertent liver biopsy in a patient with a raised right hemidiaphragm has been reported.[68] This, however, did not lead to any significant morbidity. A few milliliters of blood oozing from the puncture site can be encountered, but significant bleeding has not been reported, even in procedures performed in anticoagulated patients.[49,68] Transient bacteremia occurring 6 h after the procedure with prompt defervescence following antibiotic therapy has been described. However, the incidence of fever and bacteremia has been debated, and no firm recommendations about antibiotic prophylaxis exist.[70,71] Following TBNA of a subcarinal mass, one patient developed purulent pericarditis with polymicrobial mouth flora and required pericardiocentesis and catheter drainage. The patient survived the tamponade and infection but succumbed to metastatic melanoma.[72]

The most important complications seen with the TBNA procedure, however, are related to damage to the working channel of the bronchoscope, particularly in the earlier days when nonretractable needles were used. Scope damage has also been reported with the 19-gauge needle[73] and care needs to be taken while manipulating the catheter through the scope[74] (Fig. 17-2). In one instance, a needle became detached from the catheter but was promptly retrieved with forceps without any injury to the patient.[17]

Conclusion

The safety and the efficacy of TBNA have been proved beyond doubt. It can sample areas such as posterior carina and aortopulmonary window that cannot be sampled by the mediastinoscope. It should be considered in every patient with suspected bronchogenic carcinoma and mediastinal lymphadenopathy. It eliminates the need for mediastinoscopy in a significant number of patients and thus leads to significant cost saving and reduces patient morbidity.

The major drawback of cytology needle aspiration has been the need for a qualified and experienced cytopathologist. Interpretation of cytology specimens has been further complicated by the reported incidence of false-positive results.[21,28,75–78] Performing TBNA before any other procedure and introducing the scope without suction helps minimize specimen contamination with bronchial secretions loaded with tumor cells. Attention should be directed to determining adequacy of sampling (e.g., the presence of lymphocytes). All samples with respiratory epithelial cells, scanty tumor cells, or only suspicious cells should be rejected.[51,79,80] Care should be taken in interpreting right upper-lobe lesions which abut the mediastinum, since TBNA may falsely sample lung tissue itself.[78] Similarly, micrometastasis from an ipsilateral paratracheal area

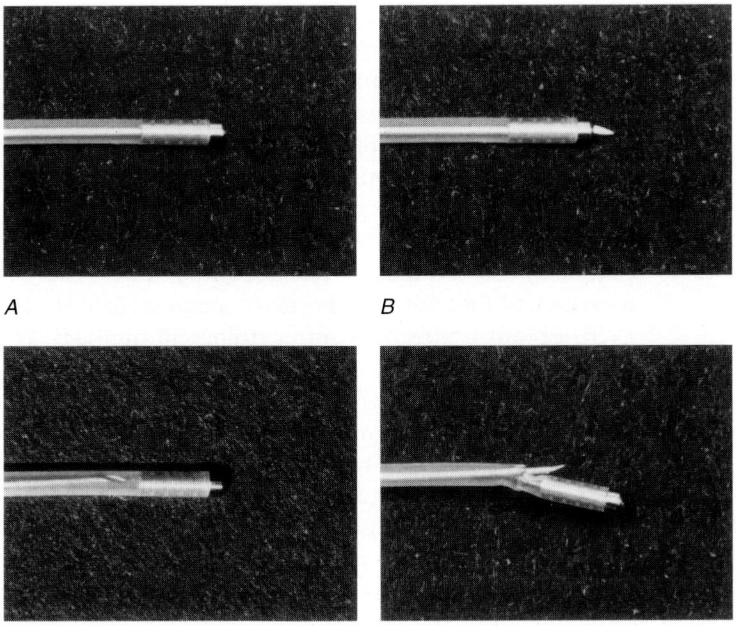

A B C D

Figure 17-2

A. Correct position of the metal needle prior to TBNA: the entire beveled end is placed inside the metal hub. *B.* Incorrect position of the metal needle: the sharp end of the needle extends beyond the metal hub and can potentially lacerate the working channel of the bronchoscope. *C* and *D.* Incorrect position of the metal needle: the needle is placed too proximal to the metal hub and can perforate its own plastic catheter during forward thrust and potentially damage the working channel of the bronchoscope. (*From Stelck MJ, et al: Maintenance of the bronchoscope and the bronchoscopy equipment. In Prakash UBS (ed): Bronchoscopy. New York, Raven, 1994:386, with permission.*)

should be interpreted with great caution in a patient with squamous cell carcinoma since surgery could still be beneficial. Futhermore, on occasion, differential diagnoses of small cell cancer, carcinoid tumor, and lymphoma could be difficult on cytologic examination.[33]

Use of the 19-gauge histology needle has circumvented some of the above limitations of the cytology needle. Lymphoma as well as sarcoidosis and other benign disorders, are now being diagnosed more readily. With increasing education and experience, TBNA yield can be significantly improved, as shown by Haponik and coworkers (21.4 to 47.6 percent; $p < .0001$), and its role in the diagnosis and the staging of cancer can be enhanced.[81] There is a learning curve, and a clinician must perform several successful aspirations with the fine gauge needle before embarking on the histology needles.

Transbronchial needle aspiration is noninvasive, requires only local anesthesia, can be done in an outpatient setting, and has the ability to sample both sides of the trachea at the time of initial bronchoscopy. Much has been done in the last 35 years, yet the outcome from lung carcinoma has changed little. However, contributions of TBNA are clearly expressed in Schieppati's[2] thoughts: "In cases of cancer of the lung or esophagus, this method, which broadens the scope of endoscopy, often permits an accurate diagnosis and prognosis, since it clearly shows the range of mediastinal invasion. This method is free of great risks and, in my opinion, its application could be extended to other diseases; i.e., mediastinal tumors, Hodgkin's disease, sarcoidosis, and lymphogranulomas. This method permits the exploration of the important lymphatic areas which are difficult to approach by any other method."

Equipment

The original Wang transbronchial needle (Mill-Rose Laboratories, Mentor, OH) had three designs: type I (W-122), single-lumen fixed needle; type II (W-222), double-lumen retractable needle; and type III (W-322), single-lumen fixed minitrocar needle. All were 22 gauge, 1.3-cm-long needles. The type I needle was used mostly for mediastinal conditions. The type II needle was used for mediastinal and peripheral lesions because it offered better protection for the scope and the airway. The type I fixed needle was more convenient to use and allowed better suction than the type II needle. The type III needle had a trocar mechanism.

To better protect the bronchoscope, all three needles were eventually modified to a retractable design. Differences still exist in the modified needles. Type I (MW-122) has better suction and is mainly used for central lesions, type II (MW-222) is more versatile and can be used for either central or peripheral lesions, and type III (MW-322) has a minitrocar to prevent plugging and is again mainly used for central lesions. A study by Gittlen and associates has indicated the efficiency of these modified needles.[85] Because the use of the versatile MW-222 needle is more complicated, a simpler MW-522 needle was developed for peripheral lesions.[86]

A newer series of needles was developed to allow easier "blowing" of the specimen onto a glass slide by the "smear technique": SW-121 for central lesions, SW-221 for central and peripheral lesions, and SW-521 for peripheral lesions. The type II SW-221 needle is automatically versatile. All SW series needles are 21 gauge and 1.5 cm long with a slightly thinner guide wire. A study showed that the SW series had favorable results compared with MW needles.[87,88]

A newer series of 20-gauge cytology needles has been evaluated with favorable results. These needles are also 1.5 cm in length. To obtain a cytology specimen for central lesions, either a second-generation MW-122 needle or a third-generation SW-121 needle can be used. For peripheral lesions, either a second-generation MW-522 needle or a third-generation SW-521 needle can be used. The third-generation SW-221 needle is the simplest and most convenient needle to use because its rigidity can be adjusted automatically.

The original histology needle, MW-418, was modified to MW-319 for better protection of the bronchoscope.[89] For histology specimens, the MW-319 is preferred for central and peripheral lesions. If the MW-319 cannot be passed into difficult branches of the airway, such as the apical segment or the superior segments, an MWF-319 can be used (Table 17-7).

HOW I DO IT

Before performing TBNA, the chest radiograph and the computerized tomography (CT) scan of the chest (if available) are thoroughly reviewed. Although CT scanning of the chest is not an absolute prerequisite, it is very helpful in identifying and precisely locating adenopathy and thus, planning needle placement. It is thus desirable to obtain chest CT in all patients before a planned TBNA. However, during a routine FB, if a lesion amenable to TBNA is encountered, the procedure can be carried out at the same sitting without a CT scan. Coagulation profile [prothrombin time (PT), partial thromboplastin time (PTT), bleeding time (BT), platelets] before TBNA is not necessary unless there is a history of bleeding diathesis or anticoagulant usage.

To obtain a specimen for cytological analysis, the needle is introduced through the working channel keeping the tip concealed within the metal hub. The FB is kept as straight as possible with its distal tip in the neutral position. These steps are extremely important to prevent needle damage to the working channel of the FB.[74] Once the metal hub is visible from the distal end of the FB, the needle is advanced and locked in place. The catheter is then retracted to a point where only the tip of the needle is visible. The scope is advanced to the target area and the tip of the needle anchored in the intercartilagenous space. At this stage, the goal is to penetrate the tracheobronchial wall as perpendicularly as possible.

The needle can be inserted through the bronchial wall by the following techniques (Fig. 17-3):

1. *Jabbing Method.* The needle is thrust through the intercartilagenous space with a quick firm jab to the catheter, while the scope is fixed at the nose or mouth.
2. *Pushing Method.* After the locked needle is anchored in the intercartiliganous space, the proximal end of the catheter is fixed against the insertion port using the index finger. This prevents the

Table 17-7
WANG TRANSBRONCHIAL NEEDLES

	Cytology Specimen			*Histology Specimen*		
Gauge/Use	*C*	*C + P*	*P*	*C*	*C + P*	*P*
22 gauge MW-322	MW-122	MW-222	MW-522	—	—	—
21 gauge	SW-121	SW-221[a]	SW-521	—	—	—
20 gauge	W-120	W-220	W-520	—	—	—
19 gauge	—	—	—	MW-319[a]	—	MWF-319

[a] Recommended needle for cytology and histology.

NOTE: W, WANG; MW, modified Wang or Mill-Rose Wang; SW, Spring Wang; 1, C, central:mediastinal and hilar lymph node; 2, C + P, combined central and peripheral; 3, with trocar mechanism in MW-322 and MW-319; 5, P, peripheral:lung nodules or mass; −1, one needle (i.e., SW-22-11); −4, four needles (i.e., MW-319-4).

SOURCE: Reproduced by permission from Wang KP: Transbronchial needle aspiration and percutaneous needle aspiration for staging and diagnosis of lung cancer. In: Mathur P, Beamis JF, eds. Clinics in Chest Medicine (Interventional Pulmology), Philadelphia: Saunders, 1995:544.

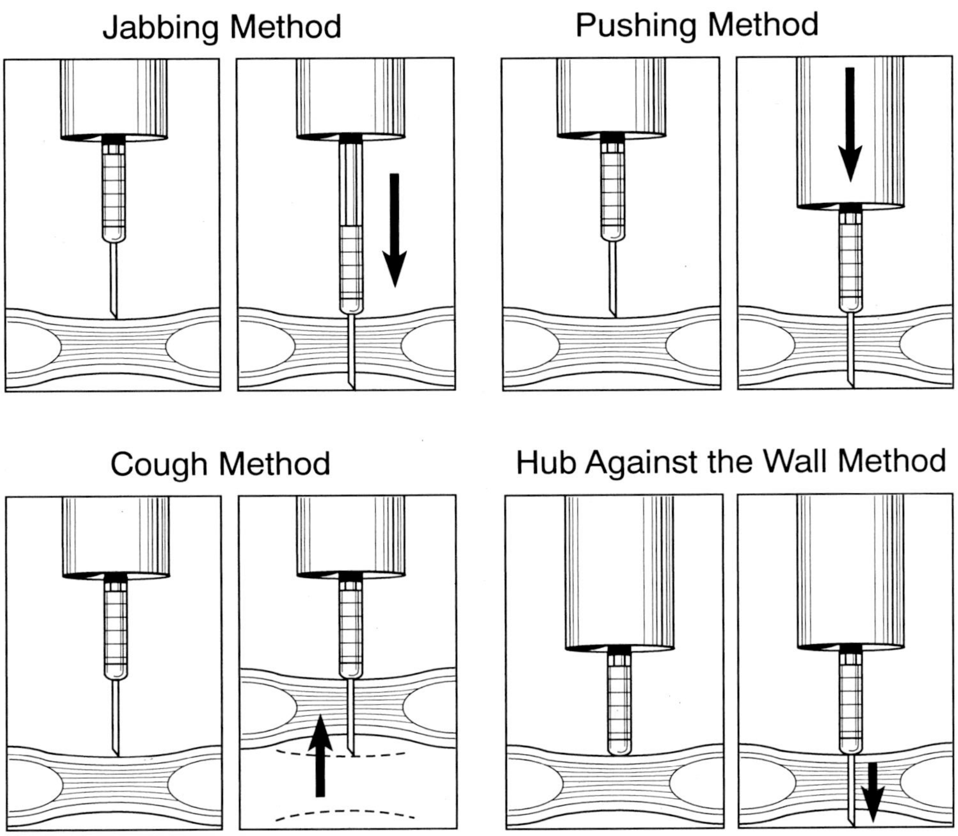

Figure 17-3

Schematic diagram of different techniques used for tracheobronchial wall penetration by TBNA. Jabbing method (*top left*). Pushing or piggyback method (*top right*). Cough method (*bottom left*). Hub against wall method (*bottom right*). [*From Dasgupta A, Mehta AC, Wang KP: Transbronchial needle aspiration. In Mathur PN, Mehta AC (eds): Seminars in Respiratory and Critical Care Medicine. New York, Thieme, 1997:571-581, with permission.*]

Figure 17-4

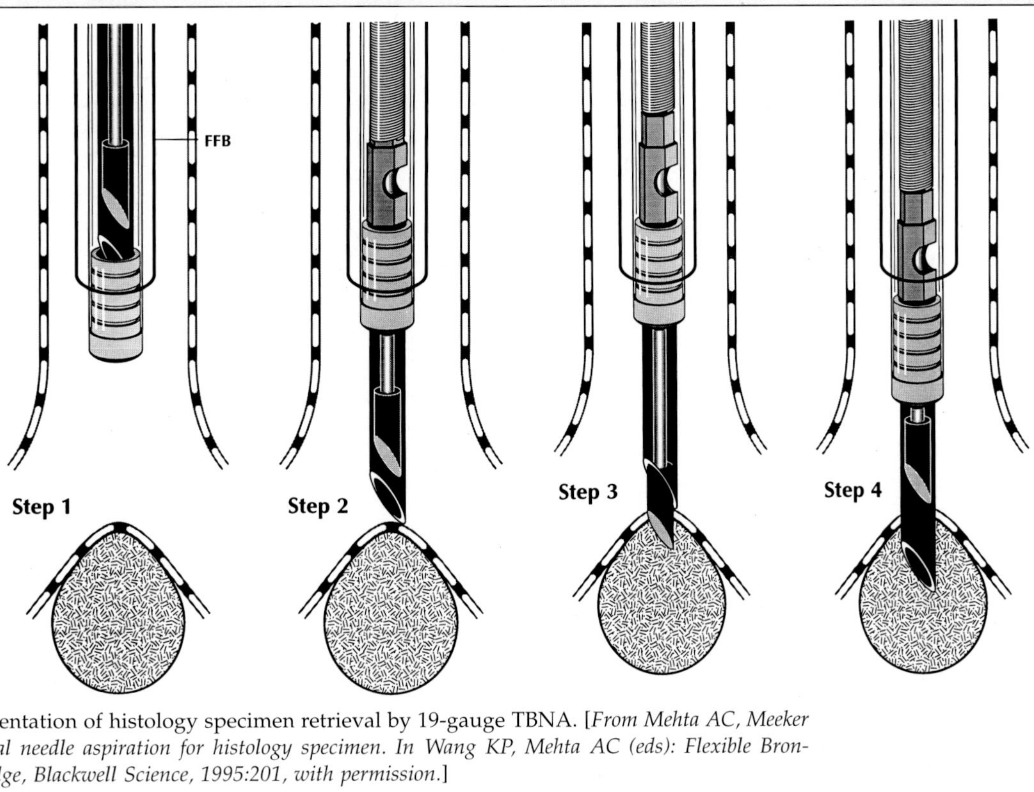

Schematic representation of histology specimen retrieval by 19-gauge TBNA. [*From Mehta AC, Meeker DP: Transbronchial needle aspiration for histology specimen. In Wang KP, Mehta AC (eds): Flexible Bronchoscopy. Cambridge, Blackwell Science, 1995:201, with permission.*]

catheter from recoiling when resistance is met. The bronchoscope and catheter are then pushed forward as a single unit until the entire needle penetrates through the tracheobronchial wall.

3. *Cough Method.* The jabbing or pushing technique is applied while the patient coughs to facilitate spontaneous penetration of the needle.[90]
4. *Hub against the Wall Method.* Occasionally, with the needle retracted, the distal end of the catheter (metal hub) can be placed directly in contact with the target and held firmly, while the needle is pushed through the tracheobronchial wall.

All of these techniques are used singly or in combination for complete penetration of the needle through the tracheobronchial wall.

Once the needle is inserted into the target site, suction is applied to the proximal side port using a 60-ml syringe. If any bloody aspirate is noted from inadvertent penetration of a major intrathoracic vessel, the needle is retracted and a new location selected.

With the suction in place, the catheter is agitated to and fro in an attempt to shear off cells from the node or the mass lesion. The needle is then pulled back out of the target site after suction is released to prevent aspiration of bronchial secretions. The tip of the FB is straightened and the catheter with the still locked needle is withdrawn through the scope in a single straight motion.

When performing TBNA for the purpose of staging, to minimize the potential for false-positive results by contamination with bronchial secretions, TBNA is performed before obtaining any washings, brushings, or biopsy specimens. The bronchoscope is introduced into the endobronchial tree without using suction. Tracheobronchial secretions at the target are washed off with saline or lidocaine before TBNA is begun. Minor modifications in technique allow for obtaining samples from peribronchial, submucosal, and endobronchial lesions. Incomplete penetration at different angles through the bronchial wall with suction helps sample submucosal lesions. Fluoroscopic guidance is needed only when sampling peripheral nodules or masses.

To prepare a smear for cytological analysis, the catheter is removed from the scope, and the specimen from the needle is blown onto a slide using air from the syringe (*smear technique*).[91] The specimen is then smeared, using another slide, and immediately placed in a 95 percent alcohol container. A few seconds' delay may result in drying artifacts on the cells. Alternatively, 3 ml of sterile normal saline or Hank's solution can be used to flush the specimen out of the needle and sent to the cytology laboratory for processing (*fluid technique*).

The TBNA technique for obtaining a histology specimen deserves special emphasis. Histology needles have a dual needle for safe specimen retrieval. Before insertion of the assembly through the working channel of the scope, the 21-gauge needle should be inside the 19-gauge needle and the 19-gauge needle tip inside the metal hub (Fig. 17-4*A*). The assembly is then inserted into the scope until the distal metal hub is just visible outside the scope, taking the same precautions as stated with the cytology needle. Once the metal hub is visualized in the trachea and the target site identified, the assistant extends the 19-gauge needle from the catheter and locks it in place (Fig. 17-4*B*). This automatically advances the 21-gauge needle which is then inserted through the tracheobronchial wall and anchored in position. The 21-gauge needle acts as a trocar for the outer 19-gauge needle and prevents plugging by bronchial tissue or cartilage. Suction is applied at the proximal end using a 60-ml syringe containing 3 ml of normal saline solution [to be certain that the needle is not entering major vascular structures]. The operator then fixes the proximal end of the catheter at the insertion port and using the "pushing method" thrusts the bronchoscope and the catheter as a single unit, advancing the needle through the tracheobronchial wall until the metal hub is flush with the wall (Fig. 17-4*C*).

The 21-gauge needle is then withdrawn into the 19-gauge needle (Fig. 17-4*D*). A core of tissue is obtained by moving the 19-gauge histology needle in and out (partially) through the tracheobronchial wall two to three times, maintaining constant suction. The 19-gauge needle is then withdrawn from the tracheobronchial wall, the assembly is removed from the scope, and the specimen is collected by flushing the needle contents into a container. On occasion the 21-gauge needle is used to push the cored tissue from the 19-gauge needle. Multiple passes are made at each target site until at least two satisfactory specimens are obtained.[33]

REFERENCES

1. Schieppati E: La puncion mediastinal a traves del espolon traqueal. *Rev As Med Argent* 1949; 663:497.
2. Schieppati E: Mediastinal lymph node puncture through the trachial carina. *Surg Gynecol Obstet* 1958; 107:243–246.
3. Brouet G, et al: La ponction pour cyto-diagnostic des adenopathies peri-tracheo-bronchiques isolees. *J Fr Med Chir Thor* 1953; 7:393–398.
4. Euler HE, et al: Zur cytodiagnostik mediastinaler Geschwulste. *Arch Ohr-Usw Heilk Hals-Usw Heilk* 1955; 167:376–383.
5. Schiessle W: La ponction transbronchique et transtracheale des adenopathies peritracheo-bronchiques. *J Fr Med Chir Thor* 1962: 16:551–569.
6. Versteegh RM, Swierenga J: Bronchoscopic evaluation of the operability of pulmonary carcinoma. *Acta Oto-laryng* 1963; 56:603–611.
7. Fox RT, et al: Transcarinal bronchoscopic needle biopsy. *Ann Thorac Surg* 1965; 1:92–96.
8. Bridgman AH, et al: An appraisal of newer diagnostic methods for intrathoracic lesions. *Dis Chest* 1968; 53:321–327.

9. Wang KP, et al: Bronchoscopic needle aspiration biopsy of paratracheal tumors. *Am Rev Respir Dis* 1978; 118:17–21.
10. Wang KP, et al: Transbronchial needle aspiration for diagnosis of lung cancer. *Chest* 1981; 80:48–50.
11. Wang KP, Terry PB: Transbronchial needle aspiration in the diagnosis and staging of bronchogenic carcinoma. *Am Rev Respir Dis* 1983; 127:344–347.
12. Shure D, Fedullo PF: Transbronchial needle aspiration of peripheral masses. *Am Rev Respir Dis* 1983; 128:1090–1092.
13. Prakash UB, et al: Bronchoscopy in North America: The ACCP survey. *Chest* 1991; 100:1668–1675.
14. Kavuru MS, Mehta AC: Applied anatomy of the airways. In Wang KP, Mehta AC (eds): *Flexible Bronchoscopy*. Cambridge, Blackwell Science, 1995: chap 2:6–17.
15. Wang KP: Staging of bronchogenic carcinoma by bronchoscopy. In Wang KP, Mehta AC (eds): *Flexible Bronchoscopy*. Cambridge, Blackwell Science, 1995; chap 14:206–214.
16. Wang KP: Flexible bronchoscopy with transbronchial needle aspiration: Biopsy for cytology specimen. In Wang KP (ed): *Biopsy Techniques in Pulmonary Disorders*. New York, Raven, 1989: chap 5:63–71.
17. Wang KP, et al: Flexible transbronchial needle aspiration: Technical considerations. *Ann Otol Rhinol Laryngol* 1984; 93:233–236.
18. Hammersley JR, Green RA: Transbronchial needle aspiration—Evaluation of penetration depth and areas of high risk use. *Am Rev Respir Disease* 1984; 129(suppl 4):43.
19. Shields TW: Surgical therapy for carcinoma of the lung. *Clin Chest Med* 1993; 14:121–147.
20. Shure D, Fedullo PF: The role of transcarinal needle aspiration in the staging of bronchogenic carcinoma. *Chest* 1984; 86: 693–696.
21. Harrow EM, et al: Transbronchial needle aspiration in clinical practice. In Wang KP, Mehta AC: *Flexible Bronchoscopy*. Cambridge, Blackwell Science, 1995: chap 16:222–234.
22. Jain P, et al: Cost-effectiveness of transbronchial needle aspiration in the staging of lung cancer. *Chest* 1996; 110(4):24s.
23. Malenka DJ, et al: Mediastinal staging in non-small cell lung cancer. *Med Decis Making* 1989; 9:231–242.
24. Wang KP, et al: Flexible transbronchial needle aspiration for staging of bronchogenic carcinoma. *Chest* 1983; 84:571–576.
25. Schenk DA, et al: Transbronchial needle aspiration in the diagnosis of bronchogenic carcinoma. *Chest* 1987; 92:83–85.
26. Utz JP, et al: The role of transcarinal needle aspiration in the staging of bronchogenic carcinoma. *Chest* 1993; 104:1012–1016.
27. Harrow E, et al: Bronchoscopic and roentgenographic correlates of a positive transbronchioal needle aspiration in the staging of lung cancer. *Chest* 1991; 100:1592–1596.
28. Schenk DA, et al: Utility of the Wang 18 gauge transbronchial histology needle in the staging of bronchogenic carcinoma. *Chest* 1989; 96:272–274.
29. Schenk DA, et al: Comparison of the Wang 19 gauge and 22 gauge needles in the mediastinal staging of lung cancer. *Am Rev Respir Dis* 1993; 147:1251–1258.
30. Schenk DA: The role of transbronchial needle aspiration in staging of bronchogenic carcinoma. In Wang KP, Mehta AC: *Flexible Bronchoscopy*. Cambridge, Blackwell Science, 1995; chap 15:215–221.
31. Shure D, Fedullo PF: Transbronchial needle aspiration in the diagnosis of submucosal and peribronchial bronchogenic carcinoma. *Chest* 1985; 88:49–51.
32. Zavala DC: Diagnostic fiberoptic bronchoscopy: Techniques and results of biopsy in 600 patients. *Chest* 1975; 68:12–19.
33. Mehta AC, Meeker DP: Transbronchial needle aspiration for histology specimens. In Wang KP, Mehta AC (eds): *Flexible Bronchoscopy*. Cambridge, Blackwell Science, 1995: chap 13: 199–205.
34. Tita JA, et al: Diagnostic utility of transbronchial needle aspiration in bronchogenic carcinoma presenting as extrinsic compression. *Chest* 1986; 89:449S.
35. Mehta AC, et al: Newer procedures using the fiberoptic bronchoscope in the diagnosis of lung cancer. *Cleve Clin J Med* 1987; 54:195-203.
36. Tsuboi E, et al: Transbronchial biopsy smear for diagnosis of peripheral pulmonary carcinoma. *Cancer* 1967; 20:687–698.
37. Wang KP, et al: Transbronchial needles aspiration of peripheral pulmonary nodules. *Chest* 1984; 86:819–823.
38. Wang KP, et al: Transbronchial needle aspiration versus transthoracic needle aspiration in the diagnosis of pulmonary lesions. *J Bronchol* 1994; 1:199–204.
39. Gasparini S, et al: Integration of transbronchial and percutaneous approach in the diagnosis of peripheral pulmonary nodules or masses. *Chest* 1995; 108:131–137.
40. Popovich J, et al: Diagnostic accuracy of multiple biopsies from flexible fiberoptic bronchoscopy. *Am Rev Respir Dis* 1982; 125: 521–523.
41. Kvale PA, et al: Diagnositic accuracy in lung cancer: Comparison of techniques used in association with flexible fiberoptic bronchoscopy. *Chest* 1976; 69:752–757.
42. Shure D, Astarita RW: Bronchogenic carcinoma presenting as an endobronchial mass: Optimal number of biopsy specimens for diagnosis. *Chest* 1983; 83:865–867.
43. Lundgreen R, et al: Comparison of transbronchial fine needle aspiration biopsy, aspiration of bronchial secretion, bronchial washing, brush biopsy and forceps biopsy in the diagnosis of lung cancer. *Eur J Res Dis* 1983; 64:378–385.
44. Buirski G, et al: Bronchial needle aspiration in the diagnosis of bronchial carcinoma. *Thorax* 1981; 36:508–511.
45. Jones DF, et al: Endobronchial needle aspiration in the diagnosis of small cell carcinoma. *Chest* 1994; 105:1151–1154.
46. Givens CD, Marini JJ: Transbronchial needle aspiration of a bronchial carcinoid tumor. *Chest* 1985; 88:152–153.
47. Puzo C, et al: Bronchoscopic needle aspiration in the diagnosis of bronchial carcinoid. *Eur Respir J* 1996; 9(suppl 23):56s.
48. York EL, et al: A value of submucous needle aspiration in the prediction of surgical resection line of bronchogenic carcinoma. *Chest* 1991; 100:1028–1029.
49. Chan CC, Mehta AC: Niche for the needle: TBNA and coagulopathy. *J Bronchol* 1996; 3:169.
50. Wang KP, et al: Rigid transbronchial needle aspiration biopsy for histological specimens. *Ann Otol Rhinol Laryngol* 1985; 94:382–385.
51. Wagner ED, et al: Transbronchial fine needle aspiration: Reliability and limitations. *Am J Clin Path* 1989; 92:36–41.
52. Ketai L, et al: Combination of flow cytometry and transbronchial needle aspiration in the diagnosis of mediastinal lymphoma. *Chest* 1985; 88:936 (letter).
53. Barzo P: Transbronchial mediastinal cystography. *Chest* 1988; 93:431–432.
54. Schwartz AR, et al: Diagnosis and treatment of a bronchogenic cyst using a transbronchial needle aspiration. *Thorax* 1986; 41:326–327.
55. Schwartz DB, et al: Transbronchial fine needle aspiration of bronchogenic cysts. *Chest* 1985; 88:573–575.
56. McDougall JC, Fromme GA: Transcarinal aspiration of a mediastinal cyst to facilitate anasthetic management. *Chest* 1990; 97:1490–1492.
57. Wang KP, et al: Transbronchial needle aspiration of a mediastinal mass: therapeutic implications. *Thorax* 1983; 38: 556–557.
58. Hirano H, et al: Transbronchial needle aspiration in the diagnosis of pulmonary sclerosing hemangioma. *Respir Med* 1993; 87:475–477.
59. Pauli G, et al: Transbronchial needle aspiration in the diagnosis of sarcoidosis. *Chest* 1984; 85:482–484.
60. Wang KP, et al: Flexible transbronchial needle aspiration for the diagnosis of sarcoidosis. *Ann Otol Rhinol Laryngol* 1989; 98:298–300.

61. Morales CF, et al: Flexible transbronchial needle aspiration in the diagnosis of sarcoidosis. *Chest* 1994; 106:709–711.
62. Baron KM, Aranda CP: Diagnosis of mediastinal mycobacterial lymphadenopathy by transbronchial needle aspiration. *Chest* 1991; 100:1723–1724.
63. Simecek C: Diagnosis of mycobacterial mediastinal lymphadenopathy by transbronchial needle aspiration. *Chest* 1992; 102:1919 (letter).
64. Sesda GJ, et al: Transcarinal needle aspiration in the diagnosis of mediastinal adenitis in a patient infected with the human immunodeficiency virus. *Thorax* 1990; 45(5):414–415.
65. Baran R, et al: Intrathoracic tuberculous lymphadenopathy; Clinical and bronchoscopic features in 17 adults without parenchymal lesions. *Thorax* 1996; 51:87–89.
66. Malabonga VM, et al: Utility of bronchoscopic sampling techniques for cryptococcal disease in AIDS. *Chest* 1991; 99: 370–372.
67. Kucera RF, et al: Hemomediastinum after transbronchial needle aspiration. *Chest* 1986; 90:466.
68. Mehta AC, et al: Bronchoscopic lever biopsy. *J Bronchol* 1994; 1:173–174.
69. Harrow EM, et al: Transbronchial needle aspiration in clinical practice: A five year experience. *Chest* 1989; 96:1268–1272.
70. Watts WJ, Green RA: Bacteremia following transbronchial fine needle aspiration. *Chest* 1984; 85:295.
71. Witt MC, et al: Incidence of fever and bacteremia following transbronchial needle aspiration. *Chest* 1986; 89:85–87.
72. Epstein SK, et al: Polymicrobial bacterial pericarditis after transbronchial needle aspiration. *Am Rev Respir Dis* 1992; 146:523–525.
73. Sherling BE: Complication with a transbronchial histology needle. *Chest* 1990; 98:783–784.
74. Mehta AC, et al: The high price of bronchoscopy. *Chest* 1990; 98:448–454.
75. Cropp AJ, et al: False-positive transbronchial needles aspiration in bronchogenic carcinoma. *Chest* 1984; 85:696–697.
76. Schenk DA, et al: Potential false positive transbronchial needle aspiration in bronchogenic carcinoma. *Chest* 1984; 86:649–650 (letter).
77. Carlin BW, et al: False-positive transcarinal needle aspirate in the evaluation of bronchogenic carcinoma. *Am Rev Respir Dis* 1989; 140:1800–1802.
78. Schenk DA, et al: Transbronchial needle aspiration staging of bronchogenic carcinoma. *Am Rev Respir Dis* 1986; 134:146–148.
79. Horsley JR, et al: Bronchial submucosal needle aspiration performed through the fiberoptic bronchoscope. *Acta Cytol* 1984; 28:211–217.
80. Baker JJ, et al: Transbronchial fine needle aspiration of the mediastinum. Importance of lymphocytes as an indicator of specimen adequacy. *Acta Cytol* 1990; 34:517–523.
81. Haponik EF, et al: Education and experience improve transbronchial needle aspiration performance. *Am J Respir Crit Care Med* 1995; 151:1998–2002.
82. Castella J, et al: Diagnosis and staging of bronchogenic carcinoma by transtracheal and transbronchial needle aspiration. *Ann Oncol* 1995; 6(suppl 3):S21–24.
83. Katis K, et al: The role of transbronchial needle aspiration in the diagnosis of peripheral lung masses or nodules. *Eur Respir J* 1995; 8:963–966.
84. Wang KP, Britt EJ: Needle brush in the diagnosis of lung mass or nodule through flexible bronchoscopy. *Chest* 1991; 100: 1148–1150.
85. Gittlen SD, et al: A new versatile transbronchial cytology needle for the staging and diagnosis of bronchogenic carcinoma. *Chest* 1988; 94:561–565.
86. Salathe M, et al: Transbronchial needle aspiration in routine fiberoptic bronchoscopy. *Respiration* 1992; 59:5–8.
87. Wang KP, et al: Transbronchial needle aspiration for cytology species. *Monaldi Arch Chest Dis* 1994; 49:265–267.
88. Wang KP: Transbronchial needle aspiration and percutaneous needle aspiration for staging and diagnosis of lung cancer. *Clini Chest Med* 1995; 16 (3):535–552.
89. Wang KP: Transbronchial needle aspiration to obtain histology specimen. *J Bronchol* 1994; 1:116–122.
90. Olsen JD, et al: Cough and transbronchial needle aspiration. *Chest* 1986; 89:315 (letter).
91. Ndukwu I, et al: Direct smear for cytological examination of transbronchial needle aspiration specimens. *Chest* 1991; 100:888 (abstr).

CHAPTER 18

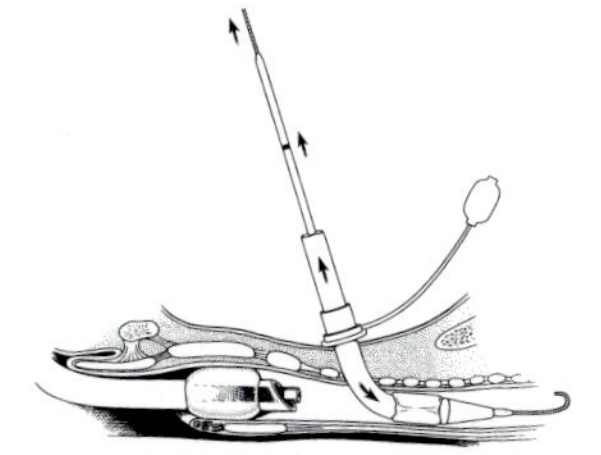

TRANSTRACHEAL OXYGEN THERAPY

Sanjiv Tewari, Kay Stelmach, and Atul C. Mehta

"As emphysema, black or brown lung, and other chronic lung diseases advance in severity, patients become dependent upon oxygen inhalation therapy for comfort and survival. Hypoxemia ravages all organ systems of the body, causing functional and psychological incompetence."[1]

—*Heimlich*

Introduction and Historical Background

In chronically hypoxemic patients, oxygen therapy improves survival and decreases morbidity. The Nocturnal Oxygen Therapy Trial[2] and the British Medical Research Council Study[3] established that the administration of oxygen to eligible patients decreases mortality. The increase in survival correlated with the number of hours that oxygen was used. Attenuation of pulmonary hypertension and improvement of right heart function may, in part, explain this benefit.[4]

In hypoxemic patients, oxygen therapy improves quality of life by decreasing the work of breathing[5] and dyspnea[6] and by improving exercise capacity.[7] Salutory effects on neuropsychiatric function[8] and sleep[9] may also be observed. At the same time, oxygen delivery by nasal cannula or mask has several limitations. Oxygen containers used with gas systems or oxygen concentrators are heavy and poorly portable. The gas irritates the nasopharynx and can impair taste, smell, and appetite (Fig. 18-1). Many patients find the apparatus aesthetically displeasing and cumbersome (Fig. 18-2). Normal daily activities such as shaving and bathing may be difficult to perform. Because of the delivery system, much of the oxygen flow delivered to the nares or mouth dissipates into the ambient air. For those patients on high flow rates of oxygen, the cost may be exorbitant. Because of these various problems, patients are often not compliant with therapy.

Realizing the beneficial effects of oxygen therapy and the inherent problems with conventional modes of oxygen delivery, Heimlich in 1982 introduced a transtracheal oxygen system for the rehabilitation of patients with chronic obstructive pulmonary disease.[1] The procedure was initially performed on intubated beagle dogs. The tips of the catheters were placed at varying levels in the endotracheal tube and the tracheobronchial tree, and pure oxygen was delivered. As the catheter was placed more distally, oxygenation consistently improved until the catheter was placed distal to the carina.

After determining that the distal trachea was the optimal catheter position, Heimlich placed catheters percutaneously through the tracheas of some of the animals. Serial bronchoscopies were performed for 1 year, and the catheters were inspected. No complications were noted. He carried out the procedure in 14 hypoxemic patients and administered oxygen through the transtracheal catheters. Following the procedure, the patients were generally less dyspneic and more alert and active, and they required significantly less oxygen to maintain normoxia.

Because of the small size of the catheter, however, flow rates in excess of 3 to 4 liters/min caused excessive back pressure in the circuit and loss of oxygen through pressure-limiting pop-off valves in the humidifiers. Christopher and others introduced an 8 Fr catheter with a larger internal diameter than the initial prototype.[10] Flow rates of up to 8 liters/min could be delivered without excessive back pressures. The tip of the catheter was designed to maximize oxygen dispersion.

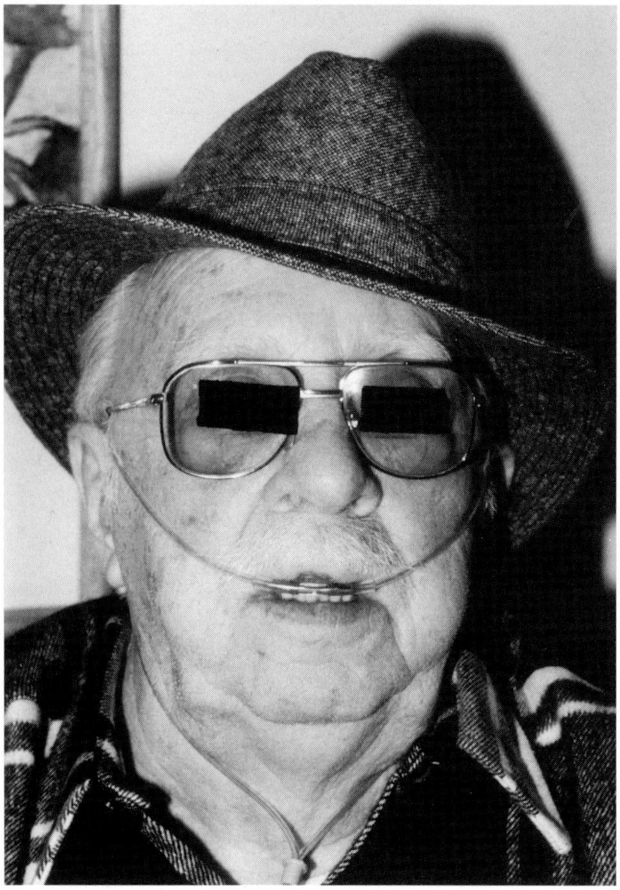

Figure 18-1

A patient on high-flow oxygen by nasal cannula with dry and irritated nares using a nasal cannula orally.

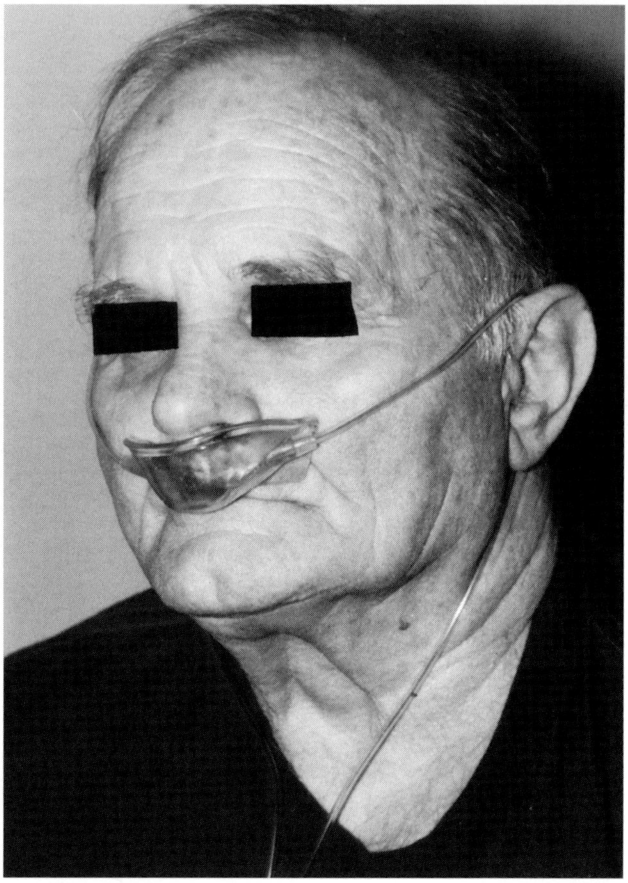

Figure 18-2

A patient using a nasal mask. These devices may be aesthetically unpleasing and may interfere with activities such as shaving and bathing.

Despite initially promising results, transtracheal oxygen therapy (TTOT) has not gained widespread acceptance as an alternative to oxygen delivery by nasal cannula. The use of an invasive procedure in relatively fragile patients, the lack of a understanding of the potential benefits, and the fear of rare, yet potentially serious, complications have dissuaded clinicians from widely adopting TTOT.

The pulmonologist caring for chronically hypoxemic patients can benefit from a detailed understanding of TTOT. This chapter is divided into three sections: a scientific review, an overview of the necessary equipment for insertion and our method of instituting TTOT, and complications of the procedure.

Scientific Review

PHYSIOLOGIC RATIONALE

Effects on Oxygenation

As compared with other oxygen delivery systems, TTOT achieves therapeutic levels of blood oxygen with lower flow rates. Heimlich observed a 57 percent reduction in oxygen requirement.[1] Using a larger-diameter catheter in eight patients with hypoxemia refractory to high-flow oxygen by nasal cannula, Christopher observed a 72 percent reduction in oxygen flow requirements and significant improvement in oxygenation.[10]

In addition to its use as rescue therapy in patients with hypoxemia refractory to oxygen by nasal cannula, TTOT may be beneficial in patients with chronic hypoxemia as an alternative to nasal cannula. In a study comparing the two modalities in patients with mean oxygen requirements of 2.7 liters/min, oxygen by the transtracheal route diminished oxygen requirements by 45 percent at rest and 39 percent with exercise.[11] The initial resolution of hypoxemia with TTOT may in 20 to 25 percent of patients be associated with a long-term increase in arterial oxygen tension.[12] This finding is not surprising given that up to 40 percent of individuals initially qualifying for oxygen therapy with nasal cannula may after a month of therapy become ineligible for such therapy by current guidelines.[13] The reasons for this improvement may relate to spontaneous improvement in the clinical condition of some patients or the beneficial effects of oxygen itself.

Transtracheal systems using pulsed oxygen delivery devices seem to further diminish oxygen requirements at rest and with exercise.[14,15] By delivering the bulk of oxygen flow during inspiration, pulsed devices decrease the amount of oxygen loss during exhalation and, thus, improve the efficiency of oxygen delivery.

Effects on Ventilation and Work of Breathing

Minute ventilation is calculated by multiplying the respiratory rate by the tidal volume. With the institution of TTOT, a portion of the patient's tidal volume is provided by the continuous flow of oxygen into the trachea. With incremental increases in transtracheal oxygen flow, less air must be entrained by the patient through the nares and mouth to maintain the same minute ventilation. Using a flow-sensing spirometer, Couser and Make demonstrated that as transtracheal flow increases, the patient's contribution to inspired minute ventilation decreases.[16,17] The exhaled minute ventilation and the arterial P_{CO_2} remain unchanged.

Owing to this reduction in inspired minute ventilation, work of breathing on inspiration using TTOT is diminished. The metabolic work performed by the inspiratory muscles and the diaphragm are both reduced.[18] In a single-blind crossover study, Benditt and others[18] measured pleural and transdiaphragmatic pressures using esophageal and gastric balloons in five patients breathing room air by mouth and receiving either air or oxygen transtracheally. The oxygen cost of breathing estimated by calculation of the pleural-pressure time index was reduced with tracheal insufflation of air or oxygen. Furthermore, the tension-time index for the diaphragm was similarly reduced with increasing transtracheal flow.

Effects on Exercise

Following institution of oxygen therapy by any route, exercise capacity is enhanced.[19] Oxygen via nasal cannula, however, requires greater flow rates as compared with TTOT to achieve adequate oxygen saturations during exercise.[20]

Exercise endurance as assessed by the 12-min walk in a double-blind fashion was greater when patients received TTOT than when they received oxygen by nasal cannula.[21] This finding was unrelated to an increase in the oxygen saturation, implying that other factors such as decreased work of breathing with TTOT are responsible.

Maximal exercise tolerance assessed by graded treadmill testing is, in contrast, no different in patients using oxygen by nasal cannula or transtracheally.[22] Using either modality, oxygenation during exercise and maximal exercise tolerance were enhanced with higher flow rates of oxygen.

Effects on Pulmonary Hypertension, Erythrocytosis, and Survival

In chronically hypoxemic patients, supplemental oxygen by nasal cannula decreases pulmonary hypertension.[4] No studies have been performed to evaluate the effect of TTOT on pulmonary pressures in this population. Delivery of oxygen transtracheally should theoretically provide the same beneficial hemodynamic benefits.

Because of a sustained improvement in oxygenation, secondary erythrocytosis is frequently ameliorated. In those patients receiving oxygen by nasal cannula with a hematocrit exceeding 45 percent, there may be significant amelioration of erythrocytosis with TTOT.[23,24] Improved compliance with therapy may account for this improvement.

TTOT may confer a greater survival benefit than does oxygen therapy by nasal cannula. A recent retrospective study of 165 patients using either TTOT or oxygen by nasal cannula, in which the groups were matched in terms of severity of illness, demonstrated a median survival of 66 and 49 months, respectively.[25] Prospective studies need to be done to validate this result.

SUBJECTIVE RATIONALE

Improvement of Dyspnea

Although the literature contains a number of anecdotal reports of patients having less dyspnea when switched from nasal cannula to TTOT, there have been no well-controlled studies performed. In a study using a quantifiable dyspnea score recorded every minute while patients were exercised, there was no difference when oxygen was delivered by nasal cannula or transtracheally.[22] The relief that some patients experience with TTOT may relate to the decreased work of breathing associated with this modality. In some patients with refractory hypoxemia despite maximal oxygen therapy with nasal cannula, transtracheal delivery may improve dyspnea by improving oxygenation.[10]

Improvement of Cosmesis and Comfort

The nasal cannula is highly conspicuous and is aesthetically displeasing to some patients. The transtracheal catheter is easily concealed from the view of others. This benefit of improved appearance although not quantifiable is important to some chronically ill patients requiring oxygen therapy.

Oxygen flow by nasal cannula particularly at high levels can cause nasal mucous membranes to become dry and irritated. The resulting loss of smell detracts from the savour that many foods have and, consequently, appetite diminishes. The nasal cannula itself provides a mechanical impediment to eating in that the act of swallowing obstructs, albeit momentarily, oxygen flow to the trachea. Some patients gain weight following the institution of TTOT.[26]

Improvement of Ambulation, Performance of Daily Activities, and Sleep

Both ambulation and activity level are greater with the use of TTOT. In a group of patients with severe chronic obstructive lung disease, Bloom and others randomized patients to oxygen therapy by transtracheal catheter or by nasal cannula. At 6 months of follow-up, patients using TTOT required significantly less assistance to care for themselves and to carry on normal activities.[23] This group also had a greater feelings of independence and a trend toward less depression and improved morale.

The reasons for this improvement in quality of life may be due to the reduced work of breathing using TTOT and improved exercise endurance. Another important factor is that patients, because of lower oxygen requirements, are liberated from heavy gas oxygen containers and can use portable and lightweight liquid oxygen cannisters for a longer duration. Despite lower oxygen requirements at rest and with exercise, patients may paradoxically use more oxygen because they are more active and more compliant with therapy.[21]

The impact of TTOT on the quality of sleep in patients without sleep apnea is unknown. In patients with severe obstructive sleep apnea and daytime hypoxemia, nocturnal transtracheal oxygen therapy reduced the frequency of sleep-disordered breathing more so than oxygen therapy with nasal cannula.[27] For patients with obstructive sleep apnea and nocturnal desaturation who cannot tolerate nasal continuous positive airway pressure (CPAP), TTOT may be a treatment option.

COST

Although there should be decreased expenditure for oxygen with TTOT, there is also increased cost for the insertion, replacement, and maintenance of the catheter. Comprehensive cost analyses comparing transtracheal oxygen therapy to nasal cannula are not available. In some patients TTOT may result in fewer days of hospitalization.[23] For most patients, TTOT does not reduce the number of admissions nor the length of stay in hospital compared with oxygen by nasal cannula.[25] Hospital costs per admission may, however, be less with transtracheal therapy.

INDICATIONS FOR TTOT

Any patient who is a candidate for long-term oxygen therapy by nasal cannula is a potential candidate for TTOT. The most clinical experience has been in patients with chronic obstructive pulmonary disease, although patients with a wide variety of interstitial lung diseases have also benefited from the procedure.

Nevertheless, the precise indications for such therapy have yet to be defined in these heterogeneous patient populations. Most clinical trials have reported clinical experiences using the transtracheal catheter rather than systematically assessing clinical factors that reliably predict improvements in dyspnea, oxygenation, exercise capacity, pulmonary hypertension, and survival. Equally important, the risk factors predicting catheter-related complications have not been extensively studied.

Table 18-1
INDICATIONS FOR TTOT FOR PATIENTS ON CONTINUOUS OXYGEN BY NASAL CANNULA

Unresolving dyspnea
Refractory hypoxemia
Excessive oxygen needs (3–4 liters/min)
Impaired exercise capacity or ambulation
Noncompliance with therapy
Intolerance to therapy (e.g., epistaxis, local irritation, skin allergy to nasal cannula)
Impaired taste and appetite
Patient preference or cosmetic reasons

Table 18-2
CONTRAINDICATIONS TO TTOT

Psychiatric disorder
Inability to communicate
Unwillingness or inability to take care of catheter
Severe co-morbid illnesses and guarded prognosis
Coagulopathy
Herniated pleura over insertion site (emphysematous patients)
Upper airway obstruction

Potential indications for the use of TTOT are outlined in Table 18-1.

CONTRAINDICATIONS TO TTOT

Transtracheal oxygen catheters should not be placed in patients in whom the initial placement would be hazardous or maintenance of the catheter would not be possible, and in situations where catheter-related complications could be fatal. The specific contraindications to TTOT are summarized in Table 18-2.

Equipment

Transtracheal catheters are generally inserted percutaneously. Tunneled catheters are surgically implanted below the skin and are rarely used. Typically, percutaneous catheters consist of a flexible polyurethane tube with proximal flanges that anchor the catheter in place at the insertion site. A chain may be inserted through fenestrations in the flanges. The chain and accompanying catheter then hang comfortably around the neck.

Many different types of percutaneous catheters are available. The Oxycath (Laboratoire Cometh, Lyon, France) is used commonly in Europe and has a long intratracheal portion with multiple fenestrations. The Microtrach (Ballard, UT) consists of a 16 gauge, 5 Fr catheter with a flanged piece which can accommodate flow rates of oxygen up to 4 liters/min. Flow exceeding this rate causes excessive back pressure in the oxygen apparatus and can release pop-off valves in the humidifier circuit. The catheter itself is inserted into the trachea using the Seldinger technique over a rigid metal needle attached to a syringe.

The SCOOP catheter (Transtracheal Systems, Denver, CO) is a 9 Fr flanged tube with a 9 or 11 cm intratracheal portion (Fig. 18-3). Flow rates of up to 8 liters/min may be delivered. The catheter insertion differs from other systems in three important ways: the catheter is inserted over a guide wire, a stent is employed to establish a transtracheal tract, and oxygen administration is delayed to avoid early subcutaneous emphysema.

HOW I DO IT

At our institution, we have used the SCOOP transtracheal system since 1986 and have inserted more than 200 such catheters. The steps for catheter insertion are well outlined in the Clinician Guide[28] that comes with the kit. The following approach reflects a combination of the manufacturer's guidelines and our modifications.

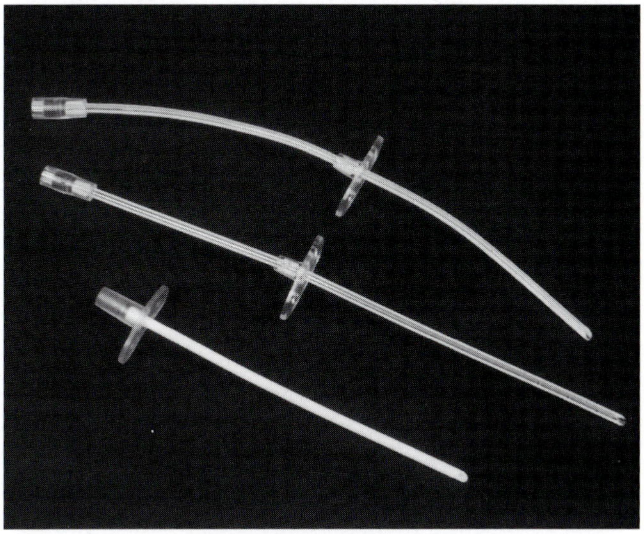

Figure 18-3

The SCOOP transtracheal system catheter. From *top* to *bottom:* the SCOOP-1 catheter, the SCOOP-2 catheter, and the stent.

Phase 1: Patient Preparation

The potential candidate for TTOT should receive the Patient Workbook and Guide that is provided with the SCOOP catheter and should view the SCOOP Patient Education and Training Video. The procedure and the potential complications are discussed in detail with the patient. All relevant questions are answered during this orientation period.

We routinely perform a complete history and physical examination and obtain a chest radiograph, spirometry, arterial blood-gas measurements, a complete blood count, and an exercise oximetry. Important points in the history include the presence of a coagulopathy, bronchorrhea, or bronchospasm. The physical examination should include a close inspection of the anatomic landmarks of the neck, noting any deformities or scars. A prior tracheostomy scar is not a contraindication to TTOT.

In examining the chest radiograph, the clinical should note pleural herniation over the tracheal insertion site, tracheal deviation, and tracheal length. The spirogram and arterial blood gas may be used to calculate a MOC score, an abbreviation for mechanical reserve, oxygenation, and carbon dioxide retention.[28] A SAL level, or score for activity level, provides an index of disability.[28]

The manufacturer suggests caution in performing the procedure in patients with poor respiratory mechanics or reserve and in severely disabled patients. Practitioners learning the procedure should avoid performing the procedure on these types of patient until they have mastered the technique.

The patient should give informed consent and should be instructed to take nothing by mouth after midnight prior to the procedure.

Phase 2: Transtracheal Procedure and "Stent Week"

The procedure consists of marking appropriate landmarks, administering local anesthetic into the soft tissues and intratracheally, and inserting the dilator and then the stent over a guide wire. With the patient sitting upright, the upper border of the thyroid cartilage is marked with a V, the adjacent cricoidothyroid cartilage is marked with a horizontal line, and the sternal notch is marked with a U. Between the cricothyroid cartilage and the sternal notch lies the cervical trachea, the site of insertion of the catheter (Fig. 18-4).

The beaded stainless steel necklace that will ultimately fit through flanges on the transtracheal catheter is placed around the neck. The length of the necklace is adjusted using a wire cutter. The necklace should fit loosely enough that two finger breadths may be accommodated and should lie over the first or second tracheal interspace. The point at which the chain crosses the midline of the trachea is where the catheter should subsequently be inserted. Cricothyroid puncture, which should be avoided, can cause hoarseness from puncture of the cricovocal ligament, poor tract development, and keloid formation.

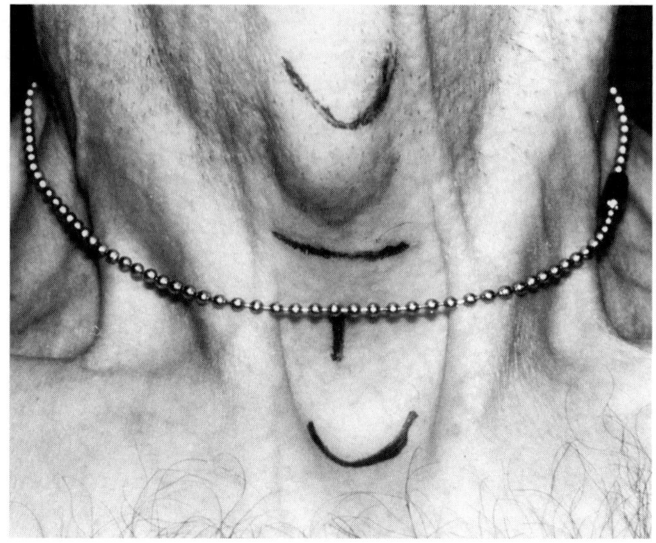

Figure 18-4

The anatomic landmarks and appropriate steel necklace length. The thyroid cartilage is marked with a V, the cricoid cartilage with a horizontal line, and the sternal notch with a U. The necklace lies over the cervical trachea at the point of subsequent catheter insertion

Following establishment of the landmarks, the clinician may perform the procedure with the patient sitting upright or lying back at a 45 degree angle. After swabbing the insertion site with alcohol, local anaesthetic is widely injected with a 27-gauge needle. The trachea is then transfixed in the midline position with the thumb and forefinger of the nondominant hand. Local anesthetic is injected deeper at the chosen insertion site. A 20-gauge needle then is inserted perpendicularly into the trachea at this site. Aspiration of air confirms that the needle is in the trachea. The patient is forewarned of a cough and, subsequently, approximately 2 ml of local anaesthetic is instilled intratracheally.

The field is then sterilized with chlorhexidine, and the neck is draped. Sterile gloves are donned by the clinician. A no. 15 scalpel is used to make a 1-cm vertical incision at the insertion site. The dermis is exposed and then the underlying fat by gently dissecting down with to and fro movements of the belly of the scalpel. An 18-gauge, 7-cm Cook needle attached to a lidocaine filled syringe is inserted perpendicular to the trachea through the intercartilagenous ligament. Air is again aspirated, confirming that the needle is in-

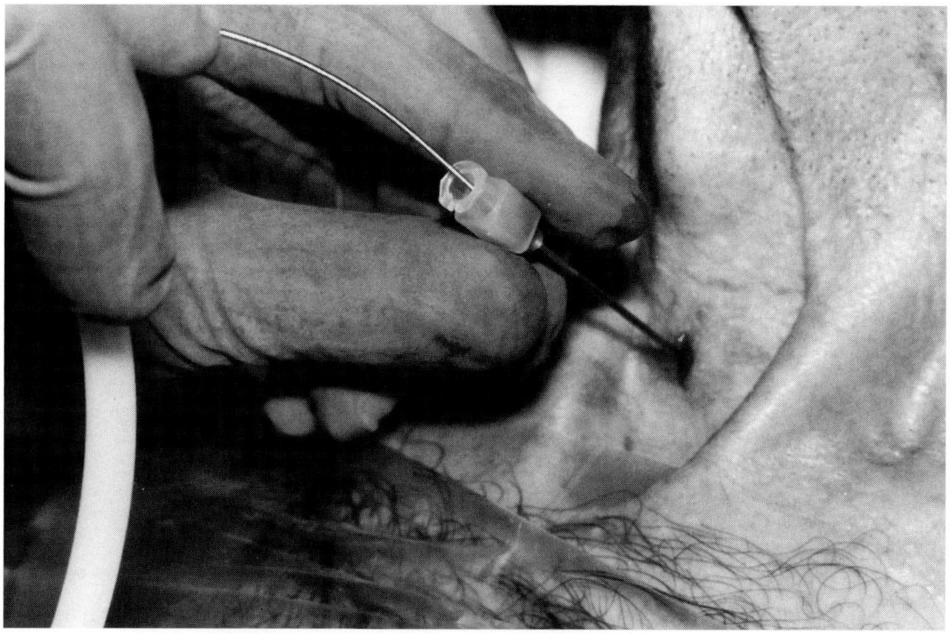

Figure 18-5

Following tracheal penetration by the 18-gauge needle, a guide wire is inserted into the trachea.

tratracheal, and local anesthetic may again be administered. A guide wire is inserted through this needle to the 11-cm reference mark (Fig. 18-5). The needle is removed over the guide wire.

An alternative approach to using the 18-gauge needle is to employ a 20-gauge Raulerson syringe to insert the guide wire[29] (Fig. 18-6). This technique may be useful when tracheal insertion with the 18-gauge needle is difficult.

A dilator is passed over the guide wire and gently rotated through the tracheal interspace (Fig. 18-7). Angling the dilator downward prevents damage to the posterior tracheal wall. The dilator should be inserted approximately 2 cm past the tracheal wall and should be left in place for at least 2 min. The dilator is removed and a lubricated stent (pre-SCOOP catheter) is placed over the guide wire into the trachea. The guide wire is then removed (Fig. 18-8). Air should be aspirated from the stent to ensure an intratracheal position. The stent is then sewn into place, and a nonocclusive dressing is applied.

Following the procedure, a chest radiograph or fluoroscopy should be used to check the catheter's position and to exclude a pneumothorax (Fig. 18-9). The patient is discharged after a period of observation. An antibiotic with coverage for skin flora, especially *Staphylococcus aureus,* is prescribed for 1 week. An analgesic, either a nonsteroidal anti-inflammatory or low-potency opiate, and a non-narcotic cough suppressant are provided. Periodic use of aqueous lidocaine through the stent can assist in suppressing cough.

During the stent week the patient continues to use oxygen through nasal prongs. This period allows the patient to become familiar with a transtracheal device and allows the tract to develop. Withholding oxygen in this early period may minimize subcutaneous emphysema.[28] The patient should clean the tract site twice daily with a cotton-tipped applicator and 3% hydrogen peroxide.

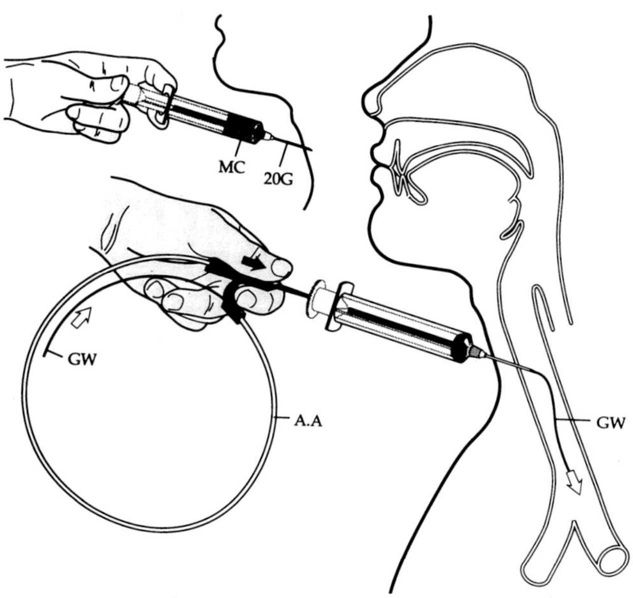

Figure 18-6

Schematic of TTOT procedure performed with use of a Raulerson syringe. A 20-gauge needle attached to the syringe is inserted into the trachea. Using an Arrow advancer (AA), a guide wire (GW) is inserted through the hollow piston and the metal cannula (MC) into the trachea. (*From Mehta AC, et al: Insertion of a pre-SCOOP transtracheal oxygen therapy catheter with use of a Raulerson syringe. Chest 1992; 101:887–888, with permission.*)

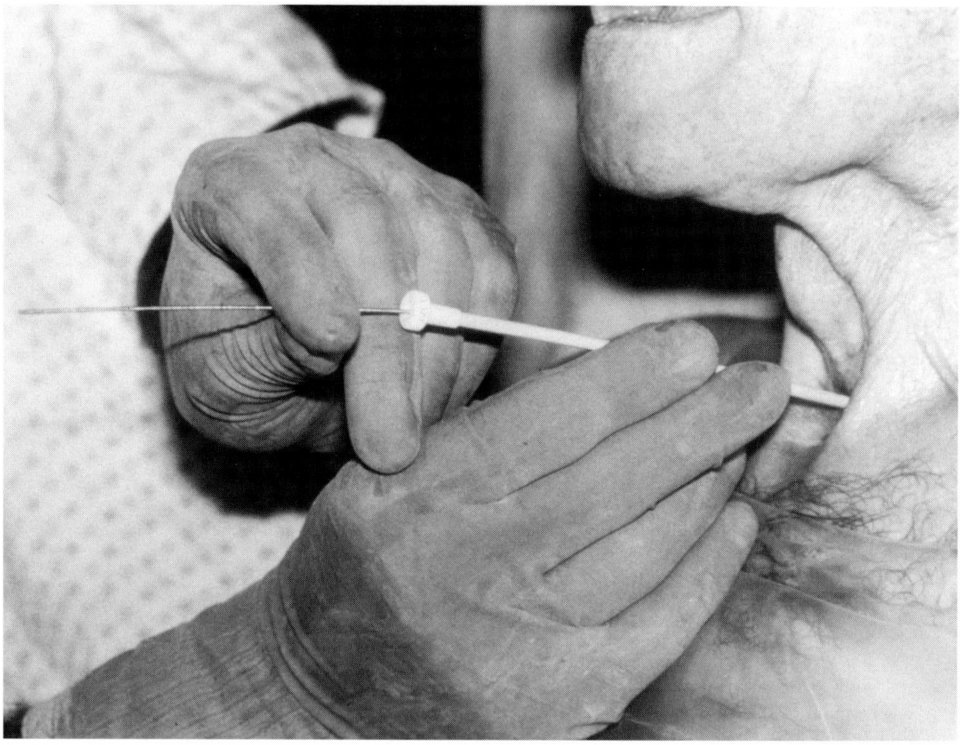

Figure 18-7

By applying gentle pressure and rotating, a dilator is placed over the guide wire into the trachea.

Phase 3: Transtracheal Oxygen with an Immature Tract

After having the stent in place for 1 week, the patient returns for insertion of a functioning SCOOP-1 catheter. The procedure is performed by administering aqueous lidocaine through the stent, removing the stent over a guide wire, and inserting the new catheter.

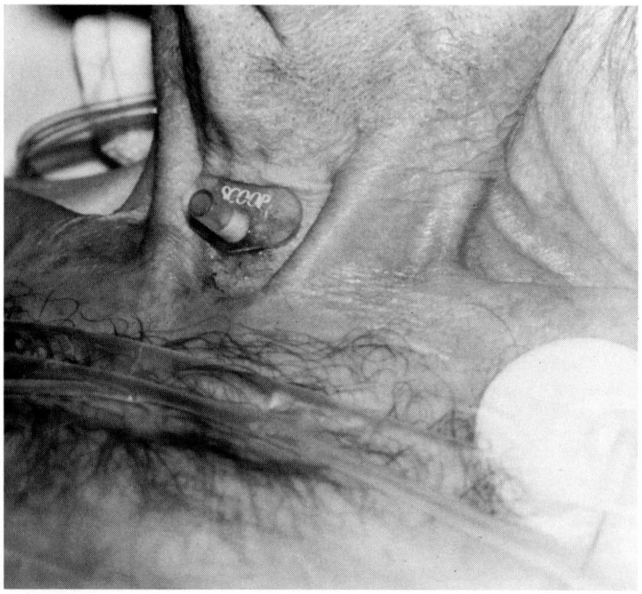

Figure 18-8

After dilation for at least 2 min, the guide wire is reinserted and the dilator is removed. A SCOOP stent is inserted over the guide wire.

The catheter is 11 cm long and, therefore, it should not reach the carina in most patients. Patients with short stature and restrictive lung disease may need shorter catheters to avoid trauma to the carina.[30] A 9-cm catheter is available, and other catheter lengths, if necessary, may be ordered.

The oxygen flow rate is titrated to the patients' needs at rest and with exercise. The patient is fitted with an oxygen hose that fits under the shirt to emerge at the waist where it is attached to a security clip on a belt. The hose then is connected to an oxygen tank. SCOOP oxygen hoses are available in different lengths, allowing for tailoring the system to the measurements of the patient.

At this point, the transtracheal tract is still immature, and dislodgement of the catheter can result in a lost tract. A piece of tape or a bandage over the right and left flanges of the catheter is used to secure the catheter in addition to the necklace.

Cleaning of the catheter becomes an important issue at this stage, since mucous plugs, which may be life-threatening, can form on the catheter. Patients are stratified in the manufacturer's guide into low, moderate, or high risk, depending on their oxygen requirements, secretion production, and MOC score.

Preventive efforts consist of cleaning the catheter in place with saline and a cleaning rod, using a humidifier, and stripping the catheter periodically over a guide wire. The intensity of such efforts and the frequency of follow-up visits are dictated by the patient's risk strata. Techniques to increase the forcefulness of coughing may help in difficult cases.[31] Patients should immedi-

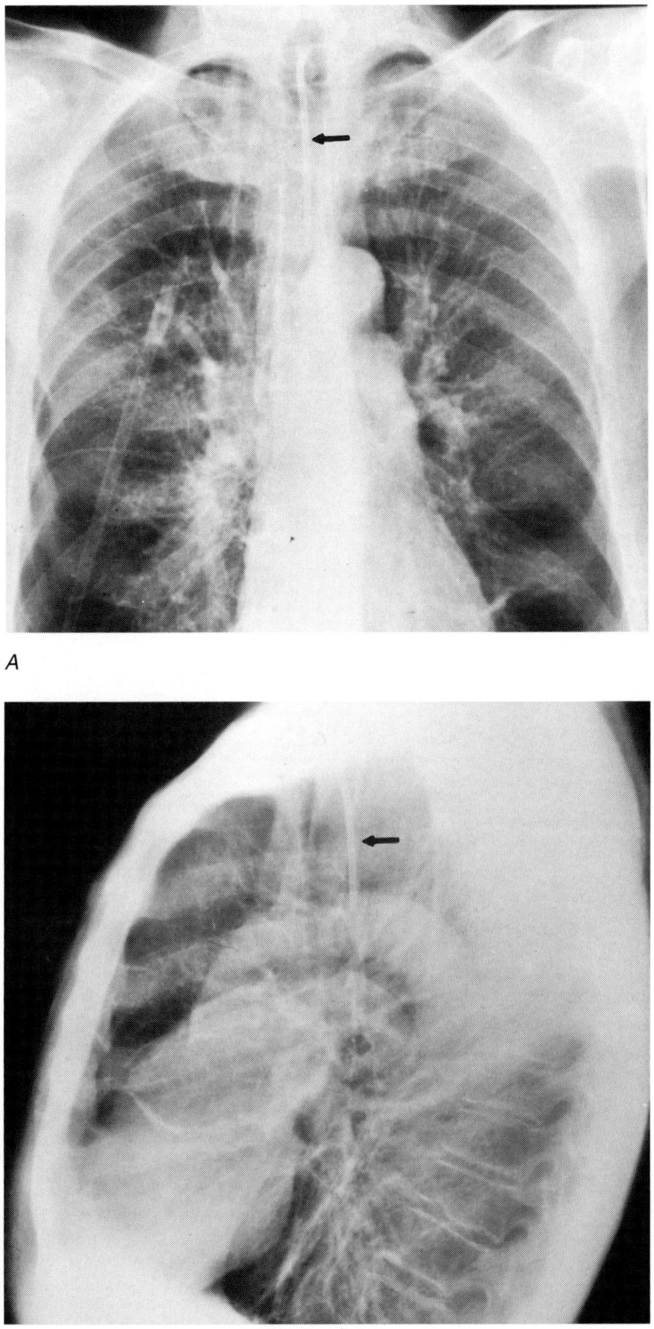

A

B

Figure 18-9

A posteroanterior (*A*) and lateral (*B*) chest radiograph showing a pre-SCOOP catheter (*arrow*) in correct position well above the carina.

ately report any new respiratory symptoms, since delay in recognition of mucous balls can prove fatal.

Phase 4: Transtracheal Oxygen with a Mature Tract

This phase begins 6 to 8 weeks after the initial insertion. The transtracheal tract is mature at this stage, meaning that the tract will not be lost with transient removal of the catheter. The patient can remove the used catheter and insert a clean one. The first catheter is then cleaned under a faucet for subsequent use. Although the tract is mature, the catheters should be exchanged quickly to avoid tract closure.

A SCOOP-2 catheter is usually inserted at this time. This catheter has multiple side ports and may be more comfortable at higher flow rates. The SCOOP-2 catheter should be removed twice per day for cleaning and to avoid mucous buildup. Patients may also clean the catheter in place in addition to or in place of removal. The SCOOP-1 catheter can also be used with a mature tract.

The SCOOP catheters should be replaced every 3 months. Routine clinical follow-up is suggested every 3 months. Objective measures of improved oxygenation and exercise such as the hematocrit and exercise oximetry, respectively, should be repeated at least once following the procedure.

Complications of TTOT

PROCEDURE-RELATED COMPLICATIONS

During the initial insertion of the transtracheal catheter, several potential complications may be encountered.[32] The catheter may be malpositioned cephalad or outside the trachea (Figs. 18-10 to 18-12). Bleeding from the insertion site and hemoptysis may occur. The latter may on occasion be significant.[33] Transient hoarseness from inadvertant puncture of the cricothyroid membrane may result. Commencing oxy-

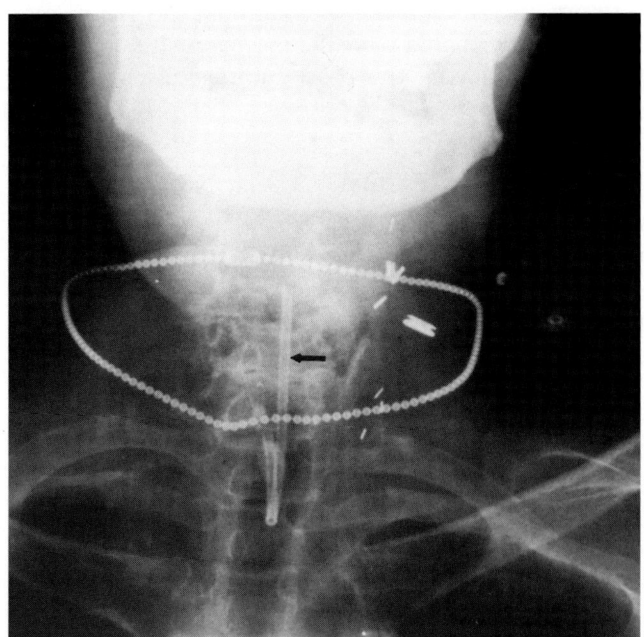

Figure 18-10

Cephalad migration of a transtracheal oxygen catheter (*arrow*).

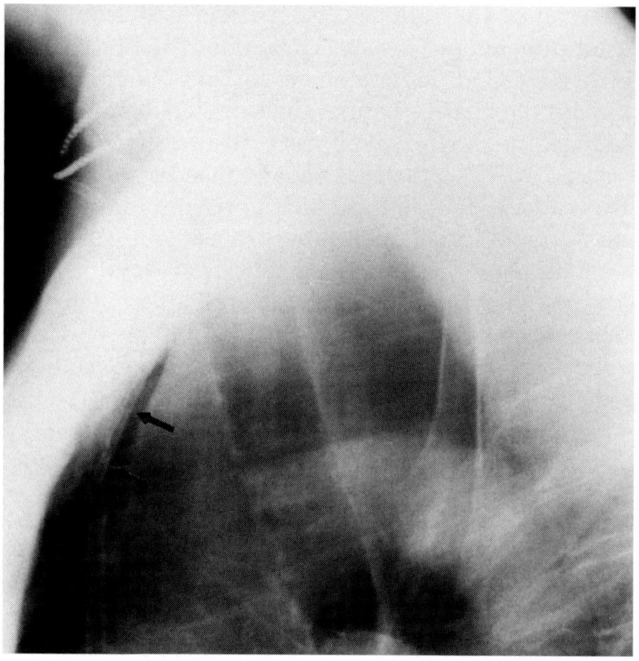

Figure 18-11

Lateral chest radiograph showing a misplaced SCOOP-2 transtracheal catheter (*arrows*) in the anterior mediastinum. (*From Adamo JP, et al: The Cleveland Clinic's initial experience with transtracheal oxygen therapy. Respir Care 1990; 35:156, with permission.*)

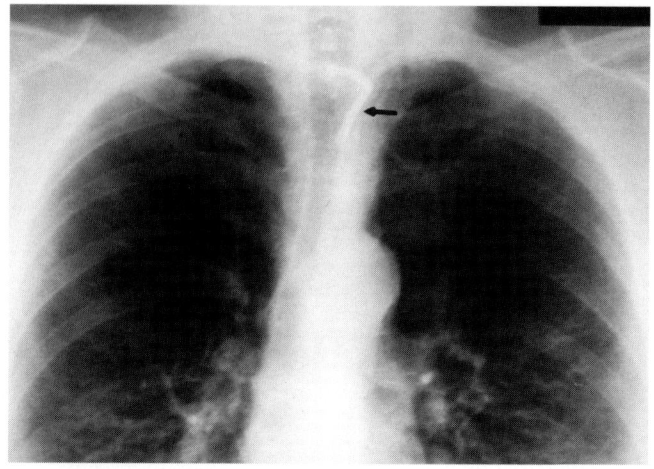

A

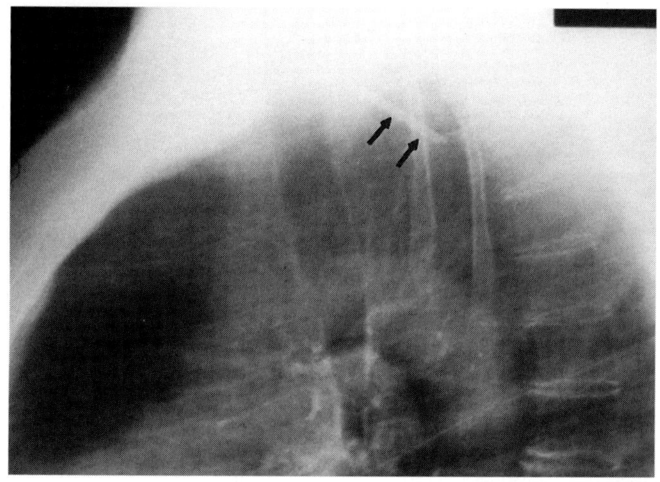

B

Figure 18-12

Posteroanterior (*A*) and lateral (*B*) chest radiograph demonstrating a misplaced transtracheal pre-SCOOP transtracheal catheter (*arrows*) in the middle mediastinum. (*From Adamo JP, et al: The Cleveland Clinic's initial experience with transtracheal oxygen therapy. Respir Care 1990; 35:156, with permission.*)

gen through the catheter just after insertion, as is done with some commercial models, can produce early subcutaneous emphysema. Bronchospasm and excessive coughing may occur and exacerbate this problem. The development of pneumothorax or pneumomediastinum should alert the clinician that the pleura may have been herniated over the insertion site. In the initial days following the procedure, cellulitis or chondritis may ensue.

POSTPROCEDURE COMPLICATIONS

With catheter systems using oxygen immediately following insertion, many problems may be noted. An example of such devices is the Micro-Trach, a 16 gauge flanged catheter inserted over a guide wire.[34] In a series of 200 patients over a 7-year span, Heimlich observed a 10 percent incidence of subcutaneous emphysema and a 1 to 2 percent incidence of local subcutaneous infection owing to the procedure.[35] There were no major complications noted nor any deaths related to the procedure. This review did not, however, systematically screen for nor quantify the number of complications. Using a 16 gauge angiocatheter attached to an inverted pediatric tracheostomy tube, a small study identified staphylococcal cellulitis and tracheobronchitis as well as catheter fracture and displacement as potential complications.[36,37] The Johnson ITO$_2$C intratracheal catheter has been associated with nearly fatal tracheal obstruction from a mucous plug.[38] Lobar collapse with respiratory failure has also been reported.[39]

The complications of catheter systems delaying the use of oxygen until the transtracheal tract is well formed have been researched more thoroughly.[25,40,41] The SCOOP catheter originally described in 1986[10] has several potential complications that are summarized in Table 18-3. The lack of reports of similar complications using other transtracheal systems may relate to the fact that they have been less extensively used and studied.

The clinician may encounter a wide variety of problems. The catheter can become displaced cephalad from its normal position or may be severed.[42] The

Table 18-3
COMPLICATIONS OF THE SCOOP CATHETER

Complication	*References*	*Frequency, %*
Technical		
Misplaced catheter	41	2
Dislodged catheter	24, 40, 41	11–22
Cephalad displacement	24, 40, 41	2–3
Severed catheter	43	2
Broken chain	44	1
Subcutaneous emphysema	24, 40, 41	0–1
Pneumomediastinum	41	1
Lost tract	24, 40, 41	7–8
Symptomatic		
Cough	40, 41	5–7
Hoarseness	24, 41	1–3
Excessive sputum production	41	4
Hemoptysis	24, 40, 41	2–5
Inspissated mucous plugs	24, 40, 41	10–25
Intolerance to high flow TTOT	41	1
Airway		
Excessive stomal granulation tissue	41, 42	6
Tracheal mucous impaction	43, 44, 45	CR
Tracheal perforation	46	CR
Infectious		
Stomal infection	24, 40, 41	1–7
Chondritis	41	1
Pneumonia	47	CR
Miscellaneous		
Unrealized expectations	24, 41	1–13
Keloid formation	24, 40	4–7

NOTE: CR, Case report(s).

chain securing the catheter can break, allowing the catheter to slip out of the trachea. If this occurs just after insertion, the tract may not be mature and may close immediately leading to a "lost tract." Subcutaneous emphysema and pneumomediastinum can occur once oxygen is administered through the catheter. A variety of symptoms can arise from the irritative effects of the catheter on the tracheal mucosa (Fig. 18-13). The expectoration of mucous plugs is common and may herald tracheal obstruction with a mucous ball (Fig. 18-14).[43-45] Tracheal obstruction with granulation tissue and tracheal perforation have also been reported.[46] Minor complications include stomal infections and chondritis. These infections usually respond well to antibiotics, although occasionally scarring and keloid formation may result.[47]

Summary

For certain patients on oxygen by nasal cannula, TTOT can reduce oxygen requirements, decrease the work of breathing, and improve exercise endurance. Dyspnea may be lessened and the quality of life increased. Survival benefit and cost savings have as yet to be definitively established.

The insertion procedure is associated with a number of early complications. Late complications arise from problems with the tract or the catheter itself. Most complications are minor, although rarely they may be life-threatening. Proper patient selection and adherence to the recommended guidelines for insertion and maintenance of the catheter minimize complications.

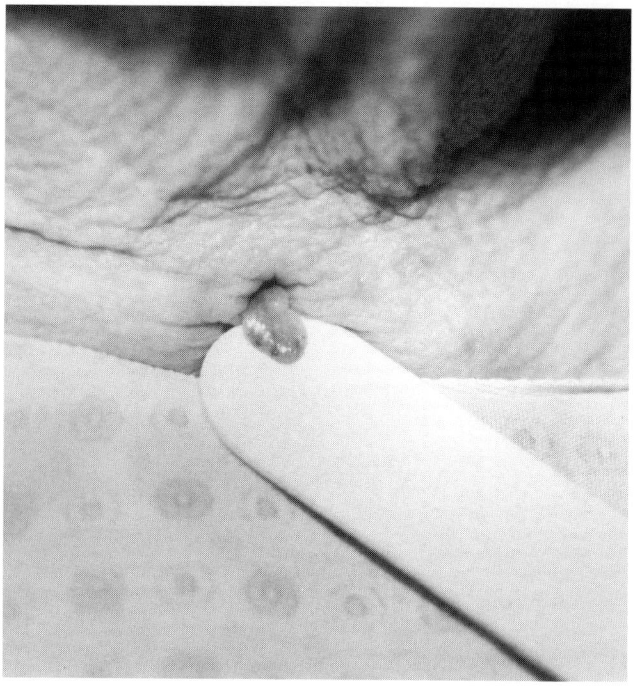

Figure 18-13

A large polypoid granuloma at the TTOT site.

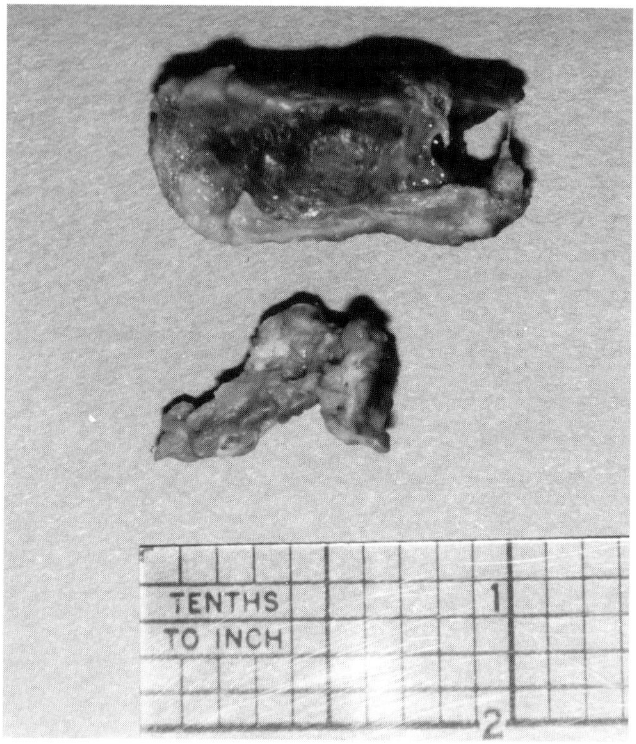

Figure 18-14

A large mucous plug which formed around the transtracheal catheter.

REFERENCES

1. Heimlich HJ: Respiratory rehabilitation with transtracheal oxygen system. *Ann Otol Rhinol Laryngol* 1982; 91:643–647.
2. Nocturnal Oxygen Therapy Trial Group: Continuous or nocturnal oxygen therapy in hypoxemic chronic obstructive lung disease: A clinical trial. *Ann Intern Med* 1980; 102:29–36.
3. Medical Research Council Working Party: Long-term domiciliary oxygen therapy in chronic hypoxic cor pulmonale complicating chronic bronchitis and emphysema. *Lancet* 1981; 1:681–686.
4. Weitzenblum E, et al: Long-term oxygen therapy can reverse the progression of pulmonary hypertension in patients with chronic obstructive pulmonary disease. *Am Rev Respir Dis* 1985; 131:493–498.
5. Tarpy S, et al: The effect of oxygen and air via nasal cannula on the oxygen cost of breathing in chronic airflow obstruction (CAO). *Am Rev Respir Dis* 1992; 145:A646 (abstr.).
6. Dean NC, et al: Oxygen may improve dyspnea and endurance in patients with chronic obstructive pulmonary disease and only mild hypoxemia. *Am Rev Respir Dis* 1992; 146:941–945.
7. Bradley BL, et al: Oxygen-assisted exercise in chronic obstructive lung disease: The effect on exercise capacity and arterial blood gas tensions. *Am Rev Respir Dis* 1978; 118:239–243.
8. Krop HD, et al: Neuropsychologic effects of continuous oxygen therapy in chronic obstructive pulmonary disease. *Chest* 1973; 64:317–322.
9. Fleetham J, et al: Sleep, arousals, and oxygen desaturation in chronic obstructive pulmonary disease: The effect of oxygen therapy. *Am Rev Respir Dis* 1982; 126:429–433.
10. Christopher KL, et al: Transtracheal oxygen therapy for refractory hypoxemia. *JAMA* 1986; 256:494–497.
11. Hoffman LA, et al: Nasal cannula and transtracheal oxygen: A comparison of patient response after 6 months of each technique. *Am Rev Respir Dis* 1992; 145:827–831.
12. O'Donohue WJ: Effect of oxygen therapy on increasing arterial oxygen tension in hypoxemic patients with stable chronic obstructive pulmonary disease while breathing ambient air. *Chest* 1991; 100:968–972.
13. Tarpy SP, Celli BR: Long-term oxygen therapy. *N Engl J Med* 1995; 333:710–714.
14. Tiep BL, et al: Pulsed nasal and transtracheal oxygen. *Chest* 1990; 97:364–368.
15. Yaeger ES, et al: Oxygen therapy using pulse and continuous flow with a transtracheal catheter and a nasal cannula. *Chest* 1994; 106:854–860.
16. Couser JI, Make BJ: Transtracheal oxygen decreases inspired minute ventilation. *Am Rev Respir Dis* 1989; 139:627–631.
17. Williams MH: Transtracheal oxygen decreases inspired minute ventilation. *Am Rev Respir Dis* 1989; 140:562 (letter).
18. Benditt J, et al: Transtracheal delivery of gas decreases the oxygen cost of breathing. *Am Rev Respir Dis* 1993; 147:1207–1210.
19. Morrison DA, Stovall JR: Increased exercise capacity in hypoxemic patients after long-term oxygen therapy. *Chest* 1992; 102:542–550.
20. Hoffman LA, et al: Patient response to transtracheal oxygen delivery. *Am Rev Respir Dis* 1987; 135:153–156.
21. Wesmiller SE, et al: Exercise tolerance during nasal cannula and transtracheal oxygen delivery. *Am Rev Respir Dis* 1990; 141:789–791.
22. Dewan NA, Bell CW: Effect of low flow and high flow oxygen delivery on exercise tolerance and sensation of dyspnea: A study comparing the transtracheal catheter and nasal prongs. *Chest* 1994;105:1061–1065.

23. Bloom BS, et al: Transtracheal oxygen delivery in patients with chronic obstructive pulmonary disease. *Respiratory Med* 1989; 83:281–288.
24. Christopher KL, et al: A program for transtracheal oxygen delivery: Assessment of safety and efficacy. *Ann Intern Med* 1987; 107:802–808.
25. Clifford D, et al: Transtracheal oxygen improves survival and reduces hospital costs. *Am J Respir Crit Care Med* 1995; 151(suppl):A681 (abstr).
26. Evans RB, et al: Transtracheal oxygen improves FEV_1 and weight. *Chest* 1989; 98(suppl):174S.
27. Farney RJ, et al: Transtracheal oxygen, nasal CPAP and nasal oxygen in five patients with obstructive sleep apnea. *Chest* 1992; 101:1228–1235.
28. Transtracheal Systems: SCOOP transtracheal oxygen therapy: Clinician guide. 1990.
29. Mehta AC, et al: Insertion of a pre-SCOOP transtracheal oxygen therapy catheter with use of a Raulerson syringe *Chest* 1992; 101:887 (letter).
30. Sciurba FC, et al: The use of a short-length transtracheal oxygen catheter in patients of small stature with restrictive lung disease. *Chest* 1992; 101:1165–1167.
31. Wesmiller SW, et al: Understanding transtracheal oxygen delivery. *Nursing* 1989; 19:43–47.
32. Shneerson J: Transtracheal oxygen delivery. *Thorax* 1992; 47: 57–59.
33. Adamo JP, et al: The Cleveland Clinic's initial experience with transtracheal oxygen therapy. *Respiratory Care* 1990; 35:153–160.
34. Heimlich HJ: Oxygen delivery for ambulatory patients: How the Micro-Trach increases mobility. *Postgrad Med* 1988; 84:68–79.
35. Heimlich HJ, Gerson CC: The Micro-Trach: A seven year experience with transtracheal oxygen therapy. *Chest* 1989; 95: 1008–1012.
36. Govan JR, Banner NR: Long term transtracheal oxygen delivery through microcatheter in patients with hypoxaemia due to chronic obstructive airways disease. *Br Med J* 1986; 293:111–114.
37. Walsh DA, Govan JR: Long term continuous domiciliary oxygen therapy by transtracheal catheter. *Thorax* 1990; 45:478–481.
38. de Groot REB, et al: A nearly fatal tracheal obstruction resulting from a transtracheal oxygen catheter. *Chest* 1993; 104(5):1634–1635.
39. Ulstad DR, Koppin J: Massive atelectasis with respiratory arrest due to transtracheal oxygen catheter-related mass formation. *Chest* 1994; 106:982 (letter).
40. Hoffman LA, et al: Transtracheal delivery of oxygen: Efficacy and safety for long-term continuous therapy. *Ann Otol Rhinol Laryngol* 1991; 100:108–115.
41. Rai NS, et al: Transtracheal oxygen therapy—Does practice make perfect? *J Bronchol* 1994; 1:205–212.
42. Punzal; PA, et al: Laser resection of granulation tissue secondary to transtracheal oxygen catheter. *Chest* 1992; 101:269–271.
43. Roth BJ, et al: Acute respiratory compromise resulting from tracheal mucous impaction secondary to a transtracheal oxygen catheter. *Chest* 1992; 101:465–466.
44. Fletcher EC, et al: Endotracheal mass resulting from a transtracheal catheter. *Chest* 1988; 93:438–439.
45. Burton GG, et al: Fatal airway obstruction caused by a mucous ball from a transtracheal catheter. *Chest* 1991; 99:1520–1523.
46. Menon AS, et al: Tracheal perforation: A complication associated with transtracheal oxygen therapy. *Chest* 1993; 104:636–637.
47. Couser JJ, Make BJ: Respiratory tract infection complicating transtracheal oxygen therapy. Chest 1992; 101:273-275.

CHAPTER 19

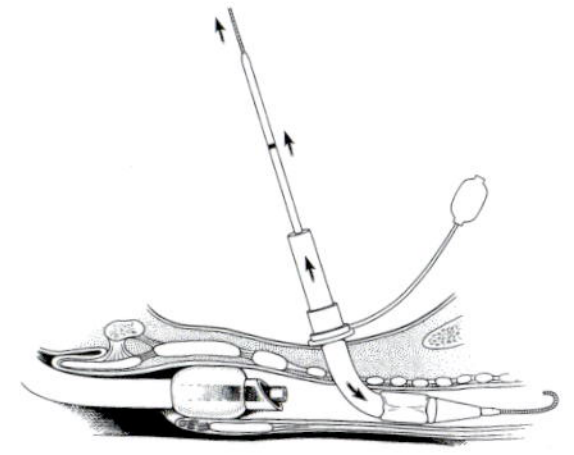

PERCUTANEOUS THORACIC NEEDLE BIOPSY

Robert D. Tarver, Lynn S. Broderick, and Dewey J. Conces, Jr.

Historical Background

Fine-needle aspiration biopsy of chest lesions has been used for more than 100 years. The first report of a thoracic needle aspiration biopsy, in 1883, reported a diagnostic biopsy of pneumonia.[1] In 1885, Menetrier was the first to make the diagnosis of lung carcinoma with a needle biopsy.[2] The technique was not popular earlier in this century because of the potential for complications. In the 1960s, Dahlgren and Nordenstrom[3] popularized the transthoracic fine-needle aspiration biopsy for diagnosing pulmonary lesions. Several factors led to the current utility of the fine-needle aspiration biopsy: improved radiographic techniques including high-resolution fluoroscopy and computed tomography, the development of small gauge needles which can provide histologic and cytologic material from lung and mediastinum, vastly improved cytologic interpretation, and improved management of complications. All these factors have contributed to making transthoracic fine-needle aspiration biopsy a safe, rapid, and accurate diagnostic test.

Fine-Needle Biopsy of Solitary Pulmonary Nodules

Solitary pulmonary nodules are common clinical problems that often require fine-needle biopsy for diagnosis (Fig. 19.1). Fine-needle biopsy is a relatively safe, simple, and accurate procedure which is easily performed. Most transthoracic fine-needle aspiration biopsies of the thorax are performed on outpatients. Outpatient biopsies can reduce health care costs and still maintain diagnostic accuracy and patient safety. In patients older than 70 or those with significant pulmonary or cardiac disease consideration should be given to performing this procedure on an inpatient basis. A thorough preprocedure evaluation, optimal patient care during the procedure, and necessary follow-up care can make a difficult problem for the patient as trouble-free as possible.[4–11]

Image-guided transthoracic fine-needle biopsy combined with expert cytopathology provides an accurate diagnosis in thoracic malignancy with an overall sensitivity of 70 to 100 percent in most series. Several papers have reported a 95 to 97 percent sensitivity for malignancy.[12–28] Histologic samples can increase the yield for malignancy above that achieved by cytology specimens alone.[24,29,30] This is particularly important when dealing with suspected lymphoma. Normal yields of 60 to 75 percent can be increased to 95 percent with the addition of histologic samples.[18,29,31] Cell type differentiation of bronchogenic carcinoma with cytologic analysis is not as accurate as the determination that the lesion is cancer. Agreement between the cytologic diagnosis and the final surgical pathology occurs between 65 and 85 percent of the time.[32,33] The most common error made is in separating poorly differentiated squamous cell carcinoma from adenocarcinoma. Cytology is very good at differentiating small cell carcinoma from non-small cell, which is all that is needed to determine treatment options. In evaluating anterior mediastinal masses, distinguishing lymphoma from thymoma may be difficult with cytology alone.[31,34]

Figure 19-1

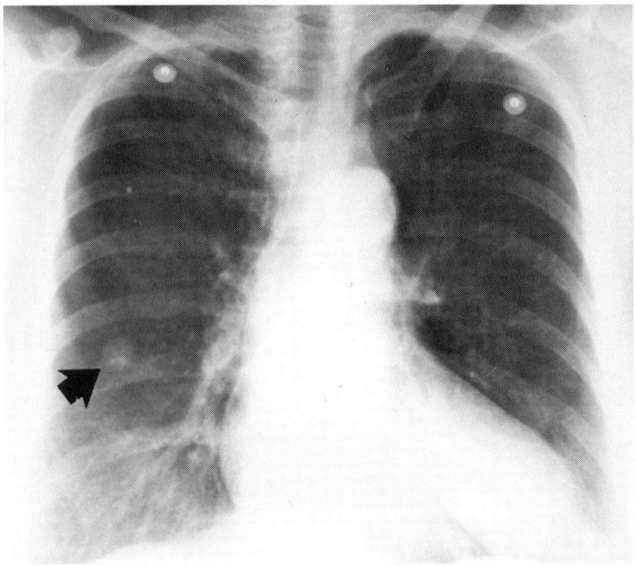

A

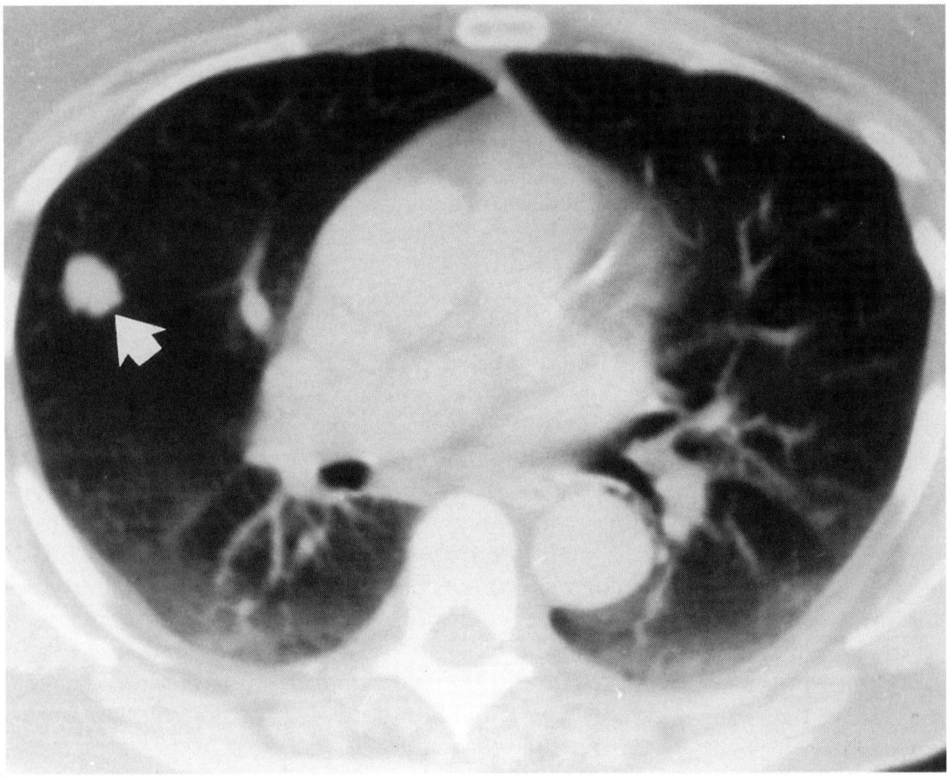

B

A. Chest radiograph showing a patient with a solitary lung nodule in the right lung (*arrow*). *B*. CT scan of the same patient showing the location of the nodule in the lateral portion of the anterior segment of the right upper lobe (*arrow*).

A major difficulty with transthoracic fine-needle aspiration biopsies is the difficulty in making specific benign diagnoses. Specific benign diagnoses can be made in 56 to 97 percent of cases.[15,16,35] The difficulty is based on a number of factors including possibility of sampling error of a malignant lesion, failure to send the specimens for appropriate stains and cultures, and the difficulty of making a specific benign diagnosis from cytology alone. Specific cytopathologic diagnoses can be made in infections, hamartoma, abscess, lipoma, lipoid pneumonia, pseudotumor, and cyst. Making a specific benign diagnosis can reduce the number of negative thoracotomies by as much as 50 percent.[36]

NODULE EVALUATION

A solitary pulmonary nodule requires a thorough preprocedure evaluation. A search for old films may show that the nodule is unchanged over a 2-year period and therefore most likely benign. Low kilovoltage films or CT of the nodule can determine if there is calcification present, which would also indicate that the nodule is probably benign. A chest and abdomen CT are necessary for the complete staging of a malignant nodule. CT of the chest can determine if there is hilar or mediastinal adenopathy, or if there are other nodules, and help to plan a biopsy route. CT may lead to a specific diagnosis that would obviate the need for a biopsy (e.g., calcified granuloma, hamartoma, arteriovenous malformation, bronchogenic cyst, rounded atelectasis). CT can also detect areas of necrosis within a mass that should be avoided during biopsy, since these areas often provide nondiagnostic material. CT of the abdomen evaluates the liver and adrenals for metastasis. Pulmonary function tests are important in the preprocedural evaluation to determine if the patient is operable, how likely the patient is to develop a pneumothorax, and how well the patient may tolerate a pneumothorax. Clotting studies are indicated before biopsy. Routine hemoglobin and hematocrit are not obtained unless excessive bleeding is expected. The patient's HIV status is not obtained, since all fine-needle aspiration biopsies are performed with universal precautions.

INDICATIONS

Fine-needle aspiration biopsy is used in a number of clinical situations. The most common indication is the evaluation of a solitary pulmonary nodule in a patient at risk for lung cancer. A new nodule in patients older than 40 is often biopsied even without a history of smoking. A solitary nodule in a patient with a nonpulmonary primary cancer is another common indication for fine-needle biopsy. Nodules in immunosuppressed patients are biopsied, since these nodules could represent infection or primary tumor. In patients with multiple pulmonary nodules, a nodule is often biopsied, since this is usually an easy source of diagnostic tissue. Nodules 1 cm and larger can routinely be biopsied. It is rare, and usually due to patient uncooperativeness or inability to accurately visualize the lesion, that a 1-cm nodule cannot be biopsied. Nodules between 1 and 0.5 cm are biopsied, but the results are not as assured as with larger nodules. Nodules less than 0.5 cm are usually not biopsied, because accurate biopsy is very difficult with fluoroscopy or CT. If the clinical situation demands that tissue be obtained from such a small nodule, it can be attempted, with the caveat that there is a less than even chance that the nodule will be sampled.

CONTRAINDICATIONS

There are few absolute contraindications to fine-needle aspiration biopsy. The inability of a patient to cooperate with breath-holding instructions is a contraindication. Bleeding diathesis is a relative contraindication, since corrections of the prothrombin time (PT), partial prothrombin time (PTT), and platelet count can be accomplished. Severe pulmonary hypertension is another relative contraindication because of the risk of bleeding is higher, especially when biopsying lesions close to the central pulmonary arteries. In patients with a forced expiratory volume in 1 s (FEV_1) of less than 1 liter, serious consideration should be given to the need for a biopsy. Pneumothorax in such patients is a risky complication. Similar consideration should also be given when biopsying a patient after pneumonectomy. In all cases, especially in patients with relative contraindications to biopsy, if the tissue diagnosis will not change the clinical course or treatment, the need for the biopsy should be questioned and discussed with the referring physician. Several other relative contraindications include positive pressure ventilation, large bullae surrounding the lesion, possible echinococcal cyst, possible pulmonary arteriovenous malformation, and intractable cough.

RISKS

Fine-needle aspiration biopsy is a fairly low risk procedure with a few well known complications which are easily treated. However, conveying the risks and complications to a worried patient can be difficult. A physician may do this every day, but to the patient this is a once-in-a-lifetime procedure. A good method of establishing rapport with the patient and family is to bring them to the procedure room when the procedure is requested, often a week before the biopsy is scheduled. At this time, reviewing the films, discussing the mechanics of the procedure, and explaining the risks and complications makes for a more informed patient. If scheduling such a meeting is difficult, at least have a similar meeting immediately before the actual biopsy. It is surprising how little patients are told about their biopsy procedure by the referring physician. An informed patient and family is much more likely to be cooperative if a complication occurs.

Pneumothorax is the most common complication of a fine-needle aspiration biopsy of a lung nodule. Approximately 30 percent of patients develop a pneumothorax during or after a biopsy.[13,16,17,22,24,28,36–46] In patients with emphysematous lungs, the rate may be as high as 50 percent. Pneumothoraces may be asymptomatic. Usually a patient complains of sharp chest pain away from the biopsy site. Fluoroscopy may detect a pneumothorax if it is large, but often the complaint of pain is a more sensitive indicator of a small pneumothorax. Remember that in a supine patient the pneumothorax is over the anterolateral costophrenic sulcus and not over the lung apex. In prone patients the findings are similar, with the pneumothorax appearing over the posterior costophrenic sulcus. The pneumothorax rate increases with long procedures, uncooperative patients, patient movement with the needle in place, larger-bore needles, patient coughing, and if fissures are crossed. Most attempts to decrease the pneumothorax rate, including injecting blood clot and fibrin into the needle tract, have not been successful. Decreased pneumothorax rates have been seen if, after biopsy, the patient lies with the needle entry site dependent. This approximates the visceral puncture site with the parietal pleura and prevents air leakage from the parenchyma into the pleural space.

Hemoptysis occurs in approximately 5 percent of patients during or immediately after a fine-needle aspiration biopsy of the lung.[12,13,15–18,20,28,35,40,47,48] In the vast majority of cases the hemoptysis is a scanty amount of blood-tinged sputum after the procedure is completed. Some patients may have hemoptysis during the procedure, especially if blood from the biopsy site can reach the major airways. This is seen especially in supine patients undergoing an anterior segment of the upper-lobe biopsy. Rarely hemoptysis can become a life-threatening complication. Any hemoptysis which is persistent or increasing should be followed closely. One should not hesitate to consult with a pulmonologist, thoracic surgeon, or angiographically trained interventional radiologist. These physicians can aid in the care of hemoptysis, especially massive hemoptysis, and they all appreciate knowing about the problem early in its course. Bronchial embolization, balloon occlusion of the affected segmental bronchus, and surgical resection are all options for the treatment of life-threatening hemoptysis and all call for the interventional chest radiologist to work closely with other consultants for the good of the patient.

Infection is always listed as a possible complication of fine-needle aspiration biopsy of lung nodules but it is very uncommon. There are no case reports of infection following a fine-needle biopsy of the lung. However it certainly is a potential complication, and as more immunocompromised patients are biopsied, infection becomes a larger potential risk.

Deaths do occur as a complication of fine-needle aspiration biopsy of pulmonary nodules. The incidence of death is approximately 1 per 5000 to 10,000 biopsies. Fatal complications include tension pneumothorax, hemorrhage in patients with pulmonary hypertension, and cerebral air embolism due to leakage of air between the needle or airway into pulmonary veins. The true incidence is not available, since fatal complications are usually not reported in the literature. Only occasional case reports of fatalities are seen. A review of the literature up to 1981 indicates that there had been nine deaths, seven of them prior to 1974, following percutaneous fine-needle aspiration biopsy. These deaths were attributed to cardiac arrest, air embolism, pneumothorax, and hemorrhage.[49] Because death is such a rare complication of fine-needle aspiration biopsy, the true fatality rate may not be accurately known until a large cooperative group study is performed.[50]

Alternatives to fine-needle aspiration biopsy of lung nodules must be discussed with patients as part of a complete informed consent. If there are no old films of the nodule and it is less than 1 to 2 cm, the nodule could be followed up with sequential films to determine if it has a malignant growth pattern. Bronchoscopy can be performed to attempt to make the diagnosis, although in peripheral nodules its yield is less than 20 percent. The patient could undergo thoracotomy for an excisional biopsy and possible further surgery. Often these alternatives have not been explained to the patient sent for a fine-needle aspiration biopsy of a lung nodule.

PATIENT PREPARATION

Well-informed patients are a must in performing interventional chest procedures. Patients with a nodule are usually aware that lung cancer is a possible diagnosis. It is helpful if the primary care physician discusses the procedure and the malignant potential of the nodule before the patient meets with the radiologist for biopsy. However, many patients come to biopsy without much forewarning about the possibility of malignancy or exactly what a biopsy encompasses. The radiologist should be available beforehand to explain to the patient and referring physician what the biopsy will entail. At this time patients and their physicians have a chance to ask questions and discuss the procedure with the radiologist. A checklist, which includes a description of the procedure, the risks and complications and preprocedure evaluations, should be sent to all referring physicians. Fine-needle aspiration biopsies can safely be performed on outpatients.[11] Patients with severe lung dysfunction should be watched in the hospital overnight, even if there is no pneumothorax present after biopsy.

Patient preparation is an important part of fine-needle aspiration biopsy. Patients are scheduled in the morning so that follow-up and complications can be dealt with before evening. Patients are told that the procedure itself may take from 30 min to 1 h and that a follow-up film will be obtained 3 h after the procedure has ended. If there is no pneumothorax or other complications and the patient is doing fine, the patient is allowed to go home after the 3-h film. Inpatients are kept in the radiology department for 1 h after the procedure and then allowed to return to the ward and wait there for a 3-h film. Patients are biopsied as outpatients if they have someone to stay with them during the evening after the biopsy, if they have a phone, and if they can easily return to the emergency room. They are given the emergency room's telephone number and the number of the radiology resident on call. Patients are instructed to call or come to the emergency room if they experience chest pain, shortness of breath, or any unusual symptoms.

Patient preparation for a fine-needle aspiration involves a nurse, radiology technologist, and the radiologist. Informed consent is obtained, and any additional questions are answered by the biopsy team. The patient's pulse and blood pressure are recorded. An intravenous catheter is started and either capped with a heparin lock or attached to normal saline at a minimal rate of infusion. The intravenous catheter is for administration of analgesic drugs if needed and for intravenous access if the patient's condition worsens during the procedure. Most patients do not require more than local anesthesia; however intravenous meperidine, midazolam, or diazepam are often needed in anxious patients. In addition, it is usually necessary to administer systemic analgesics if the patient requires the placement of a chest tube. Close monitoring of patients is improved with the use of a pulse oximeter and EKG monitor. Lung biopsy is an invasive procedure with known, potentially fatal complications. Proper patient preparation, analgesia, and monitoring help prevent complications such as pneumothorax, hypotension, or hemoptysis from becoming severe. In addition, other physicians performing similar procedures such as endoscopy and bronchoscopy all use this level of patient preparation and monitoring. Radiologists, therefore, should use the same standards of patient care when performing fine-needle aspiration biopsies.[51]

IMAGING CHOICE—CT OR FLUOROSCOPY

The decision to perform a fine-needle aspiration biopsy of a lung nodule under CT or fluoroscopic guidance is a matter of personal preference. Each modality has its proponents, with several relative advantages and disadvantages. Fluoroscopy is usually less expensive than CT. Radiologists' preferences are influenced by their experience with each modality and often are based to a large part on the availability of CT or fluoroscopy time. Fluoroscopy allows for real-time visualization of the procedure. Fluoroscopic guidance seems to be better for guiding biopsies of nodules in the lower third of the lungs where large respiratory excursions occur. It can be particularly frustrating to get patients to reproducibly hold their breath using CT guidance when biopsying small lesions in the lower lobes near the diaphragms. In addition, in a fluoroscopy room immediate chest tube placement can be performed, whereas the patient may have to be moved from a CT suite to fluoroscopy for chest tube placement. (NOTE: Chest tubes can easily be placed emergently in CT without fluoroscopic guidance.) CT guidance is particularly useful when biopsying nodules adjacent to the hila, mediastinum, or heart. CT is also useful when oblique or angled biopsy approaches are needed. CT guidance is often helpful when biopsying very small nodules. CT is often used when a lesion is visible in only one plane on radiographs or fluoroscopy. CT also adds to the satisfaction of the referring clinicians because they can see that the needle has been placed within the lesion. This aspect becomes important if the biopsy is indeterminate and following the lesion is being contemplated. The choice between CT and fluoroscopic guidance is one of personal preference, nodule location, and availability.[52]

NEEDLES

Two basic needle systems are available, the single-pass biopsy needle and the multiple-pass coaxial needle system. The single-needle system consists of a needle which is used to make one pass through the skin, into the lung and into the nodule. After the needle is in the nodule, the aspiration is performed, the needle removed, and the specimen flushed onto a slide or into a preservative. A multiple-pass coaxial system consists of a guide needle and an aspiration needle. The guide needle is placed into or adjacent to the nodule, and then the aspiration needle is placed coaxially into the lesion. Aspiration is performed with the inner needle, and only the aspiration needle is withdrawn. The specimen is flushed onto a slide or into a preservative. There are advantages and disadvantages to the single-pass system and the multiple-pass coaxial system. The single-pass system creates a smaller hole in the pleura and minimizes the time a needle is across the pleura. If more samples are needed with the single-pass system, another pass must be made across the pleura and into the lesion. The multiple-pass coaxial system allows for many samples to be obtained with a single pass of the guide needle. Multiple-pass coaxial systems usually require a larger-bore needle than single-pass systems. In addition, the guide needle remains across the pleura longer than in the single-pass system. As a rough guide, large lesions in easy to biopsy locations lend themselves to the single-pass system, whereas multiple pass coaxial systems are useful for smaller lesions or lesions which require lengthy imaging procedures to correctly place a biopsy needle. If a cytologist is present, a multiple-pass coaxial system is preferred, since multiple samples can be quickly obtained and screened.

There are several dozen types of needles designed for fine-needle aspiration biopsy of lung nodules (Fig. 19-2). Radiologists should become familiar with a few types and know which situations require specific needles. The Greene needle set, a multiple-pass coaxial system, is popular. The outer guide is available in 19 and 22 gauge with corresponding inner aspiration needles of 22 or 23 gauge and 25 gauge. Greene needles come in varied lengths, with a 10- to 15-cm outer needle and a 15- or 20-cm inner aspiration needle. The inner aspiration needles are circumferentially beveled at the tip and are otherwise similar to the Chiba needles, which are popular single-pass needles. If the lung nodule is hard or resistant to aspiration, a needle with an irregular or crown-shaped tip such as the Franseen needle is useful. Thin-slotted or core biopsy needles are available in gauges small enough to use as single-pass needles or to fit coaxially into the 19-gauge Greene needle outer guide for multiple-pass sampling. These small, 22-gauge, core biopsy needles allow for histologic specimens to be obtained. Knowledge of several of the dozens of needles available is helpful when biopsying lung nodules.[53]

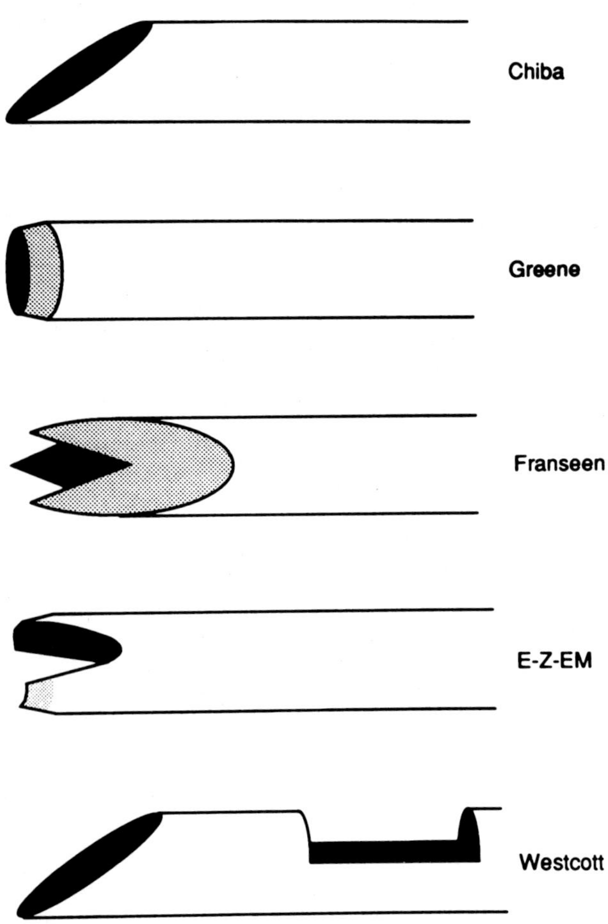

Figure 19-2

Several commonly used needles for lung biopsies. The Chiba and Greene models are used routinely for cytologic sampling. The Franseen and E-Z-EM needles are useful in biopsying more resistant or harder lesions such as hamartomas. The Westcott needle can be used to obtain cytologic as well as histologic samples. (*From Chiba, Greene, and Franseen-Cook Inc., Bloomington, Indiana, E-Z-EM-E-Z-EM, Westbury, New York, Westcott-Medi-Tech, Watertown, New York.*)

ASPIRATION TECHNIQUES

Fine-needle aspiration biopsy is a method of transferring material from a nodule to a slide or into preservative. Aspiration is usually accomplished by creating a vacuum within the needle by using a 10-cm^3 syringe attached to the aspiration needle. A small amount of air, 1 cm^3, is aspirated into the syringe before the biopsy begins. Gentle suction is applied after the tip of the needle is within the lesion. Several in and out motions can be made with the needle in the lesion during the application of suction. Before the needle is withdrawn from the lesion, suction is released. The goal of fine-needle lung nodule aspiration is to withdraw material into the tip of the needle, not to withdraw cells far up into the needle and into the hub of the syringe. Cytologists often ask that suction not be used during the first pass, since adequate tissue may be obtained by just the gentle in and out motion of the needle tip within the lesion. After the needle is removed from the patient, the needle and syringe are separated and approximately 5 to 10 cm^3 of air is drawn into the syringe. The needle and syringe are reattached, and the material from the nodule is expressed onto a slide or into a preservative. The entire procedure may be repeated with the same needle and syringe as long as sterile technique is preserved. Occasionally material may become stuck in the end of the needle; it can be pushed out of the needle tip by removing the syringe and replacing the needle stylet. The aspiration needle and syringe hub may become filled with clotted blood after several passes and prevent adequate sampling. If this occurs, a new aspiration biopsy needle should be used. At the conclusion of a coaxial-type biopsy, the outer guide needle, which may have been within the lesion, can be flushed onto a slide or into preservative.[54]

CYTOLOGIST

The cytologist has an important role in the diagnosis of lung nodules using fine-needle aspiration biopsy. The cytologist's ability to differentiate and diagnose tumors from individual cells has allowed this procedure to flourish. A portion of the aspirated material can be stained immediately and provides the cytologist with a clue as to the nature of the lesion being sampled. Having the cytologist present at the biopsy is helpful, since immediate results as to the adequacy of the specimen are available. The cytologist can halt the procedure after only one pass if an adequate specimen is obtained. Cytologists can also determine if more samples are needed and if specimens are needed for culture, flow cytometry, or electron microscopy. Care must be taken by the biopsy team not to rush into a diagnosis on the preliminary stains and slides, since the final diagnosis may be different when the permanent stains are made. The cytologist's role is to determine if adequate amounts of material have been obtained. If the cytologist can not come to the biopsy site, a cytotechnologist can be helpful in obtaining the material. In some departments the cytologist is not available to immediately process the biopsy, and material is sent from the biopsy site to cytology in a preservative. In other departments the radiologist may prepare and look at the slides during the procedure. It is the ability of the cytologist to make a specific diagnosis from a few cells that allows fine-needle aspiration biopsy of lung nodules to be a success.[55]

BIOPSY PLANNING

Using the CT of the chest, a route for biopsy is planned. Usually the shortest path to the lesion from the skin surface is chosen. However a number of factors may alter this basic tenet. Fissures should not be crossed by the biopsy needle path, since this places another hole in the pleura. If it is at all possible, a biopsy path should be chosen that passes through the visceral pleura only once. This basic rule cannot always be followed. Upper-lobe, apical lesions which can be approached anteriorly or posteriorly are often easier to biopsy posteriorly for several reasons. With a posterior approach, the patient cannot watch the procedure, which can be quite unnerving for the patient. In a posterior approach, the needle passes between the posterior ribs, which do not have as much respiratory excursion as do the anterior ribs. Biopsy paths perpendicular to the chest wall are the easiest approaches. Angled biopsy paths increase the difficulty, whether CT or fluoroscopic guidance is utilized.

FLUOROSCOPIC BIOPSY

The patient is placed prone or supine for the biopsy, according to the plan developed from the CT or from plain films. Fluoroscopy is used to determine if the nodule can be seen and to check its motion during inspiration and expiration. A rib interspace, the nodule, and a skin site are aligned during some phase of respiration using a radiopaque marker. It is best, if possible, not to place the needle during deep inspiration or expiration. If the needle is placed in one of these extremes of the respiratory cycle, the needle will spend much of its time in the patient severely angled, since most of the time the patient will be breathing quietly. Therefore midquiet inspiration is the best respiratory position in which to stick the nodule. Once a skin site has been marked, the site should be cleaned and then anesthetized with 2% lidocaine. Care should be taken not to create a pneumothorax from too deep anesthesia needle placement. If there is a question about the depth of the pleural space, the needle can be placed over a rib. The depth of the rib will give a good approximation as to the pleural depth. Practicing breathing instructions with the patient while watching the needle tip on the skin surface, the rib interspace, and the nodule will help both the patient and the radiologist get an idea of what will occur when the biopsy actually begins. It is important to warn the patient that the pleura cannot be completely anesthetized and that a small amount of pain will be felt as the pleura is crossed. A small dermatotomy is often necessary to ensure easy passage of the needle through the thick thoracic skin. The needle entry site must be in the center of the fluoroscopic screen so that parallax errors do not occur. Biopsy paths parallel with the fluoroscopic beam and perpendicular to the horizontal are the easiest biopsy paths to successfully complete. To accomplish angled approaches to lesions under ribs, the tube must be angled occasionally, but this increases the difficulty of the procedure. Occasionally, the patient must be positioned other than supine or prone, and this also usually increases the difficulty of the procedure. The depth of the lesion is usually determined from the CT, and needle depth can be determined with needles marked with centimeter marks or by marking the needle with tape at the desired depth. A needle depth marker is available on some needles, or one can be made from the small black plunger from a tuberculin syringe.

The needle should be advanced into the skin, but not into the pleural space, so that the tip of the needle, the rib interspace, and the nodule align during breath holding. If such alignment is not possible, a new skin site is chosen. Proper initial skin site is of paramount importance in making the procedure go smoothly from this point on. Proper alignment of the perpendicular needle can be difficult in patients with thin subcutaneous tissue, and the needle position may have to be checked while holding the needle perpendicular with a needle holder or the end of a syringe. Once the perpendicular needle and the nodule are aligned during suspended respiration, the needle is passed into the lung, usually during fluoroscopic guidance. If the nodule is deep within the lung, the needle can be advanced within the lung in a stepwise fashion during suspended respiration. The needle should be advanced into the lesion if a single-pass needle is used. The guide needle on a multiple pass needle system should be placed on the edge of the nodule. The change in the feel of the needle cannot always be relied on to signal that the needle tip is within the nodule. Angled fluoroscopy can be used to check the relationship between the tip of the needle and the nodule. If possible, the depth of the needle and its relationship to the nodule can be checked by rotating the fluoroscope perpendicular to the needle. Another trick is to move the needle. If the lesion moves with the needle tip, the tip is very close to the nodule. Whenever the needle is held, the patient should suspend respiration in an effort to decrease the amount of tension on and the potential tearing of the pleura. Aspiration can be performed at this time if a single-pass system is being used, or the coaxial aspiration can be performed if the guide needle has been placed. If the tissue is not obtained, repositioning of the needle is required.

Care of the patient is paramount during the entire procedure. Constant communication with the patient and monitoring of vital signs are part of good patient care. Check of the pulse and oxygenation can give an indication of the patient's condition, but talking with patients gives feedback on how they feel and how well they are tolerating the procedure. Checking for a pneumothorax with intermittent fluoroscopy is important. Small pneumothoraces will appear at the lung bases and are difficult to visualize. Often the patient will complain of pleuritic pain away from the biopsy site if a small pneumothorax develops. This sign is often more sensitive of a small pneumothorax than fluoroscopy. A large pneumothorax may develop during the procedure and will be obvious on fluoroscopy. A nurse or technologist should be in the room helping the radiologist monitor the patient's care.

CT-GUIDED BIOPSY

CT-guided fine-needle aspiration biopsy of a lung nodule is similar to fluoroscopic guidance but is not in real time. Each step must be performed and then the needle position checked with a CT scan (Fig. 19-3). Patients must be more cooperative in their respiratory control than with a fluoroscopic biopsy. First the nodule is localized and the skin entry site marked with a radiopaque marker. A scan is made with the marker in place. The skin entry site marker and the nodule should align and be present on the same scan. After the skin is cleaned and anaesthetized the biopsy needle is placed into the soft tissues of the body wall parallel to the scan plane. If a rib is encountered, a new skin entry site should be chosen instead of angling the needle to avoid dealing with a needle not parallel with the scan plane. The needle can be advanced into the nodule in a stepwise fashion checking the tip position. Once the needle tip has entered the lesion, samples may be obtained if a single-pass system is being used, or if using a multiple-pass coaxial system, the aspiration needle can be placed. A similar risk of pneumothorax exists when doing a CT-guided biopsy as with a fluoroscopic-guided biopsy. A recent paper has shown that the risk of pneumothorax in CT-guided biopsies increased with increasing lesion depth and smaller lesion size.[56] If the patient experiences any signs or symptoms of a pneumothorax, a CT scan at the biopsy site may show a pneumothorax. Additional scans through the more nondependent portions of the thorax may also show a pneumothorax if one is not seen at the level of the needle entry. On completion of the biopsy, several CT scans of the thorax serve as a temporary check for pneumothorax until a chest radiograph can be obtained.

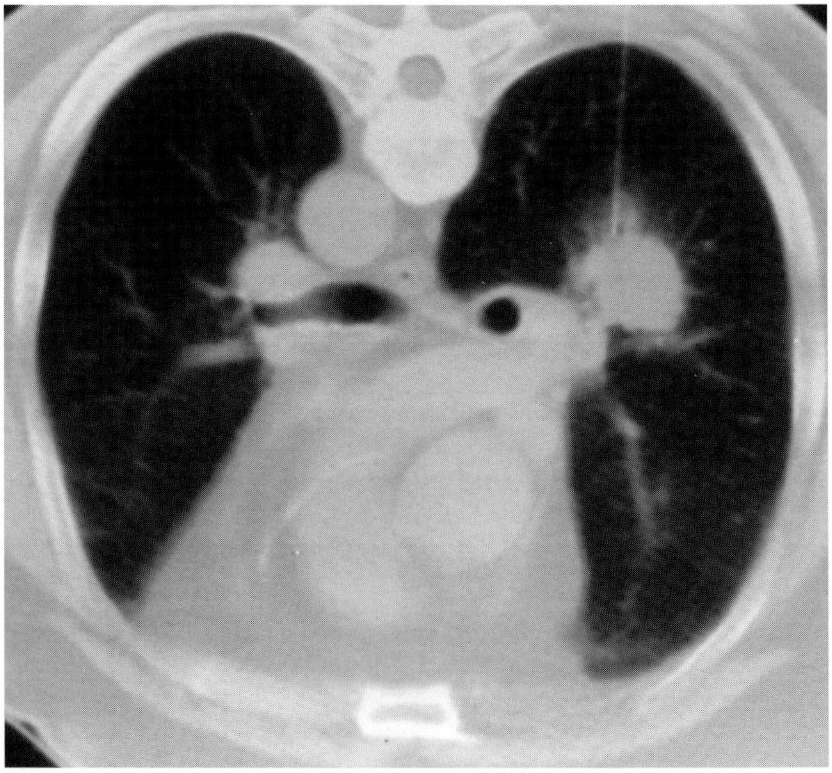

Figure 19-3

CT-guided biopsy of a right perihilar mass. Patient is in the prone position, and a guide needle has been placed into the mass. After confirmation of the needle tip location, samples are taken coaxially with an inner aspiration needle.

POSTPROCEDURE CARE, COMPLICATIONS, AND TREATMENT

The patient must be carefully monitored after a lung biopsy. The patient should lie quietly for a few minutes after the procedure. Pulse, blood pressure, oxygenation, and general well being are assessed. Patients who are stable and without complaints are turned so that the biopsy site is in the dependent position. This places the visceral pleural hole adjacent to the parietal pleura and may decrease the egress of air from the lung into the pleural space.[57] If the patient is stable and has tolerated sitting, a chest radiograph is obtained at this time. It is important that a nurse or trained technologist remain with the patient during the chest radiograph, since problems may develop when the patient stands or sits. Occasionally a very small pneumothorax, imperceptible on supine fluoroscopy, may cause a vagal reaction in an otherwise asymptomatic patient. This reaction must be recognized immediately and treated by placing the patient supine and administering fluids.

A patient who does not have a pneumothorax and has no complaints is monitored for the next 3 h. During this time a nurse monitors vital signs, breath sounds, and oxygen saturation by pulse oximetry every 15 min for the first hour and every 30 min thereafter. The patient is asked about chest pain or shortness of breath. If there is any suspicion of a new or enlarging pneumothorax, a chest film is obtained immediately. Otherwise a film is obtained 3 h after the biopsy. If there is still no pneumothorax, the patients are allowed to return home if there is someone to stay with them, they have a telephone, and there is a method of returning to the hospital quickly. Patients are instructed to proceed immediately to the emergency room should any pleuritic chest pain, hemoptysis, or shortness of breath develop. A follow-up call the next day is good medical practice. Patients appreciate the concern. Pneumothoraces can rarely develop later than 1 day after the biopsy. Waiting 4 h after the biopsy and then letting the patient go home is a policy based on a review of 673 transthoracic needle biopsies of the thorax by Perlmutt, who found that 98 percent of all pneumothoraces requiring a chest tube were detected within 1 h of the biopsy.[26] Inpatients are monitored in the radiology department for 1 h and then allowed to return to the ward until the 3-h film is obtained.

PNEUMOTHORAX

Pneumothorax is a common, expected part of performing a lung biopsy (Fig. 19-4). In most large series the incidence ranges between 5 and 30 percent.[13,16,17,22,24,28,36–43] The percentage of patients requiring treatment of pneumothorax with chest tube drainage is reported between 0 and 15 percent.[12,15–17,24,28,40,47,57,58] Factors which may increase the likelihood of a pneumothorax include advanced patient age, chronic obstructive pulmonary disease, arterial hypoxemia, intractable coughing, increased depth of the lesion, larger gauge or cutting biopsy needles, multiple pleural punctures, increased duration of the procedure, cavitary lesions, inexperience of the person performing the biopsy, and imperfect CT guidance, perhaps due to the increased number of pleural punctures.

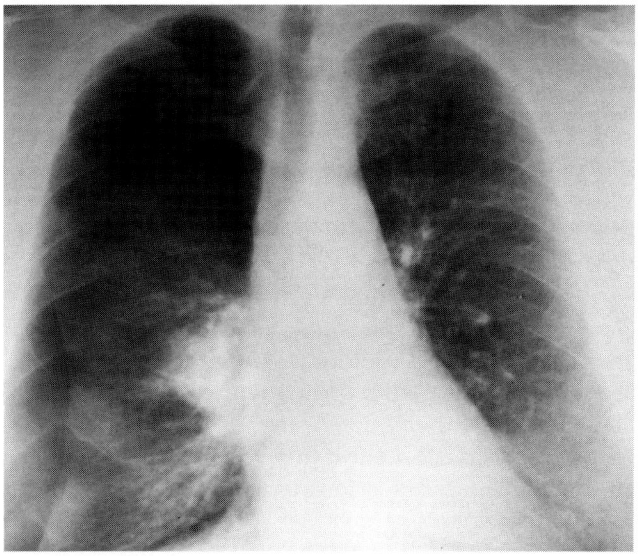

A

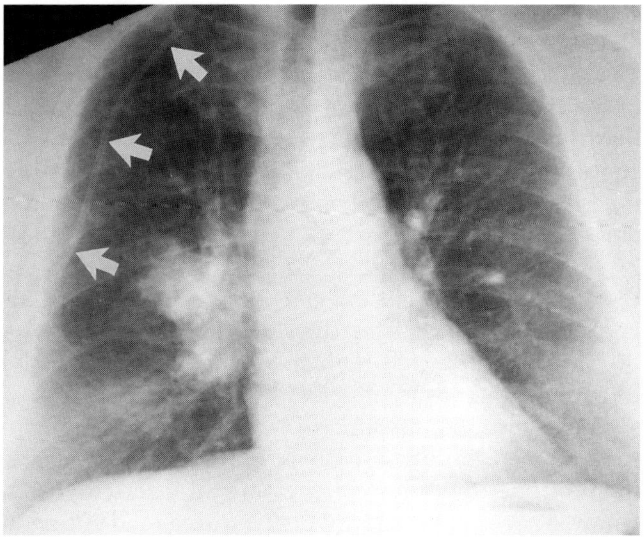

B

Figure 19-4

A. Patient with a large right pneumothorax immediately after a lung biopsy. The patient was short of breath, and a small chest tube and Heimlich valve were used. *B*. Chest radiograph after the placement of a small chest tube shows reexpansion of the lung and the course of the small tube (*arrows*).

At all times during and after the biopsy the presence of a pneumothorax should be searched for and suspected. Any patient complaint of pleuritic pain away from the biopsy site should suggest the possibility of a pneumothorax. All radiologists performing lung biopsies must be able to emergently treat a pneumothorax. Occasionally a pneumothorax must be treated immediately, and there is not enough time to call a surgeon or a pulmonologist to place a chest tube. A tension pneumothorax can develop rapidly and be fatal if not recognized and treated immediately. Small pneumothoraces can be asymptomatic. Occasionally, surprisingly large pneumothoraces can also be asymptomatic. A patient with a small pneumothorax which does not increase in size between the immediate and 3-h film should be admitted to the hospital for observation. If the pneumothorax has decreased in size or is small (less than 1 cm over the apex), patients can be allowed to go home if they have a phone, will be with someone, and can promptly return to the hospital. The reason for admission is twofold. First, it is the standard of care; no patient with a new pneumothorax would be sent from the emergency room by a surgeon. Second, if the pneumothorax enlarges, if the patient becomes symptomatic, or if a tension pneumothorax develops while the patient is in the hospital, it is a simple matter to place a chest tube. If these were to occur at home, especially a tension pneumothorax, fatal results may ensue.

A small pneumothorax should be managed conservatively with monitoring of vital signs, administration of nasal oxygen, and follow-up radiographs to confirm stability. A symptomatic or enlarging pneumothorax should be treated by the insertion of a chest tube (Fig. 19-4). It can be difficult to differentiate true shortness of breath or dyspnea from painful breathing in a patient with a relatively small pneumothorax. Patients should be given supplemental oxygen to help relieve the dyspnea. Oxygen therapy theoretically may decrease the rate of pneumothorax accumulation by allowing a higher oxygen concentration within the pleural air. The higher oxygen content intrapleural air is absorbed much faster than room air which is predominantly nitrogen. Pain medications decrease the pain of the pneumothorax and help relieve the pain associated with the insertion of the chest tube. There are several small-bore chest tubes available for the treatment of pneumothoraces. They are all inserted with a trocar, attach to a one-way flutter valve, and function well in the absence of pleural effusion. A radiologist should become familiar with one or two types and learn how to properly place and set up the tubes.

Sargent and Turner in 1970 described the rapid treatment of an iatrogenic pneumothorax in the radiology department[59] (Fig. 19-5). The ease and accuracy of percutaneous tube placement, proven effectiveness, and patient comfort of radiologically guided pneumothorax drainage with small catheters has made this the technique of choice for treatment of pneumothorax resulting from biopsy, thoracentesis, central line placement, or spontaneous pneumothorax. A few guidelines for when to place a radiologically guided catheter for pneumothorax are as follows: pneumothorax > 20 percent, pneumothorax of any size in a symptomatic patient, progressive enlargement of a pneumothorax, or development of radiographic signs of tension.[60–65]

Chest tube placement is a simple procedure; however, it is often performed in a semiemergent situation which may magnify any associated problems. The patient is placed in a supine position, and the skin over the anterior second or third rib interspace is cleansed and anesthetized. A skin entry site is enlarged with a scalpel. The chest tube is placed through the skin and into the pleural space in a nearly perpendicular position. After the chest tube and trocar assembly are within the thorax, the sharp end of the trocar can be withdrawn a few millimeters into the chest tube to prevent lung laceration. The whole assembly is angled toward the patient's lung apex and advanced at about a 45 deg angle until the tip of the chest tube is over the apex of the lung. At this time the trocar is withdrawn and the one-way valve (Heimlich) is attached to the chest tube with the interposed two- or three-way stopcock. The pneumothorax is then evacuated by having the patient cough several times. During coughing the pleural pressure is significantly higher than atmospheric pressure and the pneumothorax is rapidly evacuated. If there is a question about the intrapleural placement of the chest tube, listening to the end of the one-way valve for the sound of egressing air may confirm the intrapleural placement. If coughing does not decrease the pneumothorax, aspirating the chest tube with a syringe or connecting the efferent end of the tube to wall suction will help reduce the pneumothorax. The patient often experiences pleuritic pain when the pneumothorax shrinks and the pleural surfaces rub together again. If the tube is functioning well and is in proper position it should be sutured in place and covered with an occlusive dressing. The external chest tube and one-way valve are taped to the patient's chest. A chest radiograph is obtained, and the position and adequacy of the drainage is assessed. Small amounts of pain medicine may be required especially in the first 24 h after the placement of the chest tube. The patient is returned to the ward, and the referring physicians, nurses, and the patient are given complete instructions about the care and function of small chest tubes. If there are no complications, a repeat chest radiograph is obtained after 24 h, and if there is no pneumothorax, the stopcock is turned off, in effect clamping the chest tube. If no pneumothorax is present 12 to 24 hours later, the tube is removed. After the chest tube is removed, the patient is observed for at least 6 h before discharge.

Figure 19-5

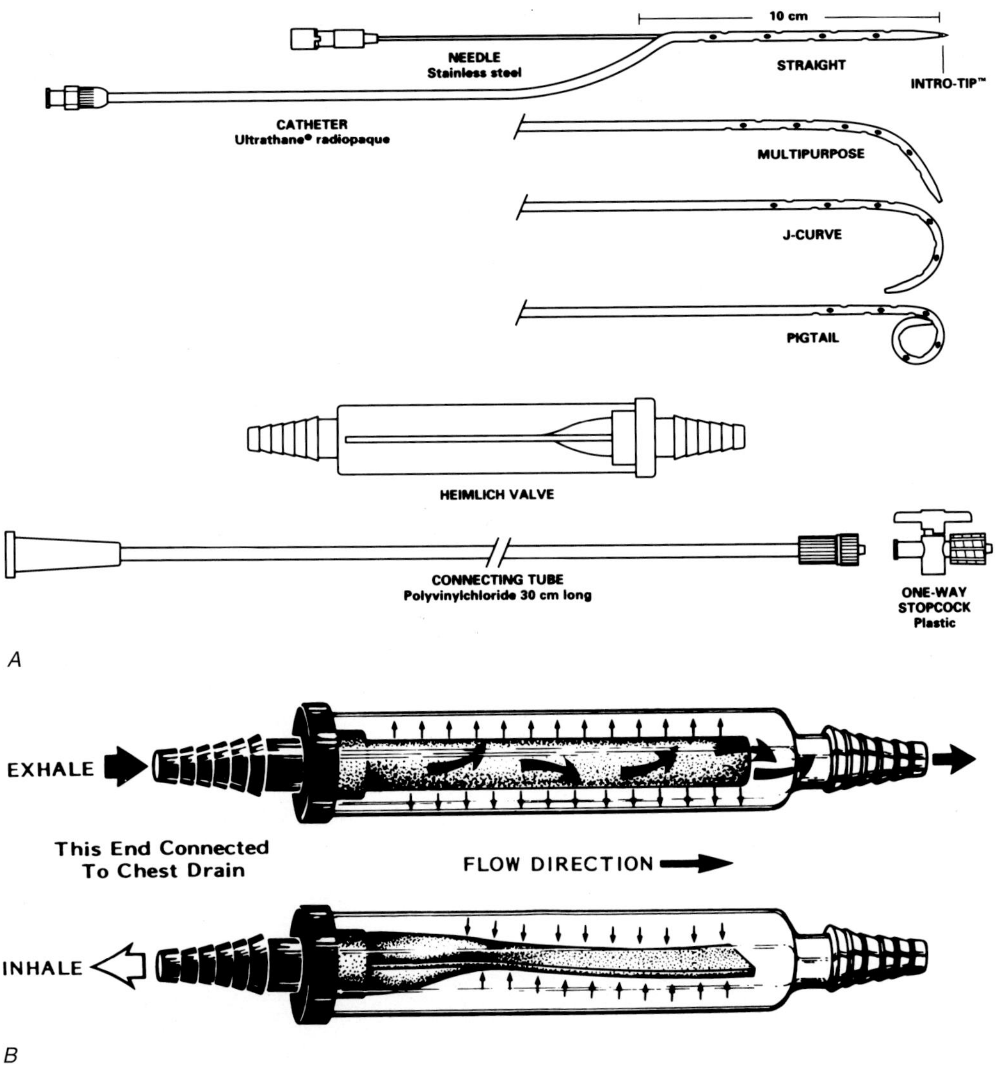

A. Schematic diagram of a Cook pneumothorax kit. As seen in the upper portion of the drawing, the catheters are available with various tip curvatures. The catheter, once inside the pleural space, is connected to the Heimlich valve via the connecting tube. *B.* Enlarged drawing of the Heimlich valve demonstrating that during exhalation the pleural pressure becomes more positive, expelling the intrapleural air from the patient and valve. During inspiration the pleural pressure becomes negative enough that the valve closes, preventing air from reentering the pleural space.

Successful treatment of pneumothoraces can be accomplished in 87 to 93 percent of patients. Treatment usually lasts between 24 and 72 h. Treatment failures are caused by catheter kinking or malposition, inadvertent withdrawal, catheter or flutter valve clogging by fluid, or the presence of a large air leak.[61–64] If the tube is functioning properly and still not evacuating the pneumothorax, it can easily be attached to the wall suction or connected to a conventional chest tube drainage apparatus. If a patient is breathing very shallowly and not generating high positive pleural pressure during expiration, the tube may fail to work properly and should be attached to suction. Small tubes have a high potential to fail if they are used in patients with pleural effusions. If a pneumothorax develops in a patient with a pleural effusion, a conventional large-bore chest tube should be considered. No serious complications have been reported from image-guided pneumothorax drainage. Potential complications include bleeding from a lacerated intercostal or internal mammary artery, infection, lung laceration, and reexpansion pulmonary edema. These complications can be diminished by inserting the trocar in the lower portion of the intercostal space, observing meticulous sterile technique, using cross table fluoroscopy during the treatment of small pneumothoraces, and slowly reexpanding long-standing collapsed lungs.

HEMOPTYSIS

Hemoptysis is the second most common complication of transthoracic needle biopsy. With the use of fine needles the incidence of significant bleeding and hemoptysis has been reduced to between 0 and 10 percent with most series reporting less than 5 percent.[12,13,15–20,35,40,47] A rare case of death from bleeding has been reported after biopsying a renal cell metastasis, and a nonfatal but massive intrapleural hemorrhage has occurred as well. Hemoptysis is usually self-limited except for patients with pulmonary hypertension (arterial or venous), underlying coagulopathy, or inadvertent laceration of the internal mammary or intercostal artery. Patients with hemoptysis should be placed with the biopsy site down to prevent aspiration of blood into other segments, and they should be reassured that the vast majority of hemorrhages after biopsy are self-limited.

MALIGNANT SEEDING

Malignant seeding of the biopsy tract from transthoracic needle biopsy has rarely been reported; however, the benefits of the procedure outweigh the risk.[66–68]

ARTERIAL AIR EMBOLISM

Arterial air embolism has been reported after a transthoracic needle biopsy. The embolism of air may lead to myocardial infarction, stroke, and death. The mechanism of systemic air embolism is presumed to be either air entry through the needle directly or the iatrogenic formation of a bronchovenous or alveolovenous fistula from the introducer needle. As little as 0.5 ml of air is sufficient to induce coronary ischemia and fatal arrhythmias. Once the symptoms of an air embolus are noticed, the patient should be placed in the left lateral decubitus position or Trendelenburg position to prevent further systemic embolization. Administering 100% oxygen promotes resorption of the air bubbles. Consideration should be given to moving the patient to a hyperbaric unit.[30,50,69–71]

Biopsy of Pulmonary Infections

Most pulmonary infections are diagnosed and treated based on clinical grounds and radiologic appearance. If the diagnosis is in question and diagnostic material is needed from the infected portion of the lung, bronchoscopy is usually performed. However, if the infection presents as a nodule, mass, or peripheral alveolar infiltrate, fine-needle aspiration biopsy is a useful diagnostic alternative to bronchoscopy. In the course of biopsying suspected malignant nodules, infection is occasionally found. At the time of biopsy the cytologist often discovers that the aspirates are not malignant and appear to have an infectious etiology.

Granulomatous infections such as tuberculosis and fungal infections are the usual etiology of the nodules. At this time extra samples are obtained and placed into the appropriate culture media. Additional slides are also made for the various microbiologic stains.[72,73]

Nodular infiltrates that are suspicious for a microbiologic cause can also be biopsied (Fig. 19-6). The procedure is exactly the same as that for fine-needle aspiration biopsy of lung nodules. Differences occur with the treatment of the aspirated material, which is placed in the appropriate growth medium, and the slides are stained for microorganisms and not malignant cells. If no material is aspirated into the aspiration needle, another sampling technique can be employed. Two to five cubic centimeters of nonbacteriostatic saline is injected into the aspiration needle with the needle tip within

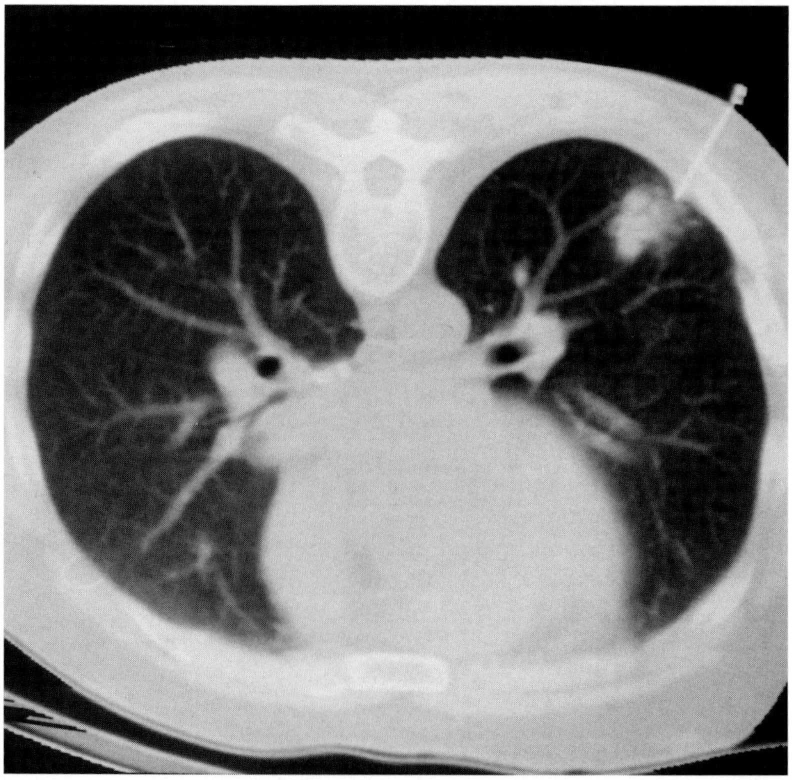

Figure 19-6

CT-guided biopsy of a nodular infectious infiltrate. *M. tuberculosis* was grown on culture.

the infiltrate, and aspiration is quickly performed. This technique often helps to gather a small amount of the infected material.

Biopsy of Chest Wall Lesions

Fine-needle aspiration biopsy of chest wall lesions offers a simple, safe, inexpensive, and rapid method for making a diagnosis. The most common chest wall lesions are rib metastases, but primary bone lesions, soft tissue tumors, and infections can be diagnosed with this technique (Fig. 19-7). The superficial location of chest wall lesions requires a shorter needle system than is needed for intrathoracic lesions. The biopsy can be performed with a simple 22-gauge hypodermic needle attached to a 10 cm^3 syringe. If the lesion is slightly deeper, a spinal needle can be used. If a coaxial system is needed, an 18-gauge hypodermic needle can serve as the guide needle and a 22-gauge spinal needle as the aspiration needle. CT or fluoroscopy can be used to guide the procedure. Fluoroscopy is a quick and simple guidance method in lesions with visible bone destruction. Ultrasound can also be used to guide biopsy of chest wall masses. For fluoroscopic guidance the patient is positioned with the biopsy site facing upward. The skin is prepared in the usual fashion. Advancing the biopsy needle perpendicular to the chest wall and parallel to the fluoroscopic beam is preferred. The curvature of the chest wall can make chest wall lesions surprisingly difficult to biopsy under fluoroscopic guidance if tangential approaches are tried. The exact depth of the lesion can be determined by first advancing the needle tip down onto the adjacent normal portion of the affected rib or bone. Once the exact depth is determined, the needle can be advanced over the suspicious area. Occasionally there is bony resistance in an area that appears to be completely destroyed by tumor. At other times no additional resistance is felt, and the biopsy depth is known only from prior testing over the uninvolved portion of the rib. Care should be taken not to enter the pleural space or lung. The patient should be treated as if a lung biopsy were being performed in regard to the development of a pneumothorax. Entering the chest wall lesion with a biopsy path that is more tangential can reduce the risk of pneumothorax but may make a fluoroscopic biopsy more difficult.[74]

CT guidance of chest wall lesions can be simpler than fluoroscopic biopsies, especially if the lesion does not involve anterior or posterior bony structures. CT guidance is easier when angled approaches are needed to avoid the shoulder girdle, when lateral approaches are needed, or when soft tissue masses without bony destruction are biopsied. CT has advantages when tangential approaches are needed to keep the needle out of the pleural space and avoid a pneumothorax. CT can depict the exact location of the needle tip as the biopsy is being performed. Radiologists should be able to perform biopsies with CT, ultrasound, and fluoroscopic guidance and become familiar with the capabilities, advantages, and disadvantages of each.

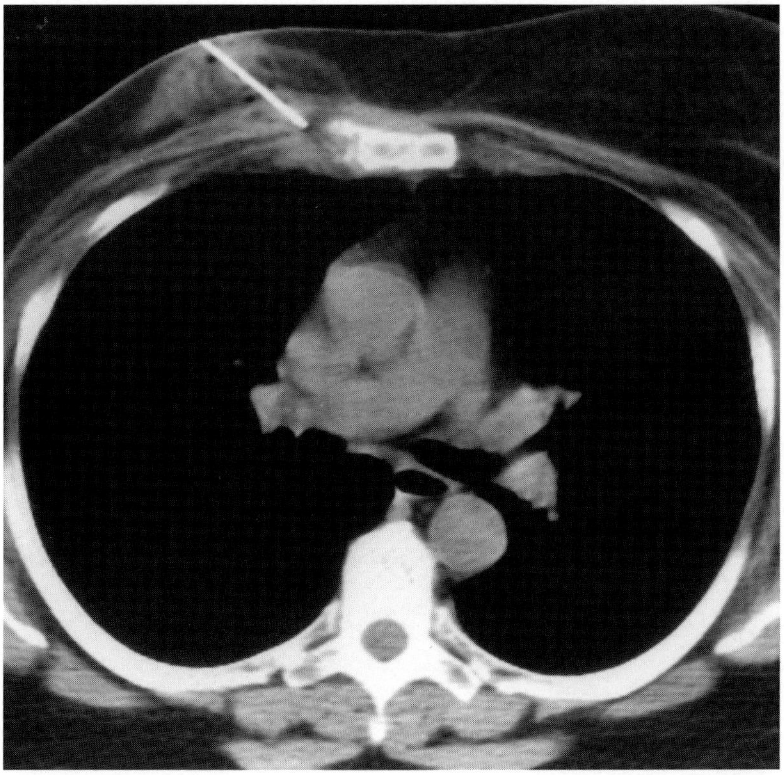

Figure 19-7

CT-guided biopsy of a soft tissue mass adjacent to the right lateral border of the sternum. Needle tip is seen within the mass. This was a metastasis from breast cancer 12 years after resection.

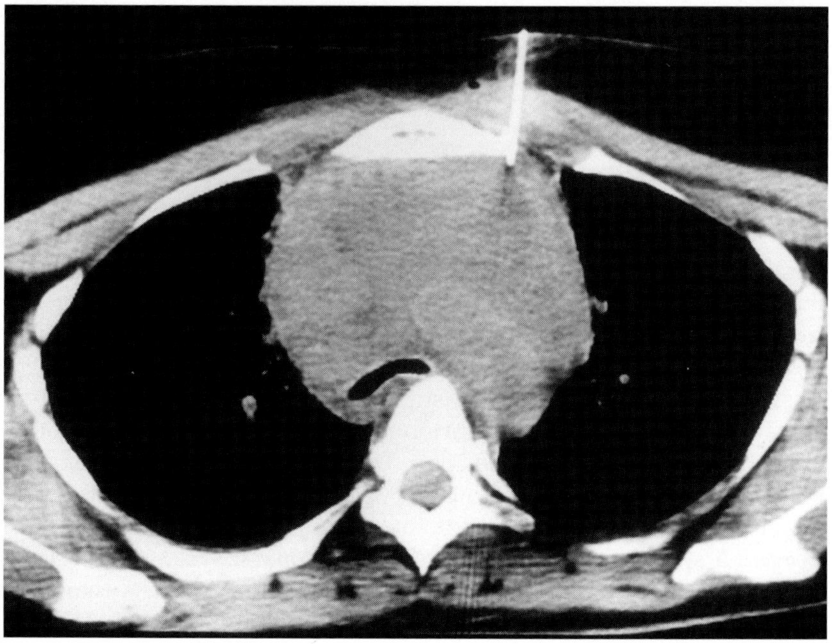

Figure 19-8

CT-guided needle biopsy of a large anterior mediastinal mass. Pathology showed the mass to be lymphoma.

Biopsy of Mediastinal and Hilar Masses

Fine-needle aspiration biopsy of mediastinal and hilar masses has become a common procedure[75–78] (Fig. 19-8). CT guidance is usually employed, but in cases where the mass is very large and CT has confirmed a safe biopsy approach, fluoroscopic or ultrasonic guidance can be utilized.[79] The question may arise as to the value of biopsying a mediastinal mass. Although many cytologists can confidently make a specific diagnosis on a fine-needle aspiration biopsy, many oncologists require a larger amount of tissue for confirmation of a specific cell type of tumor. Flow cytometry, immunologic stains, and core needle biopsies are improving the diagnostic ability of needle-type biopsies of mediastinal masses, especially the lymphoma subtypes. If the suspected diagnosis is lung cancer or recurrent lymphoma, a needle biopsy is adequate. These are choices which vary from institution to institution.[22,23]

Patient preparation, risks, needle choice, and skin site preparation are the same as for other fine-needle aspiration biopsies. Most of the biopsies of mediastinal or hilar masses are performed with CT guidance because the exact location of the mass, the normal mediastinal structures, the exact biopsy path, and the moment to moment position of the needle tip can be visualized. The exact placement of the needle within the mass can be time-consuming, so most mediastinal biopsies are performed using a coaxial needle system. Once the guide needle is placed in the correct location, no further imaging is needed, since multiple samples are taken. Once the needle is within a mediastinal mass, there is often marked transmittal of cardiac pulsations to the needle. A degree of motion of the needle of several centimeters is not unusual. Care should be taken not to handle the guide needle too much in order to keep the torque caused by transmitted cardiac motion on the needle to a minimum.

The risks of performing mediastinal fine-needle aspiration biopsies are the same as those for a lung nodule biopsy. The rates of pneumothorax, infection, and bleeding are similar. It would seem that the rate of pneumothorax should be increased, since often more pleural layers are punctured but that has not been proved. There is no reported increase in the incidence of bleeding complications, although the biopsy path is often adjacent to the great vessels or heart.

REFERENCES

1. Leyden H: Uber infectiose pneumonie. *Dtsch Med Wochenschr* 1883; 9:52–54.
2. Menetrier P: Cancer primitif du poumon. *Bull Soc Anat (Paris)* 1886; 61:643–647.
3. Dahlgren SE, Nordenstrom B: *Transthoracic Needle Biopsy.* Chicago, Year Book Medical, 1966:1–132.
4. Klein JS, Schultz S: Interventional chest radiology. *Curr Prob Diag Radiol* 1992; 21(6):223.
5. vanSonnenberg E, et al: Interventional radiology of the chest. *Chest* 1992; 102:608.
6. Weisbrod GL: Transthoracic percutaneous fine-needle aspiration biopsy in the chest and mediastinum. *Semin Interv Radio* 1991; 8:1–14.
7. Perlmutt LM, et al: Percutaneous transthoracic needle aspiration: A review. *AJR* 1989; 152:451.
8. Westcott JL: Percutaneous transthoracic needle biopsy. *Radiology* 1988; 169:593.
9. Stanley JH,et al: Lung lesions: Cytological diagnosis by fine-needle biopsy. *Radiology* 1987; 162:389.
10. Sider L, Davis TM Jr: Hilar masses: Evaluation with CT-guided biopsy after negative bronchoscopic examination. *Radiology* 1987; 164:107.

11. Poe RH, Kallay MC: Transthoracic needle biopsy of lung in nonhospitalized patients. *Chest* 1987; 92:676.
12. Charig MJ, et al: The value of a negative needle biopsy in suspected operable lung cancer. *Clin Radiol* 1991; 44:147–149.
13. Ikezoe J, et al: Sonographically guided needle biopsy of thoracic lesions. *Semin Interv Radiol* 1991; 8:15–22.
14. Sawhney S, et al: True-Cut biopsy of mediastinal masses guided by real-time ultrasound. *Clin Radiol* 1991; 44:16–19.
15. Khouri NF, et al: Transthoracic needle aspiration biopsy of benign and malignant lung lesions. *AJR* 1985; 144:281–288.
16. Stanley JH, et al: Lung lesions: Cytologic diagnosis by fine needle biopsy. *Radiology* 1987; 162:389–391.
17. Westcott JL: Direct percutaneous needle aspiration of localized pulmonary lesions: Results in 422 patients. *Radiology* 1980; 137:31–35.
18. Wittich GR, et al: Coaxial transthoracic fine-needle biopsy in patients with a history of malignant lymphoma. *Radiology* 1992; 183:175–178.
19. Ikezoe J, et al: Sonographically-guided needle biopsy for diagnosis of thoracic lesions. *AJR* 1984; 143:229–234.
20. Ikezoe J, et al: Percutaneous biopsy of the thoracic lesions: Value of sonography for needle guidance. *AJR* 1990; 154:1181–1185.
21. Yu CJ, Yang BC, Change DB, et al: Evaluation of ultrasonically-guided biopsies of mediastinal masses. *Chest* 1991; 100:399–404.
22. Yang PC, et al: Peripheral pulmonary lesions: Ultrasonography and ultrasonically-guided aspiration biopsy. *Radiology* 1985; 155:451–556.
23. Pederson OM, et al: Fine-needle aspiration biopsy of mediastinal and peripheral masses guided by real-time sonography. *Chest* 1986; 89:504–508.
24. Greene R, et al: Supplemental tissue-core histology from fine-needle transthoracic aspiration biopsy. *AJR* 1985; 144:787–792.
25. Glynn TJ Jr: Transosseous approach for transthoracic needle biopsy. *Radiology* 1990; 177:278–279.
26. Perlmutt LM, Braun SD, Newman GE, et al: Timing of chest film followup after transthoracic needle aspiration. *AJR* 1986; 146:1049–1050.
27. Fink I, Gamsu G, Harter LP: CT-guided aspiration biopsy of the thorax. *J Comput Assist Tomogr* 1982; 6:958–962.
28. Westcott JL: Percutaneous needle aspiration of hilar and mediastinal masses. *Radiology* 1981; 141:323–329.
29. Goralnik CH, et al: CT-guided cutting needle biopsies of selected chest lesions. *AJR* 1988; 151:903–907.
30. Omenaas O, et al: Cerebral air embolism after transthoracic aspiration with a 0.6 mm (23-gauge) needle. *Eur Respir J* 1989; 2:908–910.
31. Herman SJ, et al: Anterior mediastinal masses: Utility of transthoracic needle biopsy. *Radiology* 1991; 180:167–170.
32. Horrigan TP, Bergin KT: Correlation between needle biopsy of lung tumors and histopathologic analysis of resected specimens. *Chest* 1986; 90:638–640.
33. Thornbury JR, et al: Transthoracic needle aspiration biopsy: Accuracy of cytologic typing of malignant neoplasms. *AJR* 1981; 136:719–724.
34. Tikkakoski T, et al: Ultrasound-guided aspiration biopsy of anterior mediastinal masses. *J Clin Ultrasound* 1991; 19:209–214.
35. Gardner D, et al: CT-guided transthoracic needle biopsy. *Cardiovasc Intervent Radiol* 1991; 14:17–23.
36. Linder J, et al: Fine-needle aspiration biopsy of the mediastinum. *Am J Med* 1986; 81:1005–1008.
37. Sider L, Davis TM Jr: Hilar masses: Evaluation with CT-guided biopsy after negative bronchoscopic examination. *Radiology* 1987; 164:107–109.
38. Yap J, Tan KP: A comparative study of the Chiba and Turner needles in percutaneous lung biopsy. *Sing Med* 1988; 29: 14–16.
39. Quinn SF, et al: Temno biopsy needle: Evaluation of efficacy and safety in 165 biopsy procedures. *AJR* 1992; 158:641–643.
40. Morgenroth A, et al: Six years' experience with perthoracic core needle biopsy of pulmonary lesions. *Thorax* 1989; 44:177–183.
41. Torres A, et al: Diagnostic value of percutaneous lung-needle aspiration in patients with pneumonia. *Chest* 1990; 98:840–844.
42. Conces DJ Jr, et al: Thoracic needle biopsy: Improved results utilizing team approach. *Chest* 1987; 91:813–822.
43. Colquhoun SD, et al: Role of percutaneous fine-needle aspiration biopsy in suspected intrathoracic malignancy. *Ann Thorac Surg* 1991; 51:390–393.
44. Fish GD, et al: Postbiopsy pneumothorax: Estimating the risk by chest radiography and pulmonary function tests, *AJR* 1988; 150:71–74.
45. Miller KS, et al: Prediction of pneumothorax rate in percutaneous aspiration in the lung. *Chest* 1988; 93:742–745.
46. Quon D, et al: Pulmonary function testing in predicting complications from percutaneous lung biopsy. *J Can Assoc Radiol* 1988; 39:267–269.
47. DeGregorio Ariza MA, et al: Transthoracic aspiration biopsy of pulmonary and mediastinal lesions. *Eur J Radiol* 1991; 12:98–103.
48. Dolye T, Mullerworth M: Bleeding as a complication of fine needle lung biopsy. *Thorax* 1988; 43:1013.
49. Todd TRJ, et al: Aspiration needle biopsy of thoracic lesions. *Ann Thorac Surg* 1988; 32:154–161.
50. Aberle DR, et al: Fatal systemic arterial air embolism following lung needle aspiration. *Radiology* 1987; 165:351.
51. vanSonnenberg E, et al: Radiology and the law, with an emphasis on interventional radiology. *Radiology* 1993; 187:297.
52. vanSonnenberg E, et al: Difficult thoracic lesions: CT guided biopsy experience in 150 cases. *Radiology* 1988; 167:457.
53. Dahnert WF, et al: Fine-needle aspiration biopsy of abdominal lesions: Diagnostic yield for different needle tip configurations. *Radiology* 1992; 185:263.
54. Kreula J: Effect of sampling technique on specimen size in fine needle aspiration biopsy. *Invest Radiol* 1990; 25:1294.
55. Austin JHM, Cohen MB: Value of having a cytopathologist present during percutaneous fine-needle aspiration biopsy. *AJR* 1993; 160:175.
56. Kazerooni EA, et al: Risk of pneumothorax in CT-guided transthoracic needle aspiration biopsy on the lung. *Radiology* 1996; 198:371–375.
57. Moore EH, et al: Positional precautions in needle-aspiration lung biopsy. *Radiology* 1990; 175:733–735.
58. Miller KS, et al: Prediction of pneumothorax rate in percutaneous needle aspiration of the lung. *Chest* 1988; 83:742.
59. Sargent EN, Turner AF: Emergency treatment of pneumothorax: A simple catheter technique for use in the radiology department. *AJR* 1970; 109:531–535.
60. Casola G, et al: Pneumothorax: Radiologic treatment with small catheters. *Radiology* 1988; 166:89.
61. Reinhold C, et al: Treatment of pleural effusions and pneumothorax with catheters placed percutaneously under imaging guidance. *AJR* 1989; 152:1189–1190.
62. Conces DJ Jr, et al: Treatment of pneumothoraces utilizing smaller caliber chest tubes. *Chest* 1988; 94:55–57.
63. Peters J, Kubitschek KR: Clinical evaluation of a percutaneous pneumothorax catheter. *Chest* 1984; 86:714–717.
64. Perlmutt LM, et al: Transthoracic needle aspiration: Use of a small chest tube to treat pneumothorax. *AJR* 1987; 148: 849–852.
65. Mercier C, et al: Outpatient management of intercostal tube drainage in spontaneous pneumothorax. *Ann Thorac Surg* 1976; 22:163–165.
66. Berger R, et al: Dissemination of cancer cells by needle biopsy of the lung. *J Thorac Cardiovasc Surg* 1972; 63:430–432.
67. Seyfer AE, et al: Chest wall implantation of lung cancer after thin-needle aspiration biopsy. *Ann Thorac Surg* 1989; 48: 284–286.

68. Muller NL, et al: Seeding of malignant cells into the needle track after lung and pleural biopsy. *J Can Assoc Radiol* 1986; 37:192–194.
69. Tolly TL, et al: Air embolism complicating percutaneous lung biopsy. *AJR* 1988; 150:555–556.
70. Cianci P, et al: Air embolism complicating percutaneous thin needle biopsy of the lung. *Chest* 1987; 92:749–750.
71. Baker BK, Awwad EE: Computed tomography of fatal air embolism following percutaneous aspiration biopsy of the lung. *J Comput Assist Tomogr* 1988; 12:1082–1083.
72. Torres A, et al: Diagnostic value of nonfluoroscopic percutaneous lung needle aspiration in patients with pneumonia. *Chest* 1990; 98:840.
73. Scott WW Jr, Kuhlman JE: Focal pulmonary lesions in patients with AIDS: Percutaneous transthoracic needle biopsy. *Radiology* 1991; 180:419.
74. Iklard RW: A study of rib biopsy. *Chest* 1992; 102:1134.
75. Adler OB, et al: Fine-needle aspiration biopsy of mediastinal masses: Evaluation of 136 experiences. *AJR* 1983; 140:893–896.
76. Moinuddin SM, et al: Mediastinal needle biopsy, *AJR* 1984; 143:531–532.
77. Weisbrod, GL, et al: Percutaneous fine needle aspiration biopsy of mediastinal lesions. *AJR* 1984; 143:525–529.
78. Weisbrod, GL: Percutaneous fine-needle aspiration biopsy of the mediastinum. *Clin Chest Med* 1987; 8:27–41.
79. Saito T, et al: Ultrasonically guided needle biopsy in the diagnosis of mediastinal masses. *Am Rev Respir Dis* 1988; 138:697–699.

CHAPTER 20

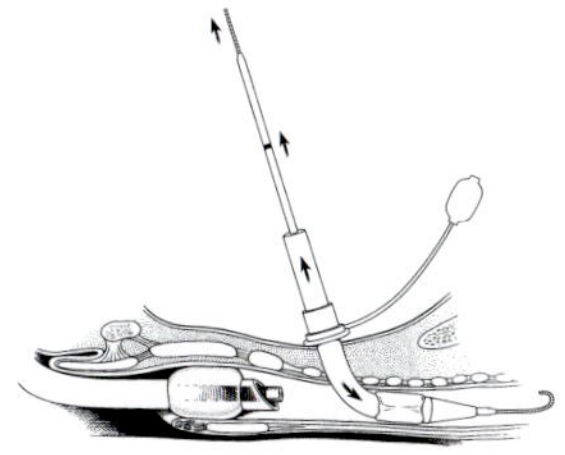

PERCUTANEOUS TRACHEOSTOMY

Paul F. Dellaripa

Percutaneous dilational tracheostomy has emerged during the past 10 years as a safe and effective alternative to standard surgical tracheostomy for patients requiring mechanical ventilation. Percutaneous techniques were introduced in 1955 by Shelden and coworkers[1] and later adopted by Toye and Weinstein[2] in 1969. Since then, the procedure has been modified using a series of dilators as described by Ciaglia and colleagues[3] and has been used widely in both medical and surgical patients. The advantages of percutaneous tracheostomy are that it avoids potentially hazardous transfer of critically ill patients to the operating room, minimizes scarring and risk of infection from larger incisions associated with standard surgical tracheostomy, and is a simpler technique that uses fewer resources than surgical tracheostomy.[4,5] Although surgical tracheostomy is usually a safe procedure, complication rates range from 6 to 66 percent.[6–14] Tracheostomy, whether percutaneous or standard surgical placement, may yield numerous benefits, including less discomfort to the patient, easier handling of secretions, prevention of laryngeal injury, and greater mobility on the part of the patient. Tracheostomy may enhance weaning from mechanical ventilation. Percutaneous tracheostomy is contraindicated if emergent airway access is necessary or when an infection is present at the surgical site. Anatomic abnormalities and an enlarged thyroid are relative contraindications, but in some groups with extensive experience percutaneous dilational tracheostomy has emerged as the treatment of choice for these conditions.[15] The presence of coagulopathy or severe thrombocytopenia is a contraindication in most settings; however, groups with significant experience in percutaneous dilational tracheostomy have performed this procedure safely in patients at risk for bleeding.[16] In general, absolute contraindications include clinical instability, high levels of positive end-expiratory pressure (PEEP), extensive neck surgery, or the presence of soft tissue infection.

Equipment for Percutaneous Dilational Tracheostomy

Three techniques have been developed for percutaneous tracheostomy: the single lead dilator technique, the dilator forceps technique, and the percutaneous dilational tracheostomy technique, which has become the standard technique used in most published series. The single lead dilator technique developed by Toye and Weinstein[17] uses a split needle technique to obtain tracheal access. A single dilator is placed through the split needle. The needle is split and removed, and a tracheostomy tube is passed over the dilator. This technique was notable for a high (6 percent) level of paratracheal insertion.[18] The dilator forceps technique used by Schachner and coworkers[19] involves use of a specially designed dilator tool that slips over the guide wire and serves to enlarge the intercartilaginous space. The percutaneous dilational tracheostomy technique developed by Ciaglia and colleagues[3] is the one most commonly used today. The two prepared kits most commonly used for this procedure are the Cook tracheostomy introducer set (Cook Critical Care, Bloomington, IN) (Fig. 20-1) and the Portex Perfit tracheostomy introducer set (Sims Medical Systems, Keene, NH) (Fig. 20-2). The main differences between the two kits are that the Cook kit uses curved dilators as opposed to straight dilators with the Perfit kit, and the Cook kit uses six dilators compared with the three dilators with the Perfit kit. Although both kits have been used extensively with similar results, the curved dilator technique is the method most commonly stud-

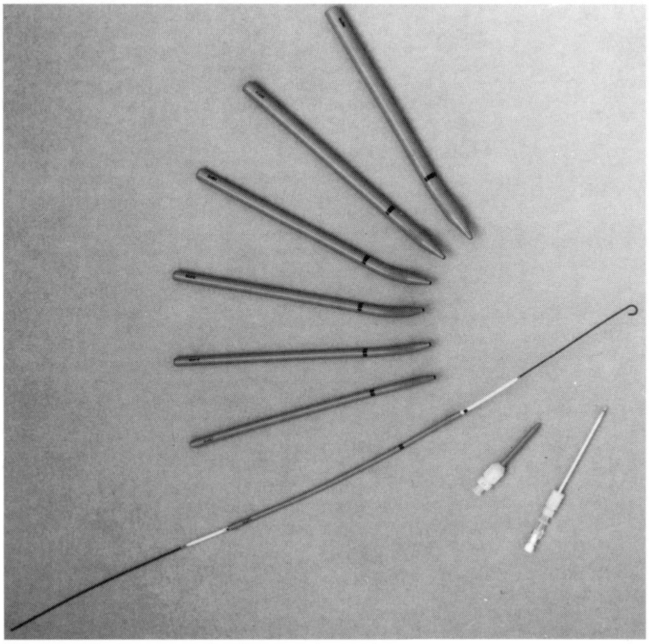

Figure 20-1

Cook tracheostomy introducer set. *(Cook Critical Care, Bloomington, IN.)*

ied in the literature and serves as the reference for discussion in the procedure section.

Included in the kit is a 15-g catheter introducer needle, a curved J-wire guide, and a guiding catheter. The dilators range in size from 12 to 36 Fr. Other equipment required includes sterile gloves, gowns, and drapes. The anesthetic agent used locally is 1% lidocaine with epinephrine. A laryngoscope and endotracheal tube should be kept on hand in the event the endotracheal tube becomes dislodged and emergent airway access is necessary.

Role of Bronchoscopy in Percutaneous Tracheostomy

The primary reason for using bronchoscopy during percutaneous tracheostomy is to avoid paratracheal insertion of the tracheostomy tube and to avoid trauma to the posterior tracheal wall during initial insertion of the needle. In addition, bronchoscopic visualization enables appropriate positioning of the endotracheal tube and helps avoid impalement of the endotracheal tube during initial insertion of the needle. The bronchoscope is especially useful during the initial learn-

Figure 20-2

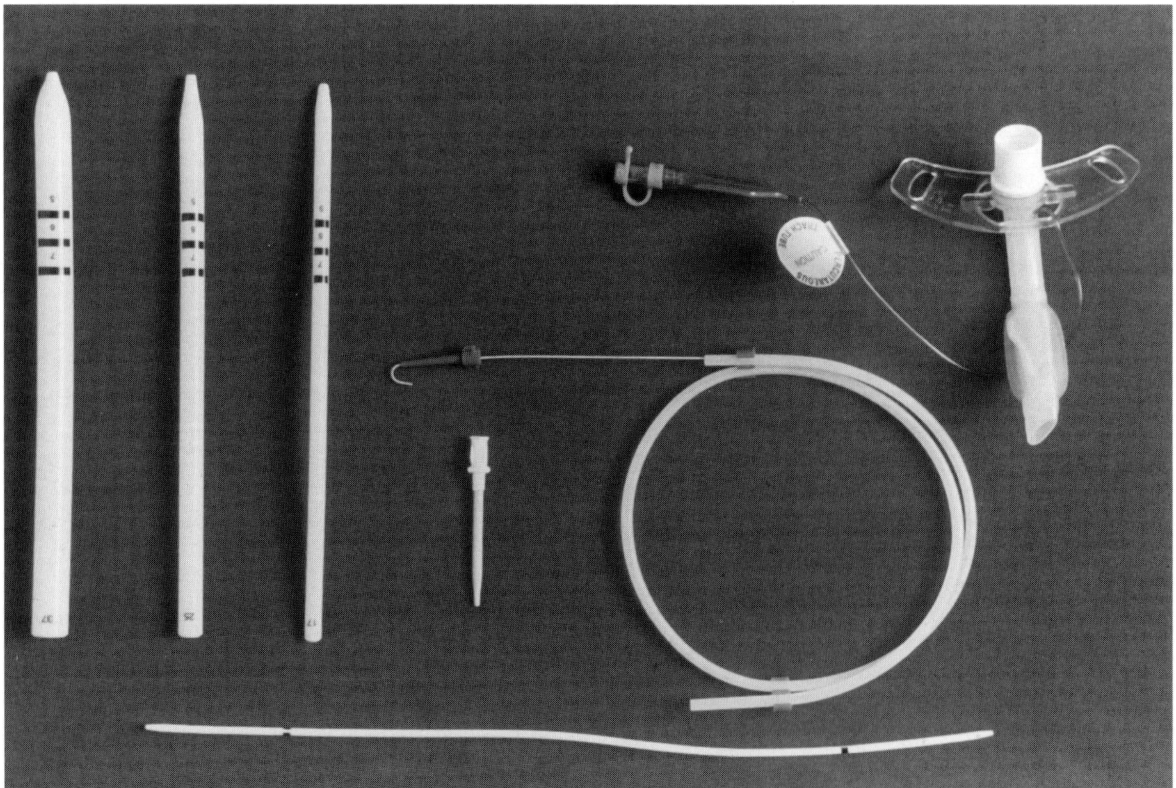

Portex Perfit tracheostomy introducer set. *(Sims Medical Systems, Keene, NH.)*

ing process and in the patient with a short or obese neck.[20–23] Many physicians used bronchoscopy early in their experience and subsequently only in difficult situations. Although use of the bronchoscope offers many advantages, including direct visualization of placement of the needle, positioning of the endotracheal tube, and placement of the tracheostomy, the presence of the bronchoscope within the endotracheal tube may result in loss of tidal volume and hypoxemia, which some authors[20] advocate warrants the use of end-tidal CO_2 monitoring. No randomized controlled trials have compared rates of complications and outcome between percutaneous tracheostomy with and without bronchoscopy.

Complications with Percutaneous Tracheostomy

The most common intraoperative and postoperative complications associated with this procedure are those that occur with tracheostomy in general: paratracheal intubation, bleeding (both major and minor), pneumothorax or subcutaneous emphysema, transient hypoxia, and death. Long-term complications include tracheal stenosis, tracheoinnominate fistula, tracheocutaneous fistula, and late hemorrhage from the tracheostomy site. Complications in the literature are divided into major and minor. Major complications include death, tension pneumothorax, major hemorrhage, and displacement of the tube leading to hypoxia. Comparing complications from one study with another can be difficult because authors' definitions of what constitutes a major or minor complication may vary. The complication rates associated with percutaneous tracheostomy among the major nonrandomized studies[15,17,19–22,24–28] available in the literature to date are summarized in Table 20-1. In the largest study to date, Marx and coworkers[20] reviewed their experience with 254 patients, four of whom had major complications, including one death, tension pneumothorax, tube displacement, and left main-stem intubation. In another study, Ivatury and colleagues,[25] using the dilator forceps technique (Rapitrach method) of percutaneous tracheostomy, performed this procedure on 61 patients with three major complications, including one fatal cardiac arrest, severe bronchospasm requiring conversion to surgical tracheostomy, and significant postoperative bleeding in a patient with end-stage cirrhosis. Toursarkissian and coworkers[15] performed percutaneous tracheostomy in 141 patients with one intraoperative death secondary to severe bronchospasm during insertion of the guide wire. Postoperatively, there were three instances of significant bleeding requiring transfusions. Marelli and colleagues[21] used endoscopic guidance in 61 patients with one intraoperative death as a result of arrhythmia and six minor complications, for a total major and minor complication rate of 4.9 and 11.4 percent, respectively. Schachner and coworkers[18] performed percutaneous tracheostomy on 80 patients using a specially designed kit and experienced one major complication of ventricular fibrillation with prompt resolution and 13 other minor complications, including damage to the tracheal rings, ruptured tracheostomy cuff, subcutaneous emphysema, and minimal bleeding. In a study of 100 patients, 94 of whom underwent percutaneous tracheostomy and six of whom underwent percutaneous cricothyroidotomy, Toye and Weinstein[17] used a single dilator technique that is no longer commonly employed and reported one death secondary to loss of the tracheostomy tube and inability to resecure the airway. There were six instances of paratracheal insertion, four instances of subcutaneous emphysema, and one instance each of pretracheal cellulitis and bilateral pneumothorax, for a major complication rate of 1 percent and a minor complication rate of 14 percent.

Other reported complications have included intrapleural placement of the tracheostomy tube, malposition leading to delayed weaning, hypercarbia leading to raised intracranial pressure, tracheal cartilage dislodgement and fracture, and skin tethering the stomal site.[29–33] In one case report,[34] profuse life-threatening hemorrhage developed 11 days after percutaneous tracheal placement in a young man with aspiration pneumonia and oliguric renal failure. Bleeding was due to lateral displacement of an aberrant anterior jugular vein and continued contact with the tracheostomy tube, leading to erosion of the vessel wall.

Avoidance of many of these complications involves particular attention to warning signs during the procedure. Difficulty in passing the dilator may indicate that the guide wire has impaled the endotracheal tube or that the guide wire is positioned in an extratracheal or paratracheal position. The problem of bleeding can be minimized with the use of epinephrine in lidocaine and avoidance of superficial veins. Pressure should be maintained between dilations. If bleeding occurs, the procedure should proceed because placement of the tracheostomy will serve to tamponade the site of bleeding. Using of bronchoscopy serves to avoid the pitfalls of paratracheal insertion and impalement of the endotracheal tube, although the operator must be vigilant for loss of minute volume, desaturation, and hypercarbia.

Late Outcomes in Percutaneous Tracheostomy

Late complications that may occur in either surgical or percutaneous tracheostomy include granuloma formation at the stomal site, laryngotracheal stenosis, late hemorrhage either from a bleeding granuloma or rup-

Table 20-1
COMPLICATION RATES IN PERCUTANEOUS TRACHEOSTOMY

Author and Year	*No.*	*Deaths [no.(%)]*	*Major Complications [no.(%)]*	*Minor Complications [no.(%)]*	*Paratracheal Insert [no.(%)]*	*Long-Term Complications*
Toye and Weinstein, 1986	100	1 (1)	2 (2)	8 (8)	6 (6)	0 (19)
Schachner et al., 1989	80	0 (0)	1 (1.25%)	13 (16%)	0 (0)	0/10
Marelli et al., 1991[a]	61	1 (1.6)	2 (3.2)	6 (9.8)	0 (0)	0/13
Griggs et al., 1991	153	0 (0)	2 (1.3)	4 (2.6)	0 (0)	NA
Ivatury et al., 1992	61	1 (1.6)	3 (4.9)	7 (11.4)	0 (0)	1/20
Manara, 1994	77	0 (0)	2 (2.6)	4 (5.2)	0 (0)	0/2
Friedman et al., 1996	100	1 (1)	4 (4)	6 (6)	1 (1)	5/10
Winkler, 1994[a]	71	0 (0)	0 (0)	4 (5.6)	1 (1.4)	2/12
Toursarkissian et al., 1994	141	1 (0.7)	5 (3.5)	13 (9.2)	3 (2.1)	3/76
Fernandez et al., 1996[a]	162	0 (0)	1 (0.6)	8 (4.9)	3 (0.6)	0/29
Marx et al., 1996[b]	254	1 (0.3)	4 (1.6)	7 (2.8)	3 (1.2)	3/254

[a]Endoscopy.

[b]Endoscopy in last 30 patients. Major complications include death, severe bronchospasm with desaturation, pneumothorax, major bleeding, stomal infection leading to systemic illness. Minor complications include stomal infection, subcutaneous emphysema, tracheal ring fracture, cuff defect leading to tracheostomy change, tube obstruction without hemodynamic or respiratory consequence. Long-term complications include tracheal stenosis, tracheoesophageal fistula, persistent stoma.

ture of an innominate artery or tracheoesophageal fistula, tracheocutaneous fistula, and a depressed scar that results in a suboptimal cosmetic appearance. Injury to the trachea may occur distally at the tip of the tracheostomy tube, at the cuff site, or at the level of the stoma. Marx and coworkers[20] noted one instance each of persistent cellulitis at the stoma and displacement of the tube. In an autopsy study, van Heurn and colleagues[35] examined the tracheas of 12 patients who underwent percutaneous tracheostomy. The puncture site was subcricoid in two patients and below the third tracheal ring in three patients, the ideal placement being between the first and second or second and third tracheal rings. Both patients with subcricoid puncture had experienced fracture of the cricoid cartilage, and fracture of the tracheal ring was noted in 11 patients overall.[35]

In another review,[36] a standardized scoring system using subjective findings, physical examination of the stoma, and tracheoscopic findings was employed in 16 patients who underwent percutaneous tracheostomy. All 16 patients had no subjective evidence of tracheal damage, and 10 of the patients who consented to tracheostomy showed no laryngeal damage. Five other patients were studied on autopsy and showed no evidence of tracheomalacia or stenosis.

Comparison of Percutaneous Tracheostomy and Surgical Tracheostomy

Three randomized studies have compared percutaneous tracheostomy versus surgical tracheostomy. Hazard and coworkers[37] randomized 12 patients to surgical tracheostomy and 12 patients to percutaneous tracheostomy. The principal finding showed a significantly decreased intraoperative duration of procedure (4.3 ± 2.2 min with percutaneous tracheostomy versus 13.5 ± 7.3 min with surgical tracheostomy) as well as a decreased rate of stomal infection (33 percent with surgical tracheostomy versus 4 percent with percutaneous tracheostomy). The differences in frequency of hemorrhage and pneumothorax were not statistically significant between the two groups. Overall, 58 percent of the standard surgical tracheostomy procedures were associated with an adverse event compared with 25 percent in the percutaneous tracheostomy group. Of all the patients, 19 survived to decannulation, and tracheal stenosis developed in five of eight patients in the surgical tracheostomy group, whereas tracheal stenosis developed in 2 of 11 patients in the percutaneous tracheostomy group, a statistically significant difference.[37]

Friedman and colleagues[27] performed a similar randomized prospective trial involving 27 patients randomized to surgical tracheostomy and 26 patients to percutaneous tracheostomy. The duration of procedure time was shorter in the percutaneous tracheostomy group (8.2 ± 4.9 min versus 33.9 ± 14.0 min for surgical tracheostomy group). Postprocedural complications rates were 12 and 41 percent, respectively, for the percutaneous tracheostomy group versus the surgical tracheostomy group. There were no statistically significant differences in intraoperative adverse events.[27] In a third study, Crofts and coworkers[38] randomized 28 patients undergoing surgical tracheostomy and 25 patients undergoing percutaneous tracheostomy. The complication rates in both groups were low and minor, with no significant difference between the two groups, and no deaths reported. No long-term data were provided in this study.[38] In a nonrandomized prospective study, Griggs and colleagues[24] prospectively compared 153 percutaneous tracheostomies with 74 surgical tracheostomies, and noted a total complication rate of 3.9 percent in the percutaneous tracheostomy group compared with 18.9 percent in the surgical tracheostomy group.

Cost Considerations of Percutaneous Tracheostomy versus Surgical Tracheostomy

In general, costs per procedure for percutaneous tracheostomy are significantly less than for surgical tracheostomy. The elimination of anesthesia charges, operating room time, and need for transfer represent the major source of savings when comparing the two procedures. Imami and coworkers[39] prospectively observed 88 patients and found that total charges for percutaneous tracheostomy were more than 50 percent less than for surgical tracheostomy ($2093 versus $4536). In their[39] study, four instances of minor bleeding, one tracheal injury, two pneumothoraces, one pneumopericardium, and one tracheoinnominate fistula were noted, for an overall complication rate of 10 percent and a 1 percent mortality rate. In another study, Barba and colleagues[23] showed a net difference of $3335 between surgical tracheostomy and percutaneous tracheostomy. In a retrospective cost analysis of 65 patients, Cobean and coworkers[40] showed a savings of an average of $1645.

Other Indications for Percutaneous Tracheostomy

Percutaneous tracheostomy has generally not been used in younger patients because the trachea is more pliable and more susceptible to collapse with the pressure of the dilation procedure. Also, landmarks may be more difficult to palpate in younger patients because the larynx lies higher in the neck. However, a small study was performed in older children and young adults (ages 10 to 20 years) with one intraoperative and one postoperative complication occurring in the same patient—stomal infection and premature removal of the guide wire. Of the nine patients decannulated, there was no sign of tracheal stenosis during a follow-up period of 39 weeks.[41]

Summary

Overall, percutaneous tracheostomy is a safe procedure that can be performed conveniently in the intensive care unit. It is cost-effective compared with surgical tracheostomy. In general, surgeons have performed this procedure, but experienced nonsurgical interventionists and anesthesiologists have also performed this procedure safely. In all such procedures, the operator must be skilled in airway management and in emergent tracheostomy techniques for the rare but potential need to convert to an open procedure.

HOW I DO IT

Personnel for the procedure include a surgeon or main operator, an assistant, and a respiratory therapist. If bronchoscopy is used, a physician or anesthesiologist skilled in bronchoscopy should be present.

The patient is prepared for percutaneous tracheostomy as for a minor surgical procedure. Adequate sedation is obtained with a short-acting benzodiazepene and, depending on the activity of the patient, a neuromuscular blocker may be employed. Some physicians place the patient on a mobile stretcher in the event conversion to a surgical tracheostomy is needed. F_{IO_2} 1.0 is maintained throughout the procedure. The patient is positioned by extending the head and placing a rolled towel between the scapulas. The endotracheal tube tape is loosened, and the patient is monitored with continuous pulse oximetry and blood pressure monitoring. Some authors[20] use end-tidal CO_2 monitoring attached to the endotracheal tube. In addition, many physicians[20–22] advocate the use of bronchoscopy throughout the entire procedure to assess the correct placement of the introducing needle and guide wire placement. This is discussed in detail later.

The anterior neck is palpated, locating the landmark structures, including the thyroid cartilage and cricoid cartilage (Fig. 20-3). The neck is prepared and draped in a sterile fashion. The head is fixed in the midline, and the trachea is immobilized between the operator's fingers. Access is obtained either between the first and second tracheal interspace or between the second and third tracheal interspace. Lidocaine, 1%, is introduced locally, and a vertical incision is made below the level of the cricoid cartilage, approximately 1 cm long. A small clamp may be used for blunt dissection and more optimal palpation of the correct position for placement of the tracheostomy. After the point of placement has been identified, the endotracheal tube is pulled back above the level of tracheostomy placement, and an introducer needle with a lidocaine-filled syringe is used to puncture the anterior trachea, pointing posterior and caudad (Fig. 20-4). Verification of correct entry can be accomplished by bronchoscopic visualization or by aspiration of air in the syringe. If the needle has impaled the endotracheal tube, moving the endotracheal tube back and forth will result in concomitant movement of the needle. Additional lidocaine can be injected into the trachea, and the needle is removed as the outer Teflon sheath is advanced (Fig. 20-5). Airflow is confirmed, the syringe is removed, and a 1.32-mm J-wire guide is advanced into the trachea. The Teflon sheath is removed while the wire remains in the tracheal lumen. While the distal J-wire marking is being maintained at the skin level, the 11 Fr introductory sheath is advanced by using a twisting motion over the J wire to dilate the access site. The dilator is removed, again maintaining the distal wire mark at skin-level (Fig. 20-6). After the initial dilation has been completed, the 8-0 Fr Teflon guiding catheter is advanced over the guide wire and positioned so that the proximal end of the guiding catheter is aligned with the mark on the proximal end of the J wire. This step is important to prevent the distal end of the guiding catheter from overriding the J wire and potentially damaging the posterior wall of the trachea. The safety ridge of the guiding catheter should then be positioned at the skin level. With the guide wire and guiding catheter in place, a series of dilations are performed (Fig. 20-7). Dilation begins with the 12 Fr dilator advanced over the guiding catheter–guide wire assembly. The dilator is positioned correctly by matching the proximal end of the dilator with the dilator positioning mark on the guiding catheter. This permits the distal end of the dilator to rest at the safety ridge at the skin level. The relationship of the wire, wire catheter, and dilator is maintained, and the entire unit is advanced with a twisting motion to the skin level mark on the dilator; this is repeated several times. The initial dilation process is continued as described with successively larger dilators; the number of dilators used varies from three to six. The tracheal entrance is slightly overdilated to enable the balloon portion of the tracheostomy tube to pass through the tracheal entrance. The appropriate size overdilation needed for the desired tracheostomy tube is estimated as follows:

Tracheostomy Tube Inner Diameter, cm	*Appropriate Dilator for Overdilation, Fr*
6	24
7	28
8	32
9	36

After overdilation has been completed, the tracheostomy tube is fitted over the appropriate size dilator (Fig. 20-8). The dilator is lubricated sufficiently, and the tracheostomy tube is positioned so that the tip is 2 cm back from the distal end of the dilator. The tracheostomy tube is also lubricated and advanced with the appropriate introductory dilator to the safety ridge of the guiding catheter, and the entire unit is advanced so that the proximal end of the tracheostomy tube is flush with the skin level. The dilator, wire, and guiding catheter are then removed.

Tracheostomy Tube Inner Diameter, cm	*Appropriate Dilator for Introduction, Fr*
6	18
7	21
8	24
9	28

Figure 20-3

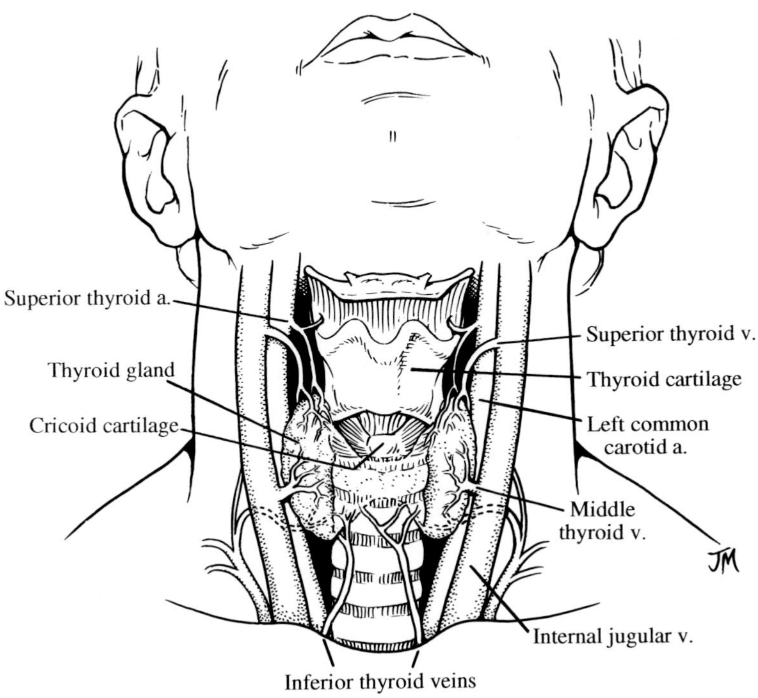

Anatomic relationship of thyroid cartilage, cricoid cartilage, and the tracheal interspace. Ideal placement is below either the first or second tracheal cartilage.

Figure 20-4

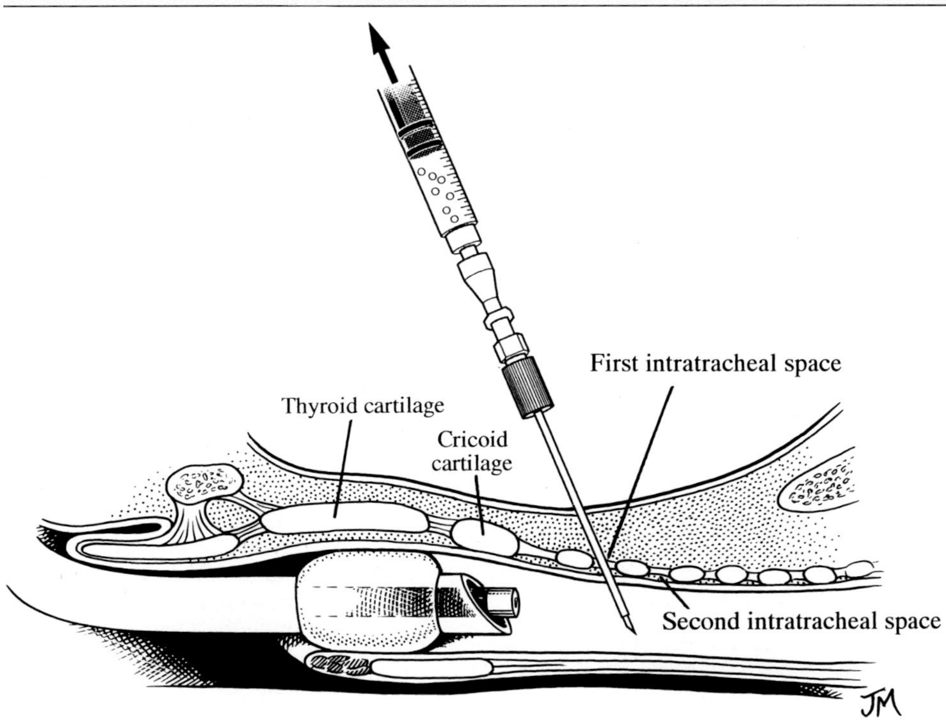

The endotracheal tube is withdrawn to just below the vocal cords. The trachea is entered either below the first or second intratracheal cartilage. Air bubbles aspirated within the syringe confirm intratracheal location. Correct placement may be confirmed by bronchoscopy.

Figure 20-5

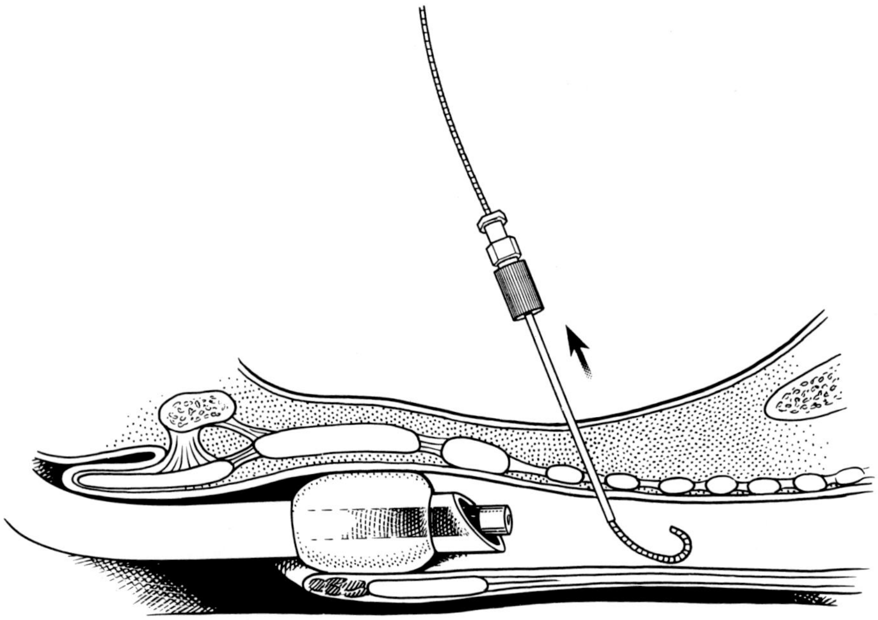

The introducer catheter is advanced into the trachea, the needle is removed, and the J wire is advanced through the catheter into the trachea. The introducer is then removed.

Figure 20-6

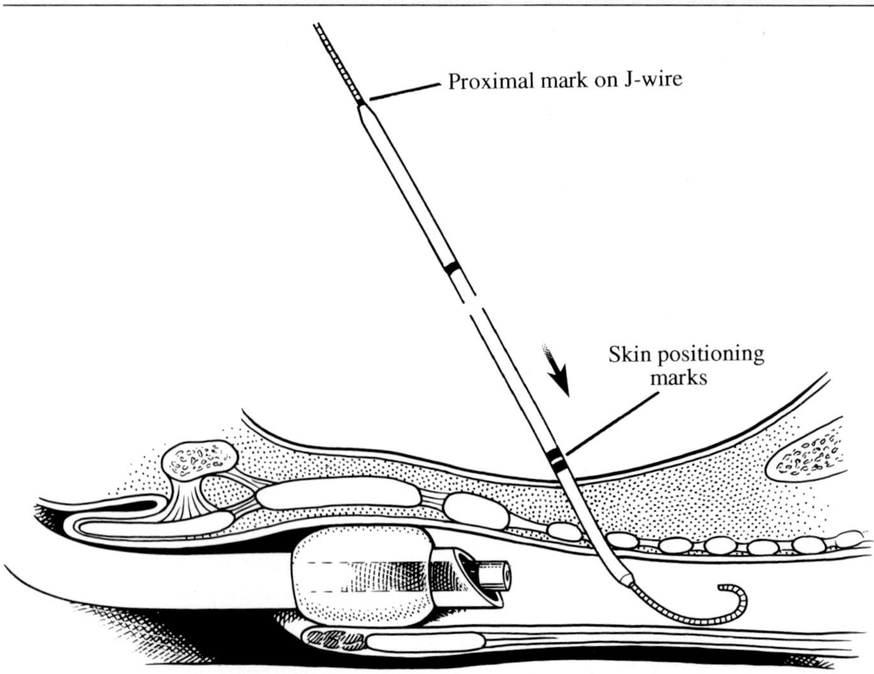

A short dilating catheter is advanced over the guide wire followed by the guiding catheter. The double black skin positioning marks are maintained at skin level. The proximal end of the guiding catheter is aligned with the mark on the proximal end of the J wire.

Figure 20-7

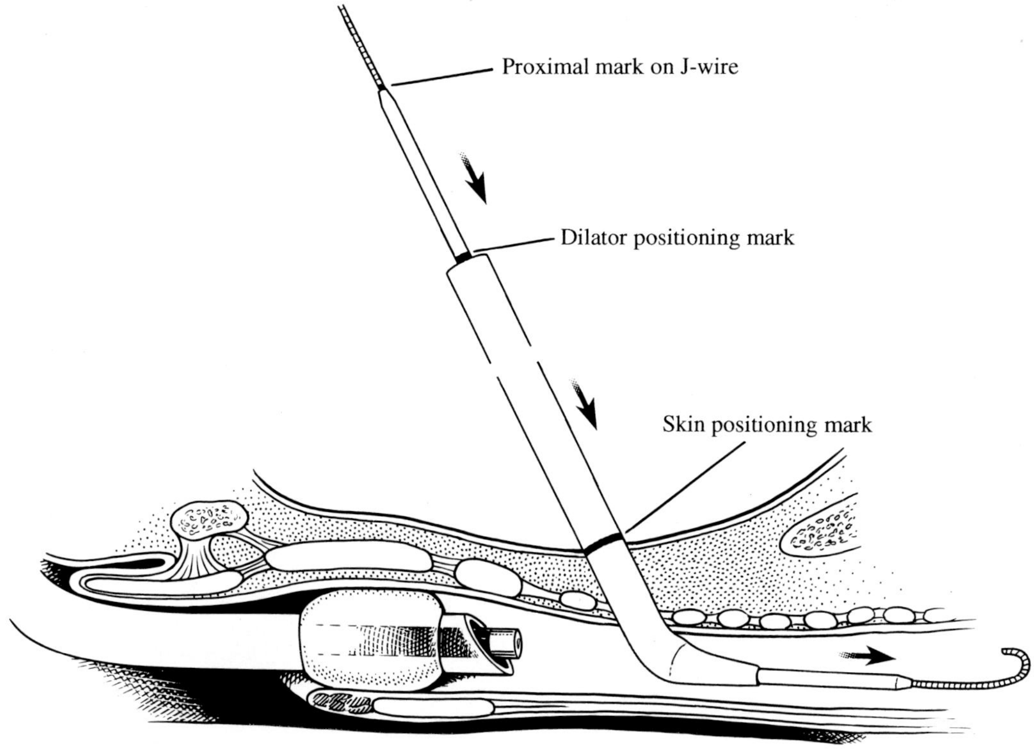

Dilators of successive sizes are positioned over the guiding catheter so that the proximal end of the dilator matches the dilator positioning mark on the guiding catheter. The distal tip of the dilator will rest at the skin level matched with the double black line of the guiding catheter. The relationship of the wire, guiding catheter, and dilator is maintained, and the entire unit is advanced so that the skin positioning marks on the dilator reach skin level.

Figure 20-8

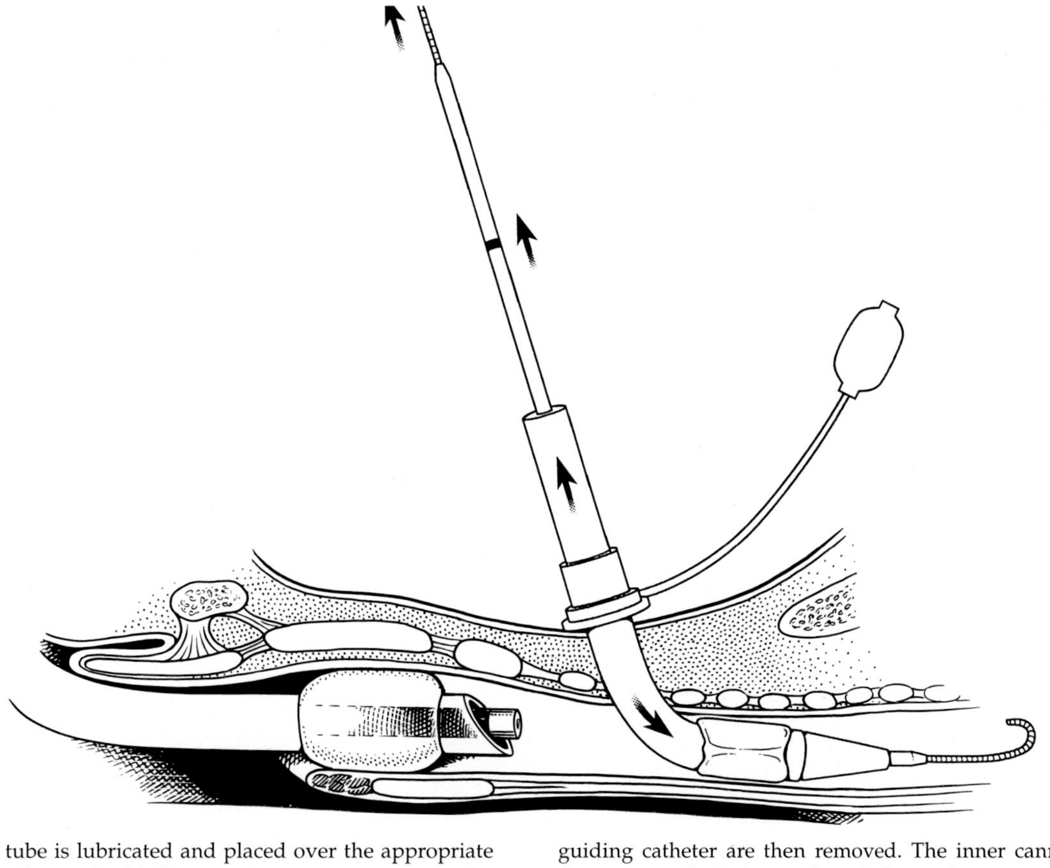

A tracheostomy tube is lubricated and placed over the appropriate size dilator and advanced with firm continuous pressure over the wire-guiding catheter unit into the trachea. The dilator, wire, and guiding catheter are then removed. The inner cannula of the tracheostomy tube is inserted, and the tracheostomy cuff is inflated.

If a dual cannula tracheostomy tube is used, the inner cannula should be removed during introduction. It is then re-placed, and the ventilator tubing is attached, the balloon on the tracheostomy cuff is inflated, and the patient is observed for adequate ventilation, at which time the endotracheal tube can be removed. The tracheostomy is sutured on each side, and a band is attached around the neck to the tracheostomy tube so that the tracheostomy tube is secured firmly.

REFERENCES

1. Shelden CH, et al: A new method for tracheotomy. *J Neurosurg* 1955; 12:428–431.
2. Toye FJ, Weinstein, JD: A percutaneous tracheostomy device. *Surgery* 1969; 65:384–389.
3. Ciaglia P, et al: Elective percutaneous dilational tracheostomy. A new simple bedside procedure; preliminary report. *Chest* 1985; 87:715–719.
4. Indeck M, et al: Risk, cost, and benefit of transporting ICU patients for special studies. *J Trauma* 1988; 28:1020–1025.
5. Smith I, et al: Mishaps during transport from the intensive care unit. *Crit Care Med* 1990; 18:278–281.
6. Stock MC, et al: Perioperative complications of elective tracheostomy in critically ill patients. *Crit Care Med* 1986; 14:861–863.
7. Stauffer JL, et al: Complications and consequences of endotracheal intubation and tracheotomy. A prospective study of 150 critically ill adult patients. *Am J Med* 1981; 70:65–76.
8. Chew JY, Cantrell RW: Tracheostomy. Complications and their management. *Arch Otolaryngol* 1972; 96:538–545.
9. Skaggs JA, Cogbill CL: Tracheostomy: Management, mortality, complications. *Am Surg* 1969; 35:393–396.
10. Rogers LA: Complications of tracheostomy. *South Med J* 1969; 62:1496–1500.
11. Yarington CT Jr, Frazer JP: Complications of tracheotomy. *Arch Surg* 1965; 91:652–655.
12. Dugan DJ, Samson PC: Tracheostomy: Present day indications and technics. *Am J Surg* 1963; 106:290–306.
13. Glas WW, et al: Complications of tracheostomy. *Arch Surg* 1962; 85:56–63.
14. Meade JW: Tracheotomy: Its complications and their management. A study of 212 cases. *N Engl J Med* 1961; 265:519–523.
15. Toursarkissian B, et al: Percutaneous dilational tracheostomy: Report of 141 cases. *Ann Thorac Surg* 1994; 57:862–867.
16. Guzman J, et al: Percutaneous dilational tracheostomy: A safe technique in patients at risk for bleeding. *Am J Respir Crit Care Med* 1995; 151:A489.
17. Toye FJ, Weinstein JD: Clinical experience with percutaneous tracheostomy and cricothyroidotomy in 100 patients. *J Trauma* 1986; 26:1034–1040.
18. Schachner A, et al: Rapid percutaneous tracheostomy. *Chest* 1990; 98:1266–1270.
19. Schachner A, et al: Percutaneous tracheostomy: A new method. *Crit Care Med* 1989; 17:1052–1056.
20. Marx WH, et al: Some important details in the technique of percutaneous dilatational tracheostomy via the modified Seldinger technique. *Chest* 1996; 110:762–766.
21. Marelli D, et al: Endoscopic guided percutaneous tracheostomy: Early results of a consecutive trial. *J Trauma* 1990; 30:433–435.
22. Fernandez L, et al: Beside percutaneous tracheostomy with bronchoscopic guidance in critically ill patients. *Arch Surg* 1996; 131:129–132.
23. Barba CA, et al: Bronchoscopic guidance makes percutaneous tracheostomy a safe, cost-effective, and easy-to-teach procedure. *Surgery* 1995; 118:879–883.
24. Griggs WM, et al: A prospective comparison of a percutaneous tracheostomy technique with standard surgical tracheostomy. *Intensive Care Med* 1991; 17:261–263.
25. Ivatury R, et al: Percutaneous tracheostomy after trauma and critical illness. *J Trauma* 1992; 32:133–140.
26. Manara AR: Experience with percutaneous tracheostomy in intensive care: The technique of choice? *Br J Oral Maxillofac Surg* 1994; 32:155–160.
27. Friedman Y, et al: Comparison of percutaneous and surgical tracheostomies. *Chest* 1996; 110:480–485.
28. Winkler WB, et al: Bedside percutaneous dilational tracheostomy with endoscopic guidance: Experience with 71 ICU patients. *Intensive Care Med* 1994; 20:476–479.
29. Noden JB, Kirkpatrick T: Intrapleural percutaneous tracheostomy. *Anaesthesia* 1995; 50:91 (letter).
30. Rigg CD, Edmondson L: Percutaneous dilational tracheostomy. Malposition leading to delayed weaning. *Anaesthesia* 1995; 50:724–725.
31. Reilly PM, et al: Occult hypercarbia. An unrecognized phenomenon during percutaneous endoscopic tracheostomy. *Chest* 1995; 107:1760–1763.
32. Sun KO: Fracture and dislodgement of tracheal cartilage during percutaneous tracheostomy. *Anaesthesia* 1995; 50:370 (letter).
33. Whittet HB, et al: Skin tethering after dilatational percutaneous tracheostomy. *Anesthesia* 1995; 50:892–894.
34. Bernard SA, et al: Percutaneous dilatational tracheostomy complicated by delayed life-threatening haemorrhage. *Aust N Z J Surg* 1992; 62:152–153.
35. van Heurn LW, et al: Pathologic changes of the trachea after percutaneous dilatational tracheotomy. *Chest* 1996; 109:1466–1469.
36. Fischler MP, et al: Late outcome of percutaneous dilatational tracheostomy in intensive care patients. *Intensive Care Med* 1995; 21:475–481.
37. Hazard P, et al: Comparative clinical trial of standard operative tracheostomy with percutaneous tracheostomy. *Crit Care Med* 1991; 19:1018–1024.
38. Crofts SL, et al: A comparison of percutaneous and operative tracheostomies in intensive care patients. *Can J Anaesth* 1995; 42:775–779.
39. Imami ER, et al: Percutaneous dilational tracheostomy: Risks and benefits of bronchoscopy. A prospective randomized study. *Crit Care Med* 1994; 22:A67.
40. Cobean R, et al: Percutaneous dilatational tracheostomy: A safe, cost-effective bedside procedure. *Arch Surg* 1996; 131:265–271.
41. Toursarkissian B, et al: Percutaneous dilational tracheostomy in children and teenagers. *J Pediatr Surg* 1994; 29:1421–1424.

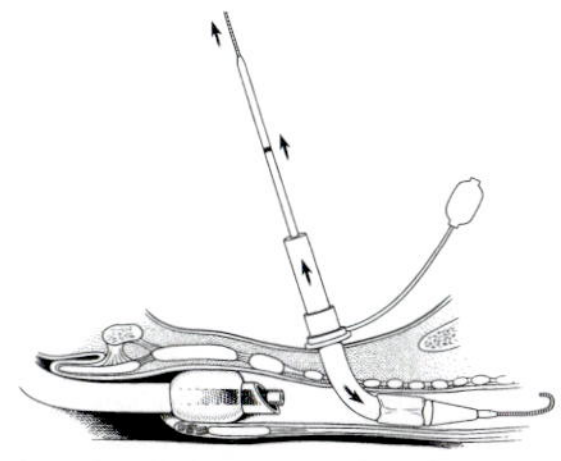

ANESTHESIA FOR ENDOSCOPIC PROCEDURES OF THE AIRWAY

Michael H. Entrup

The management of patients undergoing endoscopic procedures of the airway is a team effort, requiring a high degree of communication and cooperation among the endoscopist and members of the anesthesia care team, nursing staff, and ancillary personnel. There are few surgical procedures in which the operative approach has as great an influence on the anesthetic management of the patient, while at the same time the anesthetic management has as direct an impact on the ability of the surgeon to perform a successful operation. Operative procedures involving the airway dictate that the airway be shared by the endoscopist and the anesthesiologist. The role of the anesthesiologist in the intraoperative management of patients undergoing airway procedures cannot be overstated. The preoperative evaluation and preparation as well as the immediate postoperative care of these patients are also vital elements in ensuring a smooth perioperative course and minimizing perioperative morbidity and mortality.

Preoperative Evaluation and Preparation

The preoperative anesthetic assessment familiarizes the anesthesiologist with the pathophysiology of the patient's airway disease, as well as any coexisting disease states as they relate to anesthetic management. Information is obtained during the preoperative visit and interview by a careful history and focused physical examination, in addition to interpretation of laboratory and diagnostic data. It is during the preoperative interview that the anesthesiologist has the opportunity to discuss anesthetic options with the patient, formulate an anesthetic plan, obtain informed consent, and establish a patient-physician relationship. If a "Do Not Resuscitate" (DNR) order is in place, this directive should be reassessed before surgery.[1,2] During the preoperative interview, the anesthesiologist can allay the patient's anxiety concerning the upcoming surgical procedure. The interview has been shown to have a demonstrable calming effect on patients before operation.[3,4]

The anesthetic review of systems and physical examination focuses on the degree of cardiorespiratory compromise and reserve, and assesses the ease of controlled ventilation, laryngoscopy, and intubation. Evidence of vertebrobasilar insufficiency, gastroesophageal reflux, coagulation abnormalities, and neurologic or musculoskeletal dysfunction is also investigated. Patients with small cell carcinoma of the lung may have an associated Lambert-Eaton myasthenic syndrome.[5] Social history, use of medications, adverse reactions to medications, and anesthetic/surgical history are reviewed. Obtaining a family history of difficulties during administration of anesthetics may be important in the diagnosis and management of patients with disorders such as malignant hyperthermia, plasma cholinesterase deficiency, or porphyrias. Previous anesthetic records should be reviewed with particular attention to difficulties with laryngoscopy and intubation and adverse or prolonged effects of drugs and anesthetic agents.

The need for laboratory and diagnostic studies should be individualized and is determined by the age of the patient, the pathophysiology of the lesion, and the identification and severity of coexisting diseases. A baseline arterial blood gas analysis is helpful in guiding both intraoperative and postoperative respiratory management.[6] Tracheal tomography, spirometric flow-volume loops, magnetic resonance imaging, and computed tomography may further characterize the location, extent, dynamics, and severity of the obstructing lesion. The findings during recent direct visualization of the airway (i.e., flexible bronchoscopy) are of great importance to the anesthesiologist in formulating the anesthetic approach.

The anesthetic approach to the patient undergoing endoscopic procedures of the airway is determined by the anatomic location of the obstructing lesion, the severity of airway compromise, and the planned interventional approach. The impact of coexisting diseases on anesthetic management and the anesthesiologist's assessment regarding ease of laryngoscopy and intubation are important factors in determining the method of induction of anesthesia, maintenance of anesthesia, control of ventilation and oxygenation, and the need for postoperative ventilatory support.[7] The impact of disease on the general well-being of the patient is categorized using the American Society of Anesthesiologists classification of physical status (Table 21-1).[8]

A close correlation exists between the physical status classification and operative and anesthetic mortality.[9–11] A thorough discussion regarding the preoperative risk assessment and the proposed anesthetic and endoscopic techniques should take place between the endoscopist and the anesthesiologist before induction of anesthesia.

Although it is preferable to optimize the condition of the patient before induction of anesthesia and surgery, this is not always possible. Patients may have life-threatening obstructing airway lesions that warrant immediate intervention. Thus, many times the anesthesiologist is faced with the task of anesthetizing a patient with severe airway compromise when time does not permit adequate assessment or optimization of other medical conditions. A high degree of communication and cooperation between the anesthesiologist and the endoscopist are essential.

Anesthetic Management

The intraoperative anesthetic management of patients undergoing endoscopic procedures of the airway is one of the most challenging operations facing the anesthesiologist. Malignancies are the most frequent lesion, and many times the procedures are palliative and not curative.[12–15] The profile of the patient who is being operated on is typically an elderly patient with a compromised airway and marginal respiratory reserve. The patient frequently has a history of tobacco use and varying degrees of hypoxemia, infection, reactive airway disease, and chronic obstructive pulmonary disease. Many patients have concomitant cardiovascular disease.

The anesthesiologist may be called on to provide anesthesia services for diagnostic and therapeutic procedures, including laser bronchoscopy, brachytherapy, cryotherapy, balloon dilation, or placement of tracheal or bronchial stents. No standard approach to the anesthetic management of these patients exists. Each aspect of anesthetic management (Table 21-2) must be individualized to meet the needs of the patient and the operating team. There are a variety of ways to manage each aspect of the anesthetic care of these patients. The approach must be flexible enough to be modified

Table 21-1
AMERICAN SOCIETY OF ANESTHESIOLOGISTS CLASSIFICATION OF PHYSICAL STATUS

Class	*Description*
Class I	A normal healthy patient
Class II	A patient with mild systemic disease
Class III	A patient with severe systemic disease that limits activity but is not incapacitating
Class IV	A patient with an incapacitating systemic disease that is a constant threat to life
Class V	A moribund patient not expected to survive 24 h with or without operation
E	In the event of an emergency operation, precede the number with an "E"

Table 21-2
ANESTHETIC MANAGEMENT OF PATIENTS UNDERGOING ENDOSCOPIC SURGERY OF THE AIRWAY

Preoperative evaluation and preparation	Methods of ventilation
Preoperative medication	Management of complications
Preparation of the operating/bronchoscopy suite	Postanesthetic care
Monitoring of the patient	
Anesthesia	
Induction	
Maintenance	
Emergence	

Table 21-3
COMPLICATIONS ASSOCIATED WITH ENDOSCOPIC LASER SURGERY OF THE AIRWAY[6,12,13,16–33]

Hypoxemia	Esophageal fistula
Hypoventilation	Fire and burns
Hypertension	Bronchospasm
Tachycardia	Laryngospasm
Hypotension	Smoke-induced pneumonitis
Myocardial ischemia	Local anesthetic toxicity
Dysrhythmias	Patient awareness and recall
Hemorrhage	Gas embolization
Pneumothorax	Death
Pneumomediastinum	

throughout the course of the operation in response to the clinical setting. Communication among members of the operative team is essential.

The goals of anesthetic management are to provide optimal operating conditions for the endoscopist while minimizing the risk of complications associated with anesthesia, operative laryngoscopy and bronchoscopy, and the use of the laser (Table 21-3). These complications may not present during the course of the procedure but may only be recognized during the postoperative period.

Although the duration of these procedures is relatively short, lasting 45 to 60 min, the procedures nonetheless present a major challenge to the anesthesiologist who must anesthetize a potentially critically ill patient with coexisting disease states that may not be adequately assessed or treated. In addition, the airway must be shared between the anesthesiologist and the endoscopist. Although modern anesthetic techniques and methods of ventilation permit the safe conduct of these procedures, there must continue to be a high level of vigilance and coordination among all members of the operating team.

The anesthesiologist must provide the endoscopist with a motionless operative field to perform an adequate resection. He or she must be prepared to recognize and treat life-threatening complications should they occur. The anesthetic care must be conducted in a manner that depresses airway reflexes, minimizes the stress response caused by bronchoscopy or operative laryngoscopy while maintaining hemodynamic stability, optimizes oxygenation and ventilation of the patient, and reduces the risk to the patient and operating room personnel, especially during the use of the laser.

The properties of the laser provide the endoscopist with a powerful, precise tool that permits resection of airway lesions with controlled hemostasis, less trauma to healthy tissue and less edema, and reduced postoperative pain experienced by the patient. The use of the laser also brings to the operation a number of safety concerns (Table 21-4). These safety issues affect the operating team and operating room personnel, as well as the patient. It is imperative for the endoscopist to have proper training and be experienced in the use of the specific laser wavelength in use and in laser safety principles. Health-care facilities that incorporate the use of lasers should implement a formal laser safety program overseen by a laser safety committee. The laser safety committee credentials physicians for the use of specific laser wavelengths. This committee is also responsible for institutional safety standards, the education of personnel associated with the use of the laser, and the monitoring of maintenance of laser ma-

Table 21-4
HAZARDS ASSOCIATED WITH USE OF LASERS

Direct effect of laser beam energy	Hazards of laser usage
Damage to tissues	Atmospheric contamination by laser plume[34–40]
Perforation	Gas embolism[18,19,33]
Eye injuries[34,35]	Electrocution[41]
Burns	
Fires	

chines at proper intervals.[42] An anesthesiologist should be a standing member of this committee, especially at facilities where laser procedures are performed with patients under general anesthesia.

The principles of safe laser resection of airway diseases have been described elsewhere in this text and in the literature.[15,21,43–45] Ossoff[46] compared the incidence of laser-related complications in a group of otolaryngologists who participated in a hands-on laser surgery course with another selected group of otolaryngologists, surveyed by Fried,[47] who were members of a senior otolaryngology society. The hands-on course stressed safety precautions in the use of the laser. The rate of laser-related complications was reduced in the group attending the course.

The safety and success of operations involving laser application of the airway are dependent on all services involved in the perioperative care of the patient. The anesthesiologist and operating room personnel should also be knowledgeable regarding laser safety and the management of complications associated with the use of the laser. This point cannot be overemphasized, especially when the procedure involves the use of an endotracheal tube. This application will be discussed later in this chapter.

Anesthetic drugs, both intravenous and gaseous, are potent cardiorespiratory depressants. At the conclusion of these procedures, rapid recovery from anesthesia is desired so that depressant effects are minimized and the patient is breathing spontaneously with adequate respiratory exchange and intact upper airway reflexes. The anesthesiologist now has available a number of potent, receptor-specific, short-acting anesthetic agents and neuromuscular blocking agents that permit this goal to be accomplished.

ANESTHETIC PREMEDICATION AND NPO STATUS

The administration of premedications to the patient before operation serves a number of functions (Table 21-5). Several classes of drugs are available to achieve these effects. The use, dosage, and timing of anesthetic premedications depend on the age and condition of the patient, the desired effect, and the planned operation and anesthetic technique. In addition to anesthetic premedications, patients should continue to take all cardiovascular and bronchodilatory medications until the time of surgery.

Patients with minor degrees of airway compromise often have their operation performed on an ambulatory basis. Premedication may be administered intravenously just before entering the operating room. The use of preoperative medications in patients with severe airway compromise or limited respiratory reserve should be approached with caution. It is probably more prudent to withhold premedications with cardiorespiratory depressant effects in these patients while on the ward or in the intensive care unit. These drugs may be administered intravenously as needed in the preoperative holding area or in the operating room or bronchoscopy suite where the patient can be monitored continuously and medicated while under the supervision of a physician.

Table 21-5
GOALS OF PREOPERATIVE MEDICATION

Anxiolysis	Facilitation of induction of anesthesia
Amnesia	Reduction in anesthetic requirement
Analgesia	Attenuation of autonomic reflexes
Sedation	Allergy prophylaxis
Antisialogogue	
Aspiration prophylaxis	
Antiemesis	
Preemptive analgesia	

The major reasons for premedication in patients undergoing endoscopic procedures of the airway are to reduce anxiety and airway secretions. Patients undergoing operative procedures for malignancy frequently have increased levels of anxiety. The barbiturates were commonly used to reduce preoperative anxiety; however, the effect was more of sedation and not anxiolysis. The benzodiazepines are currently the most frequently employed drugs used in the preoperative period for pharmacologic reduction of anxiety in patients. Midazolam is an ideal drug in the setting of airway interventions. It has a short elimination half-life and is a potent amnestic agent. Antegrade amnesia is an effect of midazolam that is particularly attractive during procedures in which the anesthetic technique does not employ the use of volatile anesthetic gases or where the patient's condition warrants lighter levels of anesthesia. The incidence of operative awareness and recall has been reported to range from 4 to 32 percent during bronchoscopy.[29–31,48] Duckett and coworkers[48] reported 3 of 12 patients with recall of operative events while receiving total intravenous anesthesia with infusion or an intermittent bolus of alfentanil and propofol during laser bronchoscopy with a rigid bronchoscope and Sanders jet ventilation. Until a reliable monitor of depth of anesthesia is in routine clinical use,[49,50] operating room noise pollution should be kept to a minimum, and conversations around the "asleep" patient should be limited and focused on the care of that patient.

Midazolam also raises the seizure threshold and may protect against seizures associated with local anesthetic toxicity. The dose of midazolam should be reduced in elderly patients since they exhibit an increased sensitivity to the drug.[51,52] The elimination half-life of midazolam is prolonged in the elderly.[53]

The preoperative requirement for analgesic medications used to treat acute pain is not common in patients scheduled for endoscopic airway interventions. The sedative and respiratory and cardiovascular depressant effects of the sedative/hypnotic and narcotic analgesic classes of drugs may be additive or synergistic when used in combination. Should the patient require analgesics in the preoperative period, these should be administered under close monitoring. An alternative is to administer nonopioid analgesic drugs, such as nonsteroidal anti-inflammatory agents.

The use of anticholinergic agents is useful in reducing airway secretions. Historically, these drugs were routinely used to reduce respiratory tract secretions and prevent bradycardia and vagally mediated reflexes associated with anesthesia and surgery. The anesthetics in use today are less likely to cause these undesirable effects. The anticholinergic drugs are still frequently used intraoperatively to antagonize the muscarinic effects of anticholinesterase drugs used to reverse the effects of nondepolarizing neuromuscular blocking drugs.

In addition to an antisialogogue effect, the anticholinergic drugs relax bronchial smooth muscle and increase respiratory dead space.[54,55] The magnitude of this effect depends on preexisting bronchomotor tone. Anticholinergic drugs may attenuate the effects of fiberoptic bronchoscopy on pulmonary mechanics.[56,57]

Before the availability of midazolam, scopolamine was frequently used to achieve sedation and amnesia. The benzodiazepines appear to be more reliable in preventing operative recall, however, and the anticholinergic drugs may result in postoperative confusion in the elderly.[58,59] Other undesirable effects of the anticholinergics include an increase in heart rate, central cholinergic syndrome, and mydriasis. Glycopyrrolate is a quaternary ammonium compound less likely to cross the blood-brain barrier and, therefore, is less likely to produce central nervous system effects.

In recent years, NPO recommendations have been liberalized for healthy patients before anesthesia for elective surgical procedures. Traditional NPO guidelines were based on early animal studies that showed that a gastric fluid volume greater than 0.4 ml/kg and a pH less than 2.5 were necessary to produce significant aspiration pneumonitis. The traditional preoperative fast does not ensure that these parameters will not be exceeded. The risk of clinically significant pulmonary aspiration is low and is associated with known risk factors, which include emergency surgery, obstetric procedures, increasing American Society of Anesthesiologists physical status, difficulty managing a patient's airway, recent intake of solid foods, gastroesophageal reflux, gastrointestinal obstruction, and the use of narcotics.[60,61]

Recent clinical studies and editorials have challenged the practice of prolonged preoperative fasting and have recommended permitting healthy patients without aspiration risk factors to ingest unlimited clear liquids up to 3 h before induction of anesthesia. These recommendations do not apply to milk, pulp-containing liquids, and solid foods since they significantly increase gastric emptying time.[62–64]

Although no studies have specifically addressed fasting in patients before anesthesia for endoscopic interventions of the airway, these patients should be considered at risk for aspiration and be kept NPO following traditional guidelines. They frequently are American Society of Anesthesiologists physical status III or IV and may experience coughing and gagging during the procedure. Airway management may be difficult in these patients. Anesthetics also depress protective airway reflexes. Aspiration of gastric contents in patients with airway disease may result in disastrous consequences.

MONITORING

The standards of basic anesthesia monitoring have been defined by the American Society of Anesthesiologists.[65] These standards apply to all general anesthetics, regional anesthetics, and monitored anesthesia care whether the anesthetic is administered in the operating room or in nonoperating room anesthetizing locations.[66] The standards require the continual evaluation of oxygenation, ventilation, circulation, and temperature of the patient undergoing anesthesia.

The use of monitoring during anesthesia and surgery contributes to the care and safety of the patient. The anesthesiologist uses both clinical observation and available technology to obtain information regarding patient physiology and the proper functioning of anesthetic equipment. Monitors and alarms do not replace or lessen the level of vigilance required on the part of the anesthesiologist during the conduct of an anesthetic. Monitoring enables early detection of adverse changes not always easily recognizable by clinical observation alone. In addition, anesthesiologists and surgeons apply monitoring to view areas that do not provide easy access or visibility. This pertains especially to endoscopic interventions of the airway where the airway must be shared by the anesthesiologist and the endoscopist. The use of closed circuit television monitor during bronchoscopic procedures under general anesthesia with assisted or controlled ventilation enables the anesthesiologist to observe the operative field and time ventilation appropriately to endoscopic maneuvers, such as the use of the laser or the removal of necrotic tissue. The operative team can also view the success of endoscopic resection or placement of stents, as well as adverse events such as hemorrhage or fire in the airways.

The technology, indications, use, and complications of monitoring during anesthesia and surgery have been described in a number of texts.[67–69] Specific monitors used during anesthesia for endoscopic procedures of the airway deserve special attention (Table 21-6). The challenges presented by the endoscopic procedure may require the adaptation or elimination of monitoring equipment and anesthetic techniques routinely used during nonairway procedures.

The most important function of the pulse oximeter is the early detection of hypoxemia. Clinical signs alone are unreliable in detecting hypoxemia.[70–73] In a multicenter study of 20,802 patients undergoing anesthesia, Moller and coworkers[74,75] found a 19-fold higher incidence of detection of hypoxemia in patients monitored with pulse oximetry. The pulse oximeter has become a standard component of both intraoperative and early postoperative monitoring. Recently, application of the pulse oximeter has occurred in areas outside of the operating room and postanesthesia care unit. Many health-care facilities and organizations have policies making the use of a pulse oximeter mandatory during the administration of conscious sedation. Although the pulse oximeter is a reliable monitor, situations in which it may not accurately reflect arterial hemoglobin oxygen saturation include the injection of intravenous dyes, dyshemoglobins, light interference, low signal-to-noise ratio because of weak pulse or motion artifact, and low Sp_{O_2} values.[76–79]

Table 21-6

MONITORING DURING ANESTHESIA FOR ENDOSCOPIC AIRWAY INTERVENTIONS

Patient Monitoring	*Equipment Monitoring*
Observation of clinical signs	Anesthetic and respiratory gas analyzer
Pulse oximeter	Breathing circuit pressure
Arterial blood pressure	
Electrocardiogram	
Precordial stethoscope	
Respiratory and anesthetic gas analyzer	
Peripheral nerve stimulator	
Closed circuit monitor	
Temperature probe	

Intraoperatively, early detection of hypoxemia can guide the endoscopist and anesthesiologist in decisions regarding oxygen therapy, the appropriate instrument for bronchoscopy, and duration of apneic oxygenation technique. The use of a pulse oximeter can serve as a guide in maintaining the lowest inspired oxygen concentration to decrease the risk of fire in the airway.

Because of the sigmoid shape of the oxyhemoglobin dissociation curve, the pulse oximeter is relatively insensitive to changes in Pa_{O_2} at greater than 60 mmHg (Sp_{O_2}, 90%). It is very sensitive at a lower Pa_{O_2}. Because the magnitude of change in this range is much greater, as the Sp_{O_2} declines below 95% the operating team should prepare to take measures that will increase the Pa_{O_2}.

Cardiovascular monitoring, including continuous or continual arterial blood pressure and electrocardiography, is important because of the many adverse cardiovascular effects associated with anesthesia and bronchoscopy (see Table 21-3). The use of automated oscillotonometric blood pressure devices or radial artery catheterization can free up the anesthesiologist's hands to perform other services, such as manual ventilation and record keeping. An indwelling arterial catheter is also useful for blood gas analysis and can provide information regarding intravascular volume status and the effect of ventilation or dysrhythmias on perfusion pressure. A multiple-lead electrocardiograph with ST-analysis is more sensitive than single-lead systems at detecting myocardial ischemia.[80]

Other useful monitors include the precordial stethoscope and the peripheral nerve stimulator. In addition to clinical observation of chest excursion, adequacy of ventilation can be assessed with a precordial stethoscope and quantitated with capnography. Capnography is most easily achieved while using a closed or semi-closed system, such as an endotracheal tube attached to an anesthesia circuit. Using an open technique, such as the operating bronchoscope, requires adapting the monitor to permit gas sampling. A narrow metal tube may be placed down the barrel or alongside the bronchoscope. This technique may be cumbersome when a laser filament and suction catheter are also placed through the bronchoscope. The precordial stethoscope permits auscultation of ventilation distal to airway disease. For endobronchial lesions, when placed over the contralateral lung field, the stethoscope provides information regarding the adequacy of ventilation of that lung should it become necessary to advance the bronchoscope distally down the involved bronchus.

The peripheral nerve stimulator monitors the depth of neuromuscular blockade and serves as a guide for the anesthesiologist in the dosing, timing, and adequacy of reversal of neuromuscular blocking drugs. The use of the rigid bronchoscope with Venturi jet ventilation frequently requires general anesthesia and muscle relaxation. In a report by Hanowell and colleagues,[81] 10 percent of procedures involving rigid bronchoscopy for resection of tumor required reintubation in the postanesthesia care unit. All patients received neuromuscular blocking drugs and anticholinesterase reversal agents intraoperatively. The decision to extubate was based on clinical assessment by the anesthesiologist and the pulmonologist. Neuromuscular blockade monitoring is especially important in patients with small cell carcinoma of the lung who may have an associated Lambert-Eaton myasthenic syndrome. These patients have increased sensitivity to both the depolarizing and nondepolarizing muscle relaxants. Patients with Lambert-Eaton syndrome respond poorly to anticholinesterase drugs.[82–84]

One of the most potentially disastrous complications associated with the use of lasers during airway procedures is airway fire. This can be caused by ignition of an endotracheal tube or other nonmetallic materials, including the fiberoptic bronchoscope, suction catheters, and the laser filament. To decrease the risk of airway fire, the inspired concentration of oxygen should be maintained as low as possible using the pulse oximeter to guide oxygen therapy. The oxygen analyzer will not only measure the delivered oxygen concentration but will also set off an alarm when a hypoxic gas mixture is being administered to the patient. The oxygen ratio monitors and proportioning systems on modern anesthesia machines maintain fresh gas oxygen concentrations of at least 25% when used with nitrous oxide. Older anesthesia machines lack this safety feature when other gases, such as helium or air, are used.[85] Anesthetic gas monitors are used not only to quantitate the concentration of anesthetic delivered in the respiratory circuit but also to measure the end-tidal anesthetic concentration. This is helpful in assessing the effect of residual inhalation anesthetic during emergence from anesthesia.

Other monitors on the anesthesia machine include breathing circuit pressure monitors. These monitors provide the anesthesiologist with information about the compliance of the respiratory circuit, including pulmonary compliance. These monitors also serve as an alarm when high and low set pressure parameters are exceeded or excessive positive end-expiratory pressure is present during mechanical ventilation.

ANESTHETIC TECHNIQUES

Anesthesia for endoscopic procedures of the airway may be accomplished using a variety of techniques (Table 21-7). The decision regarding the most appropriate technique depends on the location, extent, and severity of the obstructing lesion; the general condition of the patient; and the planned operative approach. Patient preference may also be a contributing factor.

Table 21-7
ANESTHETIC TECHNIQUES FOR ENDOSCOPIC SURGERY OF THE AIRWAY

Local anesthesia with or without conscious sedation	General anesthesia
Topical	Intravenous
Nerve block	Inhalational
Monitored anesthesia care (MAC)	Balanced

Several classes of drugs can be administered to the patient (Table 21-8). The choice of drug depends on the anesthetic technique chosen and the desired drug effect. Drugs with a short duration of action are usually administered to minimize residual cardiorespiratory depressant effects at the conclusion of the procedure. Specific agents are available for the reversal of narcotics, benzodiazepines, and neuromuscular blocking drugs.

The effects of the intravenous anesthetic agents are dose dependent and may range from minimal sedation to general anesthesia.[86] They may be administered as an intermittent bolus or as a continuous infusion. Combinations of drugs may be used. This may require a reduced dose of each drug because there may be additive or synergistic effects on sedation and respiratory or cardiovascular depression.

Diagnostic flexible bronchoscopy and minor therapeutic procedures may be performed under topical anesthesia of the airway. One of the complications of this technique is local anesthetic toxicity. Topical local anesthetics administered to the lower airway are rapidly absorbed and have the potential to produce systemic toxicity.[87–90] This is more likely to occur in the presence of hypoxia, hypercarbia, and acidosis.[91,92] Tetracaine has a low therapeutic index. The maximum safe dose of tetracaine for topical anesthesia in a healthy 70-kg adult is 50 mg.[93] Complications, including death, during fiberoptic bronchoscopy with tetracaine topical anesthesia have been described.[22,23,26]

Topical anesthesia may be supplemented with intravenous sedatives and/or analgesics.[94–96] The American Society of Anesthesiologists has established guidelines for sedation and analgesia by nonanesthesiologists.[97] Patient monitoring should include pulse oximetry and supplemental oxygen, and resuscitative equipment should be immediately available.

During conscious sedation, the patient's level of consciousness is minimally depressed. The patient can respond appropriately to both physical stimulation and verbal command. Protective reflexes remain intact,

Table 21-8
DRUGS USED DURING ANESTHESIA FOR ENDOSCOPIC AIRWAY INTERVENTIONS

Anesthetic Agent	*Class*	*Examples*
Local anesthetics		Cocaine Tetracaine Lidocaine
Intravenous anesthetics	Barbiturates	Thiopental Thiamylal Methohexital
	Nonbarbiturates	Propofol Etomidate
	Benzodiazepines	Diazepam Lorazepam Midazolam
	Narcotics	Morphine Meperidine Fentanyl Sufentanil Alfentanil Remifentanil
Inhalation anesthetics	Nitrous oxide	
	Volatile anesthetics	Halothane Enflurane Isoflurane Desflurane Sevoflurane
Neuromuscular blocking agents	Depolarizing	Succinylcholine
	Nondepolarizing	Mivacurium Atracurium Vecuronium Cisatracurium Rocuronium

and the patient can maintain a patent airway. Procedures using conscious sedation may not be appropriate in the critically ill or uncooperative patient or when the procedure warrants deeper levels of sedation. Under these situations, the procedure may still be performed with topical anesthesia, but the anesthesiologist may be called on to provide specific anesthesia services to the patient, including the monitoring and control of vital signs and the administration of medical therapies and anesthetic agents.

Formerly known as "standby" anesthesia, monitored anesthesia care (MAC) more accurately reflects the involvement of the anesthesiologist in the care of the patient. The American Society of Anesthesiologists has adopted a position on MAC, which makes clear that reduced anesthetic services are not involved during participation in cases involving MAC.[98] The anesthesiologist is held to the same standards of care as in regional anesthesia or general anesthesia, including the performance of a preanesthetic examination and evaluation, participation in the planning and care of the patient, and the standards of basic intraoperative monitoring.

During some procedures involving the use of MAC, no additional anesthetic agents are administered. More often, the anesthesiologist provides the patient with deeper levels of intravenous sedation resulting in a more depressed level of consciousness from which the patient is not easily aroused. This is accompanied by a partial loss of protective reflexes.

General anesthesia results in a state of controlled unconsciousness. The patient does not respond purposefully to physical stimulation and verbal command. There is loss of protective reflexes, including an inability to maintain a patent airway independently. During the procedure, airway patency must be maintained with either an endotracheal tube or the rigid bronchoscope.

METHODS OF VENTILATION

A number of approaches are possible to ventilate and oxygenate the patient undergoing endoscopic procedures of the airway (Table 21-9). The technique employed depends on the anatomic location of the obstructing lesion, the planned operative approach, and the experience of the endoscopist.

Diagnostic evaluation or therapeutic resection of small lesions may be performed with a fiberoptic bronchoscope under topical anesthesia with or without intravenous sedation/analgesia. This method requires a cooperative patient. Glossopharyngeal and superior laryngeal nerve blocks are sometimes necessary to ablate the gag reflex. Monitoring of the patient includes pulse oximetry, and supplemental oxygen should be administered as a preventive measure against the development of hypoxemia.[99,100] In patients who require deeper levels of sedation, an alternative is to insert the fiberoptic bronchoscope through a laryngeal mask airway. With this technique, deeper levels of sedation or general anesthesia, either intravenous or inhalation, may be administered while ventilation is assisted or controlled.[101]

The use of general anesthesia is usually necessary when the procedure is performed through a rigid bronchoscope. Patients with more severe degrees of airway obstruction or limited cardiorespiratory reserve may be unable to tolerate the physiologic effects associated with fiberoptic bronchoscopy performed under topical anesthesia with spontaneous ventilation. These patients usually require general anesthesia with positive pressure ventilation either through an endotracheal tube or the rigid bronchoscope. The use of general anesthesia permits the endoscopist to continue treatment for longer periods of time.[102–104] This method may result in more efficacious resection of tracheobronchial lesions.[102]

Table 21-9

METHODS OF VENTILATING THE PATIENT UNDERGOING LASER SURGERY OF THE AIRWAY

During flexible bronchoscopy	
Spontaneous ventilation	Assisted or controlled ventilation
Bronchoscope alone	Laryngeal mask airway
Laryngeal mask airway	Endotracheal tube
	Apneic oxygenation
During rigid bronchoscopy	
Spontaneous ventilation	Controlled ventilation (*cont.*)
Controlled ventilation	High frequency jet ventilation
Intermittent positive pressure ventilation	Apneic oxygenation
Manual jet ventilation	

The advantages, disadvantages, and indications for fiberoptic bronchoscopy versus rigid bronchoscopy may be found in Chaps. 1, 3, and 5. Laser resection of tracheobronchial lesions using a fiberoptic bronchoscope inserted through an endotracheal tube raises a number of concerns. Lindholm and coworkers[105,106] have shown that a fiberoptic bronchoscope inserted through an endotracheal tube in mechanically ventilated patients occupies a significant percentage of the cross-sectional area of the endotracheal tube. This creates a significant increase in airway resistance and may result in the application of significant amounts of positive end-expiratory pressure (PEEP). A 5.7-mm bronchoscope inserted into variously sized endotracheal tubes (ranging from 7.0 mm internal diameter to 9.5 mm internal diameter) resulted in mean peak tracheal inhalation pressures of 33.7 ± 11.5 cmH_2O (range, 18 to 60 cm H_2O) and mean peak ventilator pressures of 52.8 ± 13.9 cmH_2O (range, 28 to 80 cmH_2O). The same size bronchoscope occupied 66 percent of the cross-sectional area of an endotracheal tube with a 7.0 mm internal diameter and resulted in the application of up to 35 cmH_2O of PEEP. These effects may result in significant cardiovascular effects or barotrauma. The high airway and ventilator pressures may exceed the pressure limits of mechanical ventilators. This, as well as vigorous suctioning during the procedure, may result in significant hypoxemia and hypercarbia. It has been recommended that when patients in the intensive care unit require fiberoptic bronchoscopy, an adequately sized endotracheal tube should be used, mechanical PEEP should be removed from the breathing circuit, patients should be ventilated manually, and suctioning should be intermittent and for brief periods of time.[107] It is this author's opinion that these recommendations be followed for all endoscopic resections of tracheobronchial lesions when a fiberoptic bronchoscope is inserted through an endotracheal tube. In a report by Warner and colleagues,[108] hypoventilation was noted in 30 of 32 mechanically ventilated patients under general anesthesia undergoing Nd-YAG laser bronchoscopy with a flexible bronchoscope inserted into an endotracheal tube.

The use of the laser in the vicinity of an endotracheal tube warrants special attention. Although an endotracheal tube need not be present for an airway fire to occur, the ignition and combustion of an endotracheal tube may worsen the degree of airway injury by release of toxic products of combustion or by a blow torch effect.[109–111] This event may occur when an intraluminal endotracheal tube flame is blown distally by positive pressure ventilation and may result in disastrous consequences, including a fatality. Ignition of an endotracheal tube may be the result of a direct or reflected application of laser energy or may be ignited by other flaming materials.[112] Potentially flammable materials in the airway include suction catheters, fiberoptic laser cables, endobronchial stents, pledgets, necrotic tissue, and the flexible bronchoscope. Whenever a laser or electrocautery is in use, the operating team must always be aware of the possibility of fire, not only within the airway but of any flammable material within the operating room or bronchoscopy suite. The laser may inadvertently be triggered or the energy beam reflected onto other flammable materials remote from the surgical site.

The operating team should be skilled and prepared to manage a fire whenever the laser or electrocautery is in use. The best treatment is prevention. Preventive measures include the elimination of ignitable/flammable materials in the area of the laser, as well as methods that decrease the chance of stray laser energy and reduce the flammability of materials. These include proper maintenance and testing of the laser, the use of nonreflective metal instruments with low specular reflectance, the use of laser contact probes, the proper selection and protection of endotracheal tubes against specific laser wavelengths, and minimizing the inspired oxygen concentration. Most important is adherence to proper laser technique and laser safety principles (see Chap. 5).

Numerous studies and reports with conflicting results attest to the safety of various types of endotracheal tubes exposed to laser energy. These studies have focused on the ignitability or flammability of endotracheal tubes under varying conditions, including different laser wavelengths, power density and mode of use, oxygen index of flammability, effect of protective wraps, effect of inhaled gases, and the products of combustion.[46,113–142] These conflicting results leave the clinician with the question of which is the best endotracheal tube to use during airway surgery involving the laser. This decision is especially important during microlaryngeal procedures when the CO_2 laser is often used in close proximity to the endotracheal tube. One should assume that any endotracheal tube, with the possible exception of a metal endotracheal tube, is flammable.

The major controversy facing the pulmonologist is the decision between fiberoptic bronchoscopy though an endotracheal tube and rigid bronchoscopy for laser resection of tracheobronchial lesions. The tip of the fiberoptic bronchoscope and laser filament are usually distal to the endotracheal tube. The Nd:YAG is the most commonly used laser because it can readily be transmitted by fiberoptic bundles. A polyvinyl chloride (PVC) endotracheal tube without markings has been shown to be the most resistant endotracheal tube to the damaging effects of the Nd:YAG laser.[114,116,125] This margin of safety may be eliminated when the PVC tube becomes soiled with blood or mucus.[122] Although a stainless steel endotracheal tube may offer more resistance to the Nd:YAG laser, the current sizes available do not have an internal diameter large enough to permit adequate ventilation after passage of a flexible bronchoscope.

Protective wraps around endotracheal tubes protect the shaft of the tube proximal to the cuff. Because the laser filament is delivered within the endotracheal tube or distal to it, a laser-resistant outer wrap offers no protection. The cuff and distal end of the endotracheal tube are left unprotected. The filling of the cuff with saline solution or methylene blue dye may act as a heat sink and may be an early indicator of cuff perforation.[131,132] In addition, the fluid may extinguish a small fire if the cuff is also perforated.

To further decrease the risk of fire, the delivered oxygen concentration should be lowered and maintained at a F_{IO_2} less than 0.3. Pulse oximetry is useful in guiding oxygen therapy. Should a higher F_{IO_2} become necessary, laser resection may be interrupted temporarily while the patient is ventilated with a higher inspired oxygen concentration. After the hemoglobin saturation rises, the F_{IO_2} may once again be lowered, and laser resection may proceed. Nitrous oxide is an oxidizing agent that can support ignition and combustion just as well as a high F_{IO_2}. The delivered oxygen concentration should therefore be diluted with air, nitrogen, or helium.[46,117,118,136] In addition to its high thermal conductivity, helium possesses a lower density that may facilitate gas flow beyond obstructing lesions.[143]

If a fire occurs within the airway, immediate steps should be undertaken to extinguish the flame and prevent further damage to the patient or operating room personnel (Table 21-10). These actions may minimize the morbidity associated with an airway fire. A fire within the airway should be treated with the same urgency as one would approach a cardiac arrest. Many of these steps should be undertaken simultaneously. Most important, the flow of oxygen-enriched gas should be interrupted immediately as the endotracheal tube and flexible bronchoscope are being removed and the fire is being extinguished. Both upper and lower airways should be examined by laryngoscopy and flexible and rigid bronchoscopy. All carbonaceous material should be removed from the airway. The decision to use steroids, antibiotics, or mechanical ventilation should be based on the degree of injury and the condition of the patient. These patients should be moni-

Table 21-10
TREATMENT OF AIRWAY FIRE DURING LASER SURGERY OF THE AIRWAY

Immediately stop ventilation and disconnect the endotracheal tube from the breathing circuit
Remove endotracheal tube and fiberoptic bronchoscope and extinguish all burning materials
Resume ventilation by mask or reintubate the patient
Examine the airway carefully, evaluate the extent of injury, and remove carbonaceous debris
Reintubation, mechanical ventilation, tracheostomy, steroids, antibiotics as needed
Close monitoring (including pulse oximetry, arterial blood gas analysis, and serial chest roentgenograms) in an intensive care setting
Supplemental oxygen with high humidity to prevent mucus plugging

tored closely in an intensive care setting. They may require serial bronchoscopic evaluation and removal of mucus plugs and necrotic tissue. An excellent article by Schramm and coworkers[111] reviewed the pathophysiology and management of laser-ignited endotracheal tube fires.

The use of the rigid bronchoscope eliminates the risk of an endotracheal tube fire. A number of approaches are available to ventilate the patient undergoing rigid bronchoscopy. The anesthesia breathing circuit may be attached directly to the side port of the ventilating bronchoscope. With the proximal end of the bronchoscope occluded, positive pressure ventilation is possible. General inhalation anesthesia may be administered, and end-tidal CO_2 may be monitored. Removal of the eyepiece or telescoping lens results in an open system. Periods of hyperventilation with a high inspired oxygen concentration should alternate with periods of apnea made necessary by the opening of the system for instrumentation by the endoscopist.

In 1967, Sanders[144] introduced a ventilating attachment for the bronchoscope. A 16-gauge cannula was attached to the proximal end of the bronchoscope. Oxygen from a high pressure (50 psi) source was intermittently jetted through the cannula. The Venturi principle, based on Bernoulli's law, created entrainment of surrounding gas and increased total gas flow. Carden and colleagues[145] modified the Sanders' system by attaching the jetting device to the side arm of the bronchoscope. With the Sanders' system, a maximal pressure of 22 cmH_2O could be generated at the distal end of the bronchoscope when a pressure source of 50 psi was used. The total flow of gases was 64 liters/min, entrained air accounting for 36 liters/min. This created a negative pressure of 16 cmH_2O at the proximal end of the bronchoscope. The Carden modification created a distal pressure up to 55 cmH_2O with only 30 psi of oxygen pressure. Entrained room air accounted for only 3 liters/min of the 106 liters/min gas flow.[145,146] This modification significantly increases the delivered oxygen concentration at the distal end of the bronchoscope and permits more efficient ventilation of patients with decreased lung compliance.[147]

Manual jet ventilation is an effective method of ventilating and oxygenating the patient undergoing bronchoscopy while enabling the endoscopist to work uninterrupted for prolonged periods of time.[147–149] Because it is an open system, anesthetic drugs must be administered by the intravenous route. Giesecke and coworkers[148] compared mechanical side arm ventilation with jet injection. The jet ventilation group had significantly lower Pa_{CO_2} values during bronchoscopy.

High frequency jet ventilation is an alternative method of ventilation, particularly in patients with tracheoesophageal or bronchopleural fistulas. This method may be applied to either rigid or flexible bronchoscopy.[150–154] Vourc'h and colleagues[154] demonstrated that manual jet ventilation was more effective than high frequency jet ventilation in ventilating patients with bronchial stenosis.

HOW I DO IT

After the anesthetic preoperative evaluation has been completed, a thorough discussion regarding the proposed operative and anesthetic approach takes place between the endoscopist and the anesthesiologist. The anesthetic options and plan are discussed with the patient, and informed consent is obtained. While the patient is in the anesthetic holding area, a large-bore intravenous catheter is inserted, and the patient is medicated with glycopyrrolate, 0.1 to 0.2 mg intravenously. Intravenous midazolam, 0.5 to 2.0 mg, is titrated to the desired effect. Midazolam is a rapid-onset benzodiazepine with a relatively short duration of action.[155] These features are desirable in the selection of anesthetic medications for these relatively short yet physiologically stressful procedures. An attractive property of midazolam is its ability to produce amnesia.[156–158] This effect is less reliably produced by other short-acting intravenous anesthetic medications, including propofol. At the Lahey Clinic, the majority of these procedures are performed through the rigid bronchoscope with controlled ventilation and the patient under general anesthesia. The use of the ventilating/operating bronchoscope precludes the use of inhalation anesthetics. Although these agents have potent amnestic effects, their use is avoided since effective scavenging of waste anesthetic gases is difficult while using an open ventilating system. Thus, the use of total intravenous anesthesia during these procedures may make operative awareness and recall more likely to occur.[159] This is of special concern in patients whose cardiovascular status does not permit deeper levels of anesthesia. The use of midazolam may lessen the likelihood of operative awareness and recall. At the same time, midazolam's relatively short duration of action will minimize the residual effects commonly seen with other intravenous induction agents or longer acting benzodiazepines.

In patients who do not exhibit severe airway compromise or limited cardiorespiratory reserve, the addition of a short-acting narcotic, such as intravenous fentanyl, 25 to 50 μg, may have additive sedative effects and may facilitate the induction of general anesthesia. The opioids also possess antitussive effects.

Patients with severe airway compromise or marginal cardiorespiratory reserve who cannot be monitored adequately are usually medicated with glycopyrrolate alone. In these patients, anesthetic medications are administered intravenously in the operating room just before the induction of anesthesia or during the course of the anesthetic.

Before the patient enters the operating room or bronchoscopy suite, all anesthetic and surgical monitors and equipment should be calibrated and inspected for proper function. The equipment necessary for the conduct of the procedure should be present in the room. The endoscopist should be in attendance before the induction of anesthesia in the event the patient's airway becomes more unstable during induction. Should this occur, immediate endoscopic or surgical intervention may be required.

The administration of 100% oxygen by means of a nonrebreathing circuit before induction will delay the occurrence of hypoxemia during periods of apnea or airway obstruction, which may follow the induction of anesthesia. This denitrogenation of the functional residual capacity of the patient and the subsequent increase in arterial oxygen content may be accomplished by having the patient breathe 100% oxygen at normal tidal volumes for 3 to 5 min.[160–163] This step usually occurs during the placement of monitors before the induction of anesthesia. This technique, as well as the inhalation of 100% oxygen during four vital capacity breaths, has been shown to be effective in increasing arterial hemoglobin oxygen saturation and Pa_{O2} in healthy awake patients, with the former technique providing a greater margin of safety against arterial desaturation.[161–163] Denitrogenation may take longer to achieve in patients with airway obstruction, and the margin of safety for the development of hypoxemia may be less for patients with severe V/Q mismatching. After anesthetic induction and adequate control of the airway are achieved, the concentration of inspired oxygen may be adjusted with air, nitrogen, or helium to decrease the risk of fire within the airway during the use of the laser or the electrocautery.

General anesthesia is usually induced with intravenous propofol and a short-acting narcotic, such as fentanyl. Propofol is a di-isopropyl phenol compound with a rapid onset of effect. It possesses a clearance rate more rapid than either sodium pentothal or methohexital and therefore produces a more rapid recovery.[164,165] Because of its rapid clearance, accumulation of drug is less likely to occur. Propofol may be administered either by intermittent bolus or continuous infusion. When used as the sole agent for maintenance of anesthesia, it must be administered at a higher infusion rate.[166] Because propofol does not possess analgesic properties, the addition of a narcotic medication will facilitate the induction of anesthesia and blunt the cardiovascular effects associated with laryngoscopy, intubation, and surgical stress.[27] A number of short-acting narcotics are available to the anesthesiologist for the conduct of these procedures. Although fentanyl and alfentanil have been used in the majority of laser bronchoscopies, the recent introduction of the ultrashort-acting narcotic, remifentanil, may make it the ideal drug for these operations, where rapid recovery and minimization of residual respiratory depressant effect are desired and postoperative pain is not significant. Unlike fentanyl and alfentanil, whose elimination is dependent on metabolic inactivation by the liver, remifentanil is inactivated by blood and tissue esterases and has a greater clearance and shorter elimination half-life.[167–172]

When the ability to control ventilation is in question, as in patients with severe upper airway obstruction, the maintenance of spontaneous respiration is desirable. Control of the airway in these patients should be obtained under local anesthesia with or without intravenous sedation/analgesia. The airway should be secured by either tracheostomy or with placement of a stainless steel ventilation cannula beyond the obstructing lesion. The latter technique has been described by Mehta and coworkers.[173,174] Alternatively, general anesthesia may be induced by mask with the patient breathing spontaneously. The volatile anesthetic agents permit induction and maintenance of anesthesia while maintaining spontaneous ventilation with high concentrations of oxygen. The inhalation agents are potent bronchodilators.[175] They sensitize the myocardium to both endogenous and exogenous catecholamines.[176] Traditionally, halothane has been chosen over isoflurane and enflurane for induction by mask because it is less pungent and less irritating to the airway. Two newer inhalation agents, sevoflurane and desflurane, possess properties that result in more rapid induction and recovery compared with halothane, isoflurane, and enflurane. These agents have many similar respiratory and cardiovascular effects. Desflurane is more pungent, resulting in coughing, breath holding, and larygospasm. Sevoflurane has replaced halothane for induction of anesthesia in many practices. Sevoflurane, a fluorinated methyl ethyl ether, was withdrawn from clinical investigation in 1980 because its metabolism resulted in high plasma fluoride concentrations. Clinical reports of transient renal dysfunction after prolonged use of sevoflurane have prompted recommendations that it not be used in patients with renal impairment. Additional information should be forthcoming on this agent as well as on the toxic effects of Compound A, a product of the breakdown of sevoflurane by commonly used CO_2 absorbents.[177]

After the induction of general anesthesia either by the intravenous or inhalation route, anesthesia is maintained by a balanced intravenous technique using combinations of intermittent boluses or continuous infusions of propofol, midazolam, and remifentanil. Some centers perform these procedures with the patient spontaneously breathing under general anesthesia. In our experience, the technique of spontaneous or assisted ventilation during rigid bronchoscopy makes it difficult to maintain the deeper levels of anesthesia required to supply the endoscopist with a motionless operative field without imposing significant respiratory and cardiovascular side effects of the anesthetic agents. We, therefore, administer neuromuscular blocking drugs and control ventilation by manual jet ventilation. Neuromuscular blocking drugs facilitate intubation, create a motionless field for the endoscopist, and improve chest wall compliance. A number of neuromuscular blocking drugs are now available that are associated with an intermediate duration of action, fewer cardiac effects, and less histamine release. As with any of the newer anesthetic agents, cost should be a factor considered when assessing any risk-benefit ratio. The neuromuscular blocking drugs are administered with the guidance of a neuromuscular blockade monitor. Although these monitors may indicate recovery of neuromuscular function, there may still be significant receptor blockade, which may not be tolerated in the patient with limited respiratory reserve. For this reason, we choose to antagonize all nondepolarizing neuromuscular blocking drugs at the conclusion of these procedures.

Before sharing the airway with the endoscopist, local anesthesia is administered, either topically or intravenously. This technique will blunt the hypertensive response associated with laryngoscopy and intubation.[178–180] It may also decrease anesthetic requirements.[181] A water-soluble topical anesthetic should be applied to the oropharynx, tongue, and trachea. Oil-based topical anesthetics are best avoided since they may be ignited by the laser pulse. The patient's eyes are protected with moistened gauze and covered with nonreflective metal foil, and a dental guard is inserted to protect the teeth.

Direct laryngoscopy performed by the anesthesiologist before insertion of the rigid bronchoscope will help assess the adequacy of the depth of anesthesia. In addition, the ability to visualize the glottis before endoscopic manipulation and potential trauma is important should the need for endotracheal intubation arise later. The patient is manually hyperventilated by mask, and the airway is shared with the endoscopist.

The trachea is intubated with the rigid bronchoscope, and the injector system is attached (Fig. 21-1). Venturi jet ventilation is performed manually at a rate of 10 to 20 breaths per minute. Adequate ventilation is assessed by clinical signs of chest excursion and auscultation. More proximal lesions may require the use of a ventilating tracheoscope if the ventilating slots of the bronchoscope lie above the glottis. Delivered oxygen concentration is adjusted with a gas blender. The Venturi technique entrains room air, thus lowering the concentration of oxygen delivered by the injector needle. If the clinical situation warrants a high $F_{I_{O_2}}$, the gas blender may be adjusted to oxygen alone. Additionally, the anesthesia circuit with oxygen may be attached to the side arm of the Venturi bronchoscope so that oxygen gas is entrained during Venturi ventilation.

Visualization of the operative field by means of closed circuit monitor and close communication with the endoscopist are critical in ensuring the appropriate timing of ventilation. Brief periods of apnea are usually well tolerated and should be followed by periods of moderate hyperventilation to avoid severe hypercarbia.[182,183] Lacking a routine, inexpensive monitoring technique reflecting Pa_{CO_2} during ventilation by means of an open system, changes in pulse oximetry are used to guide the duration of apnea. As the Sp_{O_2} declines to 90%, the operating team should be prepared to administer positive pressure ventilation until the hemoglobin oxygen saturation improves.

Figure 21-1

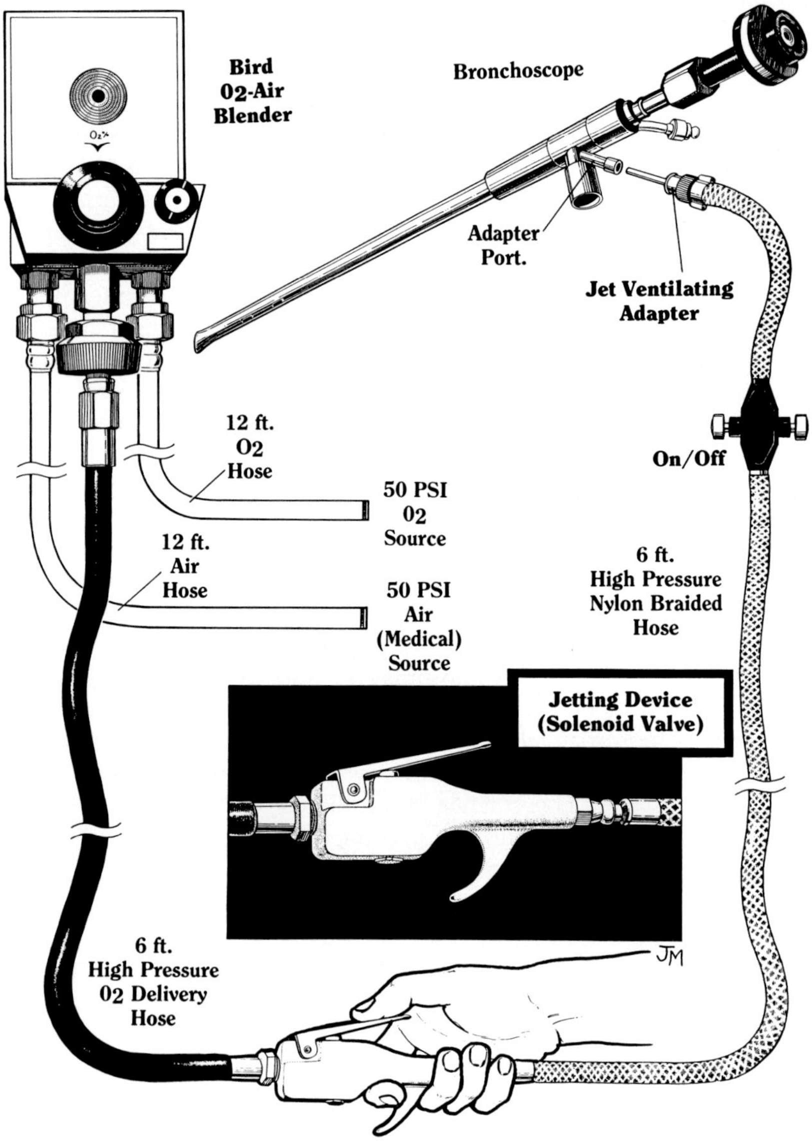

Jet ventilation system. Oxygen and air from a wall source at 50 psi through an oxygen blender where concentration of oxygen is adjusted. Ventilation is controlled manually with the jetting device. Modern jetting devices incorporate an adjustable reducing valve (*not shown*) to adjust driving pressures. An ON/OFF control at the distal end permits the endoscopist to interrupt gas flow. The jet ventilating adapter attaches to the side port of the bronchoscope.

During the procedure, episodes of hypertension are treated with deepening of anesthesia. Additionally, short-duration antihypertensive agents may be employed for the treatment of intraoperative hypertension.

At the conclusion of the procedure, the stomach contents are suctioned, and neuromuscular blockade is reversed with anticholinesterase drugs. The anesthetic agents are discontinued, and the patient is permitted to awaken. While awaiting the return of spontaneous breathing, ventilation may be controlled by means of mask, the laryngeal mask airway, or an endotracheal tube. Reintubation of the patient with airway stents is usually guided with flexible bronchoscopy.

The patient is transported to the postanesthesia care unit (PACU) breathing supplemental oxygen, and with electrocardiograph and pulse oximeter monitoring. The head of the bed is elevated during transport. Pulmonary toilet begins in the PACU.

The successful endoscopic resection of obstructing airway lesions is a team effort. It involves one of the most challenging clinical situations encountered by the anesthesiologist. Often, the procedure results in immediate symptomatic improvement for the patient. The airway trauma caused by bronchoscopy along with residual respiratory depressant effects of anesthetic drugs may not be tolerated by the patient in whom attempted resection is unsuccessful. These patients may require a period of postoperative mechanical ventilation.

REFERENCES

1. Lees DE: Preoperative ethical issues—DNR and other end of life issues and assisted suicide. American Society of Anesthesiologists 1994 Annual Refresher Course Lectures.
2. American Society of Anesthesiologists: Ethical guidelines for the anesthesia care of patients with do-not-resuscitate orders or other directives that limit treatment. Approved by the House of Delegates on October 13, 1993.
3. Egbert LD, Battit GE, Turndorf H, Beecher HK: The value of the preoperative visit by an anesthetist: A study of doctor-patient rapport. *JAMA* 1963; 185:553–555.
4. Leigh JM, Walker J, Janaganathan P: Effect of preoperative anesthetic visit on anxiety. *BMJ* 1977; 2:987–989.
5. O'Neill JH, Murray NM, Newsom-Davis J: The Lambert-Eaton myasthenic syndrome. A review of 50 cases. *Brain* 1988; 111:577–596.
6. Schiffman PL, Wilhelm J, Parisi RA: Arterial oxygen saturation during Nd:YAG laser photoresection of endobronchial tumors under local anesthesia: Use of intermittent supplemental oxygen with pulse oximetry guidance. *Chest* 1988; 94:1300–1301.
7. Stoelting RK, Dierdorf SF, McCammon RL: *Anesthesia and Co-Existing Diseases.* New York: Churchill Livingstone; 1988.
8. American Society of Anesthesiologists: New classification of physical status. *Anesthesiology* 1963; 24:111.
9. Dripps RD, Lamont A, Eckenhoff JE: The role of anesthesia in surgical mortality. *JAMA* 1961; 178:261–266.
10. Goldstein A Jr, Keats AS: The risk of anesthesia. *Anesthesiology* 1970; 33:130–143.
11. Vacanti CJ, Van Houten RJ, Hill RC: A statistical analysis of the relationship of physical status to postoperative mortality in 68,388 cases. *Anesth Analg* 1970; 49:564–566.
12. Cavaliere S, Foccoli P, Toninelli C, et al: Nd:YAG laser therapy in lung cancer: An 11 year experience with 2253 applications in 1585 patients. *J Bronchol* 1994; 1:105.
13. Beamis JF Jr, Vergos K, Rebeiz EE, Shapshay SM: Endoscopic laser therapy for obstructing tracheobronchial lesions. *Ann Otol Rhinol Laryngol* 1991; 100:413–419.
14. Dumon JF: *YAG Laser Bronchoscopy.* New York: Praeger; 1985.
15. Ramser ER, Beamis JF Jr: Laser bronchoscopy. *Clin Chest Med* 1995; 16:415–426.
16. Brutinel WM, Cortese DA, Edell ES, McDougall JC, Prakash UB. Complications of Nd:YAG laser therapy (Editorial). *Chest* 1988; 94:902–903.
17. Personne C, Colchen A, Leroy M, Vourc'h G, Toty L: Indications and technique for endoscopic laser resections in bronchology: A critical analysis based upon 2,284 resections. *J Thorac Cardiovasc Surg* 1986; 91:710–715.
18. Peachey T, Eason J, Moxham J, Jarvis D, Driver M: Systemic air embolization during laser bronchoscopy. *Anaesthesia* 1988; 43:872–875.
19. Ross DJ, Mohsenifar Z, Potkin RT, Roston WL, Shapiro SM, Aleander JM: Pathogenesis of cerebral air embolism during neodymium-YAG laser photoresection. *Chest* 1988; 94: 660–662.
20. Lukomsky GI, Ovchinnikov AA, Bilal A: Complications of bronchoscopy: Comparison of rigid bronchoscopy under general anesthesia and flexible fiberoptic bronchoscopy under topical anesthesia. *Chest* 1981; 79:316–321.
21. Dumon JF, Shapshay S, Bourcereau J, Cavaliere S, Meric B, Garbi N, Beamis J: Principles of safety in application of neodymium-YAG laser in bronchology. *Chest* 1984; 86:163–168.
22. Credle WF Jr, Smiddy JF, Elliott RC: Complications of fiberoptic bronchoscopy. *Am Rev Respir Dis* 1974; 109:67–72.
23. Suratt PM, Smiddy JF, Gruber B: Deaths and complications associated with fiberoptic bronchoscopy. *Chest* 1976; 69: 747–751.
24. Pereira W Jr, Kovnat DM, Snider GL: A prospective cooperative study of complications following flexible fiberoptic bronchoscopy. *Chest* 1978; 73:813–816.
25. Hoffman S, Bruderman I: Blood-pressure and blood-gas changes during anesthesia for bronchoscopy using a modified method of ventilation. *Anesthesiology* 1972; 37:95–98.
26. Weisel W, Tella RA: Reaction to tetracaine (pontocaine) used as topical anesthetic in bronchoscopy: A study of 1,000 cases. *JAMA* 1951; 147:218–222.
27. Wark KJ, Lyons J, Feneck RO: The haemodynamic effects of bronchoscopy: Effect of pretreatment with fentanyl and alfentanil. *Anaesthesia* 1986; 41:162–167.
28. Shrader DL, Lakshminarayan S: The effect of fiberoptic bronchoscopy on cardiac rhythm. *Chest* 1978; 73:821–824.
29. Moore JK, Seymour AH: Awareness during bronchoscopy. *Ann R Coll Surg Engl* 1987; 69:45–47.
30. Fairley HB: An evaluation of local and general anaesthesia for diagnostic bronchoscopy. *Can Anaesth Soc J* 1956; 3:366–377.
31. Barr AM, Wong RM: Awareness during general anesthesia for bronchoscopy and laryngoscopy using the apnoeic oxygenation technique. *Br J Anaesth* 1973; 45:894–900.
32. Kelly JS, Roy RC: Intraoperative awareness with propofol-oxygen total intravenous anesthesia for microlaryngeal surgery. *Anesthesiology* 1992; 77:207–209.
33. Golish JA, Pena CM, Mehta AC: Massive air embolism complicating Nd-YAG laser endobronchial photoresection. *Lasers Surg Med* 1992; 12:338–342.
34. Leibowitz HM, Peacock GR: Corneal injury produced by carbon dioxide laser radiation. *Arch Ophthalmol* 1980; 52:993.
35. Wolbarsht ML, Fligsten KE, Hayes JR. Retina: Pathology of neodymium and ruby laser burns. *Science* 1965; 150:1453–1454.
36. Freitag L, Chapman GA, Sielczak M, Ahmed A, Russin D: Laser smoke effect on the bronchial system. *Lasers Surg Med* 1987; 7:283–288.
37. Kokosa J, Eugene J: Chemical composition of laser-tissue interaction smoke plume. *J Laser Appl* 1989; 2:59.
38. Ferenczy A, Bergeron C, Richart RM: Human papillomavirus DNA in CO_2 laser-generated plume of smoke and its consequences to the surgeon. *Obstet Gynecol* 1990; 75:114–118.
39. Ferenczy A, Bergeron C, Richart RM: Carbon dioxide laser energy disperses human papillomavirus deoxyribonucleic acid onto treatment fields. *Am J Obstet Gynecol* 1990; 163:1271–1274.
40. Baggish MS, Poiez BJ, Joret D, Williamson P, Refai A: Presence of human immunodeficiency virus DNA in laser smoke. *Lasers Surg Med* 1991; 11:197–203.
41. Pashayan AG: Lasers and laser safety. In Kirby RR, Gravenstein N (eds): *Clinical Anesthesia Practice.* Philadelphia: WB Saunders; 1994:1370–1379.
42. Ball K: *Lasers: The Perioperative Challenge.* Philadelphia: Mosby-Year Book; 1990.
43. Ossoff RH, Coleman JA, Courey MS, Duncavage JA, Werkhaven JA, Reinisch L: Clinical applications of lasers in otolaryngology-head and neck surgery. *Lasers Surg Med* 1994; 15:217–248.
44. Colt HG: Laser bronchoscopy. *Chest Surg Clin North Am* 1996; 6:277–291.
45. Mehta AC, Harris RJ, DeBoer GE: Endoscopic management of benign airway stenosis. *Clin Chest Med* 1995; 16:401–413.
46. Ossoff RH: Laser safety in otolaryngology-head and neck surgery: Anesthetic and educational considerations for laryngeal surgery. *Laryngoscope* 1989; 99:1–26.
47. Fried MP: A survey of the complications of laser laryngoscopy. *Arch Otolaryngol* 1984; 110:31–34.
48. Duckett JE, McDonnell TJ, Unger M, Parr GV: General anaesthesia for Nd:YAG laser resection of obstructing endobronchial tumors using the rigid bronchoscope. *Can J Anaesth Soc J* 1985; 32:67–72.
49. Glass PS, Bloom M, Kearse L, Rosow C, Sebel P, Manberg P: Bispectral analysis measures sedation and memory effects of

propofol, midazolam, isoflurane, and alfentanil in healthy volunteers. *Anesthesiology* 1997; 86:836–847.
50. Liu J, Singh H, White PF: Electroencephalogram bispectral analysis predicts the depth of midazolam-induced sedation. *Anesthesiology* 1996; 84:64–69.
51. Bell GD, Spickett GP, Reeve PA, Morden A, Logan RF: Intravenous midazolam for upper gastrointestinal endoscopy: A study of 800 consecutive cases relating dose to age and sex of patient. *Br J Clin Pharmacol* 1987; 23:241–243.
52. Brophy T, Dundee JW, Heazelwood V, Kawar P, Varghese A, Ward M: Midazolam, a water-soluble benzodiazepine, for gastroscopy. *Anesth Intensive Care* 1982; 10:344–347.
53. Greenblatt DJ, Abernethy DR, Locniskar A, Harmatz JS, Limjuco RA, Shader RI: Effect of age, gender, and obesity on midazolam kinetics. *Anesthesiology* 1984; 61:27–35.
54. Severinghaus JW, Stupfel M: Respiratory dead space increase following atropine in man, and atropine, vagal or ganglionic blockade and hypothermia in dogs. *J Appl Physiol* 1955; 8:81–87.
55. Gal TJ, Suratt PM: Atropine and glycopyrrolate effects on lung mechanics in normal man. *Anesth Analg* 1981; 60:85–90.
56. Neuhaus A, Markowitz D, Rotman HH, Weg JG: The effects of fiberoptic bronchoscopy with and without atropine premedication on pulmonary function in humans. *Ann Thorac Surg* 1978; 25:393–398.
57. Throburn JR, James MF, Feldman C, Moyes DG, Du Toit PS: Comparison of the effects of atropine and glycopyrrolate on pulmonary mechanics in patients undergoing fiberoptic bronchoscopy. *Anesth Analg* 1986; 65:1285–1289.
58. Smith DS, Orkin FK, Gradner SM, Zakeosin G: Prolonged sedation in the elderly after intraoperative atropine administration. *Anesthesiology* 1979; 51:348–349.
59. Berggren D, Gustafson Y, Eriksson B, Bucht G, Hanson LI, Reiz S, Winblad B: Postoperative confusion after anesthesia in elderly patients with femoral neck fractures. *Anesth Analg* 1987; 66:497–504.
60. Olsson GL, Hallen B, Hambraeus-Jonzon K: Aspiration during anaesthesia: A computer-aided study of 188,358 anesthetics. *Acta Anaesthesiol Scand* 1986; 30:84–92.
61. Kallar SK: Aspiration pneumonitis: Fact or fiction? *Probl Anesth* 1988; 2:29.
62. Kallar SK, Everett LL: Potential risks and preventive measures for pulmonary aspiration: New concepts in preoperative fasting guidelines. *Anesth Analg* 1993; 77:171–182.
63. Goresky GV, Maltby JR: Fasting guidelines for elective surgical patients (Editorial). *Can J Anaesth* 1990; 37:493–495.
64. Minami H, McCallum RW: The physiology and pathophysiology of gastric emptying in humans. *Gastroenterology* 1986; 86:1592.
65. American Society of Anesthesiologists: Standards for basic anesthetic monitoring. Approved by House of Delegates on October 21, 1986 and last amended on October 23, 1996.
66. American Society of Anesthesiologists: Guideline for nonoperating room anesthetizing locations. Approved by House of Delegates on October 19, 1994.
67. Miller RD (ed): *Anesthesia.* New York: Churchill Livingstone; 1994.
68. Barash PG, Cullen BF, Stoelting RK (eds): *Clinical Anesthesia.* Philadelphia: JB Lippincott; 1989.
69. Kirby RK, Gravenstein N (eds): *Clinical Anesthesia Practice.* Philadelphia: WB Saunders; 1994.
70. Comroe JH Jr, Botelho S: The unreliability of cyanosis in the recognition of arterial anoxemia. *Am J Med Sci* 1947; 214:1–6.
71. Stephen CR, Slater HM, Johnson AL, Sekelj P: The oximeter—a technical aid for the anesthesiologist. *Anesthesiology* 1951; 12:541–555.
72. Tyler IL, Tantisira B, Winter PM, Motoyama EK: Continuous monitoring of arterial oxygen saturation with pulse oximetry during transfer to the recovery room. *Anesth Analg* 1985; 64:1108–1112.
73. Pullerits J, Burrows FA, Roy WL: Arterial desaturation in healthy children during transfer to the recovery room. *Can J Anaesth* 1987; 34:470–473.
74. Moller JT, Pedersen T, Rasmussen LS, et al: Randomized evaluation of pulse oximetry in 20,802 patients: 1. Design, demography, pulse oximetry failure rate, and overall complication rate. *Anesthesiolgy* 1993; 78:436–444.
75. Moller JT, Johannessen NW, Espersen K, et al: Randomized evaluation of pulse oximetry in 20,802 patients: II. Perioperative events and postoperative complications. *Anesthesiology* 1993; 78:445–453.
76. Scheller MS Unger RJ, Kelner MJ: Effects of intravenously administered dyes on pulse oximetry readings. *Anesthesiology* 1986; 65:550–552.
77. Barker SJ, Tremper KK: The effect of carbon monoxide inhalation on pulse oximetry and transcutaneous P_{O_2}. *Anesthesiology* 1987; 66:677–679.
78. Barker SJ, Tremper KK, Hyatt J: Effects of methemoglobinemia on pulse oximetry and mixed venous oximetry. *Anesthesiology* 1989; 70:112–117.
79. Severinghaus JW, Naifeh KH: Accuracy of response of six pulse oximeters to profound hypoxia. *Anethesiology* 1987; 67:551–558.
80. London MJ, Hollenberg M, Wong MG, Levenson L, Tubau JF, Browner W, Mangano DT: Intraoperative myocardial ischemia: Localization by continuous 12-lead electrocardiography. *Anesthesiology* 1988; 69:232–241.
81. Hanowell LH, Martin WR, Savelle JE, Foppiano LE: Complications of general anesthesia for Nd:YAG laser resection of endobronchial tumors. *Chest* 1991; 99:72–76.
82. Anderson HJ, Churchill-Davidson HC, Richardson AT: Bronchial neoplasm with myasthenia: Prolonged apnoea after administration of succinylcholine. *Lancet* 1953; 2: 1291–1293.
83. Wise RP: A myasthenic syndrome complicating bronchial carcinoma. *Anaesthesia* 1962; 17:488–504.
84. Telford RJ, Hollway TE: The myasthenic syndrome: Anaesthesia in a patient treated with 3,4 diaminopyridine. *Br J Anaesth* 1990; 64:363–366.
85. Eisenkraft JB: The anesthesia machine. In Ehrenworth J, Eisenkraft JB (eds): *Anesthesia Equipment. Principles and Applications.* St. Louis: Mosby-Year Book; 1993.
86. Bremang JA: Neurolept analgesia in ambulatory (nasal) endoscopies. *J Otolaryngol* 1991; 20:435.
87. Efthimiou J, Higenbottam T, Holt D, Cochrane GM: Plasma concentrations of lignocaine during fiberoptic bronchoscopy. *Thorax* 1982; 37:68–71.
88. Bromage PR, Robson JG: Concentrations of lignocaine in the blood after intravenous, intramuscular epidural and endotracheal administration. *Anaesthesia* 1961; 16:461–478.
89. Viegas O, Stoelting RK: Lidocaine in arterial blood after laryngotracheal administration. *Anesthesiology* 1975; 43: 491–493.
90. Wu FL, Razzaghi A, Souney PF: Seizure after lidocaine for bronchoscopy: Case report and review of the use of lidocaine in airway anesthesia. *Pharmocotherapy* 1993; 13:72–78.
91. de Oliveira LF, Heavner JE, de Jong RH: 5-Hydroxytryptophan intensifies local anesthetic-induced convulsions. *Arch Int Pharmacodyn Ther* 1974; 207:333–339.
92. Bosnjak ZJ, Stowe DF, Kampine JP: Comparison of lidocaine and bupivacaine depression of sinoatrial nodal activity during hypoxia and acidosis in adult and neonatal guinea pigs. *Anesth Analg* 1986; 65:911–917.
93. Catterall WA, Mackie K: Local anesthetics. In Hardman JG, Limbird LE (eds): *Goodman & Gilman's The Pharmacological Basis of Therapeutics*, 9th ed. New York: McGraw-Hill; 1996:341.
94. Greig JH, Cooper SM, Kasimbazi HJ, Monie RD, Fennerty AG, Watson B: Sedation for fiberoptic bronchoscopy. *Respir Med* 1995; 89:53–56.

95. Crawford M, Pollock J, Anderson K, Glavin RJ, MacIntyre D, Vernon KD: Comparison of midazolam with propofol for sedation in outpatient bronchoscopy. *Br J Anaesth* 1993; 70:419–422.
96. Shelly MP, Wilson P, Norman J: Sedation for fiberoptic bronchoscopy. *Thorax* 1989; 44:769–775.
97. American Society of Anesthesiologists: Practice guidelines for sedation and analgesia by non-anesthesiologists. A report by the American Society of Anesthesiologists task force on sedation and analgesia by non-anesthesiologists. *Anesthesiology* 1996; 84:459.
98. American Society of Anesthesiologists: Position on monitored anesthesia care. Approved by House of Delegates on October 21, 1986.
99. Dubrawsky C, Awe RJ, Jenkins DE: The effect of bronchofiberscopic examination on oxygenation status. *Chest* 1975; 67:137–140.
100. Milman N, Faurschou P, Grode G, Jorgensen A: Pulse oximetry during fiberoptic bronchoscopy in local anaesthesia: Frequency of hypoxaemia and effect of oxygen supplementation. *Respiration* 1994; 61:342–347.
101. Dich-Neilsen JO, Nagel P: Flexible fiberoptic bronchoscopy via the laryngeal mask. *Acta Anaesthesiol Scand* 1993; 37:17–19.
102. George PJ, Garrett CP, Nixon C, Hentzel MR, Nanson EM, Millard FJ: Laser treatment for tracheobronchial tumors: Local or general anaesthesia? *Thorax* 1987; 42:656–660.
103. Brutinel WM, Cortese DA, McDougall JC, Gillio RG, Bergstralh EJ: A two-year experience with the neodymium-YAG laser in endobronchial obstruction. *Chest* 1987; 91:159–165.
104. Chan AL, Tharratt RS, Siefkin AD, Albertson TE, Volz WG, Allen RP: Nd:YAG laser bronchoscopy. Rigid or fiberoptic mode? *Chest* 1990; 98:271–275.
105. Lindholm CE: Flexible fiberoptic bronchoscopy in the critically ill patient. *Ann Otol* 1974; 83:786.
106. Lindholm CE, Ollman B, Snyder JV, Millen EG, Grenvik A: Cardiorespiratory effects of flexible fiberoptic bronchoscopy in critically ill patients. *Chest* 1978; 74:362–368.
107. Ehrenworth J, Brull SJ: Anesthesia for thoracic diagnostic procedures. In Kaplan JA (ed): *Thoracic Anesthesia*, 2nd ed. New York: Churchill Livingstone; 1991:321–346.
108. Warner ME, Warner MA, Leonard PF: Anesthesia for neodymium-YAG(Nd-YAG) laser resection of major airway obstructing tumors. *Anesthesiology* 1984; 60:230–232.
109. Cozine K, Rosenbaum LM, Askanazi J, Rosenbaum SH: Laser-induced endotracheal tube fire. *Anesthesiology* 1981; 55:583–585.
110. Sosis MB: airway fire during CO_2 laser surgery using a Xomed laser endotracheal tube. *Anesthesiology* 1990; 72:747–749.
111. Schramm VL Jr, Mattox DE, Stool SE: Acute management of laser-ignited intratracheal explosion. *Laryngoscope* 1981; 91:1417–1426.
112. Hirshman CA, Smith J: Indirect ignition of the endotracheal tube during carbon dioxide laser surgery. *Arch Otolaryngol* 1980; 106:639–641.
113. Emergency Care Research Institute: Health Devices: Laser-resistant endotracheal tubes and wraps. 1990; 4:107–139.
114. Geffin B, Shapshay SM, Bellack GS, Hobin K, Setzer SE: Flammability of endotracheal tubes during Nd-YAG laser application in the airway. *Anesthesiology* 1986; 65:511–515.
115. Treyve E, Yarington CT Jr, Thompson GE: Incendiary characteristics of endotracheal tubes with the carbon dioxide laser: an experimental study. *Ann Otol Rhinol Laryngol* 1981; 90:328–330.
116. Sosis MB: What is the safest endotracheal tube for Nd-YAG laser surgery? A comparative study. *Anesth Analg* 1989; 69:802–804.
117. Wolf GL, Simpson JI: Flammability of endotracheal tubes in oxygen and nitrous oxide enriched atmosphere. *Anesthesiology* 1987; 67:236–239.
118. Pashayan AG, Gravenstein JS: Helium retards endotracheal tube fires from carbon dioxide lasers. *Anesthesiology* 1985; 62:274–277.
119. Simpson JL, Schiff GA, Wolf GL: The effect of helium on endotracheal tube flammability. *Anesthesiology* 1990; 73:538–540.
120. Hawkins DB, Joseph MM: Avoiding a wrapped endotracheal tube in laser laryngeal surgery: Experiences with apneic anesthesia and metal laser-flex endotracheal tubes. *Laryngoscope* 1990; 100:1283–1287.
121. Fried MP, Mallampati SR, Liu FC, Kaplan S, Caminear DS, Samonte BR: Laser resistant stainless steel endotracheal tube: Experimental and clinical evaluation. *Lasers Surg Med* 1991; 11:301–306.
122. Sosis M, Dillon F: Hazards of a new, clear, unmarked polyvinylchloride tracheal tube designed for use with the Nd-YAG laser. *J Clin Anesth* 1991; 3:358–360.
123. Green JM, Gonzalez RM, Sonbolian N, Rehkopf P: The resistance to carbon dioxide laser ignition of a new endotracheal tube: Xomed Laser-Shield II. *J Clin Anesth* 1992; 4:89–92.
124. Sosis MB, Dillon F: Prevention of CO_2 laser-induced endotracheal tube fires with the laser guard protective coating. *J Clin Anesth* 1992; 4:25–27.
125. Sosis MB, Dillon FX: A comparison of CO_2 laser ignition of the Xomed, plastic, and rubber endotracheal tubes. *Anesth Analg* 1993; 76:391–393.
126. Kautzky M, Fitzgerald R, Dechtyar L, Schenk P: Effects of the holmium:YAG and erbium:YAG lasers on endotracheal tubes. *ORL J Otorhinolaryngol Relat Spec* 1993; 55:105–109.
127. Sosis MB: Evaluation of five metallic tapes for protection of endotracheal tubes during CO_2 laser surgery. *Anesth Analg* 1989; 68:392–393.
128. Sosis M, Dillon F: Reflection of CO_2 laser radiation from laser-resistant endotracheal tubes. *Anesth analg* 1991; 73:338–340.
129. Sosis MB, Braverman B: Evaluation of foil coverings for protecting plastic endotracheal tubes from the potassium-titanyl-posphate laser. *Anesth Analg* 1993; 77:589–591.
130. Sosis MB: Evaluation of a technique of nitrogen insufflation to decrease plastic endotracheal tube cuff flammability during carbon dioxide laser surgery. *J Clin Anesth* 1993; 5:468–470.
131. LeJeune FE Jr, Guice C, LeTard F, Marice H: Heat sink protection against lasering endotracheal cuffs. *Ann Otol Rhinol Laryngol* 1982; 91:606–607.
132. Sosis MB, Dillon FX: Saline-filled cuffs help prevent laser-induced polyvinylchloride endotracheal tube fires. *Anesth Analg* 1991; 72:187–189.
133. Pashayan AG, SanGiovanni C, Davis LE: Positive end-expiratory pressure lowers the risk of laser-induced polyvinylchloride tracheal-tube fires. *Anesthesiology* 1993; 79:83–87.
134. Sosis MB, Pritikin JB, Caldarelli DD: The effect of blood on laser-resistant endotracheal tube combustion. *Larynogoscope* 1994; 104:829–831.
135. Green JM, Sonbolian N, Gonzalez RM, Larson CE, Rehkopf P: CO_2 laser resistance of various ointments and tapes. *Anesthesiology* 1991; 74:964–965.
136. Pashayan AG, Gravenstien JS, Cassisi NJ, McLaughlin G: The helium protocol for larynogotracheal operations with CO_2 laser: A retrospective review of 523 cases. *Anesthesiology* 1988; 68:801–804.
137. Leonard PR: The lower limits of flammability of halothane, enflurane, and isoflurane. *Anesth Analg* 1975; 54:238–240.
138. Simpson JI, Wolf GL, Rosen A, Krespi Y, Schiff GA: The oxygen and nitrous oxide indices of flammability of endotracheal tubes determined by laser ignition. *Laryngoscope* 1991; 101:981–984.
139. AlHaddad S, Brenner J: Helium and lower oxygen concentration do not prolong tracheal tube ignition time during potasium titanyl phosphate laser use. *Anesthesiology* 1994; 80:936–938.
140. Arnold JE, Allphin AL: Effect of extraluminal oxygen on carbon dioxide laser ignition of endotracheal tubes. *Arch Otolaryngol Head Neck Surg* 1992; 118:722–724.

141. Ossoff RH, Duncavage JA, Eisenman TS, Karlan MS: Comparison of tracheal damage from laser-ignited endotracheal tube fires. *Ann Otol Rhinol Laryngol* 1983; 92:333–336.
142. Terrill JB, Montogomery RR, Reinhardt CF: Toxic gases from fires. *Science* 1978; 200:1343–1347.
143. Tobias JD: Helium: applications in the practice of anesthesia and critical care. *Am J Anesth* 1997; 24:194.
144. Sanders RD: Two ventilating attachments for bronchoscopes. *Del Med J* 1967; 39:170.
145. Carden E, Trapp WG, Oulton J: A new simple method for ventilating patients undergoing bronchoscopy. *Anesthesiology* 1970; 33:454–458.
146. Carden E: Positive-pressure ventilation during anesthesia for bronchoscopy: A laboratory evaluation of two recent advances. *Anesth Analg* 1973; 52:402–406.
147. Carden E, Burns WW, McDevitt NB, Carson T, et al: A comparison of Venturi and side-arm ventilation in anesthesia for bronchoscopy. *Can Anaesth Soc J* 1973; 20:569–574.
148. Giesecke AH Jr, Gerbershagen HU, Dortman C, Lee D: Comparison of the ventilating and injection bronchoscopes. *Anesthesiology* 1973; 38:298–303.
149. Godden DJ, Willey RF, Fergusson RJ, Wright DJ, Crompton GK, Grant IW: Rigid bronchoscopy under intravenous general anesthesia with oxygen Venturi ventilation. *Thorax* 1987; 37:532–534.
150. Schlenkhoff D, Droset H, Scieszka S, Vogt H: The use of high-frequency jet ventilation in operative bronchoscopy. *Endoscopy* 1986; 18:192–194.
151. Schneider M, Probst R: High frequency jet ventilation via a tracheoscope for endobronchial laser surgery. *Can J Anaesth* 1990; 37:372–376.
152. Eriksson I, Sjostrand U: Effects of high-frequency positive-pressure ventilation (HFPPV) and general anesthesia on intrapulmonary gas distribution in patients undergoing diagnostic bronchoscopy. *Anesth Analg* 1980; 59:585–593.
153. Bor U, Eriksson I, Sjostrand U: High-frequency positive pressure ventilation (HFPPV): A review based upon its use during bronchoscopy and for laryngoscopy and microlaryngeal surgey under general anesthesia. *Anesth Analg* 1980; 59:594.
154. Vourc'h G, Fischler M, Michon F, Melchior JC, Seigneur F: Manual jet ventilation v. high frequency jet ventilation during laser resection of tracheo-bronchial stenosis. *Br J Anaesth* 1983; 55:973–975.
155. Reves JG, Fragen RJ, Vinik HR, Greenblatt DJ: Midazolam: Pharmacology and uses. *Anesthesiology* 1985; 62:310–324.
156. Hargreaves J: Benzodiazephine premedication in minor day-case surgery: Comparison of oral midazolam and temazepam with placebo. *Br J Anaesth* 1988; 61:611–616.
157. Wong HY, Fragen RJ, Dunn K: Dose-finding study of intramuscular midazolam preanesthetic medication in the elderly. *Anesthesiology* 1991; 74:675–679.
158. Shafer A, White PF, Urquhart ML, Doze VA: Outpatient premedication: Use of midazolam and opioid analgesics. *Anesthesiology* 1989; 71:495–501.
159. Bailey PL, Stanley TH: Intravenous opioid anesthetics. In Miller RD (ed): *Anesthesia,* 4th ed. New York: Churchill Livingstone; 1994:300–303.
160. Gold MI: Preoxygenation. *Br J Aneseth* 1989; 62:241–242.
161. Gold MI, Durate I, Muravchick S: Arteial oxygenation in conscious patients after 5 minutes and after 30 seconds of oxygen breathing. *Anesth Analg* 1981; 60:313–315.
162. Gambee AM, Hertzka RE, Fisher DM: Preoxygenation techniques: Comparison of three minutes and four breaths. *Anesth Analg* 1987; 66:468–470.
163. Valentine SJ, Marjot R, Monk CR: Preoxygenation in the elderly: A comparison of the four-maximal-breath and three-minute techniques. *Anesth Analg* 1990; 71:516–519.
164. Cockshott ID: Propofol ('Diprivan') pharmacokinetics and metabolism—an overview. *Postgrad Med J* 1985; 61 (Suppl 3): 45–50.
165. Hudson RJ, Stanski DR, Burch PG: Pharmacokinetics of methohexital and thiopental in surgical patients. *Anesthesiology* 1983; 59:215–219.
166. Glas PS: Prevention of awareness during total intravenous anesthesia (Letter). *Anesthesiology* 1993; 78:399–400.
167. Egan TD, Minto CF, Hermann DJ, Barr J, Muir KT, Shafer SL: Remifentanil versus alfentanil: Comparative phamacokinetics and pharmacodynamics in healthy adult male volunteers. *Anesthesiology* 1996; 84:821–833.
168. Egan TD: Remifentanil pharmacokinetics and pharmacodynamics: A preliminary appraisal. *Clin Pharmacokinet* 1995; 29:80–94.
169. Thompson JP, Rowbotham DJ: Remifentanil—an opioid for the 21st century. *Br J Anaesth* 1996; 76:341–343.
170. Dershwitz M, Hoke JF, Rosow CE, Michalowski P, Connors PM, Muir KT, Dienstag JF: Pharmacokinetics and pharmacodynamics of remifentanil in volunteer subjects with severe liver disease. *Anesthesiology* 1996; 84:812–820.
171. Dershwitz M, Randel GI, Rosow CE, Fragen RJ, Connors PM, Librojo ES, Shaw DL, Peng AW, Jamerson BD: Initial clinical experience with remifentanil, a new opioid metabolized by esterases. *Anesth Analg* 1995; 81:619–623.
172. James MK, Feldman PL, Schuster SV, Bilotta JM, Brackeen MF, Leighton HJ: Opioid receptor activity of GI 87084B, a novel ultra-short acting analgesic, in isolated tissues. *J Pharmacol Exp Ther* 1991; 259:712–718.
173. Mehta AC, Lee FY, Cordasco EM, Kirby T, Eliachar I, De Boer G: Concentric tracheal and subglottic stenosis: Management using the Nd-YAG laser for mucosal sparing followed by gentle dilation. *Chest* 1993; 104:673–677.
174. Mehta AC, Livingston DR, Levine HL, et al: Ventilatory management during neodyminum:yttrium aluminum garnet photoresection of subglottic and higher tracheal lesions. Transactions of the American Broncho-esophagological Association, 1986.
175. Hirshman CA, Edelstein G, Peetz S, Wayne R, Downes H: Mechanism of action of inhalational anesthesia on airways. *Anesthesiology* 1982; 56:107–111.
176. Johnston RR, Eger EI II, Wilson C: A comparative interaction of epinephrine with enflurane, isoflurane, and halothane in man. *Anesth Analg* 1976; 55:709–712.
177. Kharasch ED: Inhalation anesthetic toxicity: Current controversies. American Society of Anesthesiologists 1997 Annual Refresher Course Lectures, p 122.
178. Stoelting RK: Blood pressure and heart rate changes during short-duration laryngoscopy for tracheal intubation: Influence of viscous or intravenous lidocaine. *Anesth Analg* 1978; 57:197–199.
179. Jakobsen CJ, Ahlburg P, Holdgard HO, Olsen KH, Thomsen A: Comparison of intravenous and topical lidocaine as a suppressant of coughing after bronchoscopy during general anesthesia. *Acta Anaesthesiol Scand* 1991; 35:238–241.
180. Gaumann DM, Tassonyi E, Fathi F, Griessen M: Effects of topical laryngeal lidocaine on sympathetic response to rigid panendoscopy under general anesthesia. *ORL J Otorhinolaryngol Relat Spec* 1992; 54:49–53.
181. DeFazio CA, Niederlehner JR, Burney RG: The anesthetic potency of lidocaine in the rat. *Anesth Analg* 1976; 55:818–821.
182. Frumin MJ, Epstein RM, Cohen G: Apneic oxygenation in man. *Anesthesiology* 1959; 20:789–798.
183. Fraioli RL, Sheffer LA, Steffenson JL: Pulmonary and cardiovascular effects of apneic oxygenation in man. *Anesthesiology* 1973; 39:588–596.

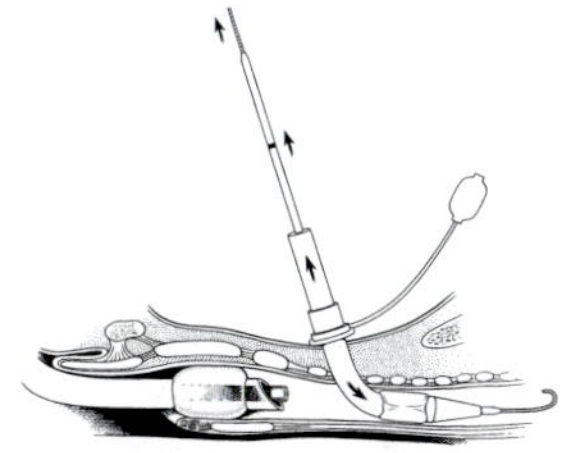

CHAPTER 22

FLUORESCENCE IMAGING FOR EARLY LUNG CANCER

Stephen Lam

In humans, lung cancer occurs after a prolonged latent period, encompassing several decades, during which the normal respiratory epithelium undergoes cellular alterations, with development of atypical changes becoming gradually more severe with time and ultimately progressing to carcinoma in situ and to invasive carcinoma.[1,2] Less than 15 percent of patients with invasive lung cancer can be cured of the disease. On the other hand, the potential for cure is essentially 100 percent in patients with early lung cancer (carcinoma in situ or microinvasive cancer) with local therapeutic measures such as photodynamic therapy,[3] cryotherapy,[4] or surgery.[5] In patients harboring premalignant lung lesions, chemopreventive agents can be used to revert or suppress the carcinogenic process from progression to full-blown malignancy. The success of cervical cytology screening, coupled with treatment of preinvasive lesions with cryotherapy or laser, in reducing the incidence and mortality of invasive cervical cancer[6] offers hope that a similar strategy may also lead to a reduction in lung cancer mortality—the most common cause of cancer mortality in North America. The challenge is how to detect and localize preinvasive lesions among individuals at risk of developing lung cancer.

Conventional White-Light Bronchoscopy

USE AND LIMITATIONS

Dysplasia and carcinoma in situ are difficult to detect by conventional white-light bronchoscopy because these lesions are only a few cell layers thick and a few millimeters in surface diameter. For this reason they may not produce any visible abnormality on conventional white-light examination. The difficulty of identifying these small preinvasive lesions is illustrated by the following observations. Serial sectioning of the bronchial tree by Auerbach and coworkers[1] in smokers whose death was not due to lung cancer showed the presence of carcinoma in situ in 4.3 percent of those who smoked one to two packs of cigarettes per day and 11.4 percent in those who smoked greater than two packs per day. In patients who died of lung cancer, carcinoma in situ was found in other parts of the bronchial tree in 15 percent of these patients.[1] A study by Sato and coworkers, using differential brushing of all segmental bronchi from B_{10} to B_1 bilaterally in patients with sputum positive or suspected positive for lung cancer, demonstrated synchronous and metachronous lung cancers in 12.6 percent and 2.8 percent of patients, respectively; prior to the use of the selected brushings the incidence had been reported to be 1.7 percent and 13.8 percent, respectively.[7] In other words, if synchronous cancers were missed prior to treatment, they would manifest themselves as second primary cancers on follow-up. Since most bronchoscopists rarely encounter patients with carcinoma in situ despite examining many patients with known or suspected lung cancer, these studies would suggest that small preinvasive lesions are often missed. The problem with missing these small preinvasive lesions is that the mortality of patients with invasive lung cancer is very high, especially for those with second primary lung cancers because the options for treatment are limited after the first surgery.[8]

Although "blind" segmental brushing may be a useful screening technique to detect bronchial cancers that are not visible bronchoscopically, the procedure has several drawbacks. (1) Multiple samples need to be taken. (2) Although it can be performed under local anesthesia it is more commonly done under general anesthesia, with or without concomitant biopsy of the segmental spurs of each lobe. (3) The entire procedure generally takes 1 to 2 h. (4) There is the problem of cross contamination, especially if nondisposable brushes are used. (5) Accurate interpretation of the numerous samples obtained from each patient requires meticulous examination of the samples by experienced cytotechnologists and cytopathologists, who can make a diagnosis by assessing the number, staining, and appearance of atypical cells. (6) If bronchial brushing shows malignant cells without a visible bronchoscopic abnormality, a repeat brushing of the same segment in a separate bronchoscopic procedure is required for confirmation before treatment can be undertaken. Clearly the task would be much easier if the lesions could be made visible for direct biopsy.

There is a misconception that roentgenographically occult lung cancers, that is, cancers that are detected by sputum cytology examination with a negative chest radiograph, represent early lung cancers. In fact, review of the pathology of several reports showed that only 20 percent of the tumors were truly in-situ carcinomas.[9,10] Thirty-nine percent had full thickness involvement or peribronchial extension. In this latter group, about one-third had N1/N2 lymph node spread, and a few patients even had systemic metastases. The size of the tumors detected by sputum cytology examination was not small. Even for carcinoma in situ, the mean surface diameter was approximately 10 mm and some of the lesions were as large as 5 cm.[10,11] For this reason, about 40 percent of roentgenographically occult lung cancers have obvious bronchoscopic abnormalities. More subtle changes that can be readily missed by less experienced endoscopists are present in approximately 30 percent of the cases. These subtle changes, however, can be mimicked by inflammation or squamous metaplasia. A study by Sato and coworkers[7] showed that only 14 percent of the bronchial biopsies from areas that showed minute abnormalities were confirmed as moderate/severe dysplasia or cancer. Therefore it would be desirable to be able to decrease the number of nonspecific biopsies by being able to differentiate benign metaplasia from significant dysplasia or cancer. Furthermore, with improvement in methods to detect preinvasive lung lesions in sputum specimens such as with automated image cytometry[12] or molecular markers,[13] a larger proportion of roentgenographically occult lung cancers will be either bronchoscopically invisible or have minute abnormality only.

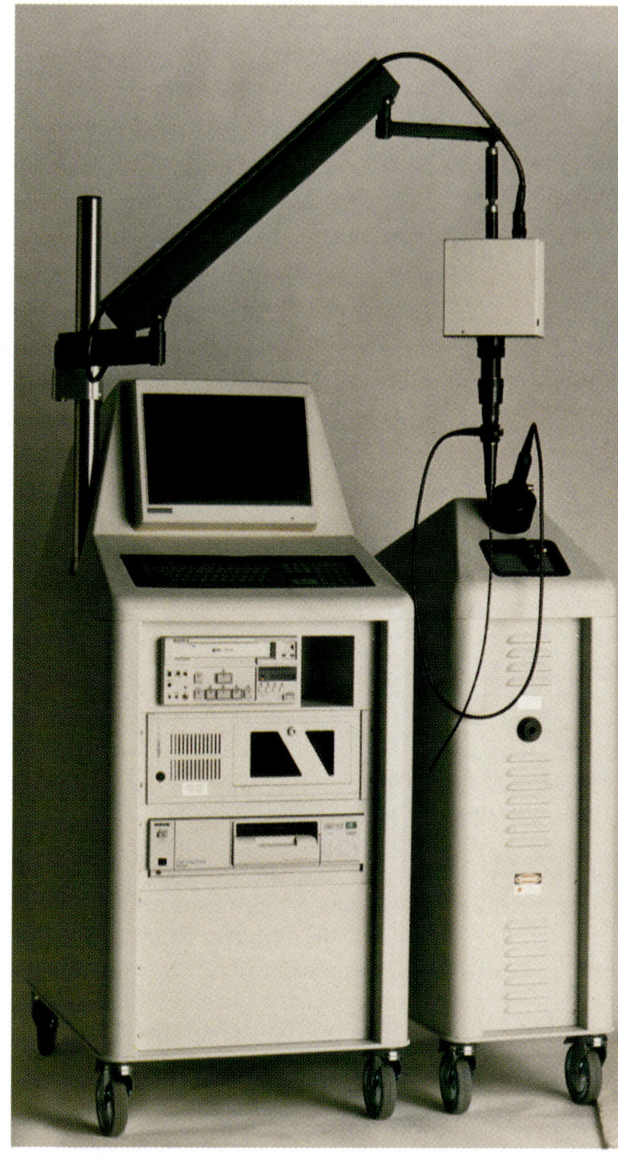

Figure 22-1

LIFE Device.

Fluorescence Bronchoscopy

HISTORY OF DEVELOPMENT

Since the bronchoscope only examines the surface of a body cavity, it is unlikely that further advances in white-light bronchoscopy can substantially improve our ability to detect precancerous lesions or early cancers. Recent studies suggest that instead of making use of reflected and scattered light, one can use light-induced tissue autofluorescence to improve significantly (by more than two times) the detection rate of early lung cancer lesions with a similar specificity.[14,15]

The concept of fluorescence detection has intrigued the minds of many since the beginning of the 20th century. In 1933, Sutro and Burman observed that when surgically excised breast tissue was exposed to Wood's light, normal breast tissue fluoresced green, while breast cancer tissue fluoresced purple.[16] In recent years, in vivo spectroscopy during bronchoscopic examination with an optical multi-channel analyzer and helium-cadmium laser (442 nm) for illumination has demonstrated a significant decrease in autofluorescence intensity, predominantly in the green region of the visible spectrum, in areas with dysplasia or carcinoma in situ compared to normal bronchial tissue.[17] The reason for the decrease in autofluorescence in premalignant tissues has not been clearly defined. Most of the fluorescence comes from the submucosa; the epithelium contributes only a small amount (a few percent) toward the overall fluorescence. It is likely that the drop in fluorescence intensity is due to both thickening of the epithelium and a loss of fluorophore concentration or efficiency.[18] Preferential diffusion of longer wavelength (red) fluorescent light horizontally from the adjacent normal mucosa into the tumor area provides further opportunity to distinguish abnormal from normal tissue. Further advances in imaging technology have made it possible to reexamine the use of tissue autofluorescence alone to detect early lung cancer and precancerous lesions.

INSTRUMENTATION

One such device, called the Lung Imaging Fluorescence Endoscope (LIFE), was developed by the British Columbia Cancer Agency research staff in collaboration with Xillix Technologies Corporation in Vancouver, Canada.

LIFE is composed of a helium-cadmium laser as a light source (442 nm), two image-intensified CCD cameras with green and red filters, respectively, a computer with an imaging board, and a color video monitor (Fig. 22-1). Two images at different (red and green) wavelengths are simultaneously captured in precise registration by the imaging board. The images are then combined and processed by the imaging board using a specially developed algorithm that allows normal tissue to be clearly distinguished from malignant tissue when displayed as a pseudocolor image on the video monitor; for example, normal tissue as green and tumor as brown or brownish red (Fig. 22-2). An abnormal area can be biopsied under direct vision for pathologic confirmation. It is important to note that fluorescence bronchoscopy using tissue autofluorescence does not require exogenous fluorescent drugs.

Equipment List for Fluorescence Bronchoscopy

Not all commercially available fiberoptic bronchoscopes are suitable for fluorescence examination. The fiberoptic bundle in some models has intrinsic fluorescence on excitation by blue or violet light. The illumination light guide in some models produces uneven illumination, resulting in a poor quality fluorescence image. The bronchoscopes that have been tested and were found to be suitable are the Olympus BF20D, BF40D, and P30D, as well as the Pentax FB-18RX. The only other equipment required is the LIFE device.

Figure 22-2

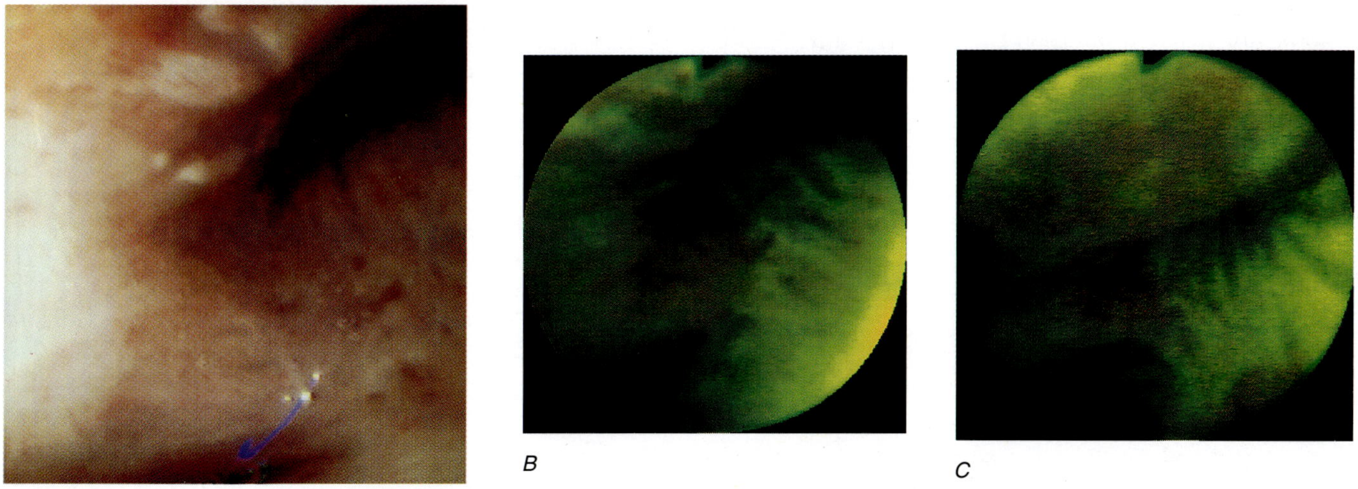

A B C

White-light (*A*) and fluorescence bronchoscopy (*B, C*) appearance of the right main-stem bronchus and right upper lobe junction in a patient with carcinoma in-situ. White-light examination showed thickening of the longitudinal folds in the right upper lobe only. Fluorescence bronchoscopy showing abnormal fluorescence (indicated by reddish-brown color) not only in the right upper lobe (*B*) but in two separate sites in the distal right main bronchus as well (*C*). Biopsy confirmed the presence of carcinoma in situ in all three areas. Normal mucosa was represented by green color.

Procedures

Conventional white-light bronchoscopy is first carried out under local anaesthesia with topical lidocaine (Fig. 22-3). A thorough examination without trauma to the bronchial mucosa from coughing, rapid breathing, and restlessness requires a calm, comfortable patient during the examination and takes an average of 30 min. This is achieved by giving midazolam (0.5 to 1.0 mg IV in titrated doses at 2- to 5-min intervals, maximum 5 mg) during administration of the topical anesthetic to produce moderate sedation and for the amnesiac effect postbronchoscopy. Alfentanil (100 to 300 μg) is given IV in titrated doses at 2- to 5-min intervals during the bronchoscopy (maximum 1500 μg) to suppress cough and to produce a light sleep. For very anxious patients, midazolam 0.5 to 1.0 mg is given IV during the bronchoscopy. One milliliter of 1% lidocaine prewarmed to body temperature is given at each lobar orifice to suppress the cough reflex. The lidocaine is instilled slowly rather than as a rapid bolus which may stimulate coughing. Oxygen (2 to 6 liters/min by nasal prongs) is routinely administered throughout the bronchoscopy with continuous oximetry monitoring to maintain the arterial oxygen saturation >92%. This is to minimize the occurrence of desaturation during the procedure which may divert the attention of the bronchoscopist. The bronchoscope tube is inserted gently in synchrony with the breathing cycle. Usually, with the exception of B_1 and B_6, up to the sixth generation bronchi can be examined with a 5.9-mm diameter bronchoscope. Careful attention is made to the surface markings such as the normal mucosal sheen, the sharpness of the circular and longitudinal folds, and the thickness of the bifurcations. A thorough knowledge of the normal anatomy and the nomenclature of the

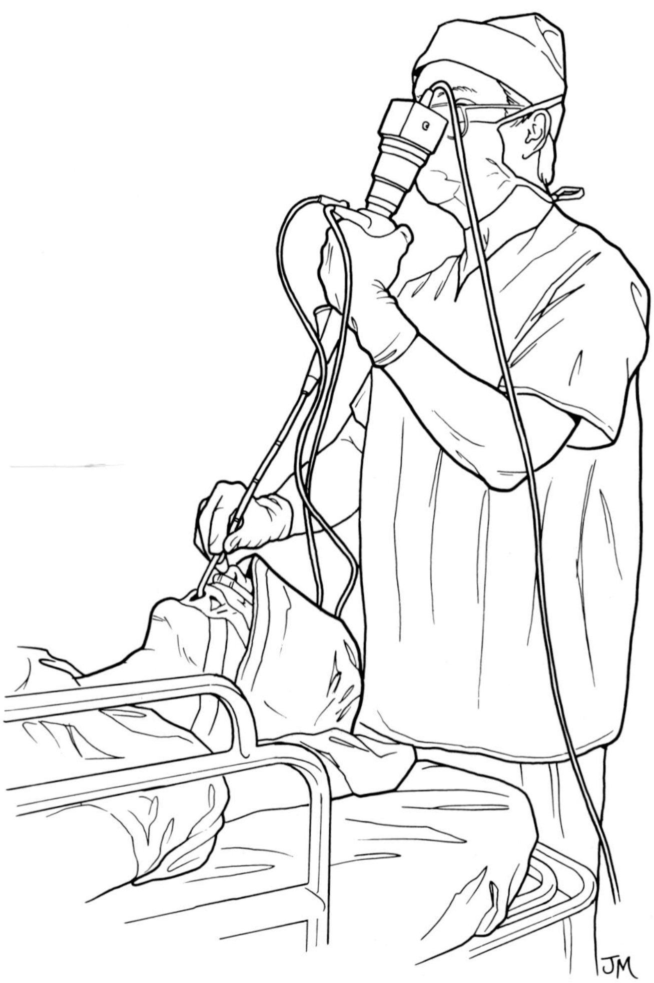

Figure 22-3

Conventional white-light bronchoscopy is performed first.

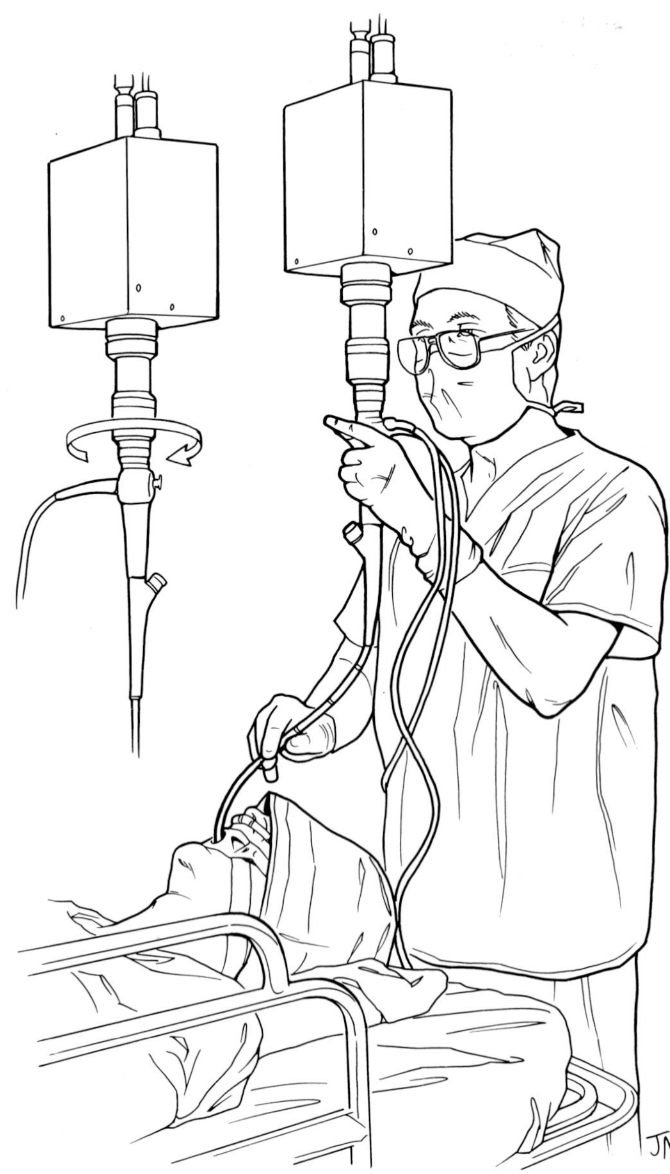

Figure 22-4

The bronchoscope eye piece is attached to the LIFE camera.

branches is required. Any abnormality suspicious for preinvasive or invasive cancer is recorded in the image management system for later biopsy. Following the white-light examination, the bronchoscope light guide is inserted into the helium-cadmium laser and the LIFE camera is attached to the bronchoscope for the fluorescence examination (Fig. 22-4). The bronchial tree is scanned again for any abnormality suspicious for preinvasive or invasive lesions (Fig. 22-5). The site(s) of abnormalities is (are) recorded in the image management system (Fig. 22-6). Following the white-light and fluorescence examination, all the areas that are suspicious for preinvasive or invasive lung cancer are biopsied for pathologic confirmation. For small lesions, the biopsies are taken under fluorescence examination.

Clinical Results

The performance of the LIFE device was tested in 223 subjects with lung cancer or at risk for developing lung cancer. Using the pathologic findings of directed and random bronchial biopsy specimens as the gold standard, the proportion of biopsy-proved moderate/severe dysplasia and carcinoma in situ detected by white-light bronchoscopy alone was 38.5 and 40 percent, respectively. With the addition of the LIFE examination, the detection rate was 73.1 and 91.4 percent, respectively. The specificity of white-light bronchoscopy was 91.1 percent. With fluorescence bronchoscopy, the specificity was 86.7 percent.[15]

Data collected in the multicenter clinical trial in the United States and Canada showed similar results.[19] In 173 subjects with suspected lung cancer, fluorescence bronchoscopy was found to be more than six times better than white-light bronchoscopy in detecting moderate/severe dysplasia or carcinoma in situ. The relative specificity was lower (0.73) compared to the pilot study probably reflecting the learning curve in a larger group of investigators. False-positive fluorescence was found to be due mainly to trauma from insertion of the bronchoscope or excessive suctioning. Infiltration of the submucosa by eosinophils and mononuclear cells may also give rise to false-positive fluorescence. Chronic bronchitis without asthma, however, did not present a problem. False-negative examination can occur from inadequate examination of the bronchial tree. It is therefore imperative that a thorough examination be made by inserting the bronchoscope as distally as possible.

Indications

Fluorescence bronchoscopy has been found to be useful in the localization of sputum-cytology-positive, ra-

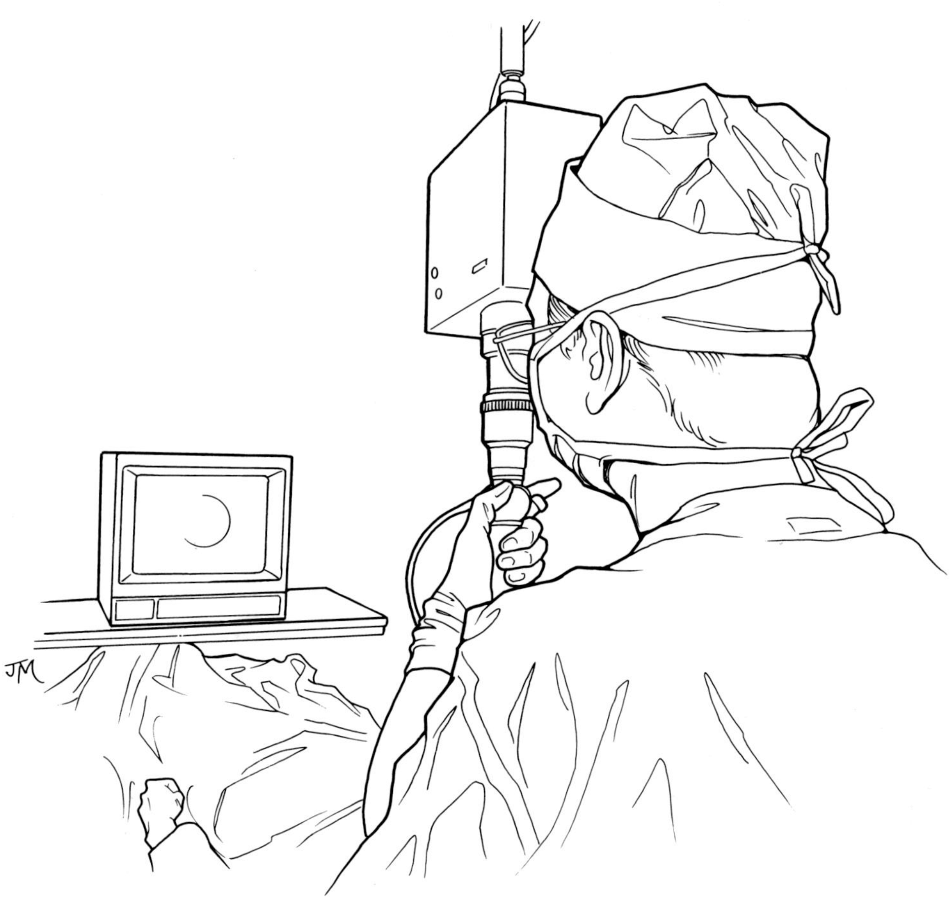

Figure 22-5

The bronchial tree is scanned for areas of abnormal fluorescence.

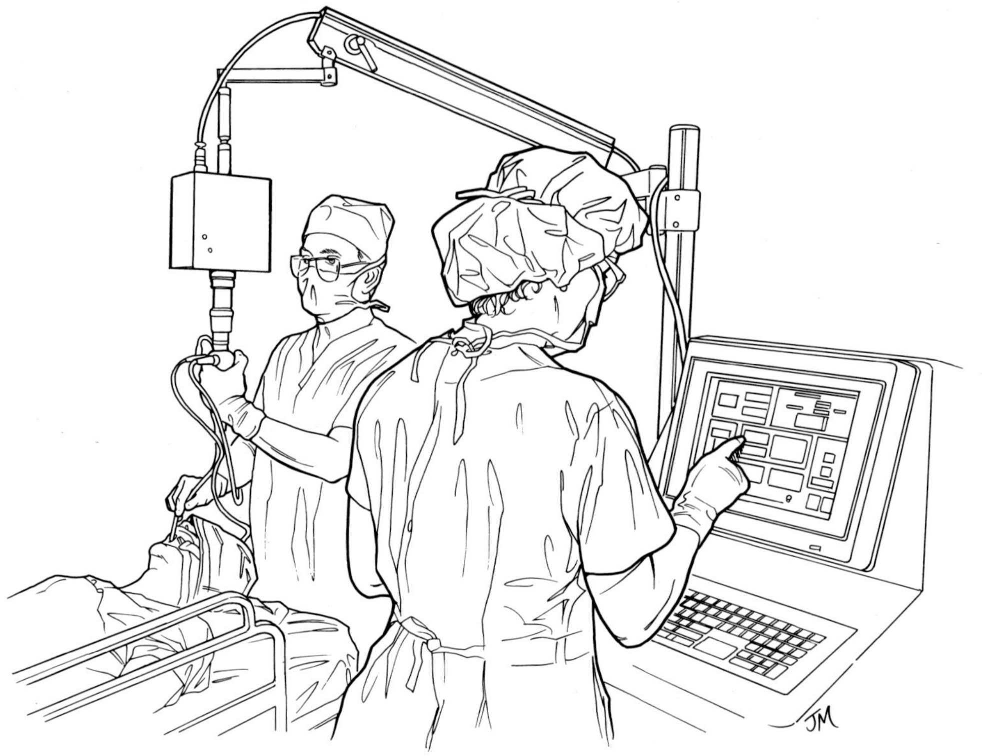

Figure 22-6

Areas suspicious for preinvasive or invasive cancer are recorded in the image management system.

diologically occult lung cancer and in the preoperative assessment of patients with lung cancer to determine the extent of the endobronchial spread and to detect synchronous dysplastic lesions or in-situ carcinoma that are invisible on conventional white-light examination. It is a useful tool to educate endoscopists in recognizing subtle bronchial lesions. If current work directed towards improving the sensitivity of sputum cytology to detect preinvasive lung lesions using quantitative image cytometry or molecular markers were successful, fluorescence bronchoscopy would become an indispensable tool for the endoscopist. As a research method, it offers the possibility of studying the pathogenesis of lung cancer and the effect of chemopreventive treatment by providing the means to localize and sample the same preinvasive lesions sequentially. By coupling sensitive diagnostic tools to new treatment modalities such as chemoprevention and various endobronchial therapies, it is hoped that the traditionally poor prognosis of patients with lung cancer can be altered in the near future.

References

1. Auerbach O, Stout AP, Hammond EC, et al: Changes in bronchial epithelium in relation to cigarette smoking and in relation to lung cancer. *N Engl J Med* 1961; 265:253–267.
2. Saccomanno G: Carcinoma in-situ of the lung: Its development, detection and treatment. *Sem Res Med* 1982; 4:156–160.
3. Lam S: Photodynamic therapy of lung cancer. *Sem Oncol* 1994; 21:15–19.
4. Ozenne G, Vergnon JM, Roulier A, et al: Cryotherapy of in situ or microinvasive bronchial carcinoma. *Chest* 1990; 98:105S.
5. Cortese DA, Pairolero PC, Bergstralh, et al: Roentgenographically occult lung cancer: A ten year experience. *J Thorac Cardiovasc Surg* 1983; 86:373–380.
6. Anderson GH, Boyes DA, Benedet JL, et al: Organization and results of the cervical cytology screening programme in British Columbia, 1995–85. *Br Med J* 1988; 296:975–978.
7. Sato M, Saito Y, Nagamoto N, et al: Diagnostic value of differential brushing of all branches of the bronchi in patients with sputum positive or suspected positive for lung cancer. *Acta Cytologica* 1993; 37:879–883.
8. Pairolero PC, Williams DE, Bergstralh EJ, et al: Postsurgical stage I bronchoscopic carcinoma: Morbid implications of recurrent disease. *Ann Thorac Surg* 1984; 38:331–338.
9. Bechtel JJ, Kelley WR, Petty TL, et al: Outcome of 51 patients with roentgenographically occult lung cancer detected by sputum cytologic testing: A community hospital program. *Arch Intern Med* 1994; 154:975–980.
10. Woolner LB, Fontana RS, Cortese DA, et al: Roentgenographically occult lung cancer: Pathologic findings and frequency of multicentricity during a 10-year period. *Mayo Clin Proc* 1984; 59:453–466.
11. Usuda K, Saito Y, Nagamoto N, et al: Relation between bronchoscopic findings and tumor size of roentgenographically occult bronchogenic squamous cell carcinoma. *J Thorac Cardiovasc Surg* 1993; 106:1098–1103.
12. Lam S, MacAulay C, Palcic B: Detection and localization of early lung cancer by imaging techniques. *Chest* 1993; 103:12S–14S.
13. Mao L, Hruban RH, Boyle JO, et al: Detection of oncogene mutations in sputum precedes diagnosis of lung cancer. *Cancer Res* 1994; 54:1634–1637.
14. Lam S, MacAulay C, Hung J, et al: Detection of dysplasia and carcinoma in-situ using a lung imaging fluorescence endoscope (LIFE) device. *J Thorac Cardiovasc Surg* 1993; 105:1035–1040.

15. Lam S, MacAulay C, LeRiche JC, et al: Early localization of bronchoscopic carcinoma. *Diagn Ther Endosc* 1994; 1:75–78.
16. Sutro CJ, Burman MS: Examination of pathologic tissue by filtered ultraviolet radiation. *Arch Pathol* 1933; 16:346–349.
17. Hung J, Lam S, LeRiche JC, et al: Autofluorescence of normal and malignant bronchial tissue. *Lasers Surg Med* 1991; 11: 99–105.
18. Qu J, MacAulay C, Lam S, et al: Optical properties of normal and carcinomatous bronchial tissue. *Appl Optics* 1994; 33: 7397–7405.
19. Lam S, Kennedy T, Unger M, et al: Localization of bronchial intraepithelial neoplastic lesions by fluorescence bronchoscopy. *Chest* 1998; 113:696–702.

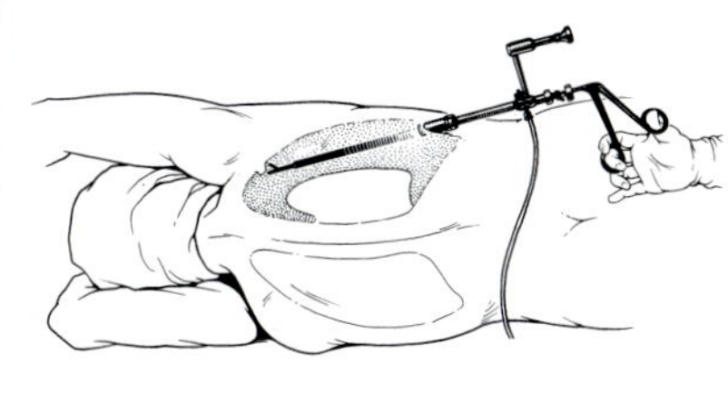

INDEX

Abrams biopsy, *186*, 189, 229–230, 233, *233*, *234*
Abscesses, 224*t*, 226–227, 247
Accessible emission limit, for lasers, 55
Adenitis, mediastinal tuberculous, 248
Adenoid cystic tumor, 50
Adenosine deaminase, 227
Adult respiratory distress syndrome, 154
Air embolism, 229, 280
Airway(s)
  fires in, 304–305, 305*t*
  mechanical dilation of, 7. *See also* Stent(s).
  obstruction of, 113–115
    diagnosis of, 114–115
    etiology of, 113–114
    types of, *114*
  potentially flammable materials in, 304
  stenosis of, benign, 29–40, 113–114. *See also* Benign airway stenosis.
Airway Wallstent. *See* Wallstent devices.
Alpha one antitrypsin deficiency, 133
Amoebic hepatic abscesses, 224*t*, 226–227
Amylase, in pleural effusions, 228
Amyloidoma, 49
Anesthesia, 12–13, 295–308
  for chest tube placement, 159–160
  complications of, 301
  cost of, 87*t*
  death associated with topical, 301
  drugs for, 301–303, 302*t*
  guidelines for, 301
  induction of, 305–308
  intraoperative management of patients given, 296, 297*t*
  for laser bronchoscopy, 52
  local, 104, 301, 302*t*
  medication prior to administration of, 298*t*, 298–299
  monitoring of, 299–301, 300*t*, 302
  oxygen prior to induction of, 306
  patients' physical status and, 295–296, 296*t*
  preoperative evaluation and preparation for, 295–296
  for rigid bronchoscopy, 22
  standby, 302
  for stent insertion, 104
  techniques for administration of, 301*t*, 301–303
  topical, 301, 301*t*
Aphonia, 34
Apnea, 22*t*
Argon laser, 48
Argon plasma coagulation, 84
Argyle Turkel safety thoracentesis system, 232, 238
Arrow-Clarke thoracentesis kit, 232, 238
Arrow Pneumothorax kit, 160
Arterial embolism, 130*t*, 280
Asbestos, 224*t*, 227
Aspergillosis, 224*t*, 226
Atelectasis, 133, 182
Attenuation coefficient, 48

Balloon dilation
  of benign airway stenosis, 129–138. *See also* Benign airway stenosis, balloon dilation of.
Baxter thoracentesis catheter, 232, 238
Benign airway stenosis, 29–40, 113–114
  adjuvant therapy for, 35–36
  balloon dilation of, 19*t*, 129–138
  atelectasis and, 133
    bronchoscope for, 6*t*
    bronchospasm and, 133
    catheters for, 131, *131*
    chest pain and, 133
    complication of, 19*t*, 133
    contraindications to, 130
    cryotherapy and, 129, 130*t*, 137
    electrocautery and, 129, 130*t*
    guide wire for, 131, *131*
    indications for, 130
    inflation syringe for, *133*
    laser resection and, 129, 130*t*, 137
    laser vaporization and, 132
    procedure for, *132*, 137–138
    radiopaque markers for, 131–132, *132*
    results of, *133*, 133–134, 134*t*, 135*t*
    stent placement and, 132
    technique for, *131*, 131–132, *132*
    visualization of, 132, *132*
  causes of, 29–31, 30*t*, 113–114, 129
  clinical manifestations of, 29
  endoscopic therapy for, 32–36, 36*t*
  endotracheal intubation and, 29

Page numbers in *italics* indicate illustrations; those followed by a *t* denote tables.

Benign airway stenosis (*Cont.*)
  evaluation of, 31–32
    chest radiography in, 31
    CT in, 31–32
    flexible bronchoscopy in, 32
    flow volume loop in, 31, *31*
    MRI in, 32
    multiplanar reconstruction in, 32, *32*
  infectious disease and, 114
  laser therapy for, 33–34, 49
  postintubation injury and, 29–30
  signs and symptoms of, 31
  stents for, 34–35
  surgical management of, 36–40
    anesthesia for, 37
    care following, 38
    dilation during, 38
    evaluation in, 37
    laser photodissection in, 37–38
    patient education for, 37
    patient follow-up after, 38
    patient selection for, 37
    team approach to, 37
    ventilation for, 37, *38*
  tracheostomy and, 29, 30, 129, 130*t*
  treatment of, 29, 32–35
    adjuvant therapies in, 35–36
    antibiotics in, 35–36
    balloon dilation in, 129–138
    corticosteroids and, 35
    dilation in, 32–33, 129–139
    intraluminal stent placement in, 34–35
    laser therapy in, 33–34
    microtrapdoor technique in, 33
    multimodality approach to, 35
    surgery in, 36–40
Berylliosis, 129, 130*t*
Biopsy, 18
  Abrams, *186*, 189, 229–230, 233, *233*, *234*
  closed pleural, 214, 229–230. *See also* Closed pleural biospy; Pleural biopsy.
  contraindications to, 198
  fine-needle, 269–282. *See also* Fine-needle aspiration biopsy.
  forceps, *198*
  of infections, *280*, 280–281
  in mesothelioma diagnosis, 191*t*
  needle. *See* Needles, for pleural biopsy.
  negative, rational for, 188
  pleural, 233–238. *See also* Pleural biopsy.
  thoracoscope-guided, 175–176
  transbronchial lung, 248
Brachytherapy, 6*t*. *See also* Endobronchial brachytherapy.
  advantages and disadvantages of, 87*t*
  for bronchogenic carcinoma, 141
  bronchoscope for, 6*t*
  complications of, 19*t*, 87*t*
  cost of, 87*t*
  with flexible bronchoscope, 19*t*
  high dose rate, 142, 143*t*, *147*
  low dose rate, 142, 143*t*, *146*
  low vs. high dose rate, 143, 144
  for occult lung cancer, 86*t*
  surgery and, 85
Bronchial artery embolization, 130*t*
Bronchial reimplantation, 129
Bronchitis, radiation, 144
Bronchogenic carcinoma, 49*t*
  brachytherapy for, 141
  cell type differentiation of, 269
  laser bronchoscopy in, 58
  prognosis for, 141
  staging of, 243–244, 246*t*
Bronchopleural fistula, 120, 154, 155*t*, 157*t*
Bronchoscope(s). *See also specific type, e.g.,* Flexible bronchoscope.
  for airway dilation, 7
  bleeding and, 5
  for brachytherapy, 6*t*
  damage to, 4, 11–15
  development of, 3
  difference between, 4–5
  Dumon-Harrell universal, *20*, *21*
  fiberoptic, 3
  flexible, 4. *See also* Flexible bronchoscope.
    rigid vs., 4, 52–54
  for laser bronchoscopy, 5, 6*t*
  open-tube, 4. *See also* Open-tube bronchoscope.
  for phototherapy, 6*t*
  rigid, 4. *See also* Open-tube bronchoscope.
    flexible vs., 4, 52–54
  selection of, 5–7, 6*t*
  for stent insertion, 6, 6*t*
  types of, 4–5
  video, 4
Bronchoscopy
  anesthesia for, 12–13
  bleeding during, 5
  cost of, 87*t*
  diagnostic, 4
  fluorescence, 314–318. *See also* Fluorescence bronchoscopy.
  fluorescence vs. white-light, *315*, 317
  history of, 3
  laser, 5
  pediatric, 4
  percutaneous tracheostomy and, 286–287
  training in, 7
  white-light, 313–314
  white-light vs. fluorescence, *315*, 317
Bronchospasm, 133, 144
Burns. *See* Thermal injury.

Cannula, jet injection, 37, *37*
Capnography, 300
Carbon dioxide laser(s), 5, 6*t*
  drawback of, 48
  eye protection against, 56
  indications for, 48
  as photocoagulator, 48
  YAG lasers vs., 33
Carcinoid tumor, 50, 85, 86*t*
  cryotherapy for, 73
  endobronchial electrocautery of, *89*

Carcinoma
bronchogenic, 49*t*. *See also* Lung cancer.
brachytherapy for, 141
cell differentiation of, 269
laser bronchoscopy in, 58
prognosis for, 141
staging of, 243–244, 246*t*
metastatic, 49*t*
stenosis and, 129, 130*t*
Cardiac arrest, 53
Cardiac arrhythmia, 53, 197, 287
Cardiogenic shock, 155*t*
Cardiopulmonary surgery, 154
Cardiovascular complications, of flexible bronchoscopy, 53
Catheters, for balloon dilation, 131, *131*
Caustic chemical inhalation, 130*t*
Cervical mediastinoscopy, 244
Cesium-137, 142
Chemical inhalation, caustic, 130*t*
Chest pain, 133
Chest radiography
after chest tube placement, 165
in benign airway stenosis diagnosis, 31
following stent placement, 123–124
prior to thoracoscopy, 177
Chest tube care, 182–183
Chest tube placement, 153–166
anesthesia for, 159–160
assessment of function following, 165–166
blunt dissection technique for, 162, *162, 163*
bronchopleural fistula and, 155*t*
cardiogenic shock and, 155*t*
catheter over needle technique for, 160
complications of, 154–155, 155*t*
contraindications to, 154, 157, 157*t*
costs of, 155
drainage after, 158–159, *159*
dressing for, 163
equipment for, 158–159
guide wire technique for, 160–162, *161*
hemorrhage and, 155*t*
for hemothorax, 157, 157*t*
history of, 153
indications for, 153–154, 157, 157*t*
infection and, 155*t*
intercostal nerve block for, 160
large vs. small caliber, 155
nerve damage and, 154–155, 155*t*
outcomes for, 155
pain and, 155*t*
for parapneumonic effusions, 157*t*
patient preparation for, 158
for pleural effusions, 157, 157*t*
for pleurodesis, 157*t*, 182–183, 195
pneumothorax and, 154, 155*t*
postoperative, 154
professionals who administer, 153
prophylactic, 154
pulmonary edema and, 155*t*
radiographic assessment of function following, 165
site for, 157–158, *158*
small bore catheter over sharp trocar technique for, 155, 156*t*
supply tray for, 159*t*
suturing for, 163, *163*
techniques for, 160–163
blunt dissection, 162, *162*, 163
catheter over needle, 160
guide wire, 160–162, *161*
trocar guided, 162–163
trocar guided technique for, 162–163
Chest tube removal, 166
Chest wall lesions, 281, *281*
Chronic obstructive pulmonary disease, 133
Chylothorax, 157, 224*t*, 228
chest tube for, 157
Closed pleural biopsy, 229–230. *See also* Pleural biopsy.
complications of, 230
contraindications to, 229
historical background for, 229
indication for, 229
needles for. *See* Needles, for pleural biopsy.
Cobalt-60, 142
CO_2 monitoring, end-tidal, 287
Computed tomography (CT)
in benign airway stenosis diagnosis, 31–32
for FNAB, 273, 276, *276, 280, 281, 282*
helical, 32, *32*, 123
multiplanar reconstruction and, 32, *32*
prior to thoracoscopy, 177
of solitary pulmonary nodules, 271
in stent placement, 123
Congenital tracheal stenosis, 29, 30*t*
Congestive heart failure, pleural effusions and, 223, 224*t*
Controlled ventilation, 22, 22*t*, 303*t*
Cook pneumothorax kit, *279*
Cook tracheostomy introducer set, 285, *286*
Cope biopsy, 169, 185, 229–230, *237*, 237–238
Corneal injury, *55*, 56
Cough, thoracentesis and, 229
Covered wallstent, *98*, 99*t*, 101, 115, *117*, 117–118, *118, 119*, 121*t*
Cryoresistance, 71
Cryosensitivity, 71
Cryosurgery
acidophilic slough of, 72, *73*
for carcinoid tumor, 73
history of, 69–70
Joule-Thomson effect and, 69
scientific basis of, *70*, 70–72
Cryotherapy, 69–80, 86
advantages and disadvantages of, 87*t*
balloon dilation and, 129, 137
chemotherapy and, 73–74
clinical basis for, 72–74
complications of, 87*t*
cooling agents for, 74–75
cryoprobes for, 75, 76*t*
endoscopic equipment for, 75, 77
equipment for, 74–75, 76*t*, 77
patient care after, 80
patient selection for, 77
preparation of patient for, 77
radiotherapy and, 74
results of, 73

Cryotherapy (*Cont.*)
  retrofreezing effect of, 75
  rigid bronchoscope with, 18, 18*t*, 19
  slough removal in, 78, *79*
  technique of, 77–78, *79*, 80
    using fiberoptic bronchoscopy, 78, 80
    using rigid bronchoscopy, 77–78, *78*, *79*
Cylindroma, 74
Cysts, mediastinal, 247

Denitrogenation, 306
Double puncture method, for thoracoscopy, 179
Drainage systems, 158–159, *159*, 164–165
  commercially prepared, 165
Dry tap, 229
Dumon-Harrell bronchoscope, *20*, *21*, 60
Dumon stent, 98, *98*, 100–101, 115
Dyspnea, 121
  airway obstruction and, 114
  laser bronchoscopy in, 58
  oxygen therapy for, 257
  stenosis and, 129
Dyspnea index, 58

Electrocautery, 15. *See* Endobronchial electrocautery.
  in pneumothorax management, 217
Electromagnetic spectrum, *44*
Electrosurgery, 15
Embolization, arterial, 130*t*, 280
Emphysema, 176
  chest tube placement and, 164
  percutaneous tracheostomy and, 287
  subcutaneous, 164
  thoracoscopy and, 197
Empyema, 157*t*, 176
Endobronchial amyloid, 49
Endobronchial brachytherapy, 6, 141–148
  bronchospasm and, 144
  catheters for, 145, *146*
  complications of, 143–144
  contraindications to, 144
  efficacy of, 142, 143*t*
  equipment for, 144–145
  exsanguination and, 143
  fistula and, 143
  hemoptysis and, 143, 144
  high dose rate, 142, 143*t*, *147*
  history of, 141–142
  indications for, 144
  low dose rate, 142, 143*t*, *146*
  low vs. high dose rate, 143, 144
  pneumothorax and, 144
  pulmonary hemorrhage and, 143
  remote afterloading system for, *145*
  stenosis and, 144
  technique for, *146*, 147–148
Endobronchial electrocautery, 83–93
  advantages and disadvantages of, 87*t*
  background and history of, 84
  balloon dilation and, 129, 130*t*
  of carcinoid tumor, *89*
  complications of, 19*t*, 84, 87*t*, 93
  cost of, 87*t*
  with fiberoptic bronchoscope, 19*t*, 85*t*, *92*, 93
  local anesthesia for, 93
  necrosis associated with, 87*t*, 93
  for occult cancer, 86*t*
  oxygen during, supplemental, 93
  palliative use of, 85*t*
  with rigid loop bronchoscope, 19*t*, 85*t*
  risk assessment for, 90
  sedation for, 93
  of squamous cell carcinoma, *89*, *90*
  technique for, 84, *90*, 90–91, *92*, 93
  YAG laser therapy vs., 91
Endobronchial radiation therapy. *See* Endobronchia brachytherapy.
Endo-GIA stapler, *216*
Endoscopic stapler, 215–216, *216*
Endoscopic therapy
  antibiotics and, 35
  for benign airway stenosis, 32–36
  complications of, 36
  corticosteroids and, 35
Endoscopy snares, 65
Endoscopy suite, 178
Endotracheal intubation. *See also* Intubation.
  complications of, 29
  stenosis and, 29, 129, 130*t*
Endotracheal tube
  fires associated with, 304–305, 305*t*
  flammability of, 304
  intubation over, 23–25, *24*
  stenosis and, 29, 129, 130*t*
End-tidal CO_2 monitoring, 287
Erythrocytosis, 257
Esophageal perforation, 224*t*, 228
Esophagoscope, 3
Esophagus, stenosis of, 3
Expandable endobronchial stents, 115–119
  complications of, 122–123
  efficacy of, 120
  indications for, 11, 121–122
  insertion and removal of, 120–121
  longevity of, 123
  palliative effects of, 121–122, *122*
  placement of, *119*, 123–126
    bronchoscopy after, 124
    chest radiography after, 123–125
    CT in, 123
    follow-up for, 123–125
    mucous impactation and, 126
  types of, 116–119

Fiberoptic bronchoscope. *See also* Flexible bronchoscope.
  camera-like device at end of, 4
  endobronchial electrocautery with, 85*t*, *92*, 93
  introduction of, 3–4
Fiberoptic bronchoscopy, cryotherapy and, 78, 80
Fibers, thoracoscopic detection of, 189, 191, 194*t*
Fibroma, 49
Fine-needle aspiration biopsy (FNAB), 269–282
  advantages of, 269

air embolism and, 280
alternatives to, 272
anesthesia for, 273
of chest wall lesions, 281, *281*
complications of, 271–272, 277–280
contraindications to, 271
CT-guided, 273, *276*, *280*, *281*
death associated with, 272
disadvantages of, 270
fluoroscopy-guided, 273, 275–276
hemoptysis and, 272, 279–280
history of, 269
imaging choice for, 273
indications for, 271
infection and, 272
of infections, *280*, 280–281
malignant seeding and, 280
needles for, 273–274, *274*
patient care after, 277
patient preparation for, 272–273
planning for, 275
pneumothorax and, 271–272, *277*, 277–279
role of cytologist in, 274–275
sensitivity of, 269
of solitary pulmonary nodules, 269
techniques for, 274

Fires, 304–305
during laser bronchoscopy, 301, 303
prevention of, 304
treatment of, 305*t*

Fistula(s), 143
bronchopleural, 120, 154, 155*t*, 157*t*
malignant, 120, *122*
percutaneous tracheostomy and, 287
tracheobronchial, 119–120

Flammable materials, 304

Flexible bronchoscope
accessories for, 15
advantages of, 53
applications of, 9
balloon dilation with, 19*t*, 131–132. *See also* Balloon dilation, technique for.
brachytherapy with, 19*t*
cleaning of, 9–10
cost of, 9
disadvantages of, 54
disinfection of, 10
effect on rigid bronchoscopy of, 17, *18*
for electrosurgery, 15
laser bronchoscopy with, 53–54, *63*, 63–65
for laser photoresection, 14–15, *15*
leak test for, 10, *10*
lubricants for, 12
patient biting of, 13, *13*
photodynamic therapy with, 19*t*
prevention of damage to, 11–15, 14*t*
proper handling of, 11–12, *12*
rigid vs., 4, 18, 19*t*, 52–54
for stent insertion, 110
sterilization of, 10–11
storage of, 11
training in use of, 7
for transbronchial needle aspiration, 13, *13*, *14*
transportation of, 11

Flexible bronchoscopy, 53–54. *See also* Flexible bronchoscope.
after stent insertion, 105
after stent placement, 124
in benign airway stenosis diagnosis, 32
cardiovascular complications of, 53
hemorrhage and, 53
myocardial infarction and, 53

Flow volume loops, 31, 58

Fluid cytology, 191*t*

Fluid technique, 252

Fluorescence bronchoscopy, 314–318
clinical results of, 317
equipment list for, 315
history of, 314–315
indications for, 317–318
instrumentation for, *314*, 315
procedures for, *316*, 316–317, *317*, *318*

Fluoroscopy, 273, 275–276

Forceps
dilator, 285
Kelly, 162, *162*, *163*
optical biopsy, *198*
stent, 111, *111*

Foreign body reaction, 129, 130*t*

Foreign body removal, 18*t*, 19

Freezing. *See also* Cryotherapy.
cellular effects of, 71–72, *72*
monitoring of, 75
tangential, 78, *79*

GAMMAMED I, 142

Gas embolism, lasers and, 297*t*

Gastroesophageal reflux, 31

Gianturco stent, 6, 34–35, 115, 116, *116*, 121*t*, 123

Gingiva, injury to, 22

Gold-198, 142

Granulomas
catheters and, 50, 265, 265*t*, *266*
stents and, 34, 116, 122

Green, Horace, 3

Guide wire, for balloon dilation, 131, *131*

Hamartoma, 49

Helium-neon gas laser, 48

Hemangioma, sclerosing, 248

Hematoporphyrin derivatives, 84

Hemoptysis
endobronchial brachytherapy and, 143, 144
fine-needle biopsy and, 272, 279–280
laser bronchoscopy in, 58
ventilation-perfusion relationships and, 58

Hemorrhage
chest tube placement and, 155*t*
control of, 50
flexible bronchoscopy and, 53
thoracentesis and, 229
thoracoscopy and, 176, 194*t*, 197

Hemothorax, 157, 157*t*

Hepatic abscesses, amoebic, 224*t*, 226–227

Hepatic lacerations, 229

Hilar masses, 282
Hood stent, *98*, 99*t*, 99–100
Human immunodeficiency virus, 56
Hypertensive episodes, 308
Hyperthermia, 84, 197
Hypotension, 197
Hypovolemia, 229
Hypoxemia, 229, 300
Hypoxia, 287

Immunotherapy, 197, 197*t*
Implantable access system, 197, 199, *199*, *200*
Infection(s)
  biopsy of, *280*, 280–281
  chest tube placement and, 155*t*
  as complication of TBNA, 248
  fine-needle biopsy and, 272, *280*, 280–281
  laser bronchoscopy and, 56
  pleurodesis and, 194
  stenosis and, 129
  TBNA in diagnosis of, 248
  thoracoscopy and, 194*t*
Inflation syringe, *133*
Injection cannula, steel jet, 37, *37*
Intercostal artery laceration, 229
Intercostal space, metastases in, *214*
Intraluminal stent placement, 34–35
  complications of, 36
Intrapleural catheter, *200*
Intrapleural therapy, 195–197
Intubation. *See also* Endotracheal intubation.
  complications of, 29
  injury following, 29
  over endotracheal tube, 23–25, *24*
  with rigid bronchoscope and laryngoscope, 25, *26*
  with rigid bronchoscopy, 23–27
Iodine-125, 142
Iridium-192, 142

Jackson, Chevalier, 3, 17
Jet injection cannula, steel, 37, *37*
Jet ventilation, 22, 22*t*, 52, *308*
  high frequency vs. manual, 305
Joule-Thomson effect, 69

Karl Storz rigid thoracoscope, 177, *177*
Karnofsky performance index, 58
Kelly forceps, 162, *162*, *163*
Killian, Gustav, 3, 17

Lambert-Eaton myasthenic syndrome, 295, 301
Laryngoscope
  intubation with rigid bronchoscope and, 25, *26*
  for stent insertion, 110–111, *111*
Laryngotracheal stenosis, 30, 33
Laser(s)
  accessible emission limit for, 55
  argon, 48
  atmospheric contamination and, 297*t*
  attenuation coefficient of, 48
  carbon dioxide, 5, 6*t*, 33, 48
  classification of, 55
  components of, *45*
  corneal injury and, *55*, 56
  eye injuries, *55*, 56, 297*t*
  gas embolism and, 297*t*
  hazards associated with, 297, 297*t*
  light source for, 43–49
  maximum permissible exposure, 55
  media for, 48
  potassium titanyl phosphate, 4, 48
  reflection characteristics of surfaces in contact with, *54*
  retinal injury and, *55*, 56
  safety of, 55–58, 57*t*
  smoke plume from, 56
  thermal injury and, 56
Laser bronchoscopy, 6*t*, 33–34, 43–67, 60–65
  balloon dilation and, 129, 130*t*, 137
  for benign airway stenosis, 33–34, 49, 49*t*
  complications of, 297, 297*t*, 301
  contraindications to, 51*t*, 51–52
  esophageal endoscopy before, 52
  fires and, 301, 303
  with flexible bronchoscope, 53–54, *63*, 63–65
  flexible vs. rigid bronchoscope for, 52–54
  indications for, 49*t*, 49–51
  infection and, 56
  for laryngotracheal stenosis, 33
  lesions for, 50*t*
  light source for, 43–49
  mechanical ventilation and, 58
  outcome of, 58–60
    tests for, 58
  palliative use of, 58–59
  radiation therapy vs., 58
  respiratory failure and, 58
  with rigid bronchoscope, 18, 19*t*, 54, 60, *61*, 62–63
  rigid bronchscope in, 54
  rigid vs. flexible bronchoscope for, 52–54
  safety priorities of, 54
  set-up for, *60*
  spirometry and, 58
  survival benefit of, 59*t*, 59–60
  techniques for, 52–54, 60, *61*, 62–65
  for tracheal stenosis, 49, 49*t*
Laser light, 43–49, *44*
  absorption characteristics following exposure to, 46, *47*
  attenuation depth of, 46, 48
  effect of exposure to, 46, *47*, 48
  generation of, *44*
  intensity of, 46
  power density of, 46, *46*
  properties of, *45*, 45–46
  tissue injury from exposure to, 46, *47*
  transverse electromagnetic mode and, 46
Laser photocoagulation, 217
Laser photodissection, 37–38
Laser photoresection, 14*t*, 14–15, *15*
Lipoma, 49
Liver cirrhosis, 223, 224*t*
Local anesthesia, 93, 301
  drugs used for, 302*t*
  for electrocautery, 93

for stent insertion, 104
toxicity associated with, 301
Lung, 182
malignant nodules on, 182
metastatic adenocarcinoma in, *172*
trapped, 186
Lung cancer, 3, 83
cytology-negative pleural effusions and, 171
incidence of, 141
Lambert-Eaton myasthenic syndrome and, 295
management of, 247
non-small cell, 141
occult, 84, 86*t*
pleural effusions and, 171, 227
prognosis for, 141
small cell, 295
staging of, 243–246, 245*t*
Lung transplantation, stenosis and, 103, 129, 130*t*, *136*
Lupus pleuritis, 224*t*, 227
Lymph nodes, 242, 242*t*, 243*t*
Lymphomas, 224*t*, 227, 247

Mackensie, Morell, 3
Magnetic resonance imaging, 32
Malignant mesothelioma. *See* Mesothelioma.
Malignant seeding, 197, 280
Maximum permissible exposure, for lasers, 55
Mechanical ventilation, 58, 223, 232, 285
Mediastinal cysts, 247
Mediastinal masses, 247–248, 282, *282*
Mediastinal tuberculous adenitis, 248
Mediastinitis, fibrosing, 114
Mediastinoscopy, cervical, 244
Mesothelioma, 189, 190*t*, 191, 219
asbestos exposure and, 227
benign vs. malignant, 227
diagnosis of, 172, 189, 191*t*, 219*t*
fluid cytology in, 191*t*
sensitivity of methods for, 191*t*
surgery in, 191*t*
thoracoscopy in, 171, 191*t*
diffuse malignant, *173*
environmental vs. occupational, 191
fibronodular diffuse malignant, *173*
nodular diffuse malignant, *173*
occupational vs. environmental, 191
pleural plaques of, *173*
pleurodesis for, 193, 196*t*
prognosis for, 189, 190*t*
staging system for, 189, 191*t*
thoracoscopic findings in, 189, 191*t*, *192*, *193*
Metastatic adenocarcinoma, *173*
Metastatic pleural malignancies, 186–189
pleurodesis for, 193, 196*t*
Micrognathia, 22
Microtrapdoor technique, 33
Monitored anesthesia care, 299–301, 300*t*, 302
Montgomery T-tube stent, 34, 50, 98, *98*, 99, *100*
Mucoepidermoid tumor, 50
Mucoid squamous tumors, 73
Mucous impactation, prevention of, 126
Mucous plugs, 265, 265*t*, *266*
Multi-chamber chest drainage, 158–159, *159*
Multiplanar reconstruction, 32, *32*
Myocardial infarction, 53

Nd:YAG laser. *See* Yttrium-aluminum-garnet lasers.
Necrosis, 87*t*, 93
Needles
for fine-needle biopsy, 273–274, *274*
for pleural biopsy, 229–230, 233, *233*, 234–235, *235*, *236*, 237–238
Nerve damage, associated with chest tube placement, 154–155, 155*t*
Nitinol stent, 117, 120, 121*t*
Nodules, solitary pulmonary, 269, *270*, 271
Novastent device, 118–119, *120*, 121*t*

O'Dwyer, Joseph, 3
Open-tube bronchoscope. *See also* Rigid bronchoscope.
flexible vs., 4, 54
indications for, 52
interventional, 8
in laser bronchoscopy, 54
training in use of, 7–8
Oscillotonometric blood pressure devices, 300
O&S needle biopsy, 234–237
components of, 235, *235*
operation of, 235, *236*, 237
rules for, 237
Oxygen, supplemental, 93, 306
Oxygen therapy
cannula for, 255, *256*
nasal mask for, 255, *256*
transtracheal, 255–266. *See also* Transtracheal oxygen therapy.

Pain
after pleurodesis, 194
chest tube placement and, 155*t*
thoracentesis and, 229
Palladium-103, 142
Palliative treatment
algorithm for decision making in, *88*
endobronchial electrocautery with, 84, 85*t*
Palmaz stent, 117, 121*t*, 123
Pancreatitis, 224*t*, 228
Papilloma, 49, 73
Papillomatosis, 114
Parapneumonic effusions, 157*t*, 224*t*, 226
Paratracheal intubation, 287
Percutaneous stent fixation, 107, *107*
Percutaneous Thal-Quick Chest Tube Set, 160
Percutaneous thoracic needle biopsy, 269–282. *See also* Fine-needle aspiration biopsy.
Percutaneous tracheostomy, 285, 290, *293*
advantages of, 285
appropriate size overdilation required for tube in, 290
bleeding and, 287
complications of, 287, 288*t*
contraindications to, 285
Cook tracheostomy introducer set for, 285, *286*
cost of, 289
death associated with, 287
dilation for, 290, *293*

Percutaneous tracheostomy (*Cont.*)
  dilator forceps technique for, 285
  emphysema and, 287
  endotracheal tube placement for, 290, *291*
  end-tidal CO_2 monitoring during, 289
  hypercarbia and, 287
  hypoxia and, 287
  indications for, 289
  late outcomes in, 287–288
  malpositon of tracheostomy tube in, 287
  overdilation for, 290, *293*
  paratracheal intubation and, 287
  percutaneous dilational tracheostomy technique for, 285
  placement of tube in, 287, 290, *291, 293*
  pneumothorax and, 287
  Portex Perfit tracheostomy introducer set for, 285–286, *286*
  preparation for, 290
  Rapitrach method of, 287
  role of bronchoscopy in, 286–287
  single lead dilator technique for, 285
  surgical vs., 288–289
  techniques for, 285, 289–290, *291–293*, 294
  tracheal stenosis and, 287
pH, of pleural effusions, 225*t*, 228
Pharmaseal Argyle thoracentesis catheter tray, 232, 238
Photocoagulator, laser as, 48, 58
Photodynamic therapy, 84
  advantages and disadvantages of, 87*t*
  complications of, 19*t*, 87*t*
  cost of, 87*t*
  with flexible bronchoscope, 19*t*
  for occult lung cancer, 86*t*
  surgery and, 85
Phototherapy, 6, 6*t*
Pleural biopsy, 233–238. *See also* Closed pleural biopsy.
  Abrams needle, *186*, 189, 229–230, 233, *233, 234*
  conventional technique for, 233–234
  Cope needle, 229–230, *237*, 237–238
  modified technique for, 234
  needles for, 229–230, 233, *233*, 234–235, *235, 236*, 237–238
  O&S needle, 234–237
  specimens from, 238
  technique for, 181–182, 233–238
    conventional, 233–234
    modified, 234
Pleural effusion(s), 223, 224*t*–225*t*, 226–228
  adenosine deaminase in analysis of, 227
  amoebic hepatic abscesses and, 224*t*, 226–227
  amylase in, 228
  antinuclear antibodies and, 227
  asbestos, 224*t*, 227
  aspergillosis and, 224*t*, 226
  breast cancer and, 224*t*
  chest tube for, 157, 157*t*
  congestive heart failure and, 223, 224*t*
  diagnosis of, 170–172
    algorithms for, 170–171
  esophageal perforation and, 224*t*, 228
  exudate, 223, 226
    transudate vs., 223
  liver cirrhosis and, 223, 224*t*
  lung cancer and, 227
  lymphoma and, 224*t*, 227
  malignant, 227
  milky, 228
  pancreatitis and, 224*t*, 228
  pH analysis of, 225*t*, 228
  pneumonia and, 224*t*, 226
  pulmonary embolism and, 227–228
  rheumatoid, *174*, 224*t*, 227
  systemic lupus erythematosis and, 224*t*, 227
  transudate, 223, 226
  tuberculosis and, 172, 174, 224*t*, 226
Pleural fluid analysis, 223, 224*t*–225*t*, 226–228
Pleural inflammation, *216*
Pleural malignancies
  diagnosis of, 172, 186
  endoscopic appearance of, 186, *186*, 186*t*, *187, 188*
  histopathology of, 188–189
  metastatic, 186–189
    pleurodesis for, 193, 196*t*
  topography of, 187–188
Pleural mesothelioma. *See* Mesothelioma.
Pleural plaques, of mesothelioma, *174*
Pleural space, defined, 153
Pleurisy, tuberculous, 172, 174, *174*, 224*t*, 226
Pleurodesis, 193, 196*t*, 213
  agents for, 195
  chest tube insertion for, 157*t*, 195
  for mesothelioma, 193, 196*t*
  in pneumothorax management, 217
  quality of, 195
  talc, 176, 182, 193–195, *195*, 196*t*
Pleurolysis, 217
Pneumoncystis carinii, 175
Pneumonia
  bacterial, 224*t*, 226
  pleural effusions and, 224*t*, 226
  postobstructive, 121
Pneumothorax, 207–218
  aspiration of spontaneous, 232–233
  brachytherapy and, 144
  chest tube for, 154, 157, 157*t*
  chronic, 209–210
  clinical presentation of, 208
  as complication of chest tube placement, 154, 155*t*
  defined, 154
  diagnosis of, thoracoscopic, 210–211, 211*t*
  fine-needle biopsy and, 271–272, *277*, 277–279
  following surgery, 154
  historical perspectives on, 207–208
  induction of, 228–230, *230*
  management of, 207–218, 277–279
    decision tree for, 214*t*
  percutaneous tracheostomy and, 287
  recurrent, 154, 213
  spontaneous, 154, 208–209, 232
    management decision tree for, 214*t*
    primary, 208–209
    secondary, 209
  TBNA and, 248
  thoracentesis and, 229, 232
  thoracoscopic management of, 207–218
    advantages of, 208*t*, 213

anesthesia for, 211–212
contraindications to, 215*t*
electrocautery in, 217
endoscopic stapler in, 215–216, *216*
equipment for, 211, *212*
indications for, 208–210, 210*t*
laser coagulation in, 217
patient preparation for, 214
pleurodesis in, 217
pleurolysis in, 217
studies of, 213*t*
technique for, 214–218
ending of, 218
trocar placement and inspection for, 215, *215*
thoracoscopy and, 222*t*, 225
traumatic, 154
Pneumothorax kit, 160, *160, 279*
Polychondritis, 114
Portex Perfit tracheostomy introducer set, 285–286, *286*
Postintubation injury, 29
Potassium titanyl phosphate laser, 5, 48
Preoperative medication, 298*t*, 298–299
Pseudochylothorax, 228
Pulmonary edema
chest tube placement and, 155*t*
reexpansion, 155*t*, 164, 229
thoracentesis and, 229
Pulmonary embolism, 227–228
Pulmonary fibrosis, 133
Pulmonary hemorrhage, 143
Pulmonary hypertension, 133
Pulmonary nodules, solitary, 269, *270*, 271
Pulmonary sleeve resection, 114
Pulse oximeter, 300, 300*t*

Radiation therapy. *See also* Endobronchial brachytherapy.
bronchitis and, 144
cryotherapy and, 74
laser bronchoscopy vs., 58
silicone stents after, 102
Radioactive seeding, 17
Radiopaque markers, for balloon dilation, 131–132, *132*
Radon-222, 142
Raj needle. *See* O&S needle biopsy.
Rapitrach method, 287
Reexpansion pulmonary edema, 155*t*, 164, 229
Renal lacerations, 229
Respiratory failure, 58
rigid bronchoscopy and, 53
talc poudrage pleurodesis and, 223
Retinal injury, *55*, 56
Rheumatoid arthritis, *174*, 224*t*, 227
Rigid bronchoscope, 4
advantages of, 19, 54
components of, 19–20, *20*
diagnostic use of, 18
endobronchial electrocautery with, 85*t*, 91, *91*, 93
flexible vs., 4, 18, 19*t*, 54
indications for, 17–19, 18*t*, 52
insertion of radioactive seeds with, 17
in laser bronchoscopy, 18, 19*t*, 54, 60, *61*, 62–63
for stent insertion, 18, 18*t*, 19*t*, 108–110, *110*
Rigid bronchoscopy, 17–27
accessory instruments for, *21*
anesthesia for, 22
cardiac arrest and, 53
complications of, 22
contraindications to, 22
for cryotherapy, 77–78, *78, 79*
effect flexible bronchoscope on, 17, *18*
future of, 23
history of, 17
indications for, 17–19, 18*t*, 52
intubation over endotracheal tube with, 23–25, *24*
intubation with, 23–27
classic technique for, 25, 27, *27*
using a laryngoscope, 25, *26*
myocardial infarction and, 53
optics for, 20
respiratory failure and, 53
techniques for, 60, *61*, 62–63
ventilation, 20, 22, 22*t*
training for, 23
ventilation techniques for, 20, 22, 22*t*
Rigid coagulation suction probe, *91*, 93
Rigid laryngoscope, 110–111, *111*
Rusch stent, *98*, 99*t*, 101, *111*

Sarcoidosis, 129, 130*t*
Schieppati, E., 241
Sclerosing hemangioma, 248
SCOOP catheters, 259, *259*, 262, 263
complications of, 265*t*
granuloma and, 265, 265*t*, *266*
mucous plugs and, 265, 265*t*, *266*
Seeding, malignant, 225, 280
Silastic stent, 6, 6*t*
silicone vs., 97
Silicone stents
after radiation therapy, 102
commercially available, *98*, 99*t*, 99–101
composition of, 97
following surgery, 102
history of, 97–99
insertion of, 103–111
anesthesia techniques for, 104
bronchoscopic assessment prior to, 103–104
complications of, 105*t*, *106*, 107–108
debulking prior to, 103–104
flexible bronchoscope for, 110
flexible bronchoscopy following, 105
indications for, 97, 101–103, 102*t*
local anesthesia for, 104
physician training for, 108
results of, 105*t*, 105–106
rigid bronchoscope for, 108–110, *110*
setting up for, 103–105
surveillance after, 108
silastic vs., 97
Single puncture method, for thoracoscopy, 179
Smear technique, 252
Smoke inhalation, 129, 130*t*
Solitary pulmonary nodules, 269, *270*, 271
Spindle cell tumor, 50

Spirometry, 58
Splenic lacerations, 229
Spongiosa graft, 120
Spontaneous assisted ventilation, 22, 22*t*, 303*t*
Spontaneous ventilation, 22, 22*t*, 303*t*
Squamous cell carcinoma, endobronchial electrocautery of, *89*, *90*
Stainless steel jet injection cannula, 37, *37*
Stapler, endoscopic, 215–216, *216*
Steel jet injection cannula, 37, *37*
Stenosis. *See also* Benign airway stenosis.
  benign airway, 29–40
  berylliosis and, 129, 130*t*
  brachytherapy and, 144
  bronchial artery embolization and, 130*t*
  bronchial reimplantation and, 129
  carcinoma and, 129, 130*t*
  congenital lesions and, 130*t*
  dyspnea and, 129
  endotracheal tube and, 29, 129, 130*t*
  esophageal, 115
  etiology of, 129, 130*t*
  foreign body reaction and, 129, 130*t*
  idiopathic, 130*t*
  in infants, 129
  lung transplantation and, 103, 129, 130*t*, *136*
  pulmonary infection and, 129
  sarcoidosis and, 129, 130*t*
  smoke inhalation and, 129, 130*t*
  stents for, 34–35, 50. *See also* Stent(s).
  tracheal, 49, 49*t*, *50*
    percutaneous tracheostomy and, 287
  tracheostomy and, 29, 30, 129, 130*t*
  trauma and, 129, 130*t*
  tuberculosis and, 129
  types of, 49–50, *50*
  Wegener's granulomatosis and, 30, 114, 129, 130*t*
Stent(s)
  airway penetration by, 116
  aphonia and, 34
  for benign airway stenosis, 34–35, 50
  complications of, 115, 116, 122–123
  Dumon, 98, *98*, 100–101, 115
  expandable endobronchial, 115–119. *See also* Expandable endobronchial stents.
  fixation of, percutaneous, 107, *107*
  Gianturco, 6, 34–35, 115, 116, *116*, 121*t*, 123
  granuloma and, 34, 116, 122
  Hood, *98*, 99*t*, 99–100
  inhalation therapy and, 100
  insertion of, 6, 6*t*, 34–35. *See also* Expandable endobronchial stent, placement of.
    balloon dilation and, 132
    complications of, 36
    rigid bronchoscope for, 18, 18*t*, 108–110, *110*
  metallic, 6, 6*t*, 115
    silicone vs., 35
  Montgomery T-tube, 34, 50, 98, *98*, 99, *100*
  nitinol, 117, 120, 121*t*
  Palmaz, 117, 121*t*, 123
  percutaneous fixation of, 107, *107*
  problems with, 34
  Reynders, 99*t*, 101
  Rusch, *98*, 99*t*, 101, *111*
  silastic, 6, 6*t*
  silicone, 97–111. *See also* Silicone stents.
    metallic vs., 35
  Strecker, *116*, 116–117, *117*, 121*t*
  tracheobronchial, 34
  tracheoesophageal fistula and, 116
Stent displacement, 34
Stent forceps, 111, *111*
Stent introducer system, 34, 109, *109*
Stent placement. *See* Stent(s), insertion of.
Storz high-frequency loop electrode, 60
Storz tracheoscope, *20*
Storz ventilating bronchoscope, 93
Strecker stent, *116*, 116–117, *117*, 121*t*
Subglottic stenosis, 30
  gastroesophageal reflux and, 31
  high grade, *38*
  idiopathic, 31
  recurrent, 38
  surgical management of, *38*
Surgery
  anesthesia during, 295–308. *See also* Anesthesia.
  arterial catheterization during, 300
  for benign airway stenosis, 36–40
  brachytherapy and, 85
  cardiovascular monitoring during, 300
  equipment monitoring during, 300*t*
  monitoring during anesthesia and, 299–301, 300*t*
  patient monitoring during, 300*t*, 301
  peripheral nerve stimulator during, 300
  photodynamic therapy and, 85
  precordial stethescope during, 300
  YAG laser, 85, 297, 297*t*
Suture thread removal, 50
Systemic lupus erythematosus, 224*t*, 227

Talc pleurodesis, 176, 182, 193–195, *195*, 196*t*
  atomizer for, *178*, *195*
  infection and, 194
  pain management following, 194
  respiratory failure and, 195
TBNA. *See* Transbronchial needle aspiration (TBNA).
Teeth, injury to, 22
Telestep delivery device, 118, 123
Thermal injury, 30, 56
Thoracentesis, 223, 226–229
  air embolism and, 229
  aspiration of spontaneous pneumothorax using, 232–233
  complications of, 228–229
  contraindications to, 223
  cough and, 229
  for debilitated and sick patients, 232
  dry tap and, 229
  equipment for, 231–232
  hemorrhage and, 229
  hypovolemia and, 229
  hypoxemia and, 229
  indications for, 223, 229
  kits for, 232, 238
  lacerations associated with, 229

mechanical ventilation and, 223, 232
pain and, 229
pneumothorax and, 229
pulmonary edema and, 229
serial, 226
technique for, 230–231, *231*
therapeutic, 229
ultrasound-guided, 232
vasovagal reactions and, 229
Thoracoscopy
accuracy of, 171
anesthesia for, 179, 200
for assessment of tumor response, 197
biopsy and, 175–176
cardiac arrhythmias and, 176, 195
catheter insertion during, *200*
chest radiography before, 177
complications of, 176, 189, 194*t*, 197
contraindications to, 176, 177, 197–198
CT before, 177
death associated with, 176, 194*t*
for detection of asbestos, 189, 191, 194*t*
diagnostic, 170–176, 185–191
accuracy of, 171
advantages of, 183
for metastatic pleural malignancies, 172, 186–189
for pleural effusion, 170–172
for *Pneumocystis carinii*, 175
sensitivity of, 171
for tuberculous pleurisy, 172, 174, *174*
value of, 186
double puncture method for, 179
emphysema and, 197
for empyema, 176
equipment for, *177*, 177–178, *178*, *198*, 198–199
examination of pleural cavity during, *202*, 202–203, *203*
hemorrhage and, 176, 194*t*, 197
history of, 169–170
hyperthermia and, 197
hypotension and, 197
indications for, 177, 197
infection and, 194*t*
mineralogic studies of, 189, 191, *193*, 194*t*
mortality rate for, 176
optical biopsy forceps for, *198*
patient position during, 200, *201*
for pneumothorax, 207–218. *See also* Pneumothorax, thoracoscopic management of.
pneumothorax and, 194*t*, 197
pneumothorax induction for, 200–202, *202*
point of entry for, 178–179, 200
procedures before, 177
room for, 178
safety of, 198
second point of entry for, 203
seeding of chest wall and, 197
sensitivity of, 171, 191*t*, 194*t*
single puncture method for, 179
technique for, 179–181, *180*, *181*, 200–203
telescope for, *198*
therapeutic, 192–197
trocar for, *198*
video-assisted thoracic surgery vs., 170
Thoracostomy placement. *See* Chest tube placement.
Thoracotomy
anterior, 244
chest drainage after, 157
complications of, 163–164
Tissue injury, 46, *47*
Tracheal stenosis, 49, 49*t*, *50*. *See also* Stenosis.
congenital, 29, 30*t*
defined, 30
percutaneous tracheostomy and, 287
thermal injury and, 30
Wegener granulomatosis and, 30
Tracheobronchial fistula, 119–120
Tracheobronchial malignancy, 48, 50
Tracheobronchial stent, 34
Tracheomalacia, 29, 34
Tracheopathia osteoplastica, 49, 114
Tracheostomy, 285
cost of, 289
percutaneous. *See* Percutaneous tracheostomy.
percutaneous vs. surgical, 288–289
stenosis and, 29, 30, 129, 130*t*
Tracheostomy tube, 287, *293*
dual cannula, 294
Transbronchial lung biopsy, 248
Transbronchial needle aspiration (TBNA), 13, *13*, *14*, 241–252
advantages of, 245–246
complications of, 248
diagnostic yield from, 245*t*
disadvantages of, 248
for endobronchial lesions, 247, 247*t*
equipment for, 249–250
forceps biopsy and, 248
function of, 242
in hemangioma diagnosis, 248
history of, 241
indications for, 244*t*
infection and, 248
location of lymph nodes for, 242*t*, 243*t*
for lung cancer management, 247
for lymphoma diagnosis, 247
for mediastinal cysts and abscesses, 247–248
micrometastatic identification by, 246
needles, 249, 250*t*
penetration methods for, 250, *251*, 252
cough, *251*, 252
hub against wall, *251*, 252
jabbing, 250, *251*
pushing, 250, *251*, 252
for peribronchial and submucosal disease, 246
for peripheral nodules or masses, 246–247, 247*t*
pneumothorax and, 248
position of metal needle prior to, *249*
predictive value of, 246
safety and efficacy of, 248
sensitivity of, 246
smear from, 252
TBLB and, 248
technique for, 250, *251*, 252

Transbronchial needle aspiration (TBNA) (*Cont.*)
TTNA vs., 246
use of, 241
Transthoracic needle aspiration (TTNA), 246
Transtracheal oxygen therapy, 255–266
ambulation and, 258
catheters for, 259, *259*
for chronic hypoxemia, 256
comfort and, 258
complications of, 263–265, 265*t*
postprocedure, 264–265
procedure-related, 263–264
contraindications to, 259, 259*t*
cost of, 258
dyspnea and, 257
equipment for, 259, *259*
erythrocytosis and, 257
exercise endurance and, 257
guide wire insertion for, 261, *261*
history of, 255–256
with immature tract, 262–263
indications for, 258*t*, 258–259
marking landmarks in preparation for, 260, *260*
with mature tract, 263
oxygenation and, 256–257
patient preparation for, 260
performance of daily activities and, 258
physiologic rationale for, 256–257
pulmonary hypertension and, 257
pulsed delivery systems for, 257
stent week for, 261, *261*
subjective rationale for, 257–258
survival and, 257
techniques for, 259–263
ventilation and, 257
work of breathing and, 257
Transverse electromagnetic mode, 46
Trapped lung, 186
Trauma, 129, 130*t*
Trocars, *198*, *202*
Tuberculosis
pleural effusion and, 172, 174, *174*, 224*t*, 226
stenosis and, 19, 114, 129
Tuberculous adenitis, mediastinal, 248
Tuberculous pleurisy, 172–173, *173*, 224*t*, 226
diagnosis of, 172, 174
early, *174*
fibrinous exudative, *174*
Tumor(s)
benign, 49, 49*t*
carcinoid, 50, 73, 85, 86*t*. *See also* Carcinoid tumor.
intraluminal, 84, 86*t*
mixed cell type, 50
mucoid squamous, 73
occult, 84, 86*t*
pedunculated, 53
recurrent, 53, 83
spindle cell, 50
superficial, 84
Tumor response, 197

Ventilation, 37, *38*
controlled, 22, 22*t*, 303*t*
jet, 22, 22*t*, 52, *308*
mechanical, 58. *See also* Mechanical ventilation.
methods of, 303–305
spontaneous, 22, 22*t*, 303*t*
spontaneous assisted, 22, 22*t*, 303*t*
techniques for, 20, 22, 22*t*
Ventilation-perfusion relationships, 58
Venturi jet adapter, *20*
Venturi-jet ventilation, 22, 22*t*
Video-assisted thoracic surgery, 170
Videobronchoscopes, 4, 9

Wallstent devices, 6, *98*, 99, 101*t*, 115, *117*, 117–118, 121*t*
American vs. European, 125*t*
delivery systems for, 118, *118*, 123
European vs. American, 125*t*
for malignant fistula, *122*
placement of, *119*, 123–127
Wang transbronchial needle, 249, 250*t*
Wegener's granulomatosis, 30, 114, 129, 130*t*

YAG lasers. *See* Yttrium-aluminum-garnet lasers.
Yttrium-aluminum-garnet lasers, 5, 6*t*, *64*
advantages and disadvantages of, 87*t*
anesthesia delivery for, 52
carbon dioxide lasers vs., 33
coaxial quartz fiber for, *64*
complications of, 87*t*
cost of, 87*t*
electrocautery vs., 91
eye protection against, 56
for granuloma, 50
guidelines for safe operation of, 57*t*
for hemorrhage control, 50
indications for, 48, 49
for occult lung cancer, 86*t*
surgery and, 85, 297, 297*t*
for suture removal, 50
for tracheobronchial malignancy, 48, 50
for vaporization of granulation tissue, 50

ISBN 0-07-005207-7

90000>

9 780070 052079